Third Edition

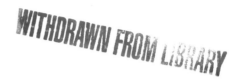

Principles of EMS Systems

Edited by

John A. Brennan, MD, FAAP, FACEP

Senior Vice President, Clinical and Emergency Services
  Director, Pediatric Emergency Medicine
  Chair, Patient Safety and Quality Committee
  Saint Barnabas Health Care System
Attending and Director, Pediatric Care Center
  Saint Barnabas Medical Center
Faculty, Emergency Medicine Residency Program
  Newark Beth Israel Medical Center
  Newark, New Jersey
EMS/EMSC Medical Consultant
  New Jersey Department of Health and Senior Services
  Office of Emergency Medical Services
Member, Board of Directors
  American College of Emergency Physicians

Jon R. Krohmer, MD, FACEP

Attending Physician
  Department of Emergency Medicine
  Spectrum Health
Director, EMS
  MERC/Michigan State University Emergency Medicine Residency
    Program
Medical Director
  Kent County EMS
  West Michigan Metropolitan Medical Response Team
  Region 6 Terrorism Response Program
  Grand Rapids, Michigan
Associate Professor
  Section of Emergency Medicine, College of Human Medicine
  Michigan State University
  East Lansing, Michigan

JONES AND BARTLETT PUBLISHERS

Sudbury, Massachusetts

BOSTON   TORONTO   LONDON   SINGAPORE

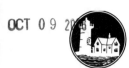

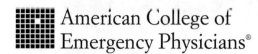
American College of
Emergency Physicians®

World Headquarters
Jones and Bartlett Publishers
40 Tall Pine Drive
Sudbury, MA 01776
978-443-5000
info@jbpub.com
www.jbpub.com

Jones and Bartlett Publishers Canada
2406 Nikanna Road
Mississauga, ON L5C 2W6
Canada

Jones and Bartlett Publishers International
Barb House, Barb Mews
London W6 7PA
United Kingdom

American College of Emergency Physicians
1125 Executive Circle
Post Office Box 619911
Dallas, TX 75261-9911
800-798-1822
www.acep.org

Thomas D. Werlinich, Associate Executive Director, Educational
   and Professional Products
Marta Foster, Director and Senior Editor, Educational and
   Professional Publications
Emma Kiewice, Project Manager
Mary Ostrowski, Editorial Assistant

Jones and Bartlett's books and products are available through most bookstores and online booksellers. To contact Jones and Bartlett Publishers directly, call 800-832-0034, fax 978-443-8000, or visit our website www.jbpub.com.
Substantial discounts on bulk quantities of Jones and Bartlett's publications are available to corporations, professional associations, and other qualified organizations. For details and specific discount information, contact the special sales department at Jones and Bartlett via the above contact information or send an email to specialsales@jbpub.com.

The American College of Emergency Physicians makes every effort to ensure that contributors to College-sponsored publications are knowledgeable authorities in their fields. Readers are nevertheless advised that the statements and opinions are provided as guidelines and should not be construed as College policy unless specifically referred to as such. The College disclaims any liability or responsibility for the consequences of any actions taken in reliance on these statements or opinions. The materials contained herein are not intended to establish policy, procedure, or a standard of care.

Production Credits
Chief Executive Officer: Clayton Jones
Chief Operating Officer: Don W. Jones, Jr.
President, Higher Education and Professional Publishing: Robert W. Holland, Jr.
V.P., Production and Design: Anne Spencer
V.P., Sales and Marketing: William Kane
V.P., Manufacturing and Inventory Control: Therese Bräuer
Publisher, Public Safety: Kimberly Brophy
Associate Editor: Janet Morris
Production Editor: Anne Spencer
Senior Photo Researcher: Kimberly Potvin
Composition: NK Graphics
Text and Cover Design: Anne Spencer
Printing and Binding: Courier Stoughton
Cover Printing: Courier Stoughton

Library of Congress Cataloging-in-Publication Data
Principles of EMS systems / edited by John A. Brennan, Jon R. Krohmer.—3rd ed.
     p. ; cm.
  Includes bibliographical references and index.
  ISBN 0-7637-3382-2 (alk. paper)
  1. Emergency medical services--United States.
  [DNLM: 1. Emergency Medical Services--organization & administration—United States. WX 215 P9632 2005] I. Brennan, John A.
II. Krohmer, Jon R. III. American College of Emergency Physicians.

RA645.5.P75 2005
362.18--dc22
                                                    2005008358

Printed in the United States of America
09 08 07 06 05   10 9 8 7 6 5 4 3 2

Contents

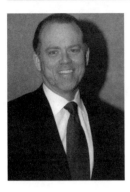

John A. Brennan, MD, FAAP, FACEP

Dr. Brennan is Senior Vice President for Clinical and Emergency Services for Saint Barnabas Health Care System, Livingston, New Jersey, where he is also Director of Pediatric Emergency Medicine and Chair of the Patient Safety and Quality Committee. He is core faculty for the emergency medicine residency program at Newark Beth Israel Medical Center, Newark, New Jersey, and the EMS/EMSC medical consultant for the New Jersey Department of Health and Senior Services. Dr. Brennan is a member of the Board of Directors of the American College of Emergency Physicians, a member of the Pediatric Emergency Medicine Subboard for the American Board of Emergency Medicine/American Academy of Pediatrics, and a national oral board examiner for the American Board of Emergency Medicine. He is a course director for both Advanced Pediatric Life Support and Pediatric Advanced Life Support, and a former liaison to the American Heart Association's Emergency Cardiac Care Committee.

In 1999, Dr. Brennan was named Outstanding Speaker of the Year by the American College of Emergency Physicians, and received its "Over the Top" speaker award in 2001. He has presented more than 150 state and national lectures on topics in emergency medicine, pediatrics, and EMS, and is the author of numerous journal articles and textbook chapters in these areas of expertise. Dr. Brennan served in the US Air Force from 1989 to 1992 and was the recipient of the US Air Force Professional Scholarship, the Air Force Commendation Medal, and a National Defense Service Medal, and was named Honorary Chief Master Sergeant. He was honorably discharged in 1992 at the rank of Major.

Dr. Brennan completed his undergraduate education at LeMoyne College, Syracuse, New York, and received his MD degree from Georgetown University School of Medicine. He completed residency training in emergency medicine at the Los Angeles County/University of Southern California Medical Center, and is board certified in emergency medicine and pediatric emergency medicine.

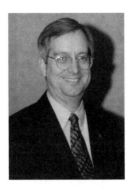

Jon R. Krohmer, MD, FACEP

Dr. Krohmer is an attending physician in the Department of Emergency Medicine at Spectrum Health and Director of EMS for the MERC/Michigan State University Emergency Medicine Residency Program. He is Medical Director for Kent County EMS in Grand Rapids, Michigan, the West Michigan Metropolitan Medical Response Team, and the Region 6 Terrorism Response Program. He is a past chair of the ACEP EMS Committee and the Trauma Care and Injury Control Committee and is currently the ACEP liaison to the American College of Surgeons Committee on Trauma. He is Past President of the Michigan College of Emergency Physicians and the National Association of EMS Physicians and is a national oral board examiner for the American Board of Emergency Medicine.

In 1998, Dr. Krohmer was named recipient of the 1998 ACEP Outstanding Contribution in EMS Award. He received the 2000 MCEP Ronald L. Krome, MD Meritorious Service Award and the 2003 Ronald D. Stewart, MD NAEMSP Leadership Award. He has presented regional, state, national, and international lectures on emergency medicine and EMS and is the author of numerous articles and chapters on EMS.

Dr. Krohmer completed his undergraduate education in pharmacy at Ferris State College, Big Rapids, Michigan, and received his MD degree from the University of Michigan Medical School. He completed his emergency medicine residency and an EMS/research fellowship at Wright State University in Dayton, Ohio. Dr. Krohmer is board certified in emergency medicine.

About the Authors

Bob W. Bailey
Former Director, Office of Emergency Medical Services
  State of North Carolina
Past President and current Associate Member, National
  Association of State EMS Directors
Steering Committee Member, National "EMS Agenda for the
  Future" project
President, Bob Bailey, Inc.
  Raleigh, North Carolina
Chapter 16, Rural EMS, with Dan Manz

Robert R. Bass, MD, FACEP
Executive Director, Maryland Institute for EMS Systems
Associate Professor of Surgery (Emergency Medicine),
  University of Maryland at Baltimore
  Baltimore, Maryland
Chapter 8, System Financing

Gordon Bergh
Assistant Director, Operations
  Austin/Travis County EMS Department
  Austin, Texas
*Chapter 7, Administration, Management, and Operations, with
  Richard Herrington*

Thomas H. Blackwell, MD, FACEP
Medical Director, The Center for Prehospital Medicine
  Department of Emergency Medicine
  Carolinas Medical Center
  Medical Director, Mecklenburg EMS Agency
  Charlotte, North Carolina
*Chapter 19, EMS Response to Terrorist Incidents and Weapons of
  Mass Destruction, with Jerry L. Mothershead, MD, FACEP*

Mary S. Bogucki, MD, PhD, FACEP
Section of Emergency Medicine
  Yale University School of Medicine
  New Haven, Connecticut
*Chapter 20, Operational EMS, with Joseph J. Heck, DO,
  FACOEP, FACEP*

John A. Brennan, MD, FAAP, FACEP, Editor
Director, Pediatric Emergency Medicine
  Saint Barnabus Health Care System
  Clinical Assistant Professor, Emergency Medicine
  Robert Wood Johnson Medical School
  New Brunswick, New Jersey
Introduction, with Jon R. Krohmer, MD, FACEP
*Chapter 15, EMS for Children, with Marianne Gausche-Hill, MD,
  FAAP, FACEP, and Robert K. Waddell II*

Theodore C. Chan, MD, FACEP
Associate Professor of Clinical Medicine, Department of
  Emergency Medicine
  University of California
  San Diego Medical Center
  San Diego, California
*Chapter 21, EMS and Public Health, with James V. Dunford, Jr.,
  MD, FACEP*

Robert M. Domeier, MD, FACEP
Saint Joseph Mercy Hospital
  Ann Arbor, Michigan
Chapter 13, Ground Interfacility and Specialty Care Transfer

James V. Dunford, Jr., MD, FACEP
Professor of Clinical Medicine and Surgery, City of San Diego
  EMS
Medical Director, Department of Emergency Medicine
  University of California
  San Diego Medical Center
  San Diego, California
*Chapter 21, EMS and Public Health, with Theodore C. Chan,
  MD, FACEP*

Peter I. Dworsky, MPH, EMT-P
Associate Director, Office of Disaster Preparedness
Director, EMTAC Ambulance
  Saint Barnabas Health Care System
  New Jersey
Assistant Director, Center for Health Care Preparedness
*Chapter 17, Disaster Response, with Stuart B. Weiss, MD, FACEP,
  FAAP, and William A. Gluckman, DO, FACEP*

Marianne Gausche-Hill, MD, FAAP, FACEP
Professor of Medicine at David Geffen School of Medicine at
  UCLA
Director, Emergency Medical Services, and
  Pediatric Emergency Medicine Fellowship
  Harbor-UCLA Medical Center
  Department of Emergency Medicine
  Torrance, California
*Chapter 15, EMS for Children, with John A. Brennan, MD, FACEP,
  and Robert K. Waddell II*
Chapter 22, Research, with Roger J. Lewis, MD, PhD

William A. Gluckman, DO, FACEP, EMT-P
Assistant Professor of Surgery, New Jersey Medical School
  Attending Emergency Physician, UMDNJ-University Hospital
EMS Medical Director, University EMS
  Newark, New Jersey
*Chapter 5, Emergency Departments and EMS, with Nancy E.
  Holecek, RN, and Neill S. Oster, MD*
*Chapter 17, Disaster Response, with Stuart B. Weiss, MD, FACEP,
  FAAP, and Peter I. Dworsky, MPH, EMT-P*

Joseph J. Heck, DO, FACOEP, FACEP
President/Medical Director, Specialized Medical Operations, Inc.
Medical Director
  Las Vegas Metropolitan Police Department
  Las Vegas, Nevada
*Chapter 20, Operational EMS, with Mary S. Bogucki, MD, PhD,
  FACEP*

Leah J. Heimbach, JD, RN
Owner, Healthcare Management Solutions, LLC and Passport
  Health of West Virginia
  Fairmont, West Virginia
*Chapter 26, Medical-Legal Concerns in EMS, with Douglas M.
  Wolfberg, Esquire*

Richard Herrington
Executive Director, Austin-Travis County EMS
  Austin, Texas
*Chapter 7, Administration, Management, and Operations, with
  Gordon Bergh*

Deb Hogue, RN, ADN, EMT-P
Health and Safety Specialist, Life EMS Ambulance
*Chapter 25, Occupational Health Issues, with Lynn Zimmerman,
  RN, BSN, Med*

Nancy E. Holecek, RN
Senior Vice President, Patient Care Services
  Saint Barnabas Health Care System
  Livingston, New Jersey
*Chapter 5, Emergency Departments and EMS, with William A.
  Gluckman, DO, FACEP, EMT-P, and Neill S. Oster, MD*

Jon R. Krohmer, MD, FACEP, Editor
Director, EMS,
Emergency Medicine Residency, Spectrum Health Downtown
Campus,
Grand Rapids, Michigan
EMS Medical Director,
Kent County Emergency Medical Services
Associate Professor,
Section of Emergency Medicine, College of Human Medicine,
Michigan State University,
East Lansing, Michigan
Recipient, 1998 ACEP Outstanding Contribution in EMS Award
Introduction, with John A. Brennan, MD, FAAP, FACEP

Roger J. Lewis, MD, PhD, FACEP
Professor of Medicine, UCLA School of Medicine
Director, Research
Harbor-UCLA Medical Center
Department of Emergency Medicine
Torrance, California
*Chapter 22, Research, with Marianne Gausche-Hill, MD, FAAP,
FACEP*

Victoria A. Maguire, EMT-P, EMD-I
Curriculum Council Chair, and Medical Curriculum Board
Chair
Senior Instructor Emergency Medical Dispatch, National
Academy of Emergency Dispatch
Communications Manager, American Medical Response
Grand Rapids, Michigan
*Chapter 10, Emergency Medical Dispatch, with James N. Pruden,
MD, FACEP*

Dan Manz
Director, Office of Emergency Medical Services and Injury
Prevention
Vermont Department of Health
Past President, National Association of State EMS Directors
Chapter 16, Rural EMS, with Bob W. Bailey

Hon. Ricardo Martinez, MD, FACEP
Clinical Professor of Emergency Medicine, Department of
Emergency Medicine
Emory School of Medicine
Atlanta, Georgia
Chapter 9, Communications, with Robert E. Suter, DO, MHA, FACEP

Greg D. Mears, MD, FACEP
State EMS Medical Director, North Carolina
Associate Professor, Department of Emergency Medicine
University of North Carolina-Chapel Hill.
Principal Investigator, National EMS Database Project (NEMSIS)
Principal Investigator, North Carolina Prehospital Medical
Information System (PreMIS)
North Carolina
*Chapter 11, Medical Record Documentation and EMS
Information Systems*

James C. Mitchiner, MD, MPH, FACEP
Attending Physician, Emergency Department
St. Joseph Mercy Hospital
Ann Arbor, Michigan
Medicare Medical Director, Michigan Peer Review Organization
Farmington Hills, Michigan
Chapter 27, EMTALA and EMS

Jerry L. Mothershead, MD, FACEP
Senior Physician Advisor
Medical Readiness and Response Group
Battelle Memorial Institute
Columbus, Ohio
Adjunct Professor
Department of Operational and Emergency Medicine
Uniformed Services University for the Health Sciences
Bethesda, Maryland
*Chapter 19, EMS Response to Terrorist Incidents and Weapons
of Mass Destruction, with Thomas H. Blackwell, MD, FACEP*

Rick Murray, EMT-P
Manager, EMS
American College of Emergency Physicians
Dallas, Texas
Chapter 2, EMS Systems, with Peter T. Pons, MD, FACEP

Susan M. Nedza, MD, MBA, FACEP
Research Faculty, Feinberg School of Medicine
Northwestern University
Chicago, Illinois
Past EMS Medical Consultant, Division of Emergency Medical
Services and Highway Safety Illinois Department of Public
Health
Past Board of Directors Member, American College of
Emergency Physicians
*Chapter 3, State and Regional EMS Systems, with Leslee Stein-
Spencer, RN, MS*

Neill S. Oster, MD
Assistant Professor Emergency Medicine
New York Methodist Hospital
Brooklyn, New York
*Chapter 5, Emergency Departments and EMS, with William A.
Gluckman, DO, FACEP, EMT-P, and Nancy E. Holecek, RN*

Jerry Overton, MPA
Executive Director, Richmond Ambulance Authority
Richmond, Virginia
*Chapter 12, Ground Transport: Ambulances, with Franklin D.
Pratt, MD, FACEP*

Peter T. Pons, MD, FACEP
Attending Emergency Physician, Denver Health Medical Center
Professor, Division of Emergency Medicine
Department of Surgery
University of Colorado Health Sciences Center
Denver, Colorado
Chapter 2, EMS Systems, with Rick Murray, EMT-P

Franklin D. Pratt, MD, FACEP
Medical Director, Los Angeles County Fire Department
Medical Director, Emergency Department
Torrance Memorial Medical Center
Torrance, California
*Chapter 12, Ground Transport: Ambulances, with Jerry
Overton, MPA*

James N. Pruden, MD, FACEP
Chairman, Department of Emergency Medicine
St. Joseph's Regional Medical Center
Paterson, New Jersey
Chairman, New Jersey State EMS Council
Deputy Medical Manager, New Jersey Urban Search and
Rescue Team
*Chapter 10, Emergency Medical Dispatch, with Victoria A.
Maguire, EMT-P, EMD-I*

Kenneth J. Robinson, MD, FACEP
Medical Director and Program Director
    LIFE STAR Helicopter Program
    Department. of EMS/Trauma
    Hartford Hospital
Associate Professor, Traumatology and Emergency Medicine
    University of Connecticut School of Medicine
President-elect, Air Medical Physician Association
*Chapter 14, Air Medical Transport, with Kenneth A. Williams, MD,
FACEP*

Jeffrey W. Runge, MD, FACEP
Administrator
    National Highway Traffic Safety Administration
    Washington, DC
Foreword

John C. Sacra, MD, FACEP
Director, Division of Emergency Medicine, and Clinical
    Associate Professor
    University of Oklahoma College of Medicine
    Tulsa, Oklahoma
Medical Director, Medical Control Board
Past President, American Trauma Society
EMS Committee Member, American College of Emergency
    Physicians
Chapter 4, Trauma Systems

Leslee Stein-Spencer, RN, MS
Chief, Emergency Medical Services and Highway Safety
    Illinois Department of Public Health
President Elect, National Association of State EMS Directors
*Chapter 3, State and Regional EMS Systems, with Susan M.
Nedza, MD, MBA, FACEP*

Ronald D. Stewart, OC, BA, BSc, MD, FRCPC, DSc
Professor and Director, Medical Humanities
    Professor, Emergency Medicine
    Professor, Anaesthesia
    Faculty of Medicine, Dalhousie University
    Halifax, Nova Scotia, Canada
Chapter 1, History of EMS: Foundations of a System

Daniel L. Storer, MD, FACEP
Adjunct Professor, Emergency Medicine
    University of Cincinnati College of Medicine
    Cincinnati, Ohio
Chapter 23, EMS Education Programs

Michel A. Sucher, MD
Acting Medical Director, Bureau of Emergency Medical Services
    Department of Health Services, State of Arizona
    Phoenix, Arizona
*Chapter 24, EMS Providers and the System Roles, with Jennifer L.
Waxler, DO, FACOEP, FACEP*

Robert E. Suter, DO, MHA, FACEP
Associate Professor, Emergency Medicine
    University of Texas-Southwestern
Medical College of Georgia
Medical Director, AMR-Dallas
Dallas, Texas
President, American College of Emergency Physicians
*Chapter 9, Communications, with Hon. Ricardo Martinez, MD,
FACEP*

Robert A. Swor, DO, FACEP
Director, EMS Programs
    Department of Emergency Medicine
    William Beaumont Hospital
Clinical Associate Professor, Department of Emergency Medicine
    Wayne State University
    Detroit, Michigan
Chapter 6, Medical Oversight and Accountability

Robert K. Waddell II
Vice President—Emergency Preparedness and Response
    Evidence Based Triage
    ThinkSharp, Inc.
Former—Director, EMS Systems
    Emergency Medical Services for Children, National Resource
    Center
    Washington, DC
President & CEO—TerraMed International, Inc
EMT-Basic, Wyoming
Paramedic, Front Range of Colorado
    Colorado EMS Training Coordinator
*Chapter 15, EMS for Children, with John A. Brennan, MD, FAAP,
FACEP, and Marianne Gausche-Hill, MD, FAAP, FACEP*

Jennifer L. Waxler, DO, FACOEP, FACEP
Chairman Emergency Department, Monmouth Medical Center,
    Regional EMS Medical Director, and EMTAC Medical
    Director
    Saint Barnabas Health Care System
Chair, MICU Advisory Board
    New Jersey
Vice-Chairman, EMS Council
*Chapter 24, EMS Providers and System Roles, with Michel A.
Sucher, MD*

Stuart B. Weiss, MD, FACEP, FAAP
Director, Center for Healthcare Preparedness
Director, Office of Disaster Preparedness
    Saint Barnabas Health Care System
Attending Emergency Physician, Newark Beth Israel Medical
    Center
    Newark, New Jersey
*Chapter 17, Disaster Response, with Peter I. Dworsky, MPH,
EMT-P, and William A. Gluckman, DO, FACEP, EMT-P*

Kenneth A. Williams, MD, FACEP
Clinical Associate Professor, Surgery
    Brown University
Associate Professor, Clinical Emergency Medicine
    University of Massachusetts
Immediate Past President, Air Medical Physician Association
Medical Consultant, Rhode Island Department of Health, EMS
    Division
USCG Liaison, RI-1-DMAT
*Chapter 14, Air Medical Transport, with Kenneth J. Robinson, MD,
FACEP*

Douglas M. Wolfberg, Esquire
Partner, Page, Wolfberg & Wirth, LLC
Former Commissioner, Commission on Accreditation of
    Ambulance Services (CAAS)
*Chapter 26, Medical-Legal Concerns in EMS, with Leah J.
Heimbach, JD, RN*

Arthur H. Yancey II, MD, MPH, FACEP
Associate Professor
    Department of Emergency Medicine
    Emory University School of Medicine
    Atlanta, Georgia
Medical Director
    Office of EMS
    Fulton County Department of Health and Wellness
    Atlanta, Georgia
Former Co-Chairman
    EMS and Transportation Subcommittee
    Atlanta Committee for the Olympic Games
Chapter 18, Emergency Medical Care at Mass Gatherings

Lynn Zimmerman, RN, BSN, Med
*Chapter 25, Occupational Health Issues, with Deb Hogue, RN,
ADN, EMT-P*

Foreword

"...on a lonely country road...considerable time may elapse after an automobile accident, before the wreck is even discovered, usually by a passing motorist. The nearest phone may be miles away, and even after reaching a telephone there is a question of whom to call... After finally contacting a proper authority, the caller must accurately describe the location...and an ambulance must travel a considerable distance from the nearest town [and may get lost] because ambulances do not have 2-way radio communications... The ambulance driver, in many cases, has no attendant to help, has had little emergency treatment training... in any event, and has little equipment in the ambulance. He arrives at the small community hospital and wheels up to the emergency room door to be greeted by a very surprised nurse who is completely unaware that the ambulance was en route. While she rushes off to phone a doctor to come in, the victims are wheeled into the room. One is DOA, having aspirated [since he had] no attendant in the back of the ambulance. The other is paralyzed due to spinal cord injuries, and will eventually be transferred [via a long ride down the highway] to a major medical facility when her condition permits.

—Captain John M. Waters, Jr., USCG, Chief, Division of Emergency Treatment and Transfer of the Injured, National Highway Safety Bureau, c. 1968

SINCE THESE WORDS WERE WRITTEN 37 SHORT YEARS AGO by Captain Waters from the predecessor to the National Highway Traffic Safety Administration, more improvements have occurred in out-of-hospital care than in all the prior millennia. As I contemplate the full spectrum of emergency medical care covered in this text, the stark contrast from what existed in 1968 is dramatic. Beginning with the publication of *Accidental Death and Disability* in 1966, there have been many stimuli for improving the emergency medical services system. Experienced wartime military medics came home to ply their trade in a street environment that was medically primitive compared to the fields of Korea and Vietnam. The first 911 call was made in Alabama in 1968. That same year, a forward-thinking group of physicians working in emergency departments met— a group that subsequently became the American College of Emergency Physicians. The National Highway Safety Act gave rise to a central agency for highway safety. Thought leaders in the states began to understand that death and injury sequelae could be reduced by extending the medical care system into the out-of-hospital realm. Surgeons who were willing to specialize in trauma and critical care fostered a fertile area of medical research.

Throughout the short history of out-of-hospital medical care, these forces have converged. The first 81-hour national standard EMT curriculum was developed by the National Highway Traffic Safety Administration, and the American Academy of Orthopaedic Surgeons published the first textbook— the "orange book." These first efforts have evolved into extensive, comprehensive training programs that have produced medical professionals who are as highly valued by the public as doctors and nurses. The isolated, rare trauma hospitals, formerly defined by where the neurosurgeon chose to practice, have evolved into statewide, organized trauma systems. A "ride to the hospital" has evolved into emergency airway control and pharmacologic physiology control, as well as treatment at the scene or in the home.

Systematic changes are the most likely to occur where the largest and easiest gains can be made. There has been much low-hanging fruit in the out-of-hospital arena over these past three decades. Yet even today emergency medical services in many areas of the United States and the rest of the world are similar to what existed in 1968. The disparities in emergency medical services between urban and rural areas, wealthy and poorer communities, and developed and developing countries need to be addressed by medical leaders and policy-makers.

The National Highway Traffic Safety Administration has provided the most consistent and long-term federal support for out-of-hospital emergency medical care, trauma system development, and EMS research since it was formed in 1970. The role of the agency has been to work closely with its other federal partners to promote, coordinate, and advocate for EMS systems that are state and community based. The National Standard EMS curricula, the EMS Agenda for the Future, the EMS National Research Agenda, the Trauma System Agenda for the Future, and the National EMS Education Agenda for the Future were produced by the agency in collaboration with its federal partners, EMS professionals, and national EMS, emergency medicine, and surgical organizations. A National EMS Information System is currently under development. Through collaboration, planning, and commitment, disparities in emergency medical services can be addressed.

At the local and state level, the responsibility for ensuring competency of EMS professionals falls squarely into the hands of physician medical directors. As medical care has expanded into the out-of-hospital setting, the responsibility for how it is practiced by "physician extenders" has not changed. But the quality and professionalism of EMS medical directors have changed dramatically over the short life of EMS. A subspecialty of emergency medicine has emerged with fellowship training and an expanding research base defining a unique body of knowledge. EMS medical directors do the job, often solely as volunteers, because they believe that quality EMS care directly translates into improved care for their patients and better outcomes, and because they see opportunities for improvements in out-of-hospital care delivery. This shared dedication by EMS professionals and EMS medical directors has led to a spirit of cooperation and collaboration that is unrivaled across the medical landscape. EMS professionals are enjoying a rapidly expanding scope of practice and procedures under the direction of local and state physician direction. Physicians are benefiting by receiving their patients into the emergency department in better shape, with treatment well underway.

Despite all of the challenges before us in the development of EMS and trauma systems, our attention has become diverted by the events of September 11, 2001. Law enforcement agencies and fire services have received unprecedented visibility. However, the public and policy-makers frequently do not recognize the importance of EMS providers. Resources are being made available to address some of the shortcomings that have been identified as a lack of preparedness. Despite significant federal funding for "first response personnel," limited federal funding has been available to support EMS preparedness.

The "age of preparedness" should be regarded in the context of the history and evolution of EMS in the United States. The EMS community has always been called upon to respond to any emergency, whether a single-victim or mass-casualty incident, regardless of the hazard—whether it is a derailed, leaking tank car of chlorine gas or a natural gas explosion. Regardless of the perils that lie ahead, EMS professionals will continue to be the front line in the post-incident management of our nation's, and indeed the world's, harmful events.

The best preparation for an EMS response to a terrorist event is for the EMS system to provide quality patient care and response for routine emergency medical events that occur across this country 24 hours a day, 7 days a week, every day of the year. The possibility of mass casualty from an act of terrorism is a fear that we all now live with. However, even as we become smarter about biological and chemical agents, we cannot allow the prospect of a mass casualty to distract us from preparing EMS systems to address our primary responsibility. Rather, EMS training should prepare its professionals to treat the everyday victim, whether in a single-victim or mass-casualty event, as they have been doing for the last generation. A patient's pathologic state following a traumatic event does not change whether the act was intentional or accidental. Treating the victims of an exploding gasoline tanker truck is no different from those injured by an improvised incendiary device.

This text will equip the EMS professional, especially the EMS medical director, for whatever comes. Let's all hope that our nation and the global community can once again reach a point where our attention is focused on the usual, everyday, come-what-may illness and injury. The National Highway Traffic Safety Administration will continue advocating for the safety and security of the American public through the prevention of traffic-related injuries, the mitigation of injuries during a crash event, and the post-incident transportation and treatment of the sick and injured, as well as the promotion of state-of-the-art EMS treatment, research, and education.

Jeffrey W. Runge, MD, FACEP, Administrator
National Highway Traffic Safety Administration
Washington, DC

Introduction

The world as we knew it has changed since September 11, 2001. The specter of disaster, whether accidental, environmental, or purposeful, was brought to our shores and into our living rooms. First responders, including out-of-hospital personnel and emergency department personnel, have always been at the leading edge of disaster preparedness. With these newly recognized threats, the public, private, and government sectors of our country are beginning to recognize the importance of EMS as an essential public service.

The authors of this textbook took great care to provide an overview of the needs of EMS systems in general as well as to discuss the lessons learned from the tragedy of September 11. It is the view of the editors that, while there were lessons to be learned specific to the September 11 tragedy, most of these "lessons" needed to be incorporated into the overall practice and viewpoint of EMS versus being a standalone chapter. Responses to large-scale events, although unique in their nature, are generally large-scale extensions of daily activities for our EMS systems.

This third edition of *Principles of EMS Systems* was written with the intent to emphasize the collaborative interaction of EMS providers, police, fire departments, emergency physicians, emergency departments, and hospitals. All of the components of the system must be in place to provide care to those in need and to ensure that the emergency medicine/health care safety net does not fail when we need it the most.

This book was written and organized to be a useful informational and reference source for EMS providers, EMS managers, and physicians providing medical oversight, as well as for EMS physician medical directors. The general overview nature of the information is intended to provide the reader with concepts and examples of issues that are critical to the daily operation of EMS systems. It is not intended as a comprehensive "how-to" manual for addressing all of those issues.

The authors of this textbook were careful to use consistent definitions and terminology throughout the book. Some of the most commonly used terms are defined below.

Out-of-hospital refers to the environment in which EMS personnel operate, inclusive of activities occurring prior to arrival at a hospital (formerly "prehospital") and those that can occur after a patient has been hospitalized (eg, interfacility activities). This term more closely reflects the scope of EMS personnel's environment.

Medical oversight is the process of ensuring the quality of care provided by EMS personnel, and formerly referred to as "medical control" or "medical direction." It includes activities performed before the time of patient contact (offline, prospective), at the time of patient contact (online, concurrent), and after patient contact (offline, retrospective).

Performance improvement refers to the development and implementation of sustainable best practices that result in improved clinical care.

Most of the EMS principles described in this textbook can be applied to local EMS systems. The reader, however, must incorporate a deep knowledge and understanding of the local and state laws, rules, and regulations that govern his or her system.

The American College of Emergency Physicians has long been committed to high-quality EMS systems and to supporting the needs of emergency physicians and out-of-hospital personnel as they provide those services. This textbook is testimony to that strong commitment. Readers are encouraged to review the ACEP Web site (www.acep.org) for current EMS policies and PREP documents and for information on the activities of the EMS Committee and the EMS Section of membership.

The EMS profession is constantly evolving. Many of the concepts discussed in this textbook follow the framework set in place by the EMS Agenda for the Future.

We hope that this textbook provides the reader with a general overview of EMS and will be both a resource for the practicing EMS provider as well as an informational resource for those readers who are beginning their EMS careers.

John A. Brennan, MD, FAAP, FACEP

Jon R. Krohmer, MD, FACEP

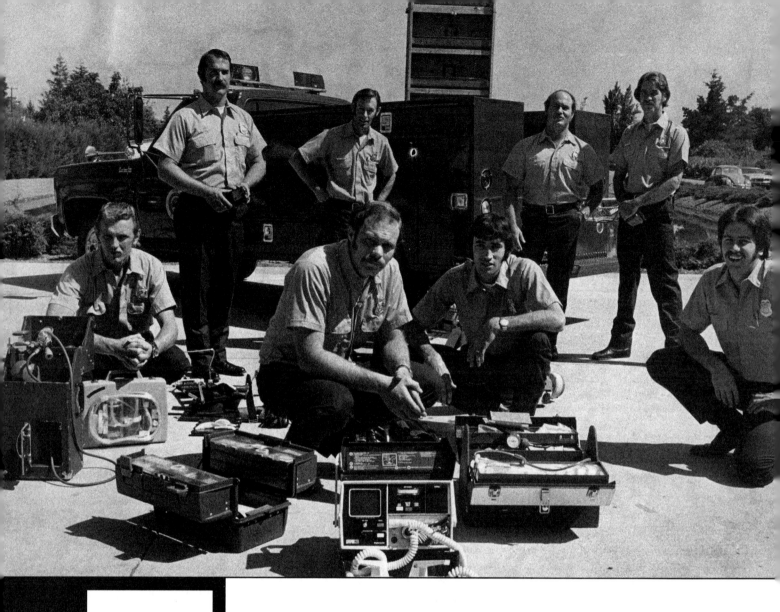

1

History of EMS:
Foundations of a System

Ronald D. Stewart, OC, BA, BSc, MD, FRCPC, DSc

Principles of This Chapter

After reading this chapter, you should be able to:

- Discuss the historical events that led to EMS systems development.
- Describe the basic building blocks of EMS systems, including clinical elements, system design/development, and legislative/public policy.
- Recall the 14 attributes of a modern EMS system.

"WHERE SHALL I BEGIN, PLEASE YOUR MAJESTY?" HE ASKED. "BEGIN AT THE BEGINNING," THE KING SAID GRAVELY, "AND GO ON TILL YOU COME TO THE END, THEN STOP."
Alice's Adventures in Wonderland, Chapter 12
Lewis Carroll (1832–1898)

THE VERY LOGICAL ADVICE GIVEN BY THE KING DURING Alice's grand adventures in Wonderland is not quite as easy to follow in considering the roots and foundations of EMS and projecting where we go from here. Simply stated, the roots are obscure and the future at times murky; we may well not be able to even *find* the beginning, let alone begin at it. And there is no end, *per se,* as of this date.

The provision of emergency medical services in communities using an organized and structured plan is of relatively recent vintage. The foundation stones upon which such systems are constructed, however, are set deeply in the bedrock of history — not all of which is medical — and are chiseled from the developments in medicine, basic science, and the changes in the philosophy and technology of military medicine. It could be argued that we could, using some imagination, trace the origins of emergency "care" to the first caveperson who had been whacked over the head, ravished by a roving saber-toothed tiger, or burned after falling into the newly discovered fire following a night of sampling the pungent juice of the prehistoric grape left for a while in a dark recess of the cave. Perhaps. But that style of immediate care was no *system;* the system came eons later, some would say only after the dawn of mass communications, even — dare we admit — with the advent of television.

The History of EMS Systems

The origin of EMS systems knows no "date" in history, no single "Eureka!" heralding a great leap forward that one would identify as "the beginning." Rather, the components of the system can be more readily identified and perhaps celebrated, the foundation of modern EMS systems being built of components derived from disciplines seemingly quite removed from things "medical." Who would think that a Russian immigrant to the United States by the name of Sikorsky would so influence the development of aeromedical systems that are now considered a standard element of EMS?[1] What possible relationship could an electrical company have to the ultimate discovery of how "hearts too good to die"[2] could be brought back to life by a machine, a machine designed by a team headed by a professor of electrical engineering who later was appointed a nonphysician professor of surgery?[3] If anything, EMS casts a wide net.

It is possible to draw descriptions of specific emergency care procedures from the well of ancient history, even though the pictures painted use imagery seen through different eyes in very different eras. Mouth-to-mouth breathing might have been described in the Bible in the language of the day as miraculous,[4] and defibrillation might have been performed in the 18th century.[5] This all might interest medical historians, but the roots of the EMS system are far more shallow — that is, more recent — than those snippets of the past might indicate. Whereas the philosophy that drives, or perhaps should drive, modern systems of EMS is wonderfully illustrated in the parable of the Good Samaritan,[6] there are serious questions as to whether that well-meaning pilgrim might have, in our modern and litigious world, ended up in a court of law.[7]

EMS: A Child of Military Medicine

It can effectively be argued that systems designed to provide immediate care of the sick and wounded were born out of the carnage of war. All components of the system might not have been, but certainly the organized plan was. In modern times, it befell Napoléon's chief surgeon Baron Dominique-Jean Larrey to put into place a system of retrieval of the wounded from the battlefield — something quite novel in late 18th century Europe and elsewhere.[8] Until that time, the wounded were considered a liability, and an organized system for their retrieval and treatment was not part of the battle plan. Baron Larrey not only selected a corps of soldiers to act as "medics" with distinctive uniforms and hierarchy, but also designed and had built a covered cart ("ambulances volontes" or "mobile dressing-stations")* designed for both the rapid delivery of supplies and surgeons to the wounded on the field, and the quick transport of wounded soldiers from the field. The lessons taught by Larrey and fostered by Napoléon were apparently lost to the next several decades of French military organizers.

The deficiencies resulting from a lack of attention to the wounded were alarmingly evident to an "accidental tourist" by the name of Jean Henri Dunant, a Swiss banker who, during a trip to Italy seeking out business opportunities related to the French Emperor, happened upon Napoléon III's attack on the Austrians at Solferino in June 1859. Struck by the suffering of the soldiers on the field and surrounding villages in the days following the battle, Monsieur Dunant went back to Geneva and, after publishing a vivid account of his experiences and observations at Solferino,[9] worked tirelessly to found a group known later as the International Committee of the Red Cross.

---

* Although this phrase might be translated from modern French into English as "flying ambulance," it is unlikely this renders the most accurate meaning in 18th century France, since use of the word "ambulance" in military terminology was reserved for hospitals or casualty treatment stations near the battlefield that were "portable" or "mobile," as late even as World War I. Use of the term *exclusively* to mean a vehicle for the transport of patients came later. In the context of 18th century military medicine, it is perhaps more accurately rendered as "mobile dressing-station," or even "mobile hospital."

After a stuttering start, military physicians on both sides of the American Civil War put into place some of the principles first used by Larrey to care for the wounded. The civilian horse-drawn ambulances appearing in the cities of Cincinnati and New York and elsewhere shortly after the Civil War grew largely from this military experience. Many of these urban "ambulances" were staffed by physicians and usually operated from hospitals. Activating these "systems" initially depended on telegraph services and word of mouth. The great invention of that century — the telephone — helped achieve a more rapid response, and Alexander Graham Bell's "talking box" could be viewed as one of the great developments in EMS history, even before 911.

Taking to the air . . .

A specialized field of EMS, aeromedical evacuation, awaited the invention of the heavier-than-air flying machine and the turn of the 20th century. Although historical rumor suggests that patients might have been carried with bags of mail in French hot-air balloons from a Paris besieged by the Prussians during the 1870–71 Franco-Prussian War, there is little to confirm this. Even if there were solid evidence that this took place, the event should be viewed more as an accident of history rather than as a stone cemented solidly in the EMS foundation.[10]

Within the decade in which the Wright brothers flew their oversized motorized kite from the dunes of Kitty Hawk, plans were proposed to the US Army for the design of an airplane that could carry a stretcher. Enthusiasm was noticeably and perhaps understandably absent in the official correspondence of the Army until the shock of World War I and its increasingly efficient killing machinery opened the eyes of some, while at the same time closed the eyes of millions of others. What was perhaps the first organized aeromedical evacuation during wartime took place in 1915, when an aircraft carried 13 wounded French soldiers during the Serbian retreat from Albania.[11]

But the advances in aeronautical technology that would eventually lead to the establishment of efficient and effective airborne rescue and aeromedical evacuation systems came about through the work of people like Igor Sikorsky. His passion for aviation became evident as early as the first decade of the 20th century in Russia when he experimented with vertical-flight machines. During the 1940s, following his immigration to the United States, his genius for invention and for solving the technical problems posed by rotor craft led to the development of the first practical helicopter capable of flying forward as well as hovering. Later versions of the same model demonstrated the ability of these machines to maneuver to permit a person to descend and even ascend ropes or rope ladders attached to the helicopter.[12] The introduction of helicopters as an essential part of military medicine awaited the Korean Conflict, and the system designed for immediate evacuation of the wounded reached the height of refinement during the Vietnam War. Results were encouraging: during that conflict, the time to definitive care was the shortest of any modern war, with resultant reductions in mortality rates from 8.5% in World War I, 4.5% in World War II, to less than 2.4% in Vietnam.[13] Both the theoretical and practical results from rapid evacuation of the wounded were not lost on those on the home front, as some were soon advocating "civilian" aeromedical systems for America.[14] The first helicopter systems for civilian use were often patchworked together with military or public safety agencies working with hospital-based personnel, the first reported having been established out of the St. Anthony Hospital system in Denver, Colorado, in 1972.[15] But the experience of Vietnam was tested as the early foundations of modern trauma systems were being laid in the United States. In the decade of the 1980s, helicopter programs expanded rapidly in almost every state.

While back on the ground . . .

But the beginnings of what we can identify as a trauma system seen in World War I were not notable for glamorous leaps forward, either in the air or elsewhere. Rather, some very simple principles and attention to detail and research provided the first inkling that early intervention in seriously injured persons might make the difference between living and dying. In what we might cite as an example of "simple principles applied," the British recognized that some 80% of soldiers in the trenches were dying from closed fracture of the femur, and medical authorities were forced to take notice. A British orthopedic surgeon, Hugh Owen Thomas, had designed and tested an immobilization device for just such an injury and had offered it to the French during the Franco-Prussian War, but it was not until World War I that its value was proved by introduction of the splint to widespread use during the vicious carnage of Flanders. A year after its use in the field, death rates in soldiers suffering fractures of the femur had fallen from 80% to 20%.[16] This may well have been the first statistical evidence that early management and a system to care for the wounded could make a

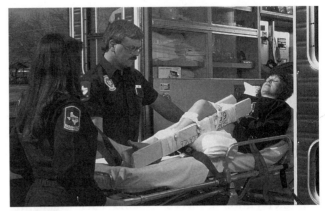

Figure 1-1 The use of the splint provided some of the first statistical evidence that early management and a system to care for the wounded could save lives.

difference and actually save lives (**Figure 1-1**). The use of the splint led Col. George W. Crile,* who in 1917 was an American surgeon in the casualty clearing stations of Flanders, to declare that the Thomas splint did more to prevent death from shock than any other single measure.[16]

Beating the clock . . . the cornerstone of trauma care

During the development of modern trauma care systems throughout the 1970s and 1980s, attention and debate focused frequently on the balance between "stay 'n' play" and "swoop 'n scoop." But the idea that time was an important factor in the trauma care equation was not a new one. In fact, during World War I, it became evident that mortality rates were directly related to the time required to deliver the wounded to

---

* This was the same Dr. George Washington Crile (1864–1943), the celebrated American surgeon and one of the founders of the Cleveland Clinic, whose experiments with external pneumatic counterpressure in the first decade of the 20th century led eventually to the "medical anti-shock trousers" of later vintage; he also was a close friend of Sir William Osler, the great Canadian physician considered by many to be the father of internal medicine, and was present at the birth in 1895 in Baltimore of Sir William's only surviving child, Edward Revere Osler. Dr. Crile attended Revere following his mortal chest wound in the trenches of Flanders in 1917, and was present when Revere succumbed to his wounds some hours later.[17] He might have been the first American to perform closed-chest cardiac compression on a patient during a cardiac arrest.[18]

definitive care. That is, the longer the time to definitive intervention, the higher the mortality rate. Looking through the retrospectoscope, all this seems rather elementary. But many of these data were new, and their importance often unappreciated. The system of casualty management evolved throughout the first World War and eventually was designed around "sorting" casualties according to severity, providing immediate first aid on the field, delivering the wounded as quickly as possible to the dressing stations, transporting victims to field hospitals for surgical intervention if necessary, and later evacuating them to tertiary care or convalescent facilities. These steps of sorting, rapidly applied "finger-in-the-dike" first measures, urgent surgical intervention, later definitive and postoperative care, and rehabilitation became the basic building blocks of a trauma care system. This basic design, with due attention to expeditiously carrying out each phase of care, has remained unchanged since first instituted in that great conflict, and from these beginnings the structure has emerged upon which most modern civilian trauma systems are based. But it took another 60 years before technologies and attitudes improved enough to save lives on the highways and byways of the home front.

Casting a Wide Net: The Struggle Against Sudden Death

Increasingly complex technology, including breakthroughs in the medical sciences, led to a broadening ability of medical care systems to stay, and in some cases to reverse, disease and injury processes, including sudden death.* Although sudden death, drowning, and "reanimation" (in modern lingo, "resuscitation") were well-known issues and evoked spurts of activity in scientific research and public activism very evident in the 18th century,[20] our ability to apply the data was limited, and at times we simply did not recognize their importance.

The search for the ABCs . . . the A and B

As has already been mentioned, attempts at bringing the "dead" back to life have been documented in an-

---

* The excellent and thoroughly researched work by Dr. Mickey Eisenberg (1997) of Seattle presents an unparalleled account of milestones in resuscitation medicine through the centuries. It has become a standard reference work, as well as an enjoyable read. It was used extensively in the preparation of this manuscript.[19]

cient writings, including the Hebrew Bible[4] and, more definitively perhaps, 18th century scientific publications.[5] In that era, perhaps the most dramatic cause of sudden loss of life, other than injury, was drowning. Ignorance of basic physiology and a lack of understanding of the process of death led to misplaced priorities; emphasis was on stimulating the nerves rather than providing air exchange. Although modern medical research focused more on attempts at artificial ventilation ("rescue breathing"), in the 18th century methods of stimulating life back into the victims of drowning ranged from the less-than-sublime to the downright repulsive, including intrarectal tobacco smoke.[5] But perhaps the greatest contribution of the 18th century was the movement to document, however unscientifically by modern standards, successful "reanimation" attempts and to organize laypersons in societies that advocated favorite methods of reviving drowned persons. Such efforts were not far removed from more recent attempts at teaching citizens CPR or the work of nongovernment organizations with specific interests in "hearts too good to die." One such group, The Royal Society for the Recovery of the Apparently Drowned, gained the patronage of George III and became the Royal Humane Society, which persists to this day.[21] The Danish equivalent of this agency published a book in 1796 that accurately described mouth-to-mouth ventilation (not for the first time), suggested chest compression, and advocated electrical shocks across the thorax.[5]

Mouth-to-mouth breathing apparently fell into disfavor, if not disrepute, in the 19th century, and it took the polio epidemic of the 1940s and 1950s to simulate the use of expired air ventilation by an American physician, James Elam. His persistent, almost evangelical, advocacy of this mouth-to-nose method of rescue breathing (he favored this over mouth-to-mouth) was backed up by his original research, which clearly demonstrated that expired air contained sufficient oxygen to sustain normal levels of blood oxygen in the victim.[22] One of his greatest successes that ensured the eventual triumph of this rediscovered technique was his convincing an Austrian immigrant and anesthetist, Peter Safar, that the "direct" method of ventilation was the only way to ventilate. The year was 1956.[23] Dr. Safar and Dr. Elam soon began to collaborate, and Dr. Safar organized the definitive demonstration that mouth-to-mouth ventilation was far superior to the then-popular and widely taught manual methods. One of the great ironies of these experiments that further demonstrated the vision of these resuscitation pioneers was that the subjects who volunteered to be anesthetized and paralyzed were medical personnel, while those ventilating them were firemen, Boy Scouts, and other volunteers from community organizations.[23] This contribution to the eventual lifesaving system that would emerge more than a decade later is often overlooked, largely because in the 21st century the participation of "lay" people in the EMS system seems to us so elementary and is taken for granted. In the 1950s, it was revolutionary.

The search for the ABCs . . . the C

So ingrained into the public's consciousness is the idea of CPR and resuscitation that it is difficult to conceive of the fact that the techniques we know and practice so well today were not always with us, nor were they "discovered" suddenly and dramatically in the manner of a breakthrough in medical science. Rather, the life-sustaining system we know as **cardio-pulmonary resuscitation,** or CPR, was woven together by many people and based on many discoveries, some going back as far as the 19th century. A German physician, Dr. Friedrich Maass, clearly described closed-chest cardiac massage in two patients who had suffered cardiac collapse secondary to chloroform anesthesia.[24] Early in the 20th century, Dr. George W. Crile performed closed-chest massage on a young woman who suffered cardiac collapse during an operation, and he correctly presumed that the pressure exerted on the chest led to an artificial pumping action of the heart that, in turn, produced peripheral blood flow.[25] But these discoveries went largely unnoticed until a team of researchers at Johns Hopkins, headed by Dr. William Kouwenhoven and at first working independently from Dr. Elam and Dr. Safar, observed a chance finding during their experiments with closed-chest defibrillation in anesthetized dogs. In the early 1950s, William Kouwenhoven, an electrical engineer, Guy Knickerbocker, also an electrical engineer, and James Jude, at the time a surgical resident at Johns Hopkins Hospital, teamed up to develop a safe and portable closed-chest defibrillator based on Kouwenhoven's earlier research in electrocution deaths that began in the 1920s. During one of their experiments on a dog, Dr. Knickerbocker observed that the pressure associated with applying the defibrillator paddles to the dog's chest caused a spike in its peripheral intra-arterial pressure. This is the closest the discoverers had come to a "Eureka!" moment. Repeated experiments refined a method to apply pressure to the chest, which was later practiced on humans. The report of their historic findings appeared in 1960.[26]

There was, initially at least, no "marriage" between the A and B of Elam and Safar and the "C" of Kouwenhoven, Knickerbocker, and Jude. In part, this disconnect occurred because it was widely thought that pressure on the chest produced some ventilation anyway, added to the fact that the two groups were working independently of each other although in the same city, and indeed the same university. That soon changed with the help of an unlikely source, the chief of the Baltimore City Fire Department, Martin McMahon. However, perhaps not too unlikely a source: Chief McMahon had been one of the volunteers recruited by Dr. Safar to conduct his ventilation experiments on the medical personnel at Johns Hopkins, and so impressed was Chief McMahon that he insisted all his firefighters be trained in the new mouth-to-mouth rescue breathing.* Chief McMahon and his firefighters might have been impressed with the new rescue breathing and closed-chest compressions; the medical establishment and official bodies were slower, indeed, to respond. The great challenge that now faced these pioneers was not "medical" *per se,* but was that of convincing a skeptical world.

The ABCs . . . the D

As the 20th century dawned with its increasing use of electricity, many workers and civilians died suddenly on coming in contact with electrical power lines. These tragedies moved Consolidated Edison, the electric company, to invest money and personnel into researching why their workers (and occasionally, customers) succumbed, often with no findings on autopsy to explain their sudden demise. Dr. Kouwenhoven began a series of experiments and observations that uncovered the cause — ventricular fibrillation — and the "cure" — a second strong electrical shock, or "countershock," from a machine called a **defibrillator.**[27] Not long after this discovery, Claude Beck, a surgeon from the Cleveland Clinic, applied an AC shock directly to the fibrillating heart of a 14-year-old boy undergoing surgery for severe pectus excavatum.[28] Defibrillation across the chest wall (closed chest) was performed first by Kouwenhoven

---

* This remarkable story, derived largely from interviews with the participants in the medical drama, is wonderfully documented in Dr. Eisenberg's book. Chief McMahon's foresight resulted in the first documented case of prehospital CPR combined with successful inhospital defibrillation in May 1960.

in the mid-1950s, but Paul Zoll, a Boston cardiologist, was the first to publish an account of his experience with closed AC-current defibrillation in 1956.[29]

Despite the early success of these "heroic" and "exotic" efforts at reversing the lethal event of ventricular fibrillation, technical problems remained, notably that the hardware was too big, too bulky, and too heavy. The technology simply didn't exist in the 1950s to make the machines (defibrillators) reasonably portable. So the rapid application of an electrical shock to the chest of the victim of sudden cardiac death had to await the improvements brought about by electrical engineering — a further example of casting a wide net in the search for the solution to this perplexing problem of cardiac arrest. The logistic problem of getting a defibrillator to a patient quickly meant that most victims of sudden cardiac death could not be helped. Many noted clinicians and researchers of the day merely assumed that the patient would be brought to the defibrillator, not vice versa. Some could not envisage such advanced treatment being carried out in anything but an operating theater or cardiology ward, let alone elsewhere in the hospital. It was beyond their comprehension that it might even be performed in homes or at roadsides. In fact, as late as 1973, the citation for the prestigious Lasker Award given to Dr. Kouwenhoven for excellence in medical research paid tribute to his devising a method (ie, closed-chest massage) that bought time "to get the patient to a defibrillator."[30] Today, in the era of portable and automated defibrillators used even by the lay public, we might find this concept strange, perhaps even difficult to understand (**Figure 1-2**).

As the pieces of the sudden death puzzle began to fit into place, one of the cornerstones of its reversal — the prompt application of a defibrillating countershock — was to be set solidly in the EMS foundation. It came out of Boston, from the work of Dr. Bernard Lown, who announced to the world in 1962 the construction and successful application of a truly portable direct-current (DC) defibrillator.[31] Although perhaps not appreciated at the time, Dr. Lown's contribution opened the door to solving the problem of out-of-hospital sudden death and must be considered a prominent milestone.

The technology of defibrillators, monitors, and other elements of out-of-hospital care improved dramatically in the 1970s and 1980s. Equipment got smaller; improvements in computer chip and other technologies permitted the development of the automated defibrillator, with its associated need for demonstrating effective outcomes while balancing

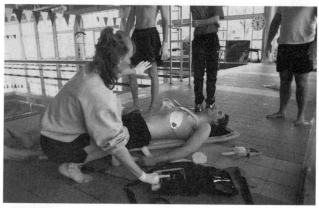

Figure 1-2 As late as the 1970s, it was assumed that the patient would be brought to a defibrillator, rather than the reverse. Most could not envisage such treatment being carried out anywhere other than in a hospital. Today defibrillators are portable and automated and can be used by the lay public.

our sometimes-eager acceptance of the promise held out by such technology. But the puzzle pieces needed to be locked together in order to ease suffering and to save life or limb in the battles we face every day. A way had to be found to bring help quickly to those who needed it — a system had to be built, but first it was necessary to realize a system was needed.

Putting it All Together: The System Emerges

Beyond the 1960s, the clinical tools were available to save the lives of many unfortunate victims of sudden death and trauma. The elements of CPR — the ABCs and D — had been developed and refined, and the improvements in military medicine, including better surgical techniques, antibiotics, and blood transfusion, began to make their mark in the jungles of Vietnam. But it was one thing to have the tools to reverse disease and even death; it was a very different thing to be able to apply them to large numbers of citizens. Getting these lifesaving measures to those who needed them begged for a system in which the chain of survival required that citizens not only have ready access to that system, but also be part of it and assume some of the responsibility for its success. Learning CPR, for example, would be the responsibility of individuals as their contribution to the community-based EMS system. Construction of a system of care was challenging and required three elements, each cemented to the other (**Figure 1-3**).

These three building blocks — clinical elements, legislative/public policy, and system design/development — form the basis of a modern EMS system.

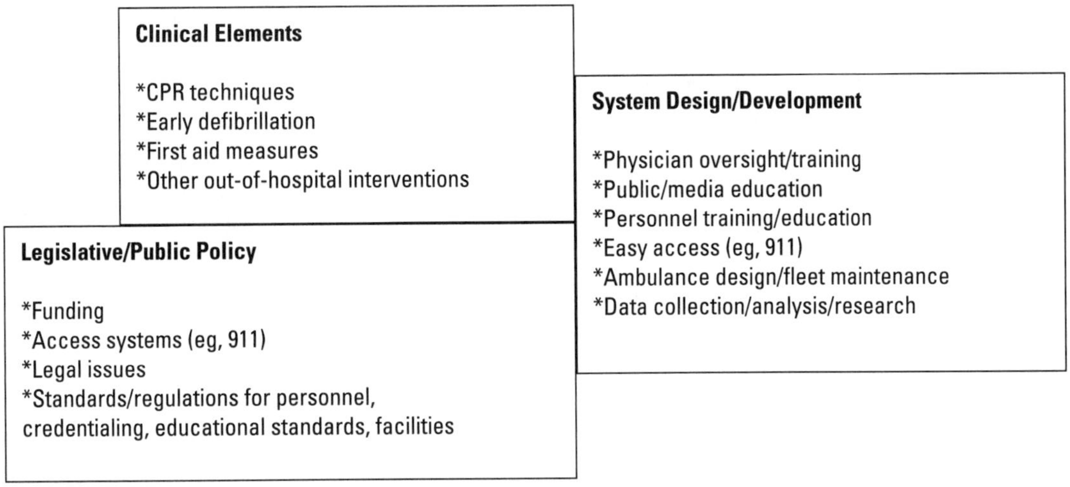

Figure 1-3 The three basic building blocks of EMS systems.

High-quality out-of-hospital care cannot adequately be delivered without regard to the other two blocks. Without public education in CPR, for example, the chain of survival[32] is broken, or at best, very weak; without 911, response times to the delivery of quality care are not optimal; without legislative action, the system might be underfunded, legal problems can ensue, available funding and research might be inadequate, and so on.

The pioneers in the development of CPR realized only too well that they had to do more than invent solutions to clinical problems or prove the scientific value of the revolutionary techniques they proposed. They recognized the importance of educating not only the public, but also their medical colleagues in various specialties and those in authority in government and nongovernment organizations. Their onerous task lasted into the next decade.

Voices in the wilderness . . .

In the evolution of human systems, the old adage "If it ain't broke, don't fix it" seems to carry special weight when it comes to things medical. The issues surrounding sudden cardiac death, the possibility of reversing that catastrophe through the use of CPR and prompt defibrillation, and the importance of a system to manage that catastrophe were taken up by the pioneers who began several decades of further research, education of their peers and the public, and efforts to inform the media of the "rightness" of their cause.

In the field of trauma care, a few lone voices were crying in the medical wilderness in the 1950s. Dr. J.D. "Deke" Farrington, a surgeon who was familiar with the advances of military medicine during both World War II and the Korean Conflict, agitated for improvement in ambulance personnel training, the design of vehicles, and better emergency department staffing.[33] Although such individuals and organizations (including the American College of Surgeons) attempted to fight the good fight, it took a candid and thoroughly researched report issued in 1966 by the National Academy of Sciences (National Research Council) to awaken the slumbering public and medical establishment.[34] This landmark document, *Accidental Death and Disability: The Neglected Disease of Modern Society,* exposed the glaring inadequacies of the "nonsystem" of trauma care and declared that they agreed with returning veterans of the Korean and Vietnam conflicts who stated that, if injured, "their chances of survival would be better in the zone of combat than on the average city street" in America.[34] The report condemned not only public apathy, but also the nonsystem of hit-or-miss ambulance care, operated for the most part by morticians. It proposed a trauma care system structure, with emphasis on prevention, education, and training, improvement of emergency departments, as well as research and outcome measurement. Reread after more than 30 years of modern EMS experience, the document was remarkably prophetic in its vision and stirred many to action.

The Irish connection . . .

A comprehensive system to combat the problem of sudden cardiac death and to reduce the risk from common cardiovascular disease, particularly acute myocardial infarction, was not "home grown." Rather, the early roots of a systems approach emerged in America from the experience of a crusty cardiologist in Belfast, Northern Ireland, Frank Pantridge. As consultants in cardiology at the Royal Victoria Hospital, Dr. Pantridge and his protégé, Dr. John Geddes, realized that, to reduce the mortality rates from cardiovascular disease — particularly the complications of acute myocardial infarction — early treatment must be delivered to patients outside the hospital. Dr. Pantridge conceived of making the coronary care unit of the hospital mobile — that is, sending his hospital physician, coronary care nurse, and ambulance attendant into the homes of those suffering from chest pain or other problems associated with heart disease. But this was not a true ambulance service, not a paramedic system as we know it today. The squad and the mobile coronary care unit were activated usually by the patient's own physician, and in the early stages an attempt was made to limit access to the service so it would not be overwhelmed.[35]

The success of the **Belfast system** was carefully documented in a study of the patients treated. In a landmark article, Geddes, Adgey, and Pantridge outlined the philosophy and solid clinical reasoning behind such a service.[36] They soon attracted attention, in particular that of several Americans who reported back to their colleagues on the other side of the Atlantic. And soon, building on the experience and shared adventure of their Irish colleagues, Dr. William Grace in New York[37] and Dr. Richard Crampton in Virginia emulated the Pantridge model after seeing first-hand the setup at the Royal Victoria Hospital in Belfast.

And on the home front . . .

The American experience took on a slightly different shading from the Belfast model. Efforts to extend coronary care beyond the confines of the hospital in other major cities in the United States tended to use resources and personnel already deployed in the streets and homes. Dr. Eugene Nagel began to train firemen and was a medical pioneer in the telemetric transmission of ECG tracings from rescue squads in Miami to hospitals that were part of the developing EMS system.[38] Dr. Leonard Cobb took a comprehensive and valuable research-oriented view of a system of out-of-hospital coronary care and originated the "Medic I" system of the Seattle Fire Department.[39] In 1969, Criley, Lewis, and Graf began a program in Los Angeles. It was built around firemen who were trained in advanced life support measures, including intravenous line placement, drug administration, and

defibrillation, and under the supervision of nurses from the county hospitals. They soon published their experience with fire-paramedics and mobile intensive care nurses.[40] But the influence of this program went far beyond the bounds of Los Angeles city and county. Television took notice of the fledgling system and created the popular television show "Emergency!" Things were never quite the same again.

During the 1970s, and with influence by the 1966 report, evidence of the value, in some patients, of mobile coronary care grew. Funding from Washington began to flow to regional EMS agencies after the passage of the **Emergency Medical Services Systems Act of 1973**. This funding enabled the development of curricula for emergency medical technicians, the training of emergency physicians in a specialty that was not recognized officially until 1978, and the purchase of communications equipment and ambulances. This was the decade in which EMS systems began to take shape throughout the United States and elsewhere. The 1966 report hit the mark, and both government and the public responded. One of the key recommendations of the report was achieved in 1968 with the founding of the American Trauma Society, which was endorsed by the American College of Surgeons, the American Association for the Surgery of Trauma, the National Safety Council, the American Medical Association, and the American Academy of Orthopaedic Surgeons. The founding of the American College of Emergency Physicians in 1968 marked the beginning of a decade-long struggle to establish an autonomous medical specialty for physicians in the not-yet-defined field of emergency medicine. Other subspecialty organizations followed — the National Association of EMS Physicians in 1984, which sought to bring together medical directors of EMS systems throughout the United States, and the National Association of EMS Educators, which followed later in the next decade.

With the advent of federal funding, and in the light of the 1966 report, EMS regions across the United States were under pressure to develop trauma systems with standards suggested by the Committee on Trauma of the American College of Surgeons and other agencies. Trauma centers were to be established, and standards were to be met. And thus began the "war of the white coats," during which hospitals and colleagues competed with each other for Level I designations, for helicopter programs, and for the loyalty of field teams (the "donut wars," as some were calling it). Adding to the frenetic pace of this era was the evidence that trauma systems actually *do* save lives.[41] But as funding declined in the 1990s, some hospitals quickly lost interest, and many academic and inner city medical centers teetered on the edge of the fiscal abyss. Some regions saw the demise of trauma systems that had required a full decade of hard work to construct. Others saw a more appropriate system evolve, with fewer players, less strife, and a less frenzied competitive environment.

Television gets into the act . . .

The fledgling pilot projects begun by Criley, Lewis, and Graf in Los Angeles in 1969[40] soon caught the eye of an inveterate fan of firefighting, Robert Cinader, who also happened to be a Hollywood producer and a chum of Jack Webb of "Dragnet" fame. Cinader frequented firehouses in the Los Angeles basin and met some of the newly minted "paramedics" at the same time Jack Webb was searching for a replacement for a waning police TV drama, "Adam-12." Cinader saw immediately the dramatic possibilities of what he actually observed on runs with the paramedics in the streets of Los Angeles. The result was "Emergency!" — a television soap opera featuring the first paramedic heroes, Johnny Gage (Randolph Mantooth) and Roy DeSoto (Kevin Tighe). Although medical types often cringed at the content of the show, and we self-styled academics looked down our ivory-tower noses at such an enterprise, the power of television cut a wide swath through the political red tape of Los Angeles county and California state budgets and swept along, tornado-like, to influence public opinion well beyond the borders of the Golden State. Public exposure of this pilot project through television, combined with the political savvy of a politician named Kenneth Hahn, was unbeatable, and soon supportive legislation and funds enabled a rapid expansion of the Los Angeles paramedic program within the county. Public perceptions and expectations, however inaccurate, were changed across the country, and there was no turning back.

The era of acceptance . . .

If the decade of the 1970s was not exactly a time of unfettered acceptance of EMS principles (however they were defined by whoever defined them), the pendulum had swung rather far from the old days of hearse ambulances. Voices urging caution in uncritical acceptance of the burgeoning systems were largely lost in the sounds of sirens and fervent testimonials. Expectations were high, as were levels of funding.

It is true that, even during this phase of EMS development and relative uncritical acceptance, lively medical debate took place. The struggle to define what were appropriate levels of training and out-of-hospital care resulted in an EMS alphabet soup — EMT, EMT-I, EMT-II, EMT-P, EMT-D, EMT-Intermediate, ALS, BLS — and on it went. Add to this the debate about "stay 'n' play" — a variation on the theme of "level of care delivered" — and "swoop 'n' scoop," which many interpreted as a return to the "old days," and the first 20 years of EMS in the United States were not, by any means, placid.

Much of the debate stemmed from the different needs of the two basic root structures from which EMS grew: a system designed to combat sudden cardiac death, and a system advocated by the 1966 white paper to reduce the toll of severe trauma. There were many common elements that would serve both goals — prevention programs; public education; easy accessibility through a universal access number (911 in the United States); dispatch using prescribed protocols; rapid response by appropriate personnel; uniform training curricula, including physician training; appropriate clinical intervention using well-defined medical protocols; high-quality standards for transport vehicles; ready communication among dispatchers, field teams, and receiving hospitals; appropriate data collection/recording; data analysis and continuous quality improvement programs; outcome measurements and research. In other words, the components of the system that would serve the needs of each element were identical. But the content of one element — clinical intervention using well-defined medical protocols — was the sticking point.

Examine the historical roots of the solution to sudden cardiac death and the management of acute myocardial infarction, which suggest that, since most deaths occur outside the confines of the hospital, treatment modalities must be taken to the patient; the patient should be "stabilized" (as the evidence from Belfast suggested) and then transported calmly and carefully to the inhospital setting. However, data from as far back as World War I suggest that, in the case of a seriously injured patient, the time to definitive care is crucial to the survival of the patient — no different from the case of someone who has suffered cardiac arrest. But there is one major difference: the definitive management of the life-threatening common path (ventricular fibrillation) in the cardiac event can be taken to the patient in the out-of-hospital environment in the form of a portable defibrillator and pharmacologic intervention.

The definitive management of a seriously injured patient likely can be provided only in a trauma unit or an operating theater. In other words, definitive management for severe trauma is "hot lights and cold steel."

The early training of paramedics in advanced procedures tended to stress skills appropriate to the management of acute myocardial infarction or cardiac arrest — the latter being a worst-case scenario and therefore a test of the system. Tools were provided at hand to do just that — portable defibrillators, intravenous lines, drugs to manage pain and dysrhythmias, measures to secure the airway (including endotracheal intubation), and more. The condition of patients who were seriously injured or in shock was not likely to be reversed by measures that could be applied in the field, as defibrillation might do to a person who suddenly collapsed in cardiac arrest. The management of the seriously injured patient tested the skill of the field team, in that, when possible, the reduction of field time had a much more prominent role both in the training of field personnel and in the protocol designed to save the lives of trauma patients. Successful EMS systems considered field time as crucial to their success and trained their personnel to apply field procedures quickly or en route to trauma centers.[42]

The era of refinement . . .

The mid-1980s and beyond were a time of reflection and refinement in EMS systems. The influence of television and the media declined somewhat and resumed its rightful place as entertainment rather than as arbiter or prominent advocate of public policy and the public good. The pendulum began to swing back toward a balanced view of what could and could not be expected of EMS systems.

But more forces were at work. Shrinking health care budgets influenced the direction and stress being brought to bear on systems that were, by medical standards, very young. In 1981, the federal EMS initiative embodied in the Emergency Medical Services Systems Act was withdrawn, and much doom was predicted. Local authorities assumed as much of the fiscal burden as possible, and insurers were tapped to pick up the slack. During this time, specialized training programs and educational materials were created, and a national curriculum update was commissioned by the National Highway Traffic Safety Administration (EMS Division). The American Heart Association and related agencies created a network for training and discussion of issues relative to cardiac resuscitation — Advanced Cardiac Life Support, or ACLS. Similar in structure and goals to ACLS was the Amer-

ican College of Surgeons' course designed to improve and standardize the management of the seriously injured — Advanced Trauma Life Support, or ATLS. Two similar programs were developed for the out-of-hospital management of trauma — Basic Trauma Life Support (BTLS) and Prehospital Trauma Life Support (PHTLS). The emergency management of children was the focus of the Pediatric Advanced Life Support (PALS) and Advanced Pediatric Life Support (APLS) programs.

Despite excellent pockets of clinical research into the outcome of patients in EMS systems, few convincing data could be cited as favorable to any particular system design in the first two decades of modern EMS history. Efforts to evaluate system outcomes in the out-of-hospital management of sudden cardiac death and cardiovascular emergencies and to standardize research language and methods culminated in 1990 in an international conference at Utstein Abbey near Stavanger, Norway.* The Utstein meeting resulted in recommendations for uniform reporting standards for cardiac events that were later published and widely accepted.[43]

The physician and EMS . . . an evolution

There can be little doubt that the seed from which modern EMS systems sprouted was planted and tended by visionary physicians who recognized, analyzed, and sought correction first of challenging clinical problems, and that these solutions were later translated to major public health needs and reinforced the link between EMS and public health activities. The recognition of ventricular fibrillation as a reversible event led researchers (in this case, physicians and electrical engineers, as well as others) to search for treatment modalities that could be readily applied to large populations. The realization that early trauma care was sorely deficient led to the 1966 report, and steps were taken as the system evolved. Crucial to all of this was the physician, whose involvement was both intimate and keenly felt. In part, such involvement stemmed from the need to analyze data to determine outcomes; most early mobile coronary care projects were pilot studies growing out of the creation of coronary care units in hospitals.

Central to these early systems was physician leadership, usually in the form of a charismatic, eager,

---

* This was the home city of Asmund S. Laerdal, the Norwegian dollmaker whose friendship with Dr. Peter Safar helped lead to the educational materials and manikins essential to mass training in CPR techniques.[23]

and at times larger-than-life doc whose professional (and sometimes personal) life revolved around the pioneer ground of early lifesaving interventions. With the development of a specialty devoted to early care and systems designed for this — that is, emergency medicine — the responsibility for out-of-hospital management shifted. This shift, particularly in the case of the management of sudden cardiac death, resulted naturally from the improvement of anesthetic techniques and the prevention of the catastrophe of ventricular fibrillation in the operating theater. In other words, neither anesthesiologists nor cardiologists were the most likely physicians to see sudden cardiac death as inhospital procedures were refined and became safer. In the 1970s, focus then shifted to the out-of-hospital environment because that is where most sudden deaths occur; with the invention of the portable defibrillator, treatment now could be relatively easily accessed.

Physician involvement then underwent a transition. From eager physician researchers in clinical and basic science laboratories, the responsibility for immediate care devolved to fledgling emergency departments and physicians who were occupied in creation of a new medical specialty. The management of out-of-hospital emergencies in that same decade was given, in most communities in the United States, to public safety agencies traditionally independent, each with its own structure, and without close ties to hospitals or the health care system (**Figure 1-4**).

Beginning in the late 1970s and extending into the mid-1980s, the involvement and authority of experienced physicians waned somewhat, in part because of the fledgling nature of the specialty of emergency medicine and partly due to the relative independence of public safety and other agencies, which often viewed EMS systems as their unique responsibility. With the expansion of emergency medicine training programs and residencies, the specialty began to treat EMS as a defined field of endeavor (if not a subspecialty specific to emergency medicine). By the 1990s, the influence of organized emergency medicine, through the American College of Emergency Physicians and the National Association of EMS Physicians, began to have some effect in "reinvolving" experienced and specifically trained physicians in the field of out-of-hospital care. Residency curricula began to reflect this philosophy, and formal training programs in both paramedic and aeromedical EMS became entrenched in the specialty. The proliferation of textbooks, handbooks, and publications in the medical literature testified to the success of this trend.

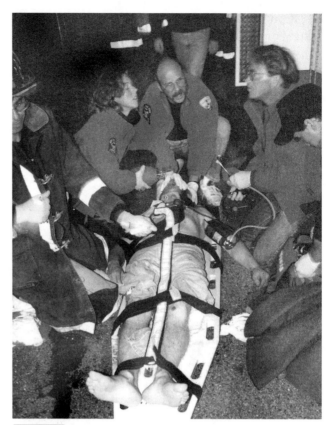

Figure 1-4 The focus of trauma care shifted to the out-of-hospital environment in the 1970s, and management of out-of-hospital care was typically provided by public safety agencies.

Thirty years after . . . an agenda for the future

The National Research Council's 1966 report, *Accidental Death and Disability: The Neglected Disease of Modern Society,* was arguably the real beginning of a public commitment to the design and development of EMS systems in the United States. It marked, in many respects, a commitment to develop standards, promote prevention, foster research, and encourage data collection and system outcome measurement. In recognition of the importance of this milestone and to build better on its legacy, NHTSA commissioned an initiative in 1995 to examine the experience of three decades of out-of-hospital emergency care systems and to present a vision of future priorities and directions. The result was the appointment of a group of experienced leaders in EMS with wide-ranging backgrounds — the fire service, government, academia, private industry, clinical care delivery, information systems, and basic research, among others. The group's report, "EMS Agenda for the Future,"[44] emphasized EMS as a component of the health care system fully integrated into and compatible with community health services.

It outlined 14 distinct attributes of modern EMS systems, as follows:

- Integration of health services
- EMS research
- Legislation and regulation
- System finance
- Human resources
- Medical direction
- Education systems
- Public education
- Prevention
- Public access
- Communication systems
- Clinical care
- Information systems
- Evaluation

The "EMS Agenda for the Future" served as a focus of discussion and debate in a series of national and regional conferences in the climate of the 1990s characterized in the health sector by major change and upheaval. The following year, NHTSA issued the "EMS Agenda for the Future: Implementation Guide"[45] that sought to set out practical methods of achieving the "agenda." Meetings and conferences of various steering committees designed to discuss methods of implementing the 14 attributes were convened over the next several years.

The "EMS Agenda for the Future" document sought to define the qualities of a modern EMS system, but it went further than that. It sought as well to predict what *might* be possible for EMS to offer to citizens in the future, a difficult mandate considering the rapidly changing nature of health care at the end of the century in almost any county or jurisdiction. The document took great pains to emphasize that EMS is but one component — although an essential one — of a modern health care system. It advocated integration into a community health services system and suggested that field teams might assume broader patient care responsibilities, at least in underserved areas. The agenda reflected the 1966 report in its commitment to prevention, public education, research, and outcome evaluation. And it restated the essential role of EMS as the public's emergency medical safety net.

Subsequent activities of this initiative have resulted in the development of the "EMS Education Agenda for the Future: A Systems Approach"[46] and the "EMS Research Agenda for the Future."[47] The former document outlines a process for reconfiguring the EMS education process to more closely reflect advances in education and to more closely align EMS education with medical education. Initial components of the education agenda are currently being developed.

The 2003 publication of the EMS research agenda attempts to provide structure and direction for establishing a research basis for out-of-hospital activities.

Our system disrupted . . .

As noted above, much of what we have learned and included in civilian EMS arose from experiences in military medicine and from lessons learned from international colleagues. Some of those colleagues were faced with the ravages of war in the form of horrendous injuries and mass-casualty events resulting from terrorist activities. It wasn't until 2001 that citizens of the United States were faced with the effects of terrorism on their homeland. Although many of the system issues that now must be faced in planning for potential terrorist events are no different from those we face on a daily basis, our perspectives and some of our planning activities have forever changed.

Alice revisited . . .

If we began by citing the experience of Alice in her Wonderland, we should conclude by remembering that Alice eventually returned to the world of reality and was apparently none the worse for wear. Many of us would liken the ups and downs of the past 30 years of EMS as a bit of a Wonderland (most of us can remember meeting our share of Cheshire Cats, Mad Hatters, a Dormouse or two . . . and attending our share of strange tea parties in our EMS journey), but we are now back in the land of reality. When all is said and done, the foundation stones and the historical principles upon which EMS is based must revolve around our commitment to the human condition and our pledge to give our best in the tradition of that Good Samaritan of old, regardless of race, creed, orientation, or blood alcohol level. May it ever be so.

References

1. Schwab CW. Helicopters and rescue: a historical overview. *Emerg Care Q*. 1986;2(3):1–12.
2. Beck CS, Leghninger DS. Death after a clean bill of health. *JAMA*. 1960;174:133.
3. Kouwenhoven WB, Langworthy OR. Cardiopulmonary resuscitation: an account of 45 years of research. *Hopkins Med J*. 1973;132:186–189.
4. The Bible, II Kings 4:32–35.
5. Herholdt JD, Rafn CG. An attempt at an historical survey of lifesaving measures for drowning persons. Copenhagen, Denmark: N Tikiob; 1796.

6. The Bible, Luke 10:30–37.

7. Stewart RD. Historical perspectives on EMS systems. In: Roush WR, ed. *Principles of EMS Systems*. 2nd ed. Dallas, Tex: American College of Emergency Physicians; 1989.

8. Larrey DJ. Mémoires de chirurgie militaire et campagnes. Paris, France. J Smith; 1812.

9. Dunant JH. Un souvenir de Solférino. Genève, Switzerland: Fick; 1862.

10. Macnab AJ. Air medical transport: "hot air" and a French lesion. *J Air Med Transport*. 1992;11:15–18.

11. Guilford FR, Soboroff BJ. Air evacuation: an historical review. *J Aviat Med*. 1947;18:601–616.

12. Boyne WJ, Lopez DS, eds. *Vertical Flight: The Age of the Helicopter*. Washington, DC: Smithsonian Institution Press; 1984.

13. Haacker LP. Time and its effects on casualties in World War II and Vietnam. *Arch Surg*. 1969;98:39–40.

14. Neel S. Army aeromedical evacuation procedures in Vietnam: implications for rural America. *JAMA*. 1968;204:99–103.

15. Cleveland HC, Bigelow DB, Dracon D, et al. A civilian air emergency service: a report of its development, technical aspects and experience. *J Trauma*. 1976; 16:452–463.

16. Jones R. Crippling due to fractures: its prevention and remedy. *Br Med J*. 1925;I:909–913.

17. Bliss M. *William Osler: A Life in Medicine*. Toronto, Ontario, Canada: University of Toronto Press; 1999: 439–440.

18. Crile GW. *Hemorrhage and Transfusion*. New York, NY: D Appleton; 1909:139.

19. Eisenberg MS. *Life in the Balance: Emergency Medicine and the Quest to Reverse Sudden Death*. New York, NY: Oxford University Press; 1997.

20. Julian DG. Cardiopulmonary resuscitation in the eighteenth century. *Heart Lung*. 1975;4:46–49.

21. Bishop PJ. A short history of the Royal Humane Society. London, England: Royal Humane Society; 1974.

22. Elam JO, Brown ES, Elder JD. Artificial respiration by mouth-to-mask method: a study of the respiratory gas exchange of paralyzed patients ventilated by operator's expired air. *N Engl J Med*. 1954;250:749–754.

23. Safar P. *Careers in Anesthesiology: An Autobiographical Memoir*. Park Ridge, Ill: Wood Library-Museum of Anesthesiology; 2000.

24. Overbeck W. Historical views concerning cardiac arrest and resuscitation. In: Stephenson HE, ed. *Cardiac Arrest and Resuscitation*. St Louis, Mo: CV Mosby; 1969: 27–40.

25. Crile GW. *Anemia and Resuscitation*. New York, NY: D Appleton; 1914. (As quoted in Eisenberg, pages 113–114.)

26. Kouwenhoven WB, Jude JR, Knickerbocker GG. Closed-chest cardiac massage. *JAMA*. 1960;173:94–97.

27. Hooker DR, Kouwenhoven WB, Langworthy OR. The effect of alternating electrical currents on the heart. *Am J Physiol*. 1933;103:444–454.

28. Beck CS, Pritchard WH, Feil HS. Ventricular fibrillation of long duration abolished by electric shock. *JAMA*. 1947;135:985–986.

29. Zoll PM, Linenthal J, Gibson W, et al. Termination of ventricular fibrillation in man by externally applied electrical countershock. *N Engl J Med*. 1956;254: 727–732.

30. Albert Lasker Clinical Medical Research Awards: Citations. *JAMA*. 1973;226:876.

31. Lown B, Amarasingham R, Neuman J. New method for terminating cardiac arrhythmias: use of synchronized capacitor discharge. *JAMA*. 1962;182:548–555.

32. Cummins RO, Ornato JP, Thies WH, et al. Improving survival from sudden cardiac death: the "chain of survival" concept. A statement for health professionals from the Advanced Cardiac Life Support Committee and the Emergency Cardiac Care Committee, American Heart Association. *Circulation*. 1991;83:1832–1847.

33. Farrington DJ. The war goes on. 1976 Presidential Address, American Association for the Surgery of Trauma. *J Trauma*. 1977;17:655–661.

34. National Academy of Sciences-National Research Council, Committees on Trauma and Shock. *Accidental Death and Disability: The Neglected Disease of Modern Society*. Washington, DC: National Academic Press; 1966.

35. Pantridge JF, Geddes JS. A mobile intensive care unit in the management of myocardial infarction. *Lancet*. 1967;2:271–273.

36. Pantridge JF, Geddes JS, Adgey AAJ. Prehospital coronary care. *Am J Cardiol*. 1969;24:666–673.

37. Grace WJ, Chadbourn JA. The first hour in acute myocardial infarction. *Heart Lung*. 1974;3:736–741.

38. Nagel EL, Hirschman JC, Meyer PW, et al. Telemetry of physiologic data: an aid to fire rescue personnel in a metropolitan area. *South Med J*. 1968;61:598–601.

39. Cobb LA, Conn RD, Samson WE, et al. Early experience in the management of sudden death with a mobile intensive coronary care unit. *Circulation*. 1970;48 (Suppl):III144.

40. Criley JM, Lewis AJ, Ailshie GE. Mobile emergency care units: implementation and justification. *Adv Cardiol*. 1975;15:9–24.

41. West JG, Trunkey DD, Lim RC. Systems of trauma care. A study of two counties. *Arch Surg*. 1979; 114:455–460.

42. Pons PT, Honigman B, Moore EE, et al. Prehospital advanced trauma life support for critical penetrating wounds to the thorax and abdomen. *J Trauma*. 1985;25:828–832.

43. Cummins RO, Chamberlain DA, Abramson NS, et al. Recommended guidelines for uniform reporting of data from out-of-hospital cardiac arrest, the Utstein style. *Ann Emerg Med.* 1991;20:861–874.

44. Delbridge TR, Bailey B, Chew JL, et al. EMS agenda for the future: where we are, where we want to be: EMS Agenda for the Future Committee. *Ann Emerg Med.* 1998;31:251-263. Also available at: http://www.nhtsa.dot.gov/people/injury/ems/agenda/emsman.html. Accessed May 28, 2004.

45. National Highway Traffic Safety Administration. EMS agenda for the future: implementation guide — moving closer to the vision. *Ann Emerg Med.* 1998;32:511–512.

Also available at http://www.nhtsa.dot.gov/people/injury/ems/agenda/index.html. Accessed May 28, 2004.

46. National Highway Traffic Safety Administration. EMS education agenda for the future: a systems approach [NHTSA Web site]. Available at: http://www.nhtsa.dot.gov/people/injury/ems/EdAgenda/final/index.html. Accessed May 28, 2004.

47. National Highway Traffic Safety Administration. EMS research agenda for the future. [NHTSA Web site]. Available at: http://www.nhtsa.dot.gov/people/injury/ems/EMS03-ResearchAgenda/preface.htm. Accessed May 28, 2004.

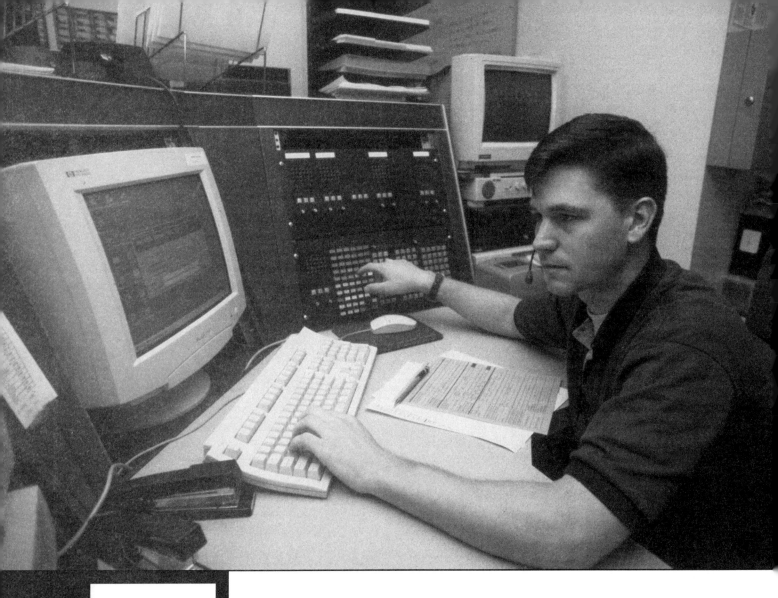

2 EMS Systems

Peter T. Pons, MD, FACEP
Rick Murray, EMT-P

Principles of This Chapter

After reading this chapter, you should be able to:

- Discuss the role of the lead agency within EMS systems.
- Recall the NHTSA statewide EMS systems evaluation components.
- Describe the integral, functional components of EMS systems — medical oversight and administrative oversight, transport agencies, dispatch, communications, clinical care protocols, receiving facilities, specialty care, training, finance, audit and quality improvement, mutual aid, and disaster planning.

WHAT IS AN EMS SYSTEM? CONSISTENT WITH THE "EMS Agenda for the Future," it is an organized, integrated program that allows for, and provides to an individual in need of acute medical assistance, the means to access and enter the health care delivery system in a timely manner. In order to do so, an EMS system must consist of, at a minimum, a communications mechanism to initiate a response, a vehicle with personnel to provide treatment and transport, and a receiving facility to which to take the patient. In a rural setting, the "system" might consist of just one ambulance and one receiving facility. In an urban area, there can be multiple agencies that provide response and transport to categorized facilities. Regardless of the size, an organized systems approach to EMS is necessary if the available resources are to be used in providing optimal patient care. Each participant in the EMS system must know his or her responsibility and how to interact with all other components.

EMS systems are developed to address the emergency medical needs of small communities, big cities, large geographic regions, or entire states. Most systems — and this discussion — are focused on the local or regional level. Most organizers of EMS do not have the luxury of developing completely new systems: they have to work with preexisting components such as hospitals and ambulances that are already providing services. Establishing oversight over these various independent providers can be extremely difficult. Unless the system can start de novo, which is unlikely, it must use and coordinate existing resources. Therefore, organizers of an EMS system must have the authority to oversee funding, contract negotiations, and medical care as well as be actively involved in developing enabling legislation.

This chapter provides an overview of the function and components of an EMS system. Many of these components are addressed in greater detail in subsequent chapters.

The EMS Agency

If a system is to carry out all of its responsibilities, there must be an administrative "lead" agency to coordinate and direct all components of the system.[1,2] This agency often exists within an existing branch of local, regional, or state government, or it is established as an independent council with authority, by contract or statute, to manage the system.[3] Wherever the agency is located, the resulting EMS plan and response system should be approved by an EMS planning authority, which can also be at the local, regional, or state level.

The EMS authority should comprise a board or council made up of a representative cross-section of the medical, out-of-hospital provider, and consumer populations of the service area. The board must have authority to establish policies for the system and must be the final authority in all disputes. Representation on the board should be broad enough to ensure that policies developed are in the best interest of patient care without undue concern over political or monetary issues. For example, the board might decide to develop joint ambulance districts involving more than one political subdivision rather than have each community provide its own dispatch, response, and transport. Such a plan might prove to be more efficient and cost-effective while providing an improved level of patient care. However, implementation of the plan might be unpopular and might even be resisted by the smaller communities that legitimately use self-determination as an argument.

In its publication "EMS Agenda for the Future," the National Highway Traffic Safety Administration (NIITSA) described the importance of EMS as part of the overall health care system and outlined the wide variations in legislation and EMS systems in the United States during its EMS technical assessments conducted in many states.[4] To date, limited funding availability has hampered efforts to enhance development, innovation, and integration of EMS systems.

Ideally, EMS lead agencies should provide technical assistance to local EMS providers, develop and support enabling legislation, integrate EMS services, and ensure direct medical involvement and oversight of all EMS activities.

Developing a Master Plan

The EMS lead agency must be responsible for developing a master plan that includes operational standards for each component of the system and provider of service. Development of this plan should rely on input from a broad-based group made up of providers and consumers. Once such a plan is implemented, the agency must maintain open communication for feedback from the same groups.

An adequate, qualified administrative staff is necessary to ensure implementation of the policies developed by the board and outlined in the master plan. The medical director, administrator, and administrative staff will be either full-time or part-time employees of the agency depending on the size and needs of the system. The agency might contract with specialists as consultants to address specific portions of the plan, for example, computer experts to help implement system audit procedures.

The EMS lead agency is responsible for overall quality improvement within the system, and each provider is responsible for the quality improvement activities of its component of the system. It must have the authority to determine who will participate within the EMS system (ie, personnel, transport agencies, and facilities). The lead agency must include the services of a physician who is responsible for establishing medical standards within the system and ensuring medical quality and accountability. It must develop clear, explicit protocols, procedures, and policies consistent with state minimum requirements, including certification or licensure requirements, but the board can also include additional requirements to address specific system needs.

Several items must be considered to ensure effective planning and development of a system's master plan. First, the agency should take inventory of system needs and of resources and services presently available within the system, although some of the resources might not be easy to quantify. For example, a hospital or community agency such as a volunteer fire department might commit significant manpower and time at very little or no cost to the system.

Questions that must be answered when surveying the local resources include: What municipal or county services are available? What segments of the population, if any, are overserved or underserved? What communications mechanisms exist? How many ambulances and rescue vehicles are available, and how are they equipped? What education programs are available? Is manpower going to be provided by volunteers, paid personnel, or both? What are the available hospital resources and their capabilities?

Second, the plan should include specific goals and objectives that can be identified and measured. Resources should be matched to the population served, as well as to the goals and objectives desired. These goals should be specific to allow meaningful assessment of the system. For example, within the service area, can basic life support (BLS) and advanced life support (ALS) be delivered within agreed-on time frames? Goals can be set that are less than ideal, but they should be specific. For example, a system might want to provide available ALS service to an expanded population: to do this, some areas will have prolonged ALS response times on some calls, but this might be considered an acceptable goal that has been identified and can be measured.

Third, methods to achieve the stated goals should be developed. This is where problem-solving must begin. This step will likely alter the list of initial goals to goals that are more desirable or realistic. Fourth, there should be a realistic time schedule in which to accomplish the stated goals. Fifth, a method to evaluate the progress toward achieving the stated goals should exist. Finally, an estimate of the cost to achieve the goals must be made and funding sources to meet those needs identified.

In summary, an EMS system master plan includes a needs assessment, data collection, and analysis of the present resources, and outlines specific goals along with improvements and innovations to be undertaken, establishes ongoing quality improvement activities, and establishes a workable budget.

Components of the EMS System

In 1973, the Emergency Medical Services Systems Act (Public Law 93–154) outlined 15 components of an

EMS system that had to be addressed in order for a system to receive federal funding under the act. States and regions no longer receive funding under this legislation, but many systems still address most of these components, as well as some others. The 15 original components were manpower, training, communications, transportation, emergency facilities, critical care units, public safety agencies, consumer participation, access to care, patient transfer, standardized record-keeping, public information and education, system review and evaluation, disaster planning, and mutual aid.

Conspicuous by its absence was the issue of medical "control" or medical oversight of EMS. The medical oversight issue was later addressed when systems applied for grant funding and in subsequent government publications, such as the "EMS Agenda for the Future." However, because EMS systems initially developed mostly without physician participation and without a firm foundation in research-verified effectiveness, catching up has been slow. Many established systems are still resistant to active and authoritative physician involvement.

Components of the modern EMS system include physician medical oversight, communications, dispatch, out-of-hospital transport agencies, interfacility transport agencies, protocols (triage, treatment, transport, and transfer), receiving facilities, specialty care units, training, audit and quality assurance, financing, public information and education, mutual aid, and disaster management.[5] With the events of September 11, 2001, the subsequent anthrax releases, and events in the United States and the world, disaster management issues have been expanded to include the activities of domestic preparedness response activities (**Figure 2-1**).

NHTSA has developed and offered for many years a program for assessment of the various components of an EMS system at a statewide level.[5] In this program, a team of experts evaluates the status of each component of the system and offers suggestions for improvement. In addition, if asked, NHTSA will follow up with a reassessment to evaluate the progress made. The components assessed during a NHTSA visit are regulation and policy, resource management, human resources and training, transportation, facilities, communication, public information and education, medical direction, trauma systems, and evaluation.

The American Ambulance Association also provides guidance regarding the functional components of an EMS system for communities seeking to contract or develop ambulance services. They have published a comprehensive guide that describes system

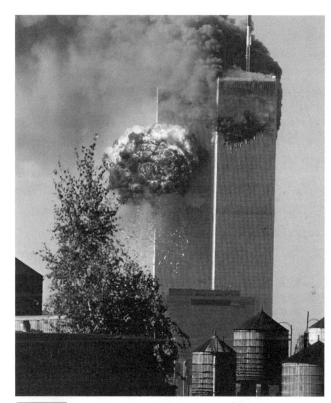

Figure 2-1 The events of September 11, 2001, created a need for the expansion of disaster management issues.

components that must be considered when contracting with a provider for EMS service.[6] Resource documents on aspects of fire service EMS are also available from the International Association of Fire Chiefs and the International Association of Fire Fighters.

Medical Oversight

Historically, there have been several terms used to describe the activities outlined in this section. Initially, the term **medical control** was used to indicate the control that physicians needed to provide over EMS personnel, as they were not independently licensed health care providers. It also referred to the **online** medical activities physicians performed when talking with EMS personnel via radio. The term **medical direction** evolved to describe these online activities and other **offline** activities such as education, quality assurance, and others. Most recently, **medical oversight** describes all of the prospective, concurrent, and retrospective activities (to be outlined later in the text) conducted by physicians (and others) assuming the ultimate responsibility and authority for the medical care provided by an EMS system and its providers. These terms are often inappropriately interchanged.

All EMS systems must be able to ensure that the medical care provided to patients is in accordance with accepted medical practice standards. This medical oversight must be the responsibility of a physician, preferably one experienced in and knowledgeable of the out-of-hospital emergency care administered to patients who are acutely ill or traumatized.[7,8] Board-certified or board-prepared emergency physicians are best suited to fill this role in most cases.

To perform this function, the physician must have specific defined authority to fulfill the following responsibilities:

- Approve participation by out-of-hospital providers who must practice under his or her supervision
- Suspend an EMS provider from medical care duties for due cause
- Establish systemwide treatment protocols, including standing orders
- Establish criteria for level of initial emergency response (ie, BLS, ALS, and so on)
- Establish criteria for determining patient destination
- Establish medical standards for dispatch procedures
- Approve online physicians or other personnel
- Establish circumstances under which nonresponse or nontransport might occur
- Establish the level of approved educational proficiency of EMS personnel of all levels, out-of-hospital care nurses, dispatchers, education coordinators, and online personnel
- Conduct effective system audits and quality improvement activities

The medical director must have unrestricted access to all relevant EMS records needed to accomplish this task.

In addition to what might be considered the administrative aspect of medical direction described above, there exists the need for immediate physician consultation or direction during an actual EMS call (**Figure 2-2**). This has commonly been referred to as **online medical direction.** The system should ensure that a communication mechanism is available whereby field providers can always obtain access to a physician for consultation. This can be to obtain a physician order, to perform a procedure or administer a drug that requires specific approval, to consult with the physician regarding difficult management issues or refusal of care, or to prepare the physician and receiving facility for an incoming patient. It is the responsibility of the EMS medical director to ensure that the physicians who serve in this capacity have appropriate knowledge and training of the out-of-hospital protocols and the use of radio equipment.

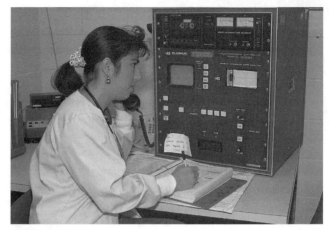

Figure 2-2 Online medical direction ensures that field providers can always obtain access to a physician for consultation.

Organizations such as the American College of Emergency Physicians (ACEP) and the National Association of EMS Physicians (NAEMSP) have long taken leadership roles in advocating for the strong involvement of knowledgeable physicians in directing the medical care activities of EMS agencies. Both organizations have prepared and published policy and position statements describing the importance of strong physician involvement and direction, as well as desired qualifications and training for these physicians.[7,9]

Transport Issues

Out-of-Hospital Transport Agencies

The EMS lead agency need not own or operate the out-of-hospital response and transport services, but it must have the authority to establish criteria for participation by these services. Most states have legislation that establishes standards for ambulance services and vehicles and permits either licensure or certification. At one time, it was thought that having this type of authority constituted restraint of trade. However, court rulings have indicated that a municipality has the authority to establish a public trust, public utility EMS, to the exclusion of all other EMS providers that would like to operate within the community.

At a minimum, the EMS lead agency must have the authority to establish operational standards for the response/transport vehicles within the system. These standards include a comprehensive equipment list, the minimal number of providers on each response, their required level of certification, and response time criteria.

All emergency transports within the EMS system should be regulated by the EMS lead agency, regardless of whether they are carried out by public, private, not-for-profit, or specialty (air and ground) transport. In some cases, critical care, interfacility, air medical, and invalid transport are also controlled and coordinated by the agency.

Interfacility Transport

In its strictest sense, interfacility transfer is not the responsibility of the EMS system, although transfer can be an integral part of a comprehensive system that uses categorized facilities. It is possible to assert that interfacility transfer constitutes emergency care and, therefore, is appropriate for an EMT or paramedic to be in attendance, but most state enabling legislation does not address this issue. Once a patient presents to a hospital's emergency department for care, that patient is the responsibility of that hospital. If the patient is transferred and his or her condition deteriorates during transport, the physician authorizing the transport could be accused of negligence and abandonment. It is now understood that the transferring physician is responsible for ensuring proper patient care during interfacility transport, unless the physician at the receiving hospital assumes that responsibility. Federal regulations such as EMTALA define the process for evaluation and stabilization of a patient prior to transfer and outline the necessary steps to ensure appropriate transfer and transport, with significant penalties for both the physician and hospital for failure to comply (see Chapter 27, "EMTALA and EMS").

Appropriately, EMS system vehicles and personnel may be used during interfacility transports. In these situations, the transferring physician is responsible for determining the level of expertise and personnel needed during the transport. When necessary, the patient should be accompanied by personnel from the sending hospital who are individually licensed (therefore, either a physician or a nurse) to provide the appropriate level of medical treatment. Under no circumstances should an EMT provide treatment or intervention in excess of his or her certification level.

To address these potential problems, some facilities have developed and maintain their own specialty transport vehicles (see Chapter 14, "Air Medical Transport," and Chapter 13, "Ground Transport: Interfacility and Specialty Care Transfers"). These can be either air or ground transport units. Hospital-based transport vehicles have evolved from general purpose ambulances to specialized critical care units with all of the appropriate equipment and personnel capable of providing extremely high-level intensive care for very specialized populations, such as pediatric, burn, or cardiac patients.

Communications to and from hospital-based specialty transport units should be coordinated by the EMS system, especially if they use radio frequencies designated for emergency medical use. These specialty units can be used in certain circumstances to respond to out-of-hospital emergency scenes. Because they are usually in a unique setting, these providers occasionally believe they are outside the direction of the regional EMS system. It must be established in advance that out-of-hospital response is the responsibility of the EMS agency and that any scene response must be approved and coordinated with all responding units. Decisions to accept the assistance of a nonsystem specialty transport unit must be the responsibility of the EMS system medical director.

Dispatch

Ideally, emergency medical response should be dispatched through a communications center that coordinates the response of all public service providers, including fire and police personnel, to better use and coordinate all available resources.

The EMS system communications center occasionally is located in an agency or political authority that is not under direct operational control of the EMS system, such as in a municipal police or fire department. In this circumstance, the dispatcher for EMS might have been assigned this responsibility in addition to his or her usual activities as dispatcher for the police or fire department. On many occasions, this person has not received additional training to properly perform the specialized and important duty of emergency medical dispatching. This is not ideal and should not occur in well-established EMS systems. Under all circumstances, the EMS agency and the medical director must have authority to establish levels of appropriate education and certification for dispatchers.[9]

Because dispatch affects patient care, the EMS agency also must have the authority to establish operational policy, including how patients access the system, prearrival instructions, and level of response and personnel capability provided. If the EMS system holds itself out as a provider of emergency service, it is obligated to respond to and evaluate the situation of any individual requesting emergency assistance. Some EMS systems have, in the past, believed their systems to be stressed by overuse and have instructed their dispatchers to screen calls and, under some circumstances, not provide an EMS response. This is not what EMS was intended to be and is fraught with great hazard, both to patients and the EMS system, when a decision that no help is needed is made in error.

Rather than attempt to determine over the telephone that no medical assistance is necessary, a formal process of questioning the caller in order to evaluate the severity of the medical problem has been adopted and implemented by many EMS systems. This standardized approach allows the dispatcher to determine not whether a response by EMS is needed, but instead the amount, level, and rapidity of the response (red lights and siren versus nonemergent). Using predefined questions and assessment tools, the person who takes the call can quickly obtain needed information and better use available resources. This process is commonly referred to as **emergency medical dispatching (EMD)**.[10]

Many EMS systems have also implemented **prearrival instructions** as part of the dispatch process. The call-taker offers instruction and assistance to the caller to begin providing medical care even before the physical arrival of responding EMS personnel. Additional information on dispatching issues is provided in Chapter 10, "Emergency Medical Dispatch."

Communications

The EMS agency must establish a comprehensive communications plan or accept a preexisting regional plan to make optimal use of available communication resources. The plan should specify how system access by the community will occur and where calls for assistance will be routed (**Figure 2-3**). Ideally, the system will adopt 911 as the universal access number.[4] In lieu of 911, a single, well-posted 7-digit number for all emergencies, medical and nonmedical, is used. Unfortunately, some communities still use different 7-digit numbers to access police, fire, and EMS. This often produces delays as citizens try to remember or find these numbers in an emergency. **Enhanced 911 systems** have been implemented in many municipalities to improve emergency response.[11] These computerized systems automatically display to the dispatcher the address and telephone number of the 911 call's origin. Thus, help can be sent even if the caller is unable to speak or provide information. This system is also routinely updated by the telephone company to maintain current information. The widespread use of cellular telephones, however, has added an impediment to the desired goal of enhanced 911. Many public safety answering systems are unable to identify the calling telephone number and, more importantly, the caller's location. As a result, enhanced 911 technology and systems are now being extended to cellular equipment to aid in identifying both the calling telephone and the caller's location.

Radio frequencies available for EMS are limited and tightly regulated by the Federal Communications Commission (see Chapter 9, "Communications"). Any provider using the medical emergency frequencies within the system must be approved to participate and abide by the rules established in the communications plan.

The plan must ensure that communications are fully coordinated and integrated with other public safety providers. To this end, the plan must designate frequency use for dispatch, disaster, online activities, intervehicle communications, and interagency communications.

To ensure that all providers, whether ground vehicles or aircraft, have appropriate communications ability, the system must define what is minimal radio equipment and develop protocols that designate appropriate frequency use. These protocols should be supplemented by education programs and QI programs to guarantee that all providers understand the procedures.

Protocols

Protocols establish the standards to be achieved under specific circumstances within the EMS system. Protocols can be developed to address any situation, medical as well as nonmedical. Procedures or policies that do not directly affect patient care should be the responsibility of administrative personnel, such as the EMS system administrator or his or her designee. Activities of the system that affect patient care must be the responsibility of the medical director. Specifically, he or she must address protocols dealing with triage, treatment, transport, transfer, and other activities as needed.

Triage in nondisaster situations addresses the level of response provided by the EMS system, as well as the level of provider capability during transport. For example, if assistance is requested for a person with a suspected wrist sprain, it might be appropriate to send a basic provider unit. But when and how this determination is made is the responsibility of the medical director. Triage protocols must be written carefully to define those specific circumstances.

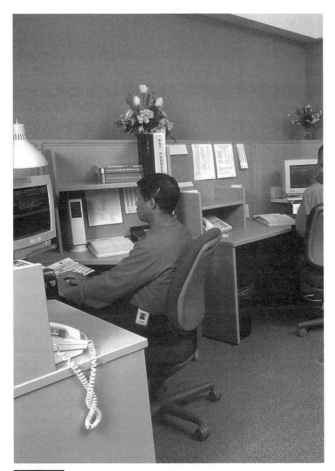

Figure 2-3 911 systems have been implemented in many municipalities to improve emergency response.

Treatment protocols are rather standard and exist for most EMS systems, but the degree of complexity varies from system to system. Standing orders are a subset of protocols and outline specific emergency actions that can be undertaken by a provider without contacting a physician for orders. The protocols or standing orders of one system might tell the provider which size needle and the maximal number of tries to start an IV, while another system's protocol might simply say, "Start an IV." Guidelines are formulated by national panels using the available evidence and consensus. Examples of these guidelines include Advanced Cardiac Life Support (**ACLS**), Basic Trauma Life Support (**BTLS**), and Prehospital Trauma Life Support (**PHTLS**). These guidelines are often used in EMS systems to develop protocols for managing patients with these problems. It should be noted that these national organizational guidelines are voluntary and do not necessarily establish the standard of care.[12]

Deviations from the EMS system protocols as written, without good reason, must be considered a breach of delegated practice authority. Any deviation from standing orders should result in an audit by the system, or the system does not truly have medical accountability. If difficult decisions must be made while caring for a patient, the system should have online communication capabilities so that consultation and direction from a physician can be obtained.

The method of transport should also be predefined. It might be appropriate to send a patient with a suspected wrist sprain to the hospital by private conveyance rather than EMS vehicle, but, again, this policy must be established by the medical director. All calls resulting in nontransport (including refusal of transport by the patient) should either involve the online physician or be critically reviewed by the medical director because a medical decision is being made that the patient is stable and does not require system transport. The potential for a wrong decision is not insignificant, thus the need for physician input or review.

Destination decisions must be made according to a predetermined, systemwide policy developed to achieve optimal patient care and protect against an unintended institutional competitive advantage or managed care plan desires or manipulation.[13] Any plan must take into account the "nearest appropriate facility" concept and might include categorization of receiving facilities based on specialized services offered by a facility, such as a burn center, hyperbaric chamber, or trauma center.

Interfacility transfers within the EMS system might be necessary to ensure that emergency patients are treated at an appropriate "definitive care facility." If the initial receiving facility does not have a neurosurgeon, for example, patients with head injuries must be transferred to a facility that does if the transferring hospital does not have the capability to provide needed care. The only requirement is that the transfer must be accomplished in an appropriate manner so the patient receives the best possible care under the circumstances. This type of transfer is medically indicated, and the transferring physician must certify that the benefit to the patient of receiving care at another facility outweighs the risks of the transfer itself.[14] Transfer situations are addressed again in Chapter 13, and in Chapter 27, "EMTALA and EMS."

Receiving Facilities

Any receiving facility within the system must have the capability to improve patient outcome by providing evaluation and stabilization of ill and injured patients. Ideally, the receiving facility is located in a hospital that has an emergency department with physician staffing 24 hours a day. The facility should have not only an emergency department but also immediately available services such as laboratory, blood bank, radiology, surgery, and critical care. In some rural areas, patients might have to be transported to emergency facilities that do not meet all of these criteria. However, relationships with other hospitals must be in place to allow transfer of those patients to an appropriate level of care as soon as possible by appropriate transfer resources.

Specialty Care

Each EMS system should identify hospitals capable of providing specialty care for the small proportion of patients who require such treatment. These units include trauma, burn, cardiac, stroke, hyperbaric, pediatric, perinatal, psychiatric, spinal, and poison treatment facilities. If these specialty services do not exist within the system, formal transfer agreements and transfer protocols should be developed with nearby resources.

If specialty care facilities exist within the EMS system, they should be used according to protocols and policies developed by the lead agency. Access to specialty care might be by direct transport from the out-of-hospital scene when appropriate or by interhospital transfer after stabilization at a receiving facility. The capability of a specialty care facility to receive patients by air medical transport is desirable.

Training

Training within the system of both new and existing personnel is a primary concern. Primary training programs that meet or exceed the national standard curricula should be established within the system. If this is not possible, it can become expensive to send providers outside of the system for their education. An alternative is to hire only certified providers who have completed training. However, this alternative has a drawback because the system has less control over the education content. If the latter option is used, the system must develop a method to ensure provider competence before employment (eg, National Registry of EMTs, entry level review, or a comprehensive test).

Primary education programs within the system should reflect additional system needs beyond the national curricula. To this end, it is appropriate for the EMS system to have input into the delivery of educa-

tion programs. On the other hand, having the education program totally controlled by the local EMS system might lead to irregularities, such as graduation of unqualified students just because of their employment status within the system. The EMS system might have some leverage with the education program located in a college or hospital because the students need a place for clinical experience to apply the skills learned during training. This is usually accomplished by a field internship, which consists of managing real patients under supervised field conditions. If the school is not responsive to the system's special needs, the system might not be supportive of the school.

Continuing education is a must for all levels of providers within the system because it is necessary for licensure or certification maintenance. Ideally, these programs are provided within the EMS system to ensure availability.

When special system needs are identified, the agency might need to conduct inservice or specialized education programs within the system. These programs should include physicians, nurses, and EMTs involved in specialty transport, as well as physicians or other personnel who will be providing online activities. Additional information on EMS education issues is provided in Chapter 23, "EMS Education Programs."

Financing

After available resources are identified and reasonably achievable goals established, a workable budget for the EMS system must be developed. If the goals cost more than the resources provide, the system will either have to alter the method of financing or lower some of the goals. Before the goals are lowered — assuming they are realistic and have a direct impact on patient care — alternative methods of funding should be considered.

Usual methods of funding include tax based, subscription, user pay, and the public utility model and its hybrid forms. There are a few systems that are 100% volunteer in that all funds are raised by donation, fundraising, and similar situations and service is provided at no cost to patients. This model was once common, but as demands for higher level response, rapid response, and education requirements have increased, this form of system funding has begun to disappear.

The **tax-based system** frequently is financed by existing revenues such as general funds, and service is provided through an existing public service agency. Another method is to have the public vote on a tax levy specifically for the provision of EMS service. This might finance an independent EMS municipal department (third service), but more frequently EMS is established within an existing service such as the fire department. This has permitted the fire service to maintain high numbers of personnel and equipment, even in the face of decreased fire suppression responses. Also, with levy-based funding, the system income is fixed and cannot respond easily to increased demand, resulting in increased operating expenses. In some systems, this has led to call screening, where some requests for emergency response are not granted to limit demand on the system. As noted earlier, call screening is an unacceptable practice.

Another form of funding is the **subscription program,** which is really another form of voluntary taxation because the user pays in advance for the service he or she might receive. In this type of funding program, an individual subscriber (or family) pays a fixed fee to the ambulance service provider that covers the charges for all ambulance service for a defined period of time, usually a year. The individual can gamble (ie, not pay) and hope that ambulance service is not required, but if it is, nonsubscribers will have to pay actual cost, which will be much higher than the subscription fee. In some cases, the user's insurance, whether private or Medicare, will cover the cost of ambulance service.

A private ambulance is the purest form of **user pay**. In this arrangement, either the patient calls the ambulance directly or the ambulance is dispatched by the EMS system, and the user pays the cost of the services provided. Sometimes the fees are regulated by the community, but the fee usually is based roughly on actual cost or the going rate paid by insurance companies or Medicare. If the private company is providing primary response to emergency situations, it must be responsive to changing demand within the community. If the company identifies an increase in the number of times it cannot answer a call because all vehicles are in service or response times are prolonged because closer units are committed and a distant ambulance had to be dispatched, it must accommodate by adding responding units or by relocating existing units. Expansion of service capability will be reflected in increased cost of emergency care.

If the volume of responses and transports is great enough, a service area might have more than one EMS provider. When emergency service is provided by private ambulance companies, free enterprise is usually allowed, and the caller may request the provider of his or her choice. In dire emergencies, the call to one private service might be passed to a competitor with a closer unit, allowing for a shorter response interval. A system in which each ambulance company has its own dispatch facility is not as effective as a system in which all emergency calls go to one dispatcher and the closest, most appropriate unit is sent.

The last method of financing is the **public utility model,** in which the EMS agency determines the goals it wishes the system to achieve and then accepts bids from providers who believe they can provide the services to meet those goals. The selected provider must then perform within specified parameters or be fined or replaced. Patients are billed for services rendered, and any difference between the bid contract and actual revenues is made up from subsidy by the community. This appears to provide a workable combination of several elements of system financing. Those who cannot pay or do not have insurance are provided service, and the community picks up the tab as in a tax-based system. If the patient is able to pay or has insurance, he or she will be billed for the service as with a private provider. The subsidy takes into account uncollectible bills and currently appears to cost less per run than either the tax-based or the private provider method.

As the cost of delivering health care has increased, government payers have sought ways of decreasing the levels of their support and monetary cost. This has extended to EMS organizations. Levels of service have been identified, and the amount of reimbursement by insurers is tied to the patient's medical condition and the need for basic or advanced care. In addition, medical necessity that an ambulance was required to accomplish the transport must be documented and substantiated to receive payment.

Following the events of September 11, 2001, and subsequent activities involving domestic preparedness response activities, the federal government has provided granting support for terrorism response capabilities. These grants initially involved support from the Department of Justice for law enforcement concerns, the Federal Emergency Management Agency for emergency management, the US Fire Administration for fire service support, the Centers for Disease Control and Prevention for public health initiatives, and the Health Resources and Services Administration for hospital planning and response activities. With the formation of the Department of Homeland Security, many of these activities are being combined. The grants are typically funneled through state-level organizations responsible for coordination and planning. Dedicated funding sources for EMS response capability growth, in many cases, have been lacking. More information on EMS system financing is presented in Chapter 8, "System Financing."

Audit and Quality Improvement

The system should perform quality review and improvement activities, evaluating all components of the system for medical accountability, appropriateness, and cost effectiveness.[15,16] To achieve this goal, the system must develop and use standardized forms to collect information on dispatches and responses, field assessment and treatment, and hospital outcome. Computer technology can be used to analyze the vast amounts of information that accumulate in this process.

To evaluate compliance, the system must first establish minimal performance standards, usually in the form of protocols. Once the standard has been established, evaluation can identify variances, and a feedback loop can be established to address problems identified within the system. Of note, however, quality improvement is focused not on the individual (although there are instances in which an individual will require corrective action), but instead on the system and how the system can improve its service delivery.[16] This often requires a major change in thought process or philosophy and the approach to quality issues, which in many health care businesses has been directed at the failure of the individual employee rather than the failure of the system. Additional information on quality improvement activities is presented in Chapter 6, "Medical Oversight and Accountability."

Public Information and Education

Public education programs are important and can be invaluable to patients by informing them of the proper way to access the system, and of first aid procedures to be performed while waiting for a response team. An educated public would know when to access the EMS system. This would reduce needless runs while increasing the likelihood that individuals in need of emergency service benefit from the system.

The agency should not have to provide all information and education programs, but it should help coordinate and encourage local volunteer agencies such as the American Heart Association, the American Red Cross, poison centers, and other similar agencies to perform these activities. The extent of the public information and education effort will depend on how informed the population is and whether there is rapid turnover or seasonal shift in population, unusual age demographics, or change in employment opportunities.

In addition, EMS agencies and providers should be actively involved in illness and injury prevention activities such as child safety seat education, bicycle helmet usage, gun safety, and seatbelt use, as well as participate in events such as community health fairs that screen patients for various preventable illnesses.

Mutual Aid

To provide EMS in the face of adversity (eg, disasters, all units out, vehicle breakdown), emergency response must also be available from outside the local system. The EMS system must make contingency plans with surrounding provider services to cross geopolitical boundaries when needed to provide assistance and patient care. These arrangements should be in the form of formal agreements and should be provided on a reciprocal basis when necessary.

Disaster Planning

In many areas, disaster planning is primarily the responsibility of the emergency management program. Although it is not the primary responsibility of the local EMS provider, the EMS system does provide the majority of initial medical response and transport units at any mass-casualty incident and must be an active participant with the rest of the emergency management community in the planning process.

Regardless of who performs the planning function, the EMS agency should ensure that a comprehensive plan exists for its service area.[17] The regional disaster preparedness plan must address coordinated central management, integration of all EMS system components, and communications during disasters (see Chapter 17, "Disaster Response"). Once a plan is developed, the EMS system must participate in disaster preparedness drills to assess performance and correct deficiencies. The drill process also educates the providers so that, when under the stress of a disaster response, they will act automatically and appropriately. The EMS system must also be a critical player in domestic preparedness planning activities, education, drills, and response.

Summary

EMS system components require organization, integration, and coordination to provide optimal patient care. The agency and the medical director must make sure that each of the necessary components is present in the system and functions as planned.

The assurance of medical accountability within an EMS system is a dynamic process, and each physician involved in medical oversight should have an intimate knowledge of the system structure and organization. The medical director usually does not have direct control over the actions and activity of the system components. However, he or she must be actively involved in all of the components, recognize weak links in the system, and correct potential problems before they occur.

References

1. Boyd DR. Emergency medical services development: a national initiative. *IEEE Trans Vehicular Technol.* 1976;VT-25:104–114.

2. Narad RA. Coordination of EMS systems: an organizational theory approach. *Prehospital Emerg Care.* 1998; 2:145–152.

3. US Department of Health, Education and Welfare. *EMS System Program Guidelines, Revised Edition.* 1979;4:17–18.

4. National Highway Traffic Safety Administration. EMS Agenda for the Future [NHTSA Web site]. Available at: http://www.nhtsa.dot.gov/people/injury/ems/agenda/emsman.html. Accessed June 1, 2004.

5. National Highway Traffic Safety Administration. *Emergency Medical Services System Development: Results of the Statewide EMS Assessment Program. Interim Report, 1994.* [For the 1995 update, see NHTSA Web site. Available at: http://www.nhtsa.dot.gov/people/injury/traffic_tech/1995/TT100.htm. Accessed June 1, 2004.]

6. American Ambulance Association. *Contracting for Emergency Ambulance Services. A Guide to Effective System Design.* McLean, Va: AAA; 1994.

7. Alonso-Serra H, Blanton D, O'Connor RE. Physician medical direction in EMS. *Prehospital Emerg Care.* 1998; 2:153–157.

8. Stone RM, Seaman KG, Bissell RA. A statewide study of EMS oversight: medical director characteristics and involvement compared with national guidelines. *Prehospital Emerg Care.* 2000;4:345–351.

9. American College of Emergency Physicians. Physician Medical Direction of Emergency Medical Services Dispatch Programs [policy statement]. Available at: http://www.acep.org/1,637,0.html. Accessed June 1, 2004.

10. Clawson JJ, for the consensus panel of the National Association of EMS Physicians. Emergency medical dispatching. *Prehospital Disaster Med.* October-December 1989.

11. Martinez R. New vision for the role of EMS. *Ann Emerg Med.* 1993;32:594–599.

12. American College of Emergency Physicians. Voluntary Guidelines for Out-of-Hospital Practices [policy statement]. Available at: http://www.acep.org/1,4861,0.html. Accessed June 1, 2004.

13. Koenig KL, Salvucci AA, Zachariah BS, O'Connor RE, for the National Association of EMS Physicians. EMS Systems and Managed Care Integration [position paper]. Available at: http://www.naemsp.org/Position%20Papers/emsystems.pdf. Accessed June 1, 2004.

14. Consolidated Omnibus Budget Reconciliation Act of 1985 (COBRA). Pub L No. 99–272, Title IX, Section 9121, 100 Stat 167 (1986).

15. Moore L. Measuring quality and effectiveness of prehospital EMS. *Prehospital Emerg Care.* 1999;3:325–331.

16. National Highway Traffic Safety Administration. *A Leadership Guide to Quality Improvement for Emergency Medical Services Systems* [NHTSA Web site]. Available at: http://www.nhtsa.dot.gov/people/injury/ems/leaderguide/. Accessed June 1, 2004.

17. Branas CC, Sing RF, Perron AD. A case series analysis of mass casualty incidents. *Prehospital Emerg Care.* 2000; 4:299–304.

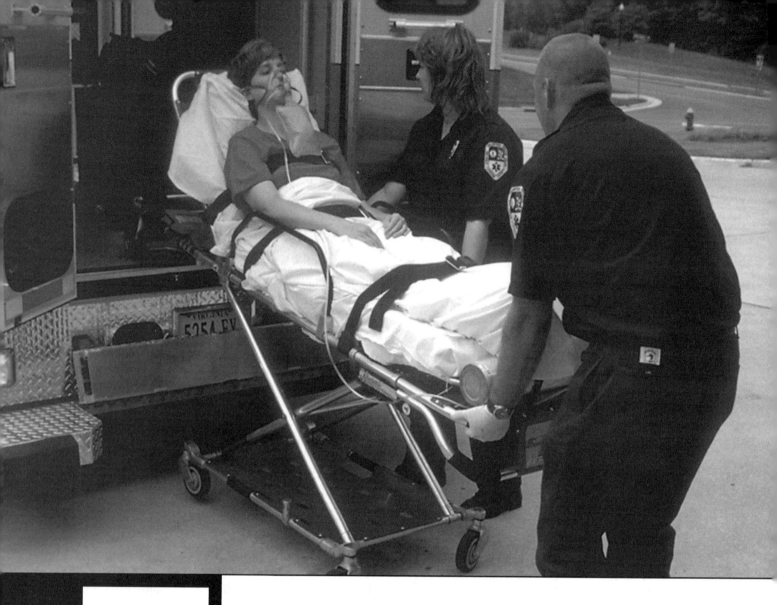

3

State and Regional EMS Systems

Susan M. Nedza, MD, MBA, FACEP
Leslee Stein-Spencer, RN, MS

Principles of This Chapter

After reading this chapter, you should be able to:

- Describe historical factors that influenced the development of state and regional EMS systems.
- Discuss the components of state EMS systems: lead agencies, the EMS director, the EMS medical director, and advisory councils.
- Recall the responsibilities of a regional EMS system.
- Discuss the challenges of EMS systems.

WHEN EMS SYSTEMS BEGAN MORE THAN 25 YEARS AGO, few could have envisioned the key position they would obtain as essential links in the health care system of every community. These systems have grown beyond the boundaries of traditional EMS services; they now are integrated into community preparedness plans and complex trauma plans and work collaboratively with local public health systems. As the number and complexity of these roles increase, an understanding of who the stakeholders in a system are, how they interact, and how systems interact with each other is required for successful participation. This knowledge is also necessary to participate in the dialogue and planning for the systems of the future. The success of meeting these present and future challenges is increasingly dependent on the ability of all stakeholders to collaborate at state and regional levels.

This chapter examines the historical factors that have influenced the development of state and regional

systems. The role of lead agencies is delineated, key leaders and stakeholders are identified, and challenges faced within these systems are explored.

The History of EMS Systems

The structure and function of modern EMS systems are the results of the interactions of the federal government, local government, providers, and scientific and private communities. These forces continue to shape the systems of today and will have significant impact on the systems of tomorrow.

The initial forces that shaped EMS developed in response to the 1966 white paper published by the National Academy of Sciences-National Research Council (NAS-NRC) entitled, *Accidental Death and Disability: The Neglected Disease of Modern Society.*

The federal government, as well as scientific and private communities, responded to the NAS-NRC report with a series of actions, including:

- The passage of the National Highway Safety Act of 1966, which identified improvement of EMS systems as a priority
- Federal government funding of EMS demonstration projects in 1971
- Robert Wood Johnson Foundation funding of EMS development projects in 1972
- Congressional hearings on EMS in 1971 and the passage of the Emergency Medical Services Systems Act of 1973 (PL 93–154),[1] which provided assistance and encouragement for the development of area-wide EMS systems

Through these activities, key principles were agreed on. The first was that the practice of concentrating on the development of individual EMS components was counterproductive, and that the development of complete systems was necessary.

The methods for providing funding mechanisms were put into place to accomplish this goal. Funds were funneled from the federal government through state governments, which also provided varying levels of oversight of the planning process. It was this funding of programs that served as the cornerstone for EMS activities through the states. Unfortunately, guaranteed federal subsidies for EMS are no longer in place, and the program funding responsibility has fallen to the states. What has remained is the methodology first used. These early initiatives set the precedent for broad stakeholder input and partnerships among a variety of government and nongovernment agencies and organizations, and they recognized the key role states have in implementation, oversight, and responsiveness to community needs.

The federal role of leadership in defining the field of EMS and identifying gaps in out-of-hospital care continues to be an important determining factor of the EMS agenda. Over the past decade, a shift has occurred from the original role of purely financial support to directed support of key projects from a variety of sources.

One such gap was recognized in the availability of quality trauma care within the health care system. Although trauma systems are covered extensively in other sections of this book, it must be recognized that state EMS agencies and their leadership have been critical to the successful adoption of trauma systems and their continued success in improving trauma care. The lessons learned in developing state trauma systems, their accreditation, their funding, and their integration into the EMS system have served as the models for other programs.

The National Highway Traffic Safety Administration (NHTSA) has exerted its influence through its support of the "EMS Agenda for the Future"[2] and standardized provider curricula.[3] These efforts drew upon the expertise of state and local leaders who were convened by the agency and charged with creating these documents. A process of stakeholder validation and comment was undertaken prior to their adoption. The role of adoption and implementation of these national goals and standards has fallen to state and local EMS agencies and providers. The greatest challenge these agencies face is finding funding, time, and manpower to implement these programs.

The national Emergency Medical Services for Children (EMSC) program, developed in 1984,[4] is another education and policy initiative. It combined both funding incentives and a national program that would partner with states and local institutions to reduce child and youth disability and death due to severe illness or injury. The program is administered through the Maternal and Child Health Bureau and NHTSA and is representative of cross-agency leadership at the federal level. It provides grants to states that support pediatric emergency care initiatives at the state and local levels. One of the most significant outcomes of this effort has been the movement to recognize or accredit hospitals and other providers who embrace efforts to improve their ability to provide care to the pediatric population. EMSC continues to collaborate closely with state EMS agencies in facility recognition and provider education and in providing targeted grants.

The Centers for Disease Control and Prevention (CDC) has also increased its support and leadership in the areas of injury control, emergency medicine data collection, trauma issues, and alcohol-related injuries. Since 2001, closer links have been forged with the EMS community to improve its ability to meet the challenges of dealing with infectious disease outbreaks such as anthrax and severe acute respiratory syndrome (SARS) and other biological threats.

The most significant event affecting EMS systems clearly has been the terrorist attacks of September 11, 2001. EMS and the nation's emergency departments have become recognized as front-line providers in community preparedness and bioterrorism response. Opportunities for funding and expanding roles and collaboration have increased dramatically since that time. Funding sources include the Department of Homeland Security, the Health Resources and Services Administration (HRSA), the CDC, the Department of Justice (DOJ), and the Federal Emergency Management Agency (FEMA). Unfortunately, EMS health care providers must compete with public health agencies, the fire service, police, and other local entities for these funds. State EMS agencies are being asked more often to partner with these other agencies.

The interactions between the federal government and local entities will continue to evolve. The common thread remains that of a national vision embraced through the collaboration of federal and state agencies, experts, and the stakeholder community. Once the agenda is recognized, the lead EMS agency in the state serves as the convener and defines the parameters and local needs with stakeholder input. It acts as the administrator of grants and, finally, is responsible for successful implementation in the most appropriate manner at the local level. The responsibility for sustainability clearly resides at state and local levels.

State EMS Systems

A comparison of state EMS systems reveals many unique approaches to emergency medical care. In passing the 1973 EMSS Act,[1] Congress recognized that each locality has unique geography, politics, and resources, which makes it impossible to mandate strict, nationwide blueprints for structures and responsibilities. This law allowed for varied system configurations while minimizing their differences.

All states have EMS legislation as a statutory basis for their EMS programs and activities. These laws serve as the legal foundation for the state EMS programs. They usually identify the activities and programs that state government will be involved in or regulate, identify the lead agency, outline the basic responsibilities of the agency, and provide the necessary authority for administration of the programs. The laws often include the authority to establish minimum standards and set penalties for noncompliance. These statutes are not static, and in many cases they serve as the method for codifying the role of the agency as it expands. A recent example is the increasing oversight of public-access defibrillation programs. One of the challenges faced by agencies is that these new responsibilities often come without dedicated funds and thus compete with other tasks the agency must accomplish.

Despite the variety of system types, common basic system components can be identified. These include a lead agency, an EMS director, and advisory councils.

Lead Agencies

The cornerstone of a state's EMS structure is the lead agency, which provides for central focus and coordination. Because an EMS system is primarily concerned with the delivery of medical care, most states have placed the lead responsibility in the state health agency. This is typically the only entity with sufficient authority, responsibility, resources, and regulatory power to organize the structure and relationships required for effective system operation.

The role of the lead agency can be broken down into three key components:

- A **regulatory role**
- A **leadership role**
- A **facilitator role**

Some of the responsibilities include licensing EMTs, obtaining and maintaining emergency response vehicles, coordinating disaster/domestic preparedness, designating trauma systems, overseeing EMSC programs (including facility recognition), approving training programs, and so on.

Regulatory Role

The regulatory role of the agency is to set minimum standards that are consistent with state laws and that safeguard quality care. Regulatory responsibilities cover an equally wide range. Major responsibilities of state agencies are licensure and certification of out-of-hospital personnel. Most states license or certify ambulance services, although some have no licensing or certification requirements, and a few delegate this responsibility to the regional or local level. Regulations specifically describe this process, including minimum standards, application, and inspection and the issuance, renewal, and revocation of licenses.

All states provide certification or licensure for out-of-hospital EMS personnel. Again, regulations identify minimum standards, education requirements, application procedures, renewal requirements, and procedures for disciplinary action. In some states, this regulatory authority over out-of-hospital EMS providers is shared with a state board of medical examiners or similar licensing board. The identification of different out-of-hospital certification levels is also a responsibility of the state. This involves the identification of training curricula and the scope of practice for various levels of providers. Recently, oversight has increased to include EMS dispatchers and EMS first responders.

Many states also are involved in facility designation and categorization. Activity in this area likely will increase as a result of new federal guidelines and funding to promote trauma system development and EMSC improvements. Coordination of these and other programs such as poison centers is a key regulatory role for the agencies.

Leadership Role

EMS agencies also facilitate improvements across the breadth of the system; the EMSC recognition process previously mentioned is an example. The agency establishes "stretch goals" or higher standards that providers are encouraged to reach toward. The incentives for these improvements come in many forms, such as grants for the purchase of equipment; public recognition programs that provide positive public relations opportunities in the community (and, at times, competitive advantages); monetary support for those implementing new technology or programs; and expertise and data-sharing capabilities for quality improvement.

EMS agencies have taken on a strong leadership role in the adoption of information technology and data collection. Much progress has been made in the standardization of forms, data submissions, and information-sharing among providers, regions, and state agencies. These data can be used for benchmarking, independent research, or local quality initiatives. The state can also facilitate access to other public databases that provide valuable information when considered in aggregate.

State agencies also are a source for model policies, procedures, and protocols that providers can modify and implement locally. They serve as the link to agencies in other states and speed communication and the adoption of best practices.

An often unrecognized role of the agency is the recruitment and retention of providers. The need to sustain an adequate workforce with appropriate training is critical to the mission of a state EMS agency.

EMS agencies often assume a leadership role in the coordination of injury control and prevention initiatives. These efforts span a continuum, from traditional trauma injury reduction programs to identifying victims of domestic violence.

Facilitator Role

Historically, agencies have been responsible for collaborating with other state agencies. Complex issues such as transportation, licensing, and disaster preparedness fall under their purview and cross traditional agency boundaries. This responsibility has grown dramatically over the past decade.

An increasingly important role of the lead agency is coordinating EMS activities with other state and federal agencies. Much of this work falls under the heading of "planning." The state EMS agency assumes a lead role in planning to ensure that expertise required by a plan is available, that the infrastructure is in place or can be implemented immediately, and that legal authority is present. This type of planning has expanded the scope of partners beyond the traditional provider and hospital communities.

To be successful, the agency must collaborate with both traditional and nontraditional partners in the private and public sectors, branches of government, and EMS advocates. It must remain neutral when competitors for funds and other resources are at the table.

Relationships with other states involve coordinating mutual aid programs for responses across borders and providing reciprocal certification for out-of-hospital providers — a particularly useful service in light of the highly mobile nature of the young EMS provider population and the constant shortage of qualified technicians. Reciprocity agreements between states ensure that personnel are able to move freely from one jurisdiction to another and with minimal bureaucratic paper shuffling. The **National Association of State EMS Directors (NASEMSD)**[5] serves as a forum for much of this collaboration.

To carry out their responsibilities, state EMS agencies typically are staffed by personnel with varied capabilities. Key areas of expertise for department personnel include EMS, data collection and IT experience, regulatory experience, provider experience, disaster coordination experience, professional educator experience, and communication skills. As the breadth of an agency's work increases, so must the expertise of its staff and its key advisor groups.

State EMS Director

The second component of the EMS system is the state EMS director. Although specific titles vary, all states have designated individuals who serve as state EMS directors and are responsible for the administrative direction of state EMS programs.

State EMS directors work closely with NASEMSD. This organization has representation from the 50 states and six US territories. It provides leadership and guidance for effective EMS system development and represents all components of an EMS system. It also works closely with other national organizations such as the National Association of EMS Physicians (NAEMSP).[6]

State EMS Medical Director

In many states, a physician is designated as state EMS medical director. The medical director might be a full-time employee, a part-time employee, an independent contractor, or a volunteer. This person's primary function is to provide overall state-level medical supervision. Some of the responsibilities might include standing medical orders or protocol development and review, review of local expanded scope programs for EMTs, liaison with medical professional organizations, and liaison with local and regional medical directors.[7]

However, the lead agency continues to be responsible for external functions such as license actions, inspection and compliance determinations, examination and certification, and operational procedures. It also maintains responsibility for internal functions such as hiring and evaluating employees, budgeting and resource allocation, strategic and operational planning, and policy development and implementation.

The EMS medical director and EMS director should function as a team: the physician acts as advisor, is an expert in evidence-based practice, and consults on resource allocation decisions. This is essential as new technology and new pharmaceuticals are introduced into practice. This latter role is increasingly important as state administrators make cost-benefit

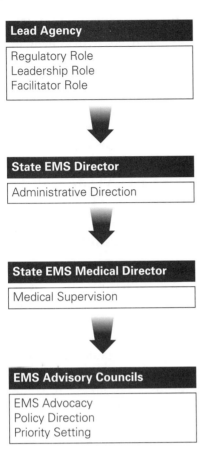

Lead Agency

Regulatory Role
Leadership Role
Facilitator Role

State EMS Director

Administrative Direction

State EMS Medical Director

Medical Supervision

EMS Advisory Councils

EMS Advocacy
Policy Direction
Priority Setting

Figure 3-1 The EMS system structure.

decisions necessary due to financial constraints. The EMS medical director also should have a key role in safeguarding EMS quality and in implementing statewide quality initiatives in collaboration with the lead agency.

Advisory Councils

The opportunity for providers and consumers to have input into an EMS system is made possible through participation in EMS advisory councils. These councils combine professionals, paraprofessionals, consumers, and public and private agencies into a body that represents all of the various special interest groups involved in the delivery of EMS. Although the specific composition of advisory councils varies by state, they typically include out-of-hospital EMS providers, EMS agencies (municipal, private, and volunteers), nurses, physicians, hospital administrators, the fire service, law enforcement, EMS educators, and the public. Each of these system stakeholders has an equal role in the development of the system, representing the issues and concerns of its special interest group in the planning process and in the de-

sign, development, and implementation of the system. The governor or executive director of the state agency appoints most council members, and most councils meet regularly. State EMS councils advise the lead EMS agencies on policy direction and priority-setting and frequently act as EMS advocates with government and private, public, and professional groups. Most importantly, these councils provide a forum for cooperative action that will result in a truly effective system (**Figure 3-1**).

The number and types of these councils have expanded as the scope of EMS has grown. Councils governing community preparedness, pediatric care, trauma care, and injury prevention are increasingly prevalent and have a key role in the collaborative processes in EMS.

The Role of Regional EMS Systems

Some states have developed comprehensive regional EMS systems that are somewhat autonomous and are a less centralized EMS system model. This development has its roots in the EMSS Act of 1973. At that time, one of the new federal requirements for distribution of funding was that the money be targeted at specific EMS regions. The "region" concept developed because it is very difficult to identify needs and implement programs that are universally appropriate and applicable throughout an entire state. Dividing states into smaller, more manageable pieces was seen as a way to ensure that funds would be targeted more appropriately and used effectively. Because of the move toward statewide integration, the concept of regionalization has been integrated into many state EMS systems. Regional EMS systems and their structures continue to be as varied as the states they serve with regard to autonomy, funding structure, governance, and scope of authority.

How EMS Regions Are Designated and Governed

The external appearance or dimensions of EMS regions were derived through several mechanisms. One common method was to define EMS regions by analyzing typical patient flow patterns. The primary central source of medical care (hospitals) became the center of the region, and the boundaries encompassed all areas from which patients normally flowed.

Occasionally, geographic considerations were also included, and physical barriers such as mountains and rivers had a role in locating boundaries. Some regions were based on political jurisdiction, such as counties or legislative districts. In a very few cases, the size and boundaries of EMS regions were determined arbitrarily. The end result was a geographic area officially designated by the state agency as an EMS region. Once the geographic boundaries of the regions were established, it was then necessary to establish the functional structure within the region. In many ways, this structure strongly resembled the state structure described earlier.

In most cases, a regional EMS advisory council is a source for provider and consumer input into the development and operation of the regional system. As with the state advisory council, the regional council comprises individuals from a variety of backgrounds, typically designated by the region's constituent political subdivisions, medical special interest groups, and consumer organizations. The council provides input on all matters of policy and procedure and is often directly involved in system planning and implementation. Council members serve as EMS advocates for their sponsoring entities and act as two-way communicators to keep local programs informed and carry local input to the regional level.

The regional EMS director provides administrative direction for the activities of the regional system. As with the state EMS director, the position titles vary, but the position itself is usually identifiable and the responsibilities essentially the same from region to region. This individual is primarily a planner, administrator, or manager. Frequently, the director is a native of the region and can apply personal knowledge to local activities.

Regional Medical Direction

In both integrated and independent regional programs, these entities tend to be highly involved with the active process of medical direction and quality improvement. The regional system usually attempts to involve the regional medical community in the medical management process and works to ensure that the medical component is fully integrated into regional activities.

The regional medical directors provide overall medical supervision and frequently act as the system's offline medical directors. In this position, the medical directors are usually involved in the provision and coordination of online medical direction and in the identification of medical direction facilities. In states where local treatment protocols are permitted by law, the regional medical director will usually be involved in their development and implementation. Finally, the regional medical director establishes the policies and mechanisms for medical accountability through case reviews, audits, and record analyses. They are increasingly involved in quality improvement initiatives and ensure medical quality when dealing with issues of resource allocation or competing local endeavors.

Regional Responsibilities

There are some responsibilities that can be universally considered as the roles of regional EMS systems, whether autonomous or integrated into a larger system. Efforts are directed toward the more concrete and specific actions related to EMS service delivery. Many regional systems are involved in recruitment, retention, and training of EMS field personnel. Regional resources are coordinated and shared to ensure effective use of manpower and education assets. Regional systems are also frequently involved in the area of transportation. This might involve the placement strategy of EMS vehicles, the assignment of response patterns, and coordination of mutual aid agreements between communities and counties.

Coordination of regional EMS communications is another responsibility of the system. Tailoring communication system capabilities to local geographic and resource constraints permits maximum effectiveness and also provides a coordinated link with the statewide communication system. Coordination and provision of public education and information programs can also be found in some regional programs. Finally, in states that have special EMS grant funding programs, the regional system coordinates and prioritizes grant applications based on the overall needs of the area.

Regional and State Collaboration

A critical service provided by regional systems is planning. This planning encompasses not only initial system design and implementation but also ongoing system evaluation. Regions often have responsibility for local collaboration of disaster planning, adoption of standardized protocols, and development of transfer agreements. The role of disaster planning has expanded at the regional level just as it has at the state level. Community preparedness plans are an integral part of regional disaster planning and have expanded to include key stakeholders outside of traditional health care entities.

The increasing demand on the emergency medical system that leads to ambulance diversion and bypass has created the need for regional diversion planning. This includes standardized criteria for bypass and systems of communication to notify providers and hospitals of high-capacity situations. This has led to the innovation of real-time Web-based systems for monitoring local emergency department and hospital bed capacity.

The EMS model of regionalization has been successfully adopted for trauma care, pediatric care, and burn care. Currently, movements exist to extend this model to other areas of specialized care, such as acute cardiac care,[8] stroke care,[9] hand injury, and hyperbaric care. All of these efforts recognize the need for community planning in providing timely access to highly specialized and resource-intensive medical interventions. The knowledge gained in designating centers, prevalence of disease in the community, monitoring quality, and determining the necessary resources in a region should provide the basis for establishing these systems. Careful thought as to the cost and maintenance of such regional efforts is necessary.

EMS System Challenges

Expansion of EMS Agenda

The scope of EMS and the complexity of its role continue to increase. This will put increasing demands on the agencies and leadership and will provide opportunities for further integration into the fabric of communities. Agencies will continue to be challenged to do more with less and to find ways to partner with providers and other agencies to fulfill their regulatory and leadership roles.

Standardization

The movement toward standardization will continue. At the education level, the adoption of national curricula and standards will require flexibility to ensure that adopting these programs locally will not have an impact on the number of providers or tax provider groups such as hospitals, physicians, and ambulance and fire services beyond their capa-

bilities. Efforts to standardize protocols for DNR, medication lists, and patient transfer will continue to expand. The greatest challenge might be in adopting technology and data collection tools that allow for use across a system, across a variety of provider settings, and across the nation. These systems must be compliant with national regulations such as the **Health Insurance Portability and Accountability Act (HIPAA)**. Agencies and their leaders must balance the need for standardization with the divergent uses of such data, methods to protect the privacy of patients and systems, the need for unique data that recognize the variations of use for the EMS data, and the need to limit the burden on providers.

Geographic Diversity

EMS systems have traditionally recognized the challenge of dealing with diverse geographic regions, local resources, and local funds. The relentless increase in cost to provide services, the shift of populations from rural to urban settings, and the loss of providers in rural settings will continue to challenge agencies in the future. As EMS becomes more technology driven and patients require access to specialized care centers, this gap will only widen. Agencies will be increasingly looked to for innovative programs in telemedicine and to monitor compliance with transfer agreements.

Manpower Issues

Experts in health policy are predicting a severe shortage in health care professionals in the next 20 years to meet the needs of the aging baby boomer population. EMS has already seen an aging of its workforce and an exodus of its volunteer providers, especially in rural communities. This trend is expected to get worse. It is not known what impact increasing flexibility and pay scales in other health care positions will have on the future EMS workforce.

Quality Agenda

The move toward adopting evidence-based practices in EMS has cast doubt on several widely accepted standards. Much of the EMS "body of knowledge" is based on consensus, and on efforts to define a research curriculum to improve scientific and health services knowledge.[10] Questions of patient consent, data sharing, and funding of such initiatives have yet to be answered.

Systems continue to be faced with the adoption

of new technology or new medications based on one or two studies that often do not look at final patient outcome but intermediate measures. The cost of this innovation in systems that are struggling to fund current staffing levels and to meet education requirements is often prohibitive. The need to undertake global cost-benefit analyses prior to the adoption of these standards and innovations will become a key task for all agencies, directors, and advisory groups.

The integration of EMS into the quality agenda of a health care system is in its infancy. Efforts to decrease medical errors, track poor outcomes due to diversion, and link out-of-hospital care to long-term patient outcome present both a challenge and an opportunity. Much of this will be accomplished through the local, regional, and state EMS systems.

Funding EMS

The greatest challenge that state and regional EMS systems face is funding. EMS systems that have no dedicated funding mechanism are vulnerable to changes in the availability of general state funds that are supported by tax and fee revenues. EMS agencies must also compete with entities that have legislative advocates, something that EMS agencies are prohibited from having. EMS does not have a natural constituency as schools, highways, and other key government services do. This leaves it vulnerable in political processes that result in the reduction of funds or decisions related to staff and budget cuts.

In light of the problems associated with the most common funding sources, states are beginning to look for innovative programs to pay for their EMS systems. For example, one trend is the creation of special funds within the state government that have independent funding sources. This offers the advantage of separating EMS funds from the highly competitive state general funds. The most common method is to attach a surcharge or fee to motor vehicle registration, driver's license applications, or motor vehicle violations, then place the funds in a special EMS account. This money is then made available to EMS programs in the form of grants to maintain and upgrade services. Other mechanisms such as taxing telephone users and collecting a portion of DUI fines have been used. The responsibility for creating special funds will become critical in the future as the cost of health care delivery continues to rise.

Summary

State and regional EMS systems developed and grew because "visionaries," more than 25 years ago, realized that a better quality of emergency medical care could be delivered if individual participants worked together in a coordinated system. The value provided by these systems speaks to the "correctness" of that vision. State EMS systems and the professionals committed to their function have moved beyond that initial vision. The integration of EMS into the health care system and the recognition of the key role it provides must continue. The collaborative efforts of state and regional agencies and providers must concentrate on educating the public on the value the system provides in their communities and to their own health. Meeting the challenges of the future will require vision, leadership, and, above all, recognition that adequate funding of EMS is a necessity — not a luxury.

References

1. Emergency Medical Services Systems Act of 1973, Pub L No. 93-154.
2. National Highway Traffic Safety Administration. EMS Agenda for the Future [NHTSA Web site]. Available at: http://www.nhtsa.dot.gov/people/injury/ems/agenda/emsman.html. Accessed January 11, 2005.
3. National standard curricula developed by the National Highway Traffic Safety Administration. List available at: http://www.nhtsa.dot.gov/people/injury/ems/nsc.htm. Accessed January 11, 2005.
4. Emergency Medical Services for Children Web site. Available at: http://www.ems-c.org. Accessed January 11, 2005.
5. National Association of State EMS Directors Web site. Available at: http://www.nasemsd.org. Accessed January 11, 2005.
6. National Association of EMS Physicians Web site. Available at: http://www.naemsp.org. Accessed January 11, 2005.
7. National Association of State EMS Directors, National Association of EMS Physicians, American College of Emergency Physicians. *The Role of State Medical Direction in the Comprehensive Emergency Medical Services System.* Falls Church, Va: NASEMSD; 2003.
8. American Heart Association. Chain of Survival: Fact Sheet [AHA Web site]. Available at: http://www.americanheart.org/presenter.jhtml?identifier=3010163. Accessed January 11, 2005.

9. American Heart Association, American Stroke Association. Stroke Treatment and Ongoing Prevention Act (STOP Stroke Act): Fact Sheet [AHA Web site]. Available at: http://www.americanheart.org/presenter.jhtml?identifier=3010190. Accessed January 11, 2005.

10. National Highway Traffic Safety Administration. EMS Research Agenda for the Future [NHTSA Web site]. Available at: http://www.nhtsa.dot.gov/people/injury/ems/EMS03-ResearchAgenda/home.htm. Accessed January 11, 2005.

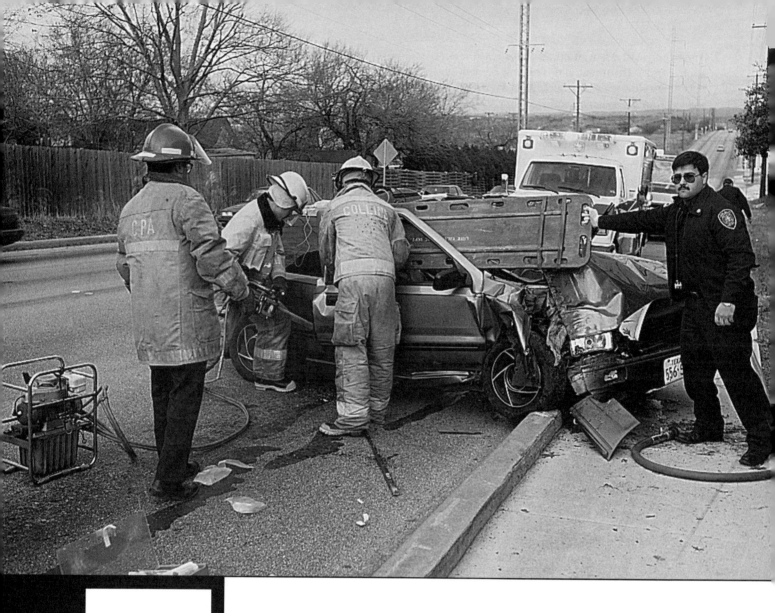

4

Trauma Systems

John C. Sacra, MD, FACEP

Principles of This Chapter

After reading this chapter, you should be able to:

- Discuss the development of our nation's trauma system.
- Describe key concepts behind the inclusive trauma care system, and explain why trauma is a public health problem.
- Explain the importance of injury prevention.
- Describe the continuum of trauma care through rehabilitation.

TRAUMA, THE MEDICAL TERM FOR BODILY INJURY, IS THIS nation's most tragic and expensive — yet correctable — national health care problem. The effects of trauma are far reaching and have an impact on a large percentage of the US population. The statistics speak for themselves.[1-3] Twenty-five percent of all emergency department visits are injury related. Trauma is the leading cause of death in children and adults younger than 45, and the fourth-leading cause of death for all ages. It also is the leading cause of disability for all ages. Each year, 150,000 deaths result from trauma. For each of these deaths, another three people are severely disabled and 75 are temporarily disabled. It is estimated that 25,000 people die needlessly each year in America due to the lack of trauma care systems.

Trauma is also the leading cause of life-years lost per death. On average, injury causes 36 life-years lost per death, while cancer causes 16, and heart disease and stroke combined are responsible for 12 years lost.[4,5] Survivors who are disabled could require a lifetime of medical treatment at society's expense. The total cost of injury in the United States approaches $260 billion per year, making it the most expensive disease process in this country.

Over the past three decades, there has been a shift from the exclusive trauma system, which focuses only on seriously injured patients, to the **inclusive trauma care system,** with an emphasis on all injured patients. The new challenge is to more fully integrate trauma systems and public health to take full advantage of the possibilities of risk factor identification and related interventions to prevent injuries in a community. This vision for trauma systems requires a national consensus to create public awareness of the problem.

The Evolution of Trauma Care in America

The need for comprehensive trauma care systems was first recognized in 1966 by the National Academy of Sciences and National Research Council in their landmark study, *Accidental Death and Disability: The Neglected Disease of Modern Society.*[6] This study called attention to the deficiencies existing in US trauma care and stressed the need for comprehensive and organized delivery of that care. Injuries were then largely perceived as random acts of fate. Out-of-hospital emergency medical care as we know it today did not exist, and few hospitals were equipped to handle seriously injured patients. This study established the need for an organization similar to the American Heart Association or American Cancer Society to focus on public awareness and prevention measures. As a result, the American Trauma Society was founded in 1968, dedicated to trauma prevention and improvement of trauma care.

Congress initiated a national effort toward trauma prevention when it passed the **Highway Safety Act of 1966.** This legislation required that states conform to national highway safety standards established by the Department of Transportation and addressed the inadequacy of the nation's delivery of medical care to injury victims.

Recognizing the need for a coordinated federal effort for implementation of a comprehensive emergency medical care delivery system, Congress passed the Emergency Medical Services Systems Acts (EMSS Acts) of 1973 and 1975. This legislation addressed the problem that, while technology in resuscitation had made meaningful advances, transportation and communication systems were fragmented and unorganized.

The EMSS Act of 1973 provided more than $20 million to state and local agencies for the purpose of upgrading equipment and developing regional approaches to communication and transportation. Although the funding was generous during the 1970s — sufficient for establishing EMS systems in many parts of the country — a comprehensive national EMS system never materialized.

During the 1980s, federal funding sources were essentially nonexistent. Although trauma centers and isolated trauma systems were demonstrating the ability to reduce unnecessary deaths, inadequate reimbursement discouraged further trauma system development. Only partial success toward the goal of implementing a system of regionalized trauma care delivery was realized. In 1985, a second report published by the National Academy of Sciences revealed little progress since the 1960s toward the goal of reducing the impact of injury in America.

The 1990s offered new opportunities. The Centers for Disease Control convened a series of consensus panels on seven aspects of injury control: violence, home and leisure injuries, occupational injuries, motor vehicle injuries, rehabilitation, acute care treatment, and acute care systems. The Acute Care Systems panel looked at the status of trauma system development in the United States, particularly on "where we have been, where we want to go, and how to get there." It recommended increased resources for injury surveillance, research, and intervention and strongly supported programs to increase public awareness of the need for injury control.

Public Law 101–590, approved by Congress in November 1990, provided new opportunities for trauma system development by supporting the concept of a trauma system that addressed the needs of all injured patients and matched them to available resources.[7] A model trauma care system plan was written by a consensus panel of experts to use in trauma system development.[8] Many states were making significant progress when Congress failed to reauthorize resources for the program in 1995.

Concurrent with government activities, significant progress was being made by professional organizations. In 1976, the American College of Surgeons Committee on Trauma (ACS/COT) published the first edition of "Optimal Resources for Care of the Severely Injured."[9] By 1999, this document had evolved into a fourth-generation publication, *Resources for Optimal Care of the Injured Patient,*[10] recognizing the needs of all injured patients and emphasizing a multidisciplinary approach to care and stressing the importance of trauma systems.

In 1987, ACS/COT developed a consultation and verification program for trauma centers using a multidisciplinary team approach. In 1988 and 1992, the American College of Emergency Physicians, recognizing that the care of injured patients required a system approach, published "Guidelines for Trauma Care Systems."[11] This document outlined the structure of a trauma care system in both urban and rural settings, defined essential system components, and described the role of providers in system management, out-of-hospital care, trauma care facilities, and rehabilitation services.

Other events accelerated the momentum toward the development of trauma systems. The Skamania Symposium was held in July 1998. Invited participants were trauma experts representing many different specialties and all areas of the United States.[12] The purpose of this meeting was to review the medical literature to quantify the current understanding of trauma system effectiveness and propose a plan for research in trauma. One of the recommendations from this conference reads as follows: "Using a national consensus process involving a spectrum of national organizations and committees interested in trauma care and prevention, construct a 'Trauma System for the Future' document including current status, a future vision, and an implementation strategy based on valid and reliable data."[12]

A 1999 study revealed significant increases in the presence of some elements of trauma system development in many states.[13] Many believed that this improvement was the result of federal assistance for trauma system development available from 1991 until 1995. The need to encourage further development has been recognized by the National Academy of Sciences Committee on Injury Prevention and Control.[14]

To meet this need, the participants of the Skamania Symposium also recommended federal funding for renewed trauma system development at the federal Health Resources and Services Administration (HRSA).

After three decades of evolution, the need for consensus regarding trauma systems development has never been more evident, and that possibility never closer. The potential design of trauma systems has been influenced by multidisciplinary groups that have described the essential components. That design concept has moved from a focus on trauma centers to trauma systems and includes the concept of inclusiveness. A research agenda has been established to strengthen medical evidence-based conclusions regarding trauma care effectiveness. A national study has been undertaken to evaluate the cost-

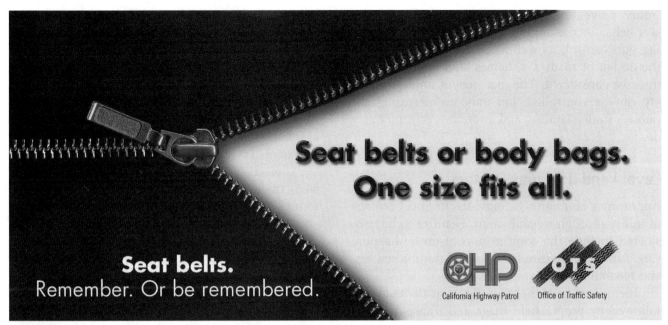

Figure 4-1 Public awareness campaigns can help reduce the human and financial costs of trauma.

effectiveness of trauma care. Based on the Skamania Symposium recommendations, the National Highway Traffic Safety Administration and the American Trauma Society are working together to develop a **trauma system vision** for our country through 2010. Developing the right coalition of policy-makers and advocates is essential to developing a successful nationwide system based on the regionalization of inclusive trauma care.

The Inclusive Trauma Care System

The primary purpose of a trauma care system is to reduce preventable deaths after injury. It is, therefore, critical to identify the major trauma patient and ensure his or her timely delivery to a designated trauma center. However, those requiring rapid and definitive surgical treatment constitute a minority of trauma patients. Changing the system focus from only the most severely injured to addressing the needs of all injured patients will result in the greatest health care benefit for the entire population. Modifying the emphasis of trauma care requires reorganization of all local resources and an inclusive approach to care for the injured.

Injuries range from minor to severe and include those to patients at risk for having unrecognized severe injuries. Many of these injuries are potentially disabling and require aggressive, early treatment and rehabilitation to ensure optimal outcome. The inclusive trauma care (ITC) system better uses existing resources by de-

livering each patient, in a timely manner, to a facility appropriately matched to the severity of injury.

The concept of ITC also promotes regionalization of trauma care systems so that people in all areas of the country will receive the best care possible. More importantly, an ITC system identifies high-risk behavior and patient groups at risk for injury. The system then focuses injury prevention efforts to minimize injury.

The Concept of Trauma

Most traumatic injuries do not result from "accidents." They are usually the direct result of man's interaction with energy and are predictable. Trauma has seasonal variations and trends with demographic distributions. Like heart disease and cancer, trauma has definable causes with established means of treatment and identifiable methods of prevention. Unlike heart disease, trauma is contagious: attitudes toward risk-taking behavior can spread throughout a community. Take, for example, attitudes and resulting behavior toward running red lights and driving while under the influence of alcohol.

Because all injuries represent a cost to society, injury prevention must be a focus in trauma care. Epidemiology reveals the most frequent causes of trauma to be motor vehicle crashes, the use of firearms, and falls among the elderly. Identified countermeasures can control these high-cost injuries, yet are largely ignored.

Enhanced public awareness regarding the financial and human cost of injury must be addressed (**Figure 4-1**).

Injury prevention countermeasures such as using seat belts, decreasing impaired driving, and instituting gun control, as well as engineering changes in the design of roadways, homes, and motor vehicles must be considered. The total cost of injury to society can be controlled, but only by increasing the public's understanding and awareness of injury as a disease process.

Level I and II Trauma Centers

Appropriate care must be provided from occurrence of injury through rehabilitation. Features to be considered include the coordination of out-of-hospital care, care at acute care facilities and trauma centers, and rehabilitation.

Identification of the extent of the patient's injury, followed by proper field triage and transport to an appropriately designated treatment center, is essential to any trauma system. There is no question that the most severely injured patients benefit from immediate transport to a Level I or II trauma center. Preventable death studies in exclusive trauma care systems show injury treatment at Level I or II trauma centers reduces unnecessary deaths from 25% to less than 3%.[15] But relying on only Level I or II trauma centers and not the entire system results in overtriage of less severely injured patients in order to capture all severely injured patients. A certain level of overtriage is necessary; if it is not controlled, however, overtriage leads to excessive costs, taxing both out-of-hospital and trauma center resources.[16,17]

ITC systems, through recognition of the existing capabilities of all appropriate hospitals and facilities, can develop triage criteria that match patient severity and needs to appropriate resources. Because some trauma patients have time-sensitive injuries, the triage criteria must include provisions for primary transport to a Level I or II trauma center. An ITC system allows for the smooth and rapid transport of patients based on clinical needs. Overtriage can be reduced by allowing patients at lower risk for severe injury to be evaluated at other facilities with secondary transfer later, if indicated.[18,19] Triage criteria established through a consensus in each region must be evaluated by performance improvement programs, making adjustments based on outcome studies.

Trauma Is a Team Disease

A committed and skilled trauma surgeon is essential to any properly organized trauma system and must be immediately available for definitive surgical intervention, serial evaluations, and intensive monitoring for all major trauma patients. Other health care professionals, including emergency physicians, anesthesiologists, orthopedic surgeons, and other surgical subspecialists must also be considered part of the trauma team.[19] The appropriate use of all members of the trauma team must be planned to provide quality care in a cost-effective manner.

Unnecessary activation of a full trauma team is labor intensive and results in inefficient use of personnel, the performance of unnecessary procedures, and excessive costs.[16] This approach has not been proved to be more effective than activating selected members of the team as needed.[20] The concept of an ITC system addresses the issue of full trauma team activation versus activation of selected members.

When designing the appropriate activation system, the ITC system considers all injured patients as well as those at risk for unrecognized injury. Establishing reasonable expectations for each member of the team results in high-quality and cost-effective care. Hospitals should configure the trauma team and the criteria for its activation based on outcome studies that are monitored by performance improvement programs. After reaching a consensus locally and developing appropriate activation standards, all members of the team will be more willing to accept their assigned responsibilities.

The Cost-Effectiveness of an ITC System

The current societal cost for trauma is overwhelming. Trauma centers are closing due to high costs and inadequate reimbursement. Because of the lack of federal and state funds for trauma system support, development of comprehensive trauma care systems is occurring in only a few states. A coalition of health professionals, elected officials, special interest groups, and others is essential to correct this problem.

With the total cost of trauma approaching $260 billion each year, combined with changes in health care financing, any system unable to decrease actual costs is certain to fail. An ITC system, with its emphasis on prevention, offers the best chance for success. Enhanced public awareness and increased individual responsibility are essential. Injury surveillance to identify high-risk groups and the development of prevention countermeasures are important parts of an ITC system.

Appropriate care for the major trauma patient is expensive: the charge for the average trauma admission is two to four times greater than for the average general admission. However, because trauma centers significantly improve survivability and reduce disability, they remain cost-effective. The amount paid in federal, state, and local taxes by a rehabilitated trauma patient who returns to work will exceed the cost of care many times.

Because of a higher level of commitment in personnel and resources, Level I and II trauma centers have higher costs than other facilities. Increased levels of reimbursement are, therefore, necessary for these centers of excellence to continue.

Changing patterns of health care payment, combined with fewer federal and state dollars dedicated to health care, demand a different approach to financing trauma systems. Trauma financing pools in each state or region, established for overall system support as well as for improving reimbursement to accredited trauma centers, should become part of an ITC system. By identifying high-cost injuries and high-risk groups, money could be obtained through fair increases in taxation and fees. Examples include additional taxation on alcohol, firearms, and ammunition, and fines for moving traffic violations, including impaired driving violations. Additional fees might be levied on all motor vehicle licenses or tags.[21-23]

Trauma systems and trauma centers are essential components of the public health safety net and are associated with high standby costs. Communities have long accepted the reality of standby costs associated with law enforcement and fire. Communities choose to purchase appropriate firefighting equipment and staff fire stations with firefighters who can respond within a moment's notice. It is understood that equipment, facilities, and personnel are needed 24 hours a day, 7 days a week, regardless of whether response is necessary. The cost of not having this safety net is just too high.

Funds are needed beyond revenue from traditional patient care sources. State funding for standby costs is appropriate because the system serves everyone in the state.

Level I and II trauma centers commit to continuous availability of personnel and resources. Emergency physicians, trauma surgeons, and other dedicated personnel must be on site to respond to time-sensitive events. The cost of this availability, as well as the cost of paying neurosurgeons, orthopedists, and other specialty physicians for standby, are staggering and potentially crippling for trauma centers.

Only through an innovative approach to comprehensive financing and reimbursement can trauma care systems be fiscally sound and capable of long-term success.

Interrelated Components of ITC Systems

A trauma care system must be part of the overall EMS system and not an independent or separate system. To avoid duplication and to integrate existing resources, the capabilities of the existing EMS system must be taken into consideration when developing a trauma/EMS system. The trauma/EMS system should, through a coordinated team effort, provide a continuum of care that includes injury prevention, acute care, and rehabilitation while addressing specialized patient needs such as pediatric care, burns, and spinal cord injuries. The system must coordinate trauma care with surrounding regions and, when indicated, adjoining states.

There is general agreement among the American College of Emergency Physicians, the American College of Surgeons Committee on Trauma, the American Trauma Society, and the National Highway Traffic Safety Administration regarding the essential components of comprehensive ITC systems. The system providers — administrators and clinicians alike — must learn to work with local and national policymakers to provide input at all stages of trauma system development. Activities by the system providers must focus on injury prevention, coordinated trauma care, and comprehensive rehabilitation.

System management provides the infrastructure for the delivery of care as well as the direction to facilitate needed changes. Managers must be actively involved in promoting the passage of enabling legislation to develop and implement comprehensive care. Administrative responsibility also requires the managers to generate sufficient financial support to ensure continued functioning of the system. Additional responsibilities include developing aggressive injury prevention programs, ensuring that education programs are provided to train adequate numbers of personnel, and designing the continuous quality improvement programs to monitor success.

The out-of-hospital care providers and trauma care facilities provide direct patient care after injury. They should be involved in the planning stages of each system component. Planning for trauma care must include an organized response by all personnel. Essential elements of planning provide for accurate identification of injured patients, adequate communication and transport capabilities, matching patients to the appropriate level of care, and returning injured patients to productive work through rehabilitation. Such planning also must consider the unique setting in which the care is to be delivered. In most cases, for example, the model for urban trauma care cannot be successfully applied to rural areas. Factors such as geography, population density, time and distance to trauma centers, expertise of personnel, current referral patterns, and levels of commitment should all be considered when designing an ITC system.

Growth of the ITC System

Legislation

The authority to develop and implement a comprehensive trauma/EMS system within a state should be vested in a state lead agency that addresses both EMS and trauma issues. If the system is to be implemented in an existing state agency, additional enabling legislation should be developed to address the unique needs of trauma care. This legislation should grant the formal authority to support an ITC delivery system, allowing the regulatory process to further define and develop the specific details. The enabling legislation should provide for:

- Designation of a lead agency
- Integration of trauma care into the EMS system
- Categorization of facilities
- Development of an injury prevention program
- Adoption of standards for trauma care
- Organization of data collection and systems evaluation
- Maintenance of confidentiality and protection of identity
- Authorization for dedicating sources of trauma funding

The provision for sufficient funding for the lead agency to carry out these responsibilities must also be included within the enabling legislation. The appropriated funds should be placed in a special account, and spending should be restricted to EMS or trauma programs. Potential sources of funds include:

- General user fees
- Taxes on cigarettes or alcohol
- Surcharges on motor vehicle registrations
- Penalties on traffic violations
- Taxes on the sale of weapons or ammunition

Additional examples of suggested legislation at the state level include many types of legal reform, including tort and reimbursement reform. A preferential payment system that would provide specialized centers with sufficient reimbursement to cover their costs and appropriate improvements for the care of major trauma patients should be considered. Other suggested legislative reforms include the creation of financial incentives for accepting interfacility transfers of major trauma patients and specialty care patients.

Leadership

Trauma system leadership can be facilitated nationally through a lead agency to advocate for system development. This agency should promote regional trauma system development and establish national standards for all aspects of trauma systems. A research and performance improvement agenda should be developed by this federal lead agency in conjunction with clinical specialty groups.

At the regional level, a lead agency with the authority and resources to accomplish the overall goals must be designated. The agency might be housed in a branch of government, or it could be a separate entity if the requisite authority is provided by statutes. It must possess the necessary expertise and commitment to carry out the following functions:

- Organize and develop minimum performance standards
- Coordinate existing resources
- Develop a consensus from providers and users through advisory committees
- Establish consistent policies
- Coordinate the trauma system with existing regional health care delivery systems
- Ensure financial viability
- Establish appropriate quality improvement programs

Existing standards for trauma and EMS such as those developed by the American College of Emergency Physicians and the American College of Surgeons Committee on Trauma[10] should be adapted to the existing resources as necessary. However, some resources might need to be created or bolstered to meet essential requirements.

Regional trauma/EMS systems should consider overall system needs, and regional councils should be appointed to develop standards that satisfy local requirements while meeting minimum statewide standards.

The trauma/EMS agency requires legal authority to regionalize EMS and to categorize facilities, including the designation of appropriate trauma centers. A consensus will be necessary to achieve the system's overall goals, and the lead agency should set a realistic time frame for system implementation. Advisory committees to the agency, consisting of both health care providers and consumers, should be established to develop recommendations and review proposed modifications.

System Development

Integration of existing resources at the regional level should be considered when a regionalized ITC system is designed. The planning process begins with an assessment of the system's current needs. Factors to be considered include:

- The magnitude of the trauma problem
- The current availability of resources within the region
- Existing patient flow and referral patterns, regardless of political boundaries

The National Highway Traffic Safety Administration has developed an excellent guide to assist in the development of state and community trauma systems.[24]

Another essential component of an ITC system is the development of a database that allows analysis of the following items:

- The percentages of moderate, major, and fatal injuries
- The distribution pattern of injuries
- The magnitude of preventable injuries
- The impact of trauma on long-term disability

As the needs assessment and development of a patient database are being conducted, it is extremely important to establish a realistic time frame for the implementation of each component of the ITC system. Appropriate steps in the implementation of the overall system include:

- Creating a system design
- Developing a policy for the integration of trauma care into the EMS system
- Reviewing and adopting guidelines and standards for trauma care
- Developing a request for proposal for facility designation
- Establishing a system to collect data from each of the acute care facilities for further evaluation

The trauma/EMS agency should be ultimately responsible for the planning process. However, successful implementation will depend on motivated efforts of all participants. The overall working environment should be one of cooperation and partnership with the use of existing community coalitions and networks. The adoption of appropriate system standards and trauma care guidelines is essential.

Finance

When trauma care is recognized as a subset of the EMS system, cost-effectiveness and quality care can often be provided without unnecessary duplication through the use of existing resources. For example, a communications system and inventory system will already be present in an organized EMS system. When added expenditures are considered to implement trauma care, the benefits must be carefully weighed against the expense to demonstrate cost-effectiveness to the system and society. Examples of this documentation include a comparison of the additional lives saved or injured persons returned to productive lifestyles against the costs incurred in implementing and maintaining a regional trauma system. It will be necessary to develop a broad consensus in support of the ITC system approach.

Overall financing will include administrative costs in both the planning and implementation stages, as well as for ongoing support of the lead agency and a data collection system. Additional costs might be incurred to reimburse the system providers — the out-of-hospital, hospital, physician, and rehabilitation personnel who render care and are otherwise not adequately compensated.

The financing plan must include a mechanism to identify and secure potential sources of funding, along with provisions for occasional alternative financing. The single greatest out-of-pocket expense is incurred by the tertiary regional trauma centers, which commit the greatest resources to provide acute and comprehensive care. The development of trauma financing pools should be considered to subsidize such centers for costs they cannot otherwise cover. Expansion of Medicare and Medicaid coverage for major trauma patients must be promoted.

The plan must also be capable of allocating funds for the creation of a public information and education program, a data collection and analysis program, and a study to document the cost-effectiveness of the trauma system. These can be developed by providing dedicated resources linked closely to the needs assessments and priorities as prescribed by the lead agency.

Public Information, Education, and Prevention

A well-planned public information and education program designed to reduce preventable injury and help generate funding is an integral component of any effective ITC system. This component can potentially result in the greatest cost savings to society by teaching the public how to access the trauma/EMS system and how to provide assistance to trauma victims before emergency medical assistance arrives.

Another function of the information program is to use the collected data as documentation of the need for prevention programs and to support additional legislative efforts. Three general strategies for prevention programs include:

- Persuasion and education programs
- Promoting relevant legislation and regulations and their monitoring and enforcement
- Providing protection by either altering behavior or the environment — active versus passive protection

The ultimate goal of the ITC system is to reduce the cost of injury, both financially and in physical and emotional suffering. To do this effectively, the community must be aware of the epidemiology and causes of injury, and there must be a systematic approach to identifying high-risk groups and preventing injuries.

Data regarding prevalence of trauma can be created from EMS, hospital, and trauma center data or by linking these data sets with public safety, public health, Worker's Compensation, and other databases. Once problem areas have been identified, countermeasures can be implemented through community coalitions of medical, civic, and government agencies.

Human Resources

The system needs enough trained personnel to maintain an organized trauma team. Using all personnel in positions consistent with their skills and knowledge is not only cost-effective but also allows each team member to perform his or her assigned responsibilities.

Policies and programs should be adopted to ensure the basic education preparation, continuing education, and recruitment and retention of qualified personnel. Programs such as Advanced Trauma Life Support, Advanced Cardiac Life Support, Certified Emergency Nurse, Critical Care Registered Nurse, and Trauma Nurse Core Curriculum should be instituted.

Out-of-Hospital Care and Communications

An efficient communication network capable of providing coordination among all system components is essential. To be efficient, it must provide for both statewide and interstate coverage. System access through 911 and dispatching of appropriate out-of-hospital personnel should be organized in each region with the goal of facilitating a coordinated systemwide emergency response (**Figure 4-2**). A trauma/

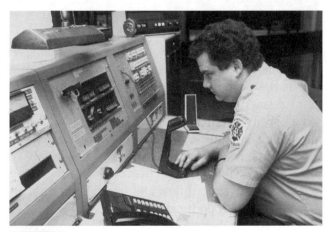

Figure 4-2 Efficient communication among all system components, through 911 and dispatch, is essential to coordinating systemwide emergency response.

EMS response plan with dispatchers trained to provide prearrival instructions is also important.

As with any EMS system, the communication system should be capable of linking dispatch with the ambulance, hospital, and other agencies such as fire, police, and disaster. It should also be capable of ambulance-to-hospital and hospital-to-hospital connections.

Out-of-Hospital EMS Medical Direction

A regional EMS system medical director is essential and should be knowledgeable in trauma system planning. This person might also be referred to as the **administrative, or offline, medical director**. He or she assumes responsibility for the development of clinical standards (protocols), as well as policies and procedures required to ensure medical accountability within the region. The EMS agency should establish a medical advisory committee with appropriate representation from EMS, consumers, and other health care personnel to provide guidance to the medical director on trauma/EMS issues. The regional director must consider recommendations and directives from the state lead agency medical advisory committee. He or she must assume responsibility for regional trauma care planning activities either personally or by designating another physician to this task. Trauma planning activities should include the involvement of medical directors from adjacent regions to ensure consistent care.

Offline medical direction requires both **prospective and retrospective performance improvement** (PI) activities. Prospective PI includes establishing standards for training and testing; hiring qualified personnel; certifying providers; developing protocols for treatment, transport, and triage; and approving operations policies when they relate to medical care. Retrospective PI includes medical audits and EMS run reviews to analyze the appropriateness of care delivered. Many offline medical direction duties can be handled by committees functioning under the supervision of the medical director.

Online, or concurrent, medical direction is essential to the operation of an ITC system and refers to the medical direction given to out-of-hospital personnel by a physician providing direct supervision on the scene or by radio or telephone.

Triage

Triage is the classification of patients according to their medical treatment needs. Triage protocols for trauma victims should be inclusive and take into consideration such factors as extent of injury, time and distance to designated trauma centers, and appropriate use of resources at these centers. Triage protocols should be sensitive enough to identify patients with major injury and specific enough not to burden the system with overtriage of minor injuries.

Major trauma patients are those who either have a severe injury or are at risk to have sustained an unrecognized severe injury. On initial evaluation, major trauma patients typically have abnormal vital signs or significant anatomic injury. However, triage is often inexact due to the patient's variable physiologic response to trauma. In some patients, what appear to be minor injuries can result in morbidity or mortality due to the patient's age or comorbid factors, while in other patients, there might be a delayed physiologic response to trauma. Patients involved in high-energy events such as a major car crash or a fall from a significant height are at risk to have sustained severe injury. Despite normal vital signs and no apparent anatomic injury on initial evaluation, some of these patients will have a significant injury discovered after a full evaluation or serial observations.

One characteristic of an ITC system is triage that matches a patient's severity of injury to an appropriate facility in a timely manner. A systems approach will consider factors that activate the regional ITC system, including injury severity, risk for severe injury, and time and distance from site of injury to definitive care, as well as potential for interhospital transfers using guidelines for immediate transport to tertiary care versus postintervention transfer.

Triage criteria for major trauma patients should include:

- Patients with multisystem, blunt, or penetrating trauma and unstable vital signs
- Patients with known or suspected anatomic injuries despite stable or normal vital signs
- Patients involved in high-energy events with risk for severe injuries despite stable or normal vital signs

Triage of trauma victims should occur at both the out-of-hospital stage (transport the patient to the nearest appropriate facility) and hospital level (transfer the patient, if needed, to a tertiary care facility). This allows further flexibility in the system to match hospital resources with changing patient needs.

Out-of-Hospital Triage

Out-of-hospital triage must consider patient acuity as well as time and distance and must identify patients who might need to bypass the nearest acute care facility and be transported to a designated trauma center. In addition, out-of-hospital triage criteria must allow for the activation of the trauma system from the field, including a team response from the designated trauma center (see Appendix 1, "Model Trauma Triage Algorithm, Out-of-Hospital," at the end of this chapter).

Level III and IV Trauma Center Triage

Criteria must be developed to identify patients who require immediate postintervention transfer (ie, requiring initial stabilization and rapid transfer to a more comprehensive trauma center) and those who can be safely held in a Level III or IV center for further evaluation and serial observations. An example of the latter is a patient who might have sustained unrecognized severe injury but who has stable or normal vital signs and no obvious anatomic injury (see Appendix 2, "Model Trauma Triage Algorithm, Level III/IV Trauma Center").

Level I and II Trauma Center Triage

Patients who require a full trauma alert or who should be evaluated initially by a member of the trauma team, with subsequent consultation by a trauma surgeon or subspecialist, should be sent directly to a Level I or II center (see Appendix 3, "Model Trauma Triage Algorithm, Level I/II Trauma Center").

Triage criteria recognize the unique requirements of individual trauma systems as well as the importance of clinical judgment. What constitutes unstable vital signs, significant anatomic injuries, or a high-energy event is best defined by the individual trauma system's protocols. Medical direction and continuous quality improvement can individualize triage criteria to provide the best and most cost-effective care. Deviations from established protocols based on clinical judgment may be allowed in some cases, but each case of deviation must be reviewed.

The distinction between patients with minor or moderate injuries and those with severe injury or who are at risk for a severe injury might change within a given trauma system. Individual variations in trauma systems might occur due to differences in the maturity or requirements of the particular system, including level of education and experience of professionals, or unique characteristics such as demographics or geography. Close cooperation among all members of the ITC system will be required to establish the appropriate response for individual system components. For a systems approach to work properly, triage protocols devised and supported by all members of the trauma system must be in place and followed.

Out-of-Hospital Transport

The transport system must strive for timely delivery of patients to the appropriate designated facilities using the most expedient and appropriate means of transport. The transport system must allow for the smooth transition from field to definitive care. Factors other than actual transport mode must also be considered because they affect the elapsed time to definitive care. These factors include public awareness of and access to the EMS system, the response time of the transport component, the level of training of the responding personnel, and the time and distance to definitive care.

The trauma plan must include regulations for personnel and equipment and protocols for triage matching injury severity to facility capability. Triage and transport protocols must consider geography, topography, available resources, population density, and the location of definitive care facilities within a region. Initial planning should include an assessment of numbers and types of vehicles, the type of equipment and personnel available, and the characteristics of the area to be served. The goal is to reach a balance between the economics of availability and utilization, as well as between actual demand and patient care requirements. The capabilities of all emergency facilities must be known by the EMS agency, and this information must be used by out-of-hospital personnel according to a triage plan to expedite the best transport decisions.

Air medical transport is an important component of trauma care and is particularly beneficial in reducing transport time in rural areas. Coordination of ground and air transport is essential. Helicopters might be used for primary scene response in certain locations, or they could be used for rendezvous with ground units at predetermined sites. Typically, helicopters are used in urban areas only when ground transport times are excessive due to environmental or external factors or in multicasualty events.

Finally, there must be a routine system for collecting data on the use and performance of transport services.

Definitive Care and Trauma Facilities

Definitive care facilities must be identified, categorized according to capability and commitment, and coordinated in order to provide a continuum of care from occurrence of injury through rehabilitation. A system that integrates all facilities within a region is essential to achieving the goal of providing cost-effective and quality trauma care. Factors that should be considered include geography, hospital distribution, population density, estimated patient volumes, transport capabilities, and times and distances within the region to definitive care.

Each comprehensive ITC system should establish appropriate standards for trauma facilities that are individualized for the particular needs of the region. The ACS/COT document, *Resources for Optimal Care of the Injured Patient,* is the best guideline for creating such standards.[10] The standards should be modified when appropriate.

Level I Facilities
A Level I facility is a valuable resource for the entire regional system and should have the capability of providing comprehensive care, including rehabilitation, to all patients. Level I facilities are typically university-based teaching hospitals with a commitment to education, research, and system leadership. An important part of the responsibility of such a facility includes public education and trauma prevention programs, as well as continuing medical education for medical professionals. Not all trauma care systems have a Level I facility.

Level II Facilities
A Level II facility has less extensive research programs than a Level I facility but provides the same standard of patient care. In most systems, Level II facilities handle most trauma patients identified

through field triage. The public education and injury prevention programs of a Level II facility could be essentially the same as those of a Level I.

Level III Facilities

A Level III facility generally does not have the resources to provide the same intensity of care as a Level I or II facility. However, it is usually capable of providing prompt assessment, resuscitation, emergency surgery, stabilization, and definitive care for many patients. A Level III facility must have a commitment commensurate with its available resources and must develop transfer agreements with Level I or II facilities for patients who need higher levels of care.

Level IV Facilities

A Level IV facility provides initial care to the severely injured despite its limited resources and provides trauma care to the most remote areas of the state or region. Consensus treatment protocols for initial stabilization and prearranged transfer agreements are essential. Most patients with less severe injuries can be properly cared for at Level IV facilities.

The ITC system must actively solicit the involvement of Level III and IV facilities. All hospitals must provide accurate data on trauma/EMS patients to achieve system integration through a comprehensive analysis of trauma care throughout the region. Each hospital within a region must recognize the need to transfer some patients. Therefore, formal letters of agreement among all facilities within the region are advisable.

Integration also requires providers in Level III and IV facilities to be committed to the development of an ITC system. The rotation of Level III and IV facility personnel through the Level I and II facilities can be instrumental in achieving this goal.

Specialized facilities that concentrate on certain areas of expertise must also be considered. Such concentration can prevent the unnecessary duplication of both capital and personnel. Examples of specialized facilities include centers for pediatric care, burn care, spinal cord injuries, eye injuries, and limb reimplantation.

Definitive Care and Interfacility Transfer

The smooth and efficient movement of trauma patients between hospitals will be facilitated by having systemwide transfer protocols and agreements. Criteria for patient transfer should be based on predetermined clinical indicators that address patient needs and the transferring and receiving facilities' ca-

pabilities. These criteria should follow existing regional triage and transfer guidelines. Transfer protocols should comply with **Emergency Medical Treatment and Labor Act (EMTALA)** requirements[25] and provide for appropriate transport methods, including the needed types and number of personnel, and should specify who will assume responsibility for medical direction. Transfer agreements should also include a requirement for the receiving hospital to provide information regarding patient outcome.

Definitive Care and Rehabilitation

A comprehensive rehabilitation program is often the most neglected part of a trauma system, yet it is as important as any of the other ITC system components. Rehabilitation might be the longest and most difficult stage in a trauma patient's recovery. Rehabilitation should begin as soon as possible following injury; each trauma care facility must have a mechanism to begin rehabilitation as soon as a patient is admitted, as well as a policy regarding subsequent transfer to specialized rehabilitation facilities. Standards for such services have been developed by the Commission on Accreditation of Rehabilitation Facilities.[26]

Evaluation

A comprehensive and well-defined performance improvement (PI) program is essential. Exclusive trauma systems have historically relied on facility-based PI programs that examine individual patient care and outcome at a specific institution. By contrast, an ITC system must have PI programs that examine performance of the entire system, including all providers and components, as well as the transition of care from one component to another. System PI also evaluates management issues such as financing, injury prevention, and outcome indicators.

The PI program must mandate systematic hospital and emergency department reporting of information regarding the trauma victim. The first step in developing a PI program is to identify the data to be collected by a **trauma registry**. This allows for systemwide monitoring of trends and patterns of injury, identification of high-risk populations, and development and evaluation of injury prevention programs.

The trauma registry should allow for correlation of data collected by the trauma/EMS system and facility-based PI programs. A minimum set of data should be collected to permit examination of an individual facility's performance as well as the overall effectiveness of the system. To facilitate data collection and improve compliance by system providers, the data to be compiled should be limited to that considered essential to the evaluation process. Similar data might be collected by each component of the system, but its analysis might differ depending on individual needs and perspectives. PI data for the out-of-hospital care component should evaluate system access, response times, effectiveness of field care, and triage and transport decisions, including scene and transport times. Differences between urban and rural settings should also be considered.

Hospital PI programs must allow each institution to evaluate its own performance. Systemwide PI should then evaluate patient outcome data from each hospital and determine every hospital's effectiveness in relation to system and national standards.

PI programs for the rehabilitation phase must evaluate the progress of all patients transferred to rehabilitation programs, skilled nursing, or residential facilities. Patients in need of rehabilitation but not referred should be identified, and the circumstances should be evaluated.

The overall design of the evaluation program is extremely important, and consensus among all participants is a goal. An essential feature of any PI program is patient confidentiality. Positive as well as negative trends should be evaluated so that conditions found to improve patient outcome can be integrated systemwide, while those that cause negative trends can be corrected.

Research is an extension of the PI process and is helpful in improving overall performance. Systems research should include an evaluation of medical care as well as the effectiveness of individual system components. The methods of treatment should continually be reevaluated to ensure optimal patient care.

Summary

The total cost of trauma, through direct cost and loss of productivity, is staggering. In an effort to improve this situation, the development of inclusive trauma care, or ITC, systems that consider all injured patients can be cost-effective.

The development of an ITC system is a complex process requiring consensus and cooperation from all system providers. A fresh look at the problem can result in a new paradigm for trauma care that moves away from major trauma overtriage and toward an ITC team philosophy system. The new paradigm will require legislation to enable creation of a trauma/

EMS system and to finance it adequately. It must build on injury prevention as a cornerstone and effectively use human resources. ITC systems, through coordination of system components and the effective use of resources, can make a difference in terms of human loss and suffering.

References

1. Rice DP, MacKenzie EJ, Jones AS, et al. *Cost of Injury in the United States: A Report to Congress.* San Francisco, Calif: Institute for Health and Aging, University of California, and Baltimore, Md: Injury Prevention Center, The Johns Hopkins University; 1989.

2. National Research Council, Committee on Trauma Research. *Injury in America: A Continuing Public Health Problem.* Washington, DC: National Academy Press; 1985.

3. National Research Council, Committee on Trauma Research. *Injury Control: A Review of the Status and Progress of the Injury Control Program at the Centers for Disease Control.* Washington, DC: National Academy Press; 1988.

4. Committee on Trauma Research, Commission on Life Sciences, National Research Council, Institute of Medicine. *Injury in America: a Continuing Public Health Problem.* Washington, DC: National Academy Press; 1985.

5. Committee to Review the Status and Progress of the Injury Control Program at the Centers for Disease Control. *Injury Control.* Washington, DC: National Academy Press; 1988.

6. National Academy of Science-National Research Council. *Accidental Death and Disability: The Neglected Disease of Modern Society.* Washington, DC: Government Printing Office; 1966.

7. Trauma Care Systems Planning and Development Act of 1990, Pub L No. 101–590.

8. US Department of Health and Human Services. *Model Trauma Care Systems Plan.* Washington, DC: Public Health Services, Health Resources and Services Administration; 1992.

9. American College of Surgeons Committee on Trauma. Optimal hospital resources for care of the seriously injured. *Bull Am Coll Surg.* 1976;61:15–22.

10. American College of Surgeons Committee on Trauma. *Resources for Optimal Care of the Injured Patient.* Chicago, Ill: American College of Surgeons; 1999.

11. American College of Emergency Physicians. Guidelines for trauma care systems. *Ann Emerg Med.* 1993; 22:1079–1100.

12. Skamania Symposium. Trauma systems evidence research action. *J Trauma.* 1999;47(3 Suppl).

13. Bass RR, Gaines PS, Carlini A. 1999 update on trauma system development in the US. *J Trauma.* 1999; 47:515–521.

14. National Academy of Sciences Committee on Injury Prevention and Control. *Reducing the Burden of Injury: Advancing Prevention and Treatment.* Washington, DC: National Academy Press; 1999.

15. Cales RH, Trunkey DD. Preventable trauma deaths: a review of trauma care system development. *JAMA.* 1985;254:1059–1063.

16. Hoff WS, Tinkoff GH, Luke JF, et al. Impact of minimal injuries on a Level I trauma center. *J Trauma.* 1992;33:408–412.

17. O'Rourke B, Bade RH, Drezner TM. Trauma triage: a nine-year experience. *Ann Emerg Med.* 1992; 21: 25–32.

18. Hedges JR, Osterud HR, Mulling RJ. Adult minor trauma patients: good outcome in small hospitals. *Ann Emerg Med.* 1992;21:402–406.

19. Eastman AB, Lewis FR Jr, Champion HR, et al. Regional trauma system design: critical concepts. *Am J Surg.* 1987;154:79–87.

20. Thompson CT, Bickell WH, Sacra JC, et al. Community hospital Level II trauma center outcome. *J Trauma.* 1992;32:336–343.

21. US Department of Transportation, National Highway Traffic Safety Administration. *Key Elements of State Trauma Legislation.* Washington, DC: DOT, Traffic Safety Programs; 1988.

22. US Department of Transportation, National Highway Traffic Safety Administration. *Comprehensive Trauma Systems Legislation: An Overview.* Washington, DC: DOT, Traffic Safety Programs; 1992.

23. Champion HR, Mabee MS. *An American Crisis in Trauma Care Reimbursement.* Washington, DC: Washington Hospital Center; 1990.

24. National Highway Traffic Safety Administration. *Development of Trauma Systems (DOTS): State and Community Guide.* Washington, DC: US Department of Transportation; 1989.

25. Consolidated Omnibus Budget Reconciliation Act of 1985 (COBRA). Pub L No. 99–272, Title IX, Section 9121, 100 Stat 167 (1986). Also Omnibus Budget Reconciliation Act of 1989 (OBRA). Pub L No. 101–239, Section 6211(h)(z), 103 Stat 2106, 1ZUSC 1395dd.

26. Commission on Accreditation of Rehabilitation Facilities. *Standards Manual for Organization Serving People with Disabilities.* Tucson, Ariz: CARF; 1989.

Appendix 1. Model Trauma Triage Algorithm, Out-of-Hospital

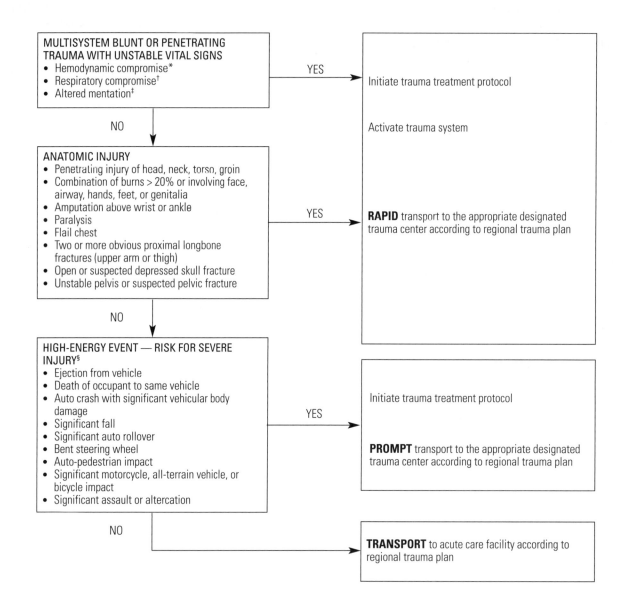

---

* In addition to hypotension: pallor, tachycardia, or diaphoresis might be early signs of hypovolemia.

† Tachypnea (hyperventilation) alone will not necessarily initiate this level of response.

‡ Altered sensorium secondary to sedative-hypnotic will not necessarily initiate this level of response.

§ High-energy event signifies a large release of uncontrolled energy. Patient is assumed injured until proved otherwise, and multisystem injuries might exist. Determinants to be considered by medical professionals are direction and velocity of impact, patient kinematics and physical size, and the residual signature of energy release (eg, major vehicle damage). Clinical judgment must be exercised and may upgrade to a high level of response and activation. Age and comorbid conditions should be considered in the decision.

Editor's Note: Appendixes 1-3 were part of an ACEP policy statement, "Guidelines for Trauma Care Systems," approved by the ACEP Board of Directors in 1992 and published in *Annals of Emergency Medicine* in 1993 (volume 22, pages 1079-1100). This policy statement was rescinded by the ACEP Board of Directors in 2000 at the recommendation of its Trauma Care and Injury Control Committee, which advised the Board that the ACEP guidelines had essentially been superseded by the ACS/COT publication *Resources for Optimal Care of the Injured Patient*. The author of this chapter has included the appendixes here, however, because their content is still current.

Appendix 2. Model Trauma Triage Algorithm, Level III/IV Trauma Center

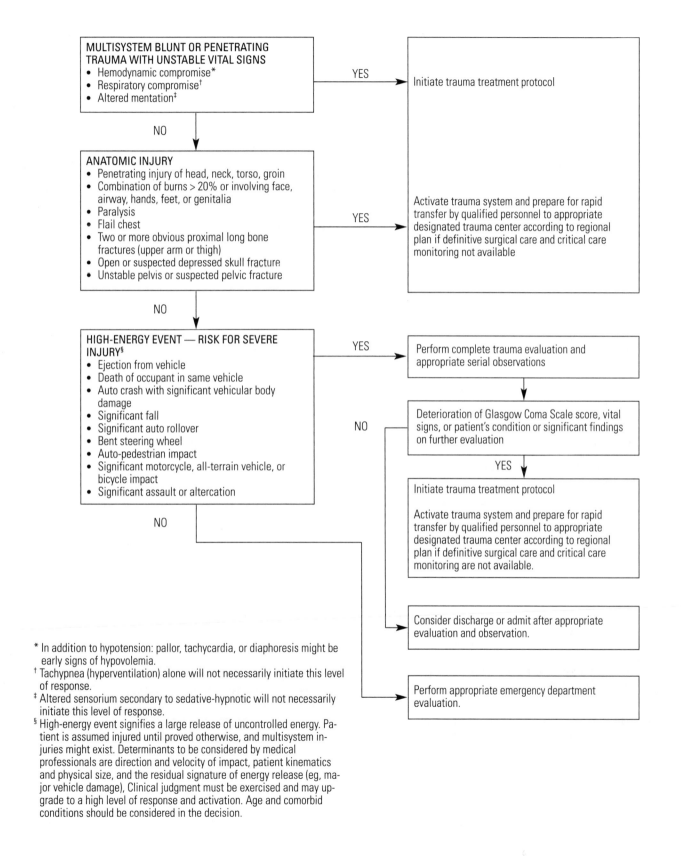

MULTISYSTEM BLUNT OR PENETRATING TRAUMA WITH UNSTABLE VITAL SIGNS
- Hemodynamic compromise*
- Respiratory compromise†
- Altered mentation‡

YES → Initiate trauma treatment protocol

NO ↓

ANATOMIC INJURY
- Penetrating injury of head, neck, torso, groin
- Combination of burns > 20% or involving face, airway, hands, feet, or genitalia
- Paralysis
- Flail chest
- Two or more obvious proximal long bone fractures (upper arm or thigh)
- Open or suspected depressed skull fracture
- Unstable pelvis or suspected pelvic fracture

YES → Activate trauma system and prepare for rapid transfer by qualified personnel to appropriate designated trauma center according to regional plan if definitive surgical care and critical care monitoring not available

NO ↓

HIGH-ENERGY EVENT — RISK FOR SEVERE INJURY§
- Ejection from vehicle
- Death of occupant in same vehicle
- Auto crash with significant vehicular body damage
- Significant fall
- Significant auto rollover
- Bent steering wheel
- Auto-pedestrian impact
- Significant motorcycle, all-terrain vehicle, or bicycle impact
- Significant assault or altercation

YES → Perform complete trauma evaluation and appropriate serial observations

↓

Deterioration of Glasgow Coma Scale score, vital signs, or patient's condition or significant findings on further evaluation

NO → YES ↓

Initiate trauma treatment protocol

Activate trauma system and prepare for rapid transfer by qualified personnel to appropriate designated trauma center according to regional plan if definitive surgical care and critical care monitoring are not available.

Consider discharge or admit after appropriate evaluation and observation.

NO → Perform appropriate emergency department evaluation.

* In addition to hypotension: pallor, tachycardia, or diaphoresis might be early signs of hypovolemia.

† Tachypnea (hyperventilation) alone will not necessarily initiate this level of response.

‡ Altered sensorium secondary to sedative-hypnotic will not necessarily initiate this level of response.

§ High-energy event signifies a large release of uncontrolled energy. Patient is assumed injured until proved otherwise, and multisystem injuries might exist. Determinants to be considered by medical professionals are direction and velocity of impact, patient kinematics and physical size, and the residual signature of energy release (eg, major vehicle damage), Clinical judgment must be exercised and may upgrade to a high level of response and activation. Age and comorbid conditions should be considered in the decision.

Appendix 3. Model Trauma Triage Algorithm, Level I/II Trauma Center

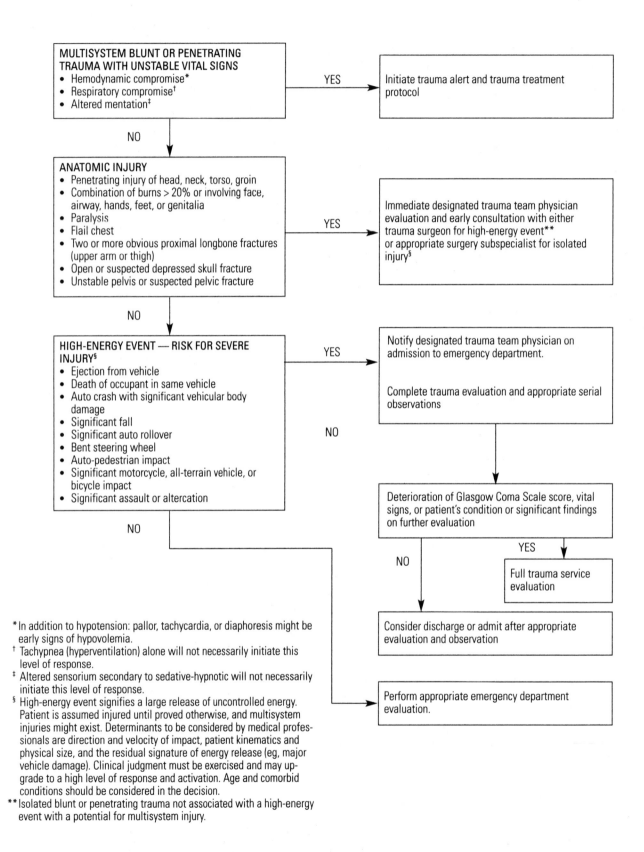

MULTISYSTEM BLUNT OR PENETRATING TRAUMA WITH UNSTABLE VITAL SIGNS
- Hemodynamic compromise*
- Respiratory compromise[†]
- Altered mentation[‡]

YES → Initiate trauma alert and trauma treatment protocol

NO ↓

ANATOMIC INJURY
- Penetrating injury of head, neck, torso, groin
- Combination of burns > 20% or involving face, airway, hands, feet, or genitalia
- Paralysis
- Flail chest
- Two or more obvious proximal longbone fractures (upper arm or thigh)
- Open or suspected depressed skull fracture
- Unstable pelvis or suspected pelvic fracture

YES → Immediate designated trauma team physician evaluation and early consultation with either trauma surgeon for high-energy event** or appropriate surgery subspecialist for isolated injury[§]

NO ↓

HIGH-ENERGY EVENT — RISK FOR SEVERE INJURY[§]
- Ejection from vehicle
- Death of occupant in same vehicle
- Auto crash with significant vehicular body damage
- Significant fall
- Significant auto rollover
- Bent steering wheel
- Auto-pedestrian impact
- Significant motorcycle, all-terrain vehicle, or bicycle impact
- Significant assault or altercation

YES → Notify designated trauma team physician on admission to emergency department.

Complete trauma evaluation and appropriate serial observations

↓

Deterioration of Glasgow Coma Scale score, vital signs, or patient's condition or significant findings on further evaluation

YES → Full trauma service evaluation

NO → Consider discharge or admit after appropriate evaluation and observation

NO → Perform appropriate emergency department evaluation.

---

* In addition to hypotension: pallor, tachycardia, or diaphoresis might be early signs of hypovolemia.

[†] Tachypnea (hyperventilation) alone will not necessarily initiate this level of response.

[‡] Altered sensorium secondary to sedative-hypnotic will not necessarily initiate this level of response.

[§] High-energy event signifies a large release of uncontrolled energy. Patient is assumed injured until proved otherwise, and multisystem injuries might exist. Determinants to be considered by medical professionals are direction and velocity of impact, patient kinematics and physical size, and the residual signature of energy release (eg, major vehicle damage). Clinical judgment must be exercised and may upgrade to a high level of response and activation. Age and comorbid conditions should be considered in the decision.

** Isolated blunt or penetrating trauma not associated with a high-energy event with a potential for multisystem injury.

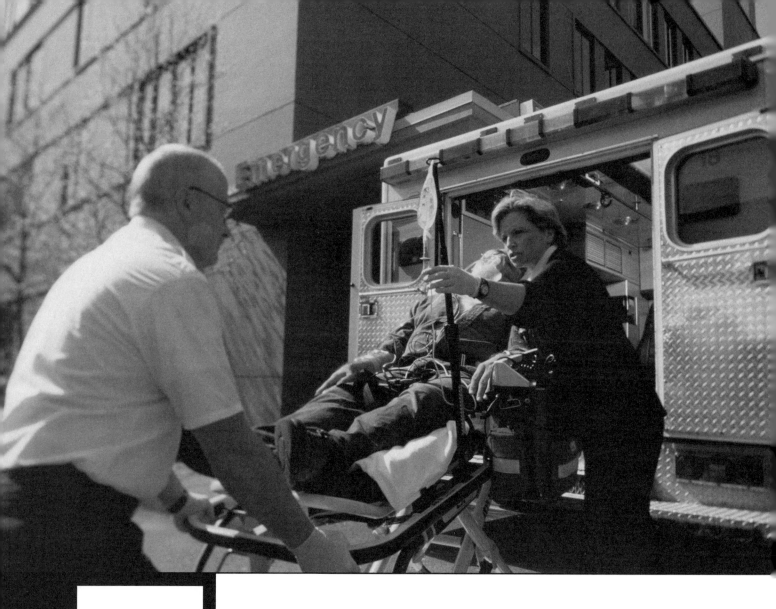

5

Emergency Departments and EMS

William A. Gluckman, DO, FACEP, EMT-P
Neill S. Oster, MD
Nancy Holecek, RN

Principles of This Chapter

After reading this chapter, you should be able to:

- Discuss how emergency departments and EMS systems are related.
- Describe how emergency departments are categorized and organized.
- Define online and offline medical direction.
- Recall EMTALA basics.
- Explain the importance of communication between the emergency department and the EMS system.

EMERGENCY DEPARTMENTS ARE THE PRIMARY ENTRY POINT for hospital admissions and a source for ambulatory care. They receive patients of all ages and provide care for a wide variety of patient complaints 24 hours a day. Many of these patients are transported by EMS. Like EMS, emergency departments don't choose the patients they receive and are required to evaluate all who present for medical care. Emergency departments and EMS systems have many similarities and, in ideal situations, complement each other to ensure optimal patient care. An understanding of emergency department organization and categorization; the various emergency department designations; and the role of physicians in medical direction, quality improvement, oversight, education, and communications is important to understanding the large, multifaceted role emergency departments have with respect to EMS.

Categorization

Emergency departments can be categorized or designated in several ways. The most common system, established by the American College of Surgeons, is the trauma center designation that rates emergency departments as Level I, II, III, or IV based on availability of resources and specialty care. To qualify for Level I status, a hospital must have a trauma surgeon in house 24 hours a day, as well as rapid access to all specialty services, most importantly, neurosurgery. In addition, there must be a commitment to education, research, and community outreach. Level II centers are similar to Level I centers but have less-extensive research and injury prevention programs. Level III centers can provide initial evaluation, resuscitation, and stabilization of trauma patients prior to transfer to a higher-level center. Some trauma patients can be cared for completely at Level III centers. Level IV centers typically serve remote areas of a state or region and provide initial stabilizing treatment to severely injured patients prior to transfer. In most cases, less severely injured patients can be cared for properly at Level IV centers.

Out-of-hospital providers must be familiar with the capabilities of the hospitals in their area and understand the trauma center designations in order to provide optimal patient care. EMS workers frequently must make decisions about where to transport patients, choosing between a specialty care center or the closest hospital when faced with a particular patient complaint or borderline unstable patient. State or local EMS system directors typically develop guidelines for the transport of patients who have special requirements. For example, EMS workers might be allowed to bypass closer hospitals for patients with conditions such as trauma, burns, high-risk pregnancy, neonatal intensive care needs, and spinal cord injury. They might be allowed to transport acute myocardial infarction (MI) patients to a center with 24-hour cardiac catheterization capability, or a stroke patient to a center that performs thrombolysis or interventional neuroradiology. These decisions typically are made according to protocols established by the EMS system's medical oversight function.

Medical Oversight

Medical oversight is essential to ensure optimal out-of-hospital care and a smooth transition of care to the emergency department. **Online medical direction** involves direct physician contact with the treating

EMS personnel (usually paramedics) by radio or phone.[1] Ideally, a board-certified emergency physician with a strong knowledge of EMS would have these duties. **Offline medical direction** includes the development of orders that are given by preset or "standing order" protocols for EMS providers to follow when specific presenting-patient criteria are met. An example of a standing order would be the initiation of an intravenous line and administration of nitroglycerine and furosemide to a person experiencing acute pulmonary edema. Strong physician input into out-of-hospital protocols allows for more appropriate care. Online medical direction allows for early physician assessment and treatment. In areas where medical direction is given from the emergency department that will be receiving the patient, good continuity of care is ensured. This also allows for immediate or near-immediate feedback to the EMS crew, as well as provider interaction and education. It is important that the physician take the time to take a verbal report and read the ambulance call report to understand what transpired in the field — the physical exam, history, treatment, and response to treatment. Sometimes an EMT obtains an important piece of history that the hospital staff would not receive otherwise. Development of relationships between emergency department staff and the out-of-hospital providers allows for a collegial work relationship, trust, understanding, and, ultimately, better patient care. Monthly meetings with formalized agendas to promote communication and provide information between the out-of-hospital providers and the emergency department staff can accomplish this. Additionally, continuing education courses and customer satisfaction initiatives are helpful.

Emergency Department Structure

Emergency departments should be structured to appropriately handle all patients who present for medical care. Walk-in entrances should be separate from EMS/ambulance entrances. Ambulatory patients can enter and be directed to triage, and from there to a treatment area or to the waiting room depending on the triage category. Ambulance entrances should be large enough to accommodate stretchers with EMS personnel walking beside them. It is difficult for a crew to squeeze through a single door with a stretcher while performing bag-mask ventilation and CPR. Automatic doors and air curtains help maintain hospital temperature and keep diesel fumes outside. Overhangs or awnings should surround the entrance to keep patients dry as they exit the ambulance. A system for rapid assessment by a triage nurse and subsequent disposition is important for patient care. It also allows the EMS unit to return to service in a timely manner. This system can sometimes be started prior to arrival based on information obtained from the radio report. Obviously, a patient with a gunshot wound to the chest is not going to the waiting room. Advance notice will allow the trauma room or other designated treatment area to be prepared and, if part of the system plan, the trauma team or other personnel to be promptly notified. An area or room should be designated for EMS crew members to write their reports. This encourages them to complete them in a timely manner and to leave them with the patient's chart for review by other medical staff.

Although there are many designs for departments, ideally, the configuration of rooms and nursing stations will allow for easy access and observation of patients, and will help keep charts and personnel close to facilitate communication. EMS radio consoles should be in an easily accessible location but not one that will interfere with daily department operations or that would cause a distraction to the staff. If 12-lead ECG transmission is part of the system, the receiving unit should be dedicated to this function and should be located close to the radio or telephone console so that the medical direction physician can retrieve it quickly.

Adequate space should be assigned for EMS equipment and linen restocking. A utility room where contaminated backboards and other equipment can be cleaned should also be provided. Some hospitals clean the equipment and place it in a clean area for pickup by the crew; others allow the space for crews to clean them at the time of patient delivery.

EMTALA

The federal **Emergency Medical Treatment and Labor Act**, or EMTALA, was passed in 1985 to regulate examination, treatment, and transfer of emergency department patients and to discourage emergency departments from "dumping" sick but uninsured patients on city or public hospitals. The scope of the regulations for EMTALA enforcement is so broad that EMS system directors and physicians involved with medical oversight must understand completely how they affect transport destination protocols for both hospital-owned and non–hospital-owned ambulances. They also must understand and comply with all rules governing interfacility transports.[2]

Interfacility transfers are either patient requested or medically indicated. With a medically indicated transfer, the treating physician must certify that the patient requires a higher level of care than can be provided at the transferring hospital. The transferring emergency department must contact the receiving hospital, and the receiving hospital must indicate that it has the capacity to care for the patient's condition (if that's the case) and accept the transfer before the patient is transported. The patient should be stabilized for transfer, and all records must be transported with the patient (nurse-to-nurse report, physician-to-physician report, and physician or nurse report should be given to the transport crew). The patient must be accompanied by appropriate personnel. Some transports require basic life support (BLS) only; thus EMTs are typically used. Critical patients will require a higher level of care en route — perhaps by paramedics. Additionally, a nurse, respiratory therapist, or physician might need to accompany a patient who requires highly specialized or advanced care.

The key point to remember is that the physician who certifies a medically indicated transfer of a patient with an emergency medical condition (as defined by law, not by common medical practice) must be sure that the transfer is effected in accordance with EMTALA regulations. Otherwise, that physician will be at risk and will put his or her hospital at risk as well. Understanding the capabilities and level of care available from the EMS system is critical in any transfer decision.

A more detailed discussion of EMTALA is presented in Chapter 27, "EMTALA and EMS."

Communications

The emergency department must be able to maintain adequate communication with out-of-hospital personnel for a variety of reasons. As mentioned earlier, online medical direction is very important. It is also important for all units to know the receiving status of a facility. Diversion, bypass, and internal disaster status must be quickly and effectively communicated to all units that might transport patients to a particular facility.[3]

When a hospital declares a critical care divert, in which it is unable to accept any more critical patients, it is imperative that this information be disseminated to EMS units. Hospitals divert when their emergency departments can no longer accept all or specific types of patients by ambulance. Emergency department diversion is a short-term, temporary approach used to make sure that patients get the right care at the right time. Diversion is a warning sign of capacity constraints under normal conditions; 62% of hospitals surveyed and three out of four urban emergency departments perceive they are at or over operating capacity. One third of all hospitals experienced emergency department diversion at a time when volumes continued to rise by 5% over the past year. The capacity problem is likely to worsen.[4]

Diversion creates a hardship for patients and for EMS personnel. Therefore, hospital administration must make every effort to avoid it. Several initiatives can be put into place to ensure all efforts are exhausted before divert or bypass is considered. These initiatives include a policy and procedure to provide structured support to the emergency department. Support should include holding criteria, triage of inpatient units, and a resource response team. The resource response team should include registration, laboratory, transport, housekeeping, and additional nurses and physicians to provide additional care. Some hospitals will have direct communication with the units by radio, pager, or cell phone, while others will rely on dispatchers or dispatch centers to make the notifications. However this is accomplished, it is important that the field units know how the hospitals are functioning.

Summary

Emergency departments and EMS systems both serve as entry points to the emergency health care system and therefore must work together to ensure optimal patient care. As such, hospitals and EMS providers must understand each other's roles, responsibilities, and capabilities. Mutual understanding is facilitated in a variety of ways. Systems of categorization, such as the trauma center designation, organize emergency departments according to their specialty and availability of resources, allowing out-of-hospital providers to make quality decisions on where to transport patients. EMS providers also receive guidance via online medical direction or direct contact with physicians, or by following established protocols when specific patient presenting criteria are met (known as offline medical direction). Effective systems of communication are especially important to ensuring medical oversight. Furthermore, emergency departments should provide quality improvement as well as education and direction to out-of-hospital providers, thus developing an ideal working relationship.

References

1. Sanders MJ. *Paramedic Textbook*. 2nd ed. St Louis, Mo: Mosby Inc; 2001:19–20.

2. Bitterman RA. *Providing Emergency Care Under Federal Law: EMTALA*. Dallas, Tex: American College of Emergency Physicians; 2001.

3. Landesman LY. *Emergency Preparedness in Health Care Organizations*. Oakbrook Terrace, Ill: Joint Commission on Accreditation of Healthcare Organizations; 1996:75-91.

4. The Lewin Group. *The Lewin Group Analysis of AHA ED Hospital Capacity Survey*; 2002:27.

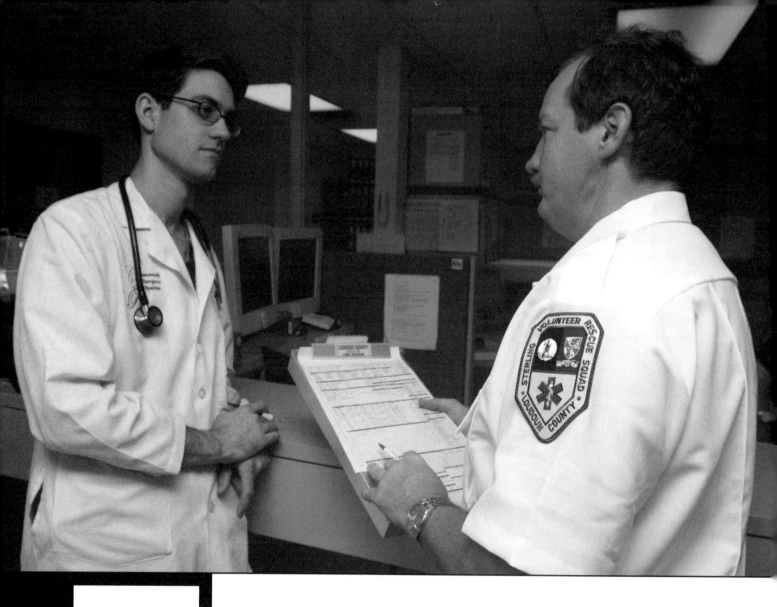

6

Medical Oversight and Accountability

Robert A. Swor, DO, FACEP

Principles of This Chapter

After reading this chapter, you should be able to:
- Define medical oversight, and explain the importance of medical (physician) accountability.
- Describe the aspects of online medical oversight.
- Describe the aspects of offline medical oversight, such as protocol development, quality assurance, and education.

THE PROVISION OF MEDICAL CARE IN THE FIELD BY PARA-medical personnel was a revolutionary concept when it was introduced in the late 1960s. Before that, emergency care for patients outside of the hospital was limited to first aid provided by bystanders and public safety personnel who were poorly trained and equipped. With the possible exception of battlefield care, the delivery of medical care by physician surrogates in the absence of a physician had no precedent. Emergency medical care in the United States has evolved dramatically. As the public has become more sophisticated regarding health care, the demand for accountability from the medical profession, and from emergency care providers in particular, has grown dramatically. Prior to the mid-1960s, care was delivered only by someone known and trusted by the patient — the private physician. As emergency care systems developed, care of the critically sick and injured was delivered more often by providers unknown to the patient. Both the public and the medical community now expect quality emergency care. Work by the prestigious Institute of Medicine has identified that errors in medical care, particularly in emergency care, are a significant public health problem.[1,2] The public increasingly expects that there is a system in place to ensure that quality care is provided.

The purpose of this chapter is to discuss and examine the relationship of the field EMS provider to the broad field of medicine.

Authority to Provide Patient Care

Medical care of patients is an activity tightly regulated by statute in the United States. Historically, this activity has been performed by individuals (physicians or nurses) or entities (hospitals and other health care facilities) licensed to do so by individual states. Furthermore, the authority to prescribe medications is restricted through state boards of pharmacy, and controlled substances are further regulated by the federal government through the Drug Enforcement Agency. The laws governing the authority to provide medical care are contained in the medical practice acts of individual states. The specifics of these statutes vary significantly from state to state.

The relationship of EMS providers to these medical practice acts depends on the level of provider and the state of licensure or certification. For most paramedics, the authority to care for patients is considered to be granted through the concept of **delegated practice.** This means that EMS personnel render care as physician surrogates acting under the supervision of a physician. EMS systems are now evolving to recognize that all EMS care is medical in origin and that dispatchers, first responders, and basic EMTs should be accountable for the care they render, as is the rest of the medical community. The demand for medical responsibility for out-of-hospital EMS care is the basis for the concept of medical oversight.

Medical control has been defined by Holroyd et al as "a system of physician-directed quality assurance that provides professional and public accountability for medical care in the prehospital setting."[3] Also called **medical command** or **medical direction** or **medical oversight,** the essence of this concept is to ensure that emergency *medical* services activities are just that — conceived, structured, and executed to ultimately provide medical benefit to patients. This rather broad mandate has resulted in a wide variety of EMS system configurations across the country, with the common purpose of providing appropriate, high-quality, out-of-hospital emergency care to patients. Medical oversight is the term — and activity — most reflective and inclusive of all the activities to ensure this mandate.

Medical oversight activities are characterized as either online or offline. **Online** (or direct) activities refer to direct voice communication with a physician (or designee) at the time care is being rendered to the patient. **Offline** (or indirect) activities are those that involve medical input into the EMS system and occur either before or after the care is delivered.

The most common mechanism for the provision of medical oversight in EMS is that of a physician who oversees a local EMS system. How this individual is selected or functions varies considerably. The federal Emergency Medical Services Systems Act of 1973, which funded and led to the development of modern EMS, wisely defined medical control and left its development to regional EMS lead agencies (303 regions in the original act).[4] This allowed for development based on each region's unique needs and resources. Initially, medical oversight of these new EMS projects was provided by one physician, the **project medical director,** who was responsible for EMS care in the region. That term has now been replaced by the more appropriate term, **EMS medical director (EMSMD)**, reaffirming that EMS systems are no longer short-term projects.

The EMSMD position has evolved considerably. Early systems were directed by physicians from a variety of disciplines: surgeons, internists, cardiologists, emergency physicians, and others. Today, the EMSMD is usually, by training or active practice, an emergency physician. In some areas (mostly rural), this role might be filled by a family physician, surgeon, or other individual with interest or expertise in EMS care. Both the American College of Emergency Physicians (ACEP) and the National Association of EMS Physicians (NAEMSP) have published position statements on the minimum criteria for the qualifications of the medical director (**Figure 6-1**).[5,6] An important component in the evolution of high-quality EMS systems has been continued involvement of high-quality medical leadership by the EMSMD.

As EMS systems have become more sophisticated, the larger medical community has been increasingly interested in the role of EMS in emergency care. Many EMS systems evolved with involvement of the trauma community, which helped develop criteria by which critical trauma patients are directed to specialized facilities. EMS systems in some commu-

Figure 6-1 Minimum criteria for the qualifications of the medical director.

Familiarity with the design and operation of out-of-hospital EMS systems

Experience in out-of-hospital emergency care

Routine participation in base-station radio control

Active involvement in the training of basic life support (BLS) and advanced life support (ALS) personnel

Active involvement in the medical audit, review, and critique of BLS and ALS personnel

Education regarding the administrative and legislative process affecting the regional and/or state EMS system

nities have expanded on that initial concept to direct other subsets of patients (pediatric, acute myocardial infarction, and stroke patients) to specialized facilities. To facilitate this input and to allow for consensus on the role of the system, most systems have developed medical oversight boards, which are composed of physicians who represent various specialties in the medical community. These boards vary dramatically in their roles and responsibilities for any given system.

Online Medical Oversight

The first EMS systems in the United States were developed with physicians actually staffing ambulances for emergency responses. Subsequent pilot programs in Miami, Columbus, and Seattle demonstrated that care delivered outside the hospital was effective, and that paramedics directly supervised by a physician could provide care effectively. The next stage in that evolution was that the physician was not physically present to supervise but was immediately available (online) to give medical directions ("medical control" at that time) via two-way radio. This included consultation for ECG interpretation using radiotelemetry. Part of the rationale for physician communication was that the physician would consult on each case and be medically accountable and responsible for the care of that patient. This concept continues today. In Michigan, for example, the EMS statute identifies that there exists a physician-patient relationship when a paramedic is on scene and calls for medical direction.[7]

The practice of online medical oversight varies significantly from region to region. There are variations in what communication devices are used and whether communications are always established with one facility, with a number of regional receiving facilities, or with one individual with a handheld radio. The provider of online consultation also varies, rendered by the EMSMD or a designee. This could be an emergency physician, a specially trained nurse (called a Mobile Intensive Care Nurse, MICN), or even a paramedic. Systems require that whoever gives online medical oversight is knowledgeable regarding emergency care and the local EMS system. One of the original purposes of the use of radio communications was that consultation could be obtained for the interpretation of ECG rhythm strips (radiotelemetry). This was initially valuable, but EMS system leaders have become comfortable with paramedic interpretations of cardiac dysrhythmias (and have also come to appreciate the costs of requiring radiotelemetry), and this specific application of radiotelemetry has become less common. (It is noteworthy that as 12-lead ECG capability has been introduced into the out-of-hospital setting, a variety of models is being used. Some systems require faxing the ECG, others require computerized interpretation, and some use only the paramedic's interpretation.)

The use of online medical oversight is not consistent around the country. Many regions require radio communications for any paramedic-patient contact, others for cases that involve ALS, and others only when specific orders are requested. Some EMS researchers have argued, however, that online medical oversight is time consuming, uses expensive personnel time, and yields few benefits. Hoffman et al, in a review of certain chief complaints (seizures, abdominal pain, altered mental status), found that few cases were affected by online medical oversight.[8] Zehnder reported that refusals of care were decreased by online medical oversight, and that potential serious illnesses could have been missed when it was not used for patients who refused care.[9] Other systems have not used online medical oversight at all, depending entirely on protocols and retrospective physician oversight of paramedic care.

Offline Medical Oversight

The central role of medical oversight is to ensure that EMS care is appropriate, timely, and of high quality. This requires medical input into virtually every facet of the EMS system. Input by the physician at the time of the emergency is useless unless structural elements are in place to ensure that the appropriate training, resources, and evaluation are available to provide high-quality EMS care. This medical input occurs in the EMS system before, during, and after each individual patient care contact and is offline, or indirect, in its effect on patient care. This does not suggest that

it is less important. In fact, it is crucial to the maturation of a quality EMS system. The most appropriate analogy is to that of administration of a hospital. A hospital has one set of individuals (hospital administration) who oversee operational and financial issues and a separate structure to manage the medical oversight (eg, medical standards of care, quality review, and physician and other provider credentialing) of patient care. These two structures work closely on all issues to make sure that both the environment and the personnel are able to provide high-quality care.

Ensuring quality in EMS and in all health care is important to the medical community. There is a wealth of literature on evaluating and improving health care services. Classic work by Donebedian has divided quality assurance of medical activities into prospective, concurrent, and retrospective activities.[10] This model also can be used to describe the scope of medical oversight activities.

Prospective Medical Oversight

The purpose of prospective medical oversight is to ensure that EMS system components are in place to provide quality medical care. These structural components should be interpreted broadly to include all aspects of patient care from access to the system to delivery of the patient to the appropriate destination. Areas to be addressed include, but are not limited to, standards for initial training, testing, credentialing, or developing of standards for credentialing of all levels of EMS providers; continuing education; protocol development; operational policy; and procedure development.[5,6] They can also include regulatory activities, including review of legislation, rules and regulations, and other policies to ensure that there are adequate minimum standards at the state level. Key elements of the system include education, operational policy, medical protocols, standard development, categorization, and disaster management.

Education

Initial education must ensure that the provider is able to perform appropriate tasks and procedures (training) and that he or she has adequate background to grow professionally (education). The education must conform to state licensure standards. It must also be integrated with the evolving body of medical knowledge as it relates to EMS. Special certification programs (eg, Basic Trauma Life Support, Advanced Cardiac Life Support, Pediatric Advanced Life Support, and others) might be required as part of initial

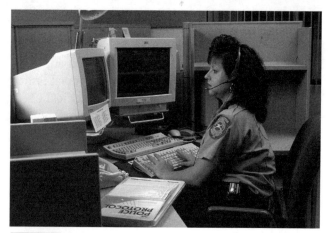

Figure 6-2 Like other out-of-hospital care providers, EMS call-takers are subject to education requirements.

training but are usually required as part of the credentialing process for an individual system. Although EMS education requirements are thought to apply to only EMTs and paramedics, they must also apply to call-takers, dispatchers, first responders, and the providers of online medical oversight (**Figure 6-2**).

Clinical education of EMS providers occurs both in the field and in a hospital. The EMS physician might need to serve as an advocate for the EMS community in its efforts to receive hospital clinical training. Specialty areas such as anesthesia for intubation training and pediatric or obstetrics are areas of critical need for initial training. These are often difficult to access by the EMS community without significant medical support.

Continuing education requirements must also be developed with medical input. They must be based on the scope of practice of EMS personnel in the community. They also include education not only specific to the individual community but also to the field of EMS as a whole. Ideally, the education program will be tied directly to those issues identified in the review of the EMS system (quality assessment). This is one method of closing the quality improvement loop.

Continuing education for providers who work on varying days and shifts is extraordinarily difficult to deliver. It is also very costly due to overtime that must be paid to allow providers to attend training sessions. One EMSMD estimated that his cost for provider overtime for continuing education was $10,000 per day of training (personal communication, 1992). In one suburban Chicago EMS system, the EMS authority conducts approximately 60 con-

ferences per month to reach all providers (personal communication with S. Zydlo, 1992). Therefore, innovative methods to provide continuing education (via videotape or the Internet or other computerized methods) are crucial components of a system's efforts.

There must be a clear administrative commitment on the part of the agency, and more importantly, on the individual paramedic to maintain a knowledge base and grow through professional education.

The **scope of practice** for each EMS system is unique. It is the sum of the initial and continuing education of the providers, the medical needs of the community, and the protocols that authorize care in the community. It is also affected by the level of emergency care provided by the hospitals in the community. For instance, a community that provides emergency angioplasty at selected hospitals might require EMS providers to evaluate myocardial infarction patients with 12-lead ECG and transport them further distances to cardiac centers. Paramedics in such a system would need additional skills (12-lead interpretation), equipment, and other adjuncts (perhaps additional pressors to treat cardiogenic shock for longer field contact times).

Operational Policy

The involvement of the EMSMD in operational EMS matters must be addressed with some sensitivity. EMS agency managers and directors, including those in the public and private sectors, have administrative responsibility for EMS agencies. EMSMDs have legal and moral responsibility for the medical care provided. Both groups must work together to ensure the success of EMS agencies. EMS systems are complex organizations that require substantial management expertise and often operate under significant financial constraints. A balance must be reached in each system between operational limitations and medical needs. EMSMDs should have significant input into a variety of operations issues, such as training and hiring standards, equipment procurement, and response time standards. Ambulance owners, fire chiefs, and other providers must similarly have a voice in the development of medical protocols and therapies to make sure they are practical as well as medically appropriate. An example would be the use an expensive drug that might have some clinical benefit but would result in significant cost overruns for the system. There are very few issues in EMS that are purely operational or purely medical (**Figure 6-3**).

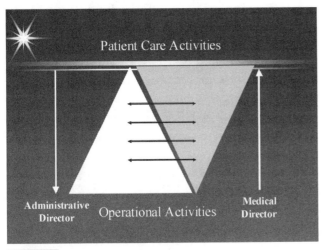

Figure 6-3 Patient care activities.

Medical Protocols

Medical protocols are the backbone of EMS field care. They dictate which procedures will be performed, which medical conditions will be treated, and how patients will be treated (eg, with nitroglycerine or furosemide for pulmonary edema). They attempt to address in a structured manner the important clinical issues that are faced by EMS providers. Some protocols are classified as **standing orders,** orders that can be performed without an online physician order and should be performed prior to any other therapy or intervention (eg, immediate defibrillation for a cardiac arrest victim, intubation for a patient with respiratory failure). Procedures that may be performed only after medical consultation vary significantly among systems. Some systems are restrictive, allowing, for example, narcotics to be given only after contact with a physician. Others require medical consultation only for administrative issues (eg, refusals). Most systems also have medical protocols for triage of trauma patients based on various physiologic (vital signs), anatomic, or mechanistic (ejection from vehicle) criteria. These triage protocols go hand in hand with the designation of hospitals that will receive seriously injured trauma patients. In addition to clinical issues, protocols (or "policies," to avoid confusion with patient care protocols) should be designed to address complex medical-legal and ethical issues (refusal of care, DNR orders, ambulance diversion, abuse and neglect). Protocols should also address when and how radio communications should be used in the system and what mode of transportation (ALS or BLS, lights and sirens, or nonemergency traffic) is used. The distinction between medical protocols and operational protocols (policies) varies among systems.

Systemwide Standard Development

In addition to development of patient care protocols, the EMS system must agree to performance standards. These must be developed through a consensus process that reviews national standards and decides which are applicable to the local EMS system. Sample standards might apply to individual providers (training requirements, continuing education and testing requirements, minimum procedural proficiency) or to the system itself (response time, staffing requirements). The process of development itself is invaluable and serves to develop a consensus on what the system expects of itself.

Categorization/Designation/Verification

The procedure of designating which hospital or hospitals are appropriate to receive individual patients is one of the more complex and politically charged issues facing medical directors and the systems they represent. Destination policies are important to the appropriate function of the EMS system because they identify to the provider which facility is most appropriate for the care of a given type of emergency. This procedure by its very nature directs patients away from certain institutions, having potential economic impact. It could be perceived as having an adverse impact on the reputation of some facilities. For that reason, and for the straightforward medical care issues, this process must be open, complete, fair, and as objective as possible. Some systems merely survey receiving facilities regarding the services they provide (eg, in-house surgery, obstetrics, availability of specialized diagnostic equipment) and allow individual providers to make decisions based on that data. Others require that receiving facilities meet fairly stringent criteria (eg, American College of Surgeons Committee on Trauma verification of trauma centers) to receive certain critical patients. Although some might argue that EMS system authority does not extend to care that is rendered inside the hospital, it is clear that patient destination has an impact on survival for certain categories of critical patients. Accordingly, the EMS system has an obligation to ensure that patients are transported to the most appropriate facility.

Most states have developed elaborate systems to care for trauma patients based on literature that shows that organized trauma systems decrease morbidity and mortality for trauma patients.[11] In these states, the designation process is much more complex and expensive. To become verified as a Level I trauma center in accordance with criteria developed by the American College of Surgeons Committee on Trauma, a hospital must have a surgeon, an anesthesiologist, and an inhospital surgical team 24 hours a day, and it must have ongoing trauma education programs and a system to evaluate the care it renders. The hospital then provides data documenting how trauma care is provided to patients, which includes specific process and outcome data. This information must also be reviewed in a formal inspection by a team of experts from outside the region or state with an onsite visit, a process called **verification.** This process, although cumbersome, ensures that not only *can* the hospital provide quality care, it *does* provide quality care. Although EMS systems do not generally have responsibility for inpatient care, they could (and should) require that EMS patients be transported to emergency facilities that do provide quality emergency care.

Disaster Management

Disaster management is clearly an important component of the EMS system. Procedures and protocols must be in place to respond and care for victims of disasters and multicasualty incidents. This topic is covered in detail in Chapter 17, "Disaster Response."

Concurrent Medical Oversight

Review of medical care at the time it is rendered is referred to as concurrent medical oversight. Feedback can be direct and specific to the individual circumstance so that patient care can be more effective. Many physicians think that reviewing care on emergency department arrival is concurrent, but it actually is retrospective. The patient who arrives in the emergency department with an endotracheal tube in the trachea might appear to be properly intubated, for instance, but the tube might have been placed after long periods of apnea and with improper technique. To be effective, concurrent evaluation must occur at the time care is provided.

In the best of all worlds, an EMSMD would be physically available at each patient encounter, would understand the limitations of the EMS environment, and would be experienced in the provision of medical care outside the hospital. Policies and protocols then could be designed with an appreciation of the limitations inherent in the field environment. But

this is rarely the case, so efforts should be made to educate the provider on scene and the physician policy-makers regarding the field environment. Scene response should be a basic responsibility of the medical director or representatives (eg, clinical supervisors). The EMSMD should be readily available to assist, assess, learn, and teach at the time care is being rendered.

Retrospective Medical Oversight

All of the topics addressed so far are important to ensure that a system is in place to provide high-quality EMS care. Equally important but less fully developed in most systems is a method of review that answers the questions, "Does the system provide quality medical care?" and "What can be done to provide better care?" This process is absolutely vital to the maturation and continued growth of EMS systems. The continued documentation of quality performance also makes the EMS system accountable to the medical community of which it is a part, and to the community it serves.

The need for **quality assurance (QA)** and **quality improvement (QI)** management methods and techniques to ensure and improve quality of EMS service are self-evident. The implementation of QA and QI appears very similar, and many EMS professionals use these terms interchangeably. They are, however, fundamentally different and have very different impacts on individual providers and systems.

Quality Assurance

QA is a method developed in the medical community to do as it says: "assure" that medical care is being provided in a quality consistent with standard medical practice. QA introduced to the medical community the concepts of a routine review of care, clear documentation of problems identified, and an emphasis on feedback to the individual practitioner. The basic assumptions of the method are that most individuals try to do a good job, want to know if mistakes are made, and will work diligently to improve their performance if a problem exists. QA also assumes that EMS and medical practice are art as well as science, and that the people best able to assess the appropriateness of care are other professional practitioners. This concept of peer review is vital to the review of care in any EMS system.

Traditionally, QA activities in EMS systems have focused on paramedic (ALS level) care. This is because early EMS laws placed only paramedics under medical control. As systems matured, it became apparent that there are multiple components to quality EMS care, and that every portion of a system should be evaluated, including (at a minimum) dispatch, first response, paramedic care, and online medical supervision.

However laudable the goals of QA programs, they suffer from a number of limitations. A review of care after an incident always has the potential of second-guessing the caregiver. Worse, retrospective reviews that look for individuals who are consistently making mistakes take on the appearance of a witch hunt, which places the entire system under strain. QA methodology makes a faulty assumption that individual providers are able to improve care rendered and are solely responsible for the success and failure of that care. A failed intubation, for instance, might be interpreted as a "problem" with the paramedic whose attempt was unsuccessful. A second shortcoming is that QA programs often identify problems but are not able to implement solutions. Because of the need to ensure public and professional accountability, QA programs will continue to be part of most EMS systems. However, evaluation in the absence of a system to use the findings of that evaluation is a frustrating, potentially damaging exercise.[12]

Quality Improvement

The medical community, EMS in particular, has searched for effective ways to improve the quality and efficiency of patient care. QI is a method that was embraced by Japanese industry after World War II and introduced to US industry in the 1970s. This revolutionary approach to management focuses on quality as measured by the customer, an emphasis on improvement of systems of care, and management's use of data (facts) to make decisions. A further emphasis is that it is the role of management to create the environment and develop the infrastructure to help frontline personnel do their jobs effectively. The emphasis on faulty processes as a major (85% of problems, in some literature) impediment to quality implies that individuals aren't given the proper tools and environment to do quality work.[13] For example, a paramedic who was unable to intubate a patient might have had problems due to poor suction equipment, no medically knowledgeable assistance on scene, and/or poor quality laryngoscopes. The concept of the customer as the one who defines quality is one that is foreign to health care providers. QI philosophy would identify anyone who uses the goods and services of an individual as a customer (**Figure 6-4**). The patient, the emergency department nurse who receives that patient, and the first responder who depends on the paramedic for patient care might all be considered to be customers, so the quality of the paramedic's function would be evaluated by all of these individuals. The emphasis on facts for decisions requires quasiscientific study and hard data on specific items that need to be improved. The focus on the *process* of care places the paramedic in a central role in EMS QI because the front-line street provider is the person who best understands and is able to evaluate EMS patient care processes. For those reasons, it is absolutely vital that paramedics be committed to and actively involved in evaluating and improving their systems. QA, QI, and other methods to ensure accountability improve patient care and increase efficiency of the EMS system and are all integral parts of EMS systems of the future.

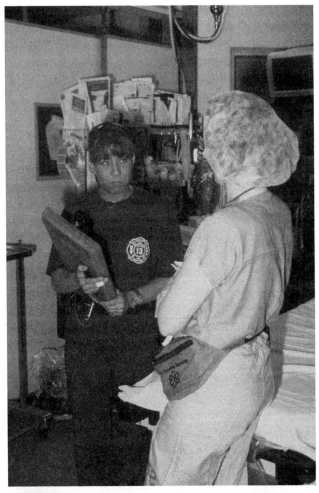

Figure 6-4 The emergency nurse who receives a patient can be considered to be a customer and therefore would evaluate the function of the paramedic.

Documentation and Data

Any review of medical care must have clear, complete data to be used to evaluate the care rendered. This usually comes from the **patient care record** (PCR), which the provider completes as part of the care of that patient. This medical record communicates initial findings and pertinent data to medical care providers in the hospital, is a legal record of the event, and is a database for the EMS system to retrospectively review individual care and the functioning of the entire system. All of these functions are important and demand that records be complete, accurate, and legible. Complete documentation is a critical part of a medical care system and is vital if the EMS system is to be able to ensure and improve quality.

Commitment

An EMS system must perform tasks to improve quality, but it also must be firmly committed to providing other things necessary to improve quality, including time, personnel, and resources. This requires an organizational commitment from everyone, from the medical director to the first responder. EMS system leaders must be willing to support improvement both philosophically and financially and integrate frontline personnel into programs to improve patient care.

The Medical Director

The EMSMD is a vital link in the provision of medical care in the field. He or she must be the physician best able to assess medical care in the context of the EMS environment. The EMSMD is expected to participate in the education of providers, communicate with the medical and hospital community, facilitate necessary hospital training available to the system, and be the local expert on EMS medical literature. In short, the medical director must ensure that the focus of the EMS system is medical and must act as the patient advocate in the system.

Future of Medical Oversight

With the maturation of emergency medicine as a specialty, a critical mass of physicians has developed a profound interest in EMS. Some EMS systems now employ full-time medical directors. Organizations such as ACEP, NAEMSP, and the Society for Academic Emergency Medicine have encouraged and supported physician interest and involvement in EMS. This interest has resulted in a wealth of EMS physician education and research, culminating in the development of specialized training programs (fellowships) for EMS physicians. By 2000, more than 100 physicians had completed EMS fellowship postgraduate training programs. These EMS subspecialists should be the leaders of the EMS industry in the years ahead and will have the interest, sophistication, and training to evaluate and improve EMS systems.

Research

The ultimate responsibility of the EMS community is to provide its patients the best possible patient care. To make that possible, the EMS system must continually work to evaluate how care is rendered and what can be done to improve it. QA and QI methods evaluate care in the context of established norms of practice. Research extends this evaluation to develop new knowledge. Research in EMS has been described by at least one knowledgeable researcher as "impressively deficient."[14] Although few medical directors and EMS providers have the interest and expertise to do quality research, it is the responsibility of all EMS providers to support efforts to improve EMS through research. (See Chapter 22, "Research.")

Summary

The opportunity to provide patient care is a privilege. Every one of us who provides emergency care is ultimately accountable for the care we provide. We are responsible to the organizations that employ us, to the medical community of which we are a part, and ultimately to the communities we serve. Medical oversight of EMS is merely a visible representation of that accountability. Medical oversight has an important role in ensuring that the ultimate goal of EMS systems, despite all other competing priorities, is quality emergency medical care.

References

1. Kohn LT, Corrigan JM, Donaldson MS. *To Err is Human: Building a Safer Health System*. Washington, DC: National Academies Press; 1999.

2. Committee on Quality of Health Care in America, Institute of Medicine. *Crossing the Quality Chasm: A New Health System for the 21st Century*. Washington, DC: National Academies Press; 2001.

3. Holroyd B, Knopp R, Kallsen G. Medical control: quality assurance in prehospital care. *JAMA*. 1986; 256:1027–1031.

4. Boyd DR. The history of emergency medical services systems in the United States of America. In: Boyd DR, Edlich RF, Micik S, eds. *Systems Approach to Emergency Medical Care.* Norwalk, Conn: Appleton-Century-Crofts; 1983.

5. Polsky S, Krohmer J, Maningas P, et al. Guidelines for medical direction of prehospital care. *Ann Emerg Med.* 1993;22:742–744.

6. Alonso-Serra H, Blanton D, O'Connor R. Physician medical direction in EMS. *Prehospital Emerg Care.* 1998;2(2):153–158.

7. Michigan Compiled Laws 333.20967 (2000).

8. Hoffman JR, Luo J, Schriger DL, et al. Does paramedic-based hospital contact result in beneficial deviations from standard prehospital protocols? *West J Med.* 1990;153:283–287.

9. Cone DC, Kim DT, Davidson SJ. Patient-initiated refusals of prehospital care: ambulance call report documentation, patient outcome, and on-line medical command. *Prehospital Disaster Med.* 1995;10(1):3–9.

10. Donebedian A. The quality of care: how can it be assessed? *JAMA.* 1988;260:1743–1748.

11. Bass RR, Gainer PS, Carlini AR. Update on trauma system development in the United States. *J Trauma.* 1999;47(3 Suppl):S15–S21.

12. Davidson SR. Closing the loop: discarding bad apples or continuously improve EMS? In: Swor RA, Rottman SA, Pirrallo RG, et al, eds. *Quality Management in Prehospital Care.* Philadelphia, Pa: Mosby-Lifeline Publishers; 1993.

13. Berwick DM, Godfrey AB, Roessner J. *Curing Health Care: New Strategies for Quality Improvement.* San Francisco, Calif: Jossey-Bass Publishers; 1990.

14. Callaham M. Quantifying the scanty science of prehospital emergency care. *Ann Emerg Med.* 1997; 30(6):785–790.

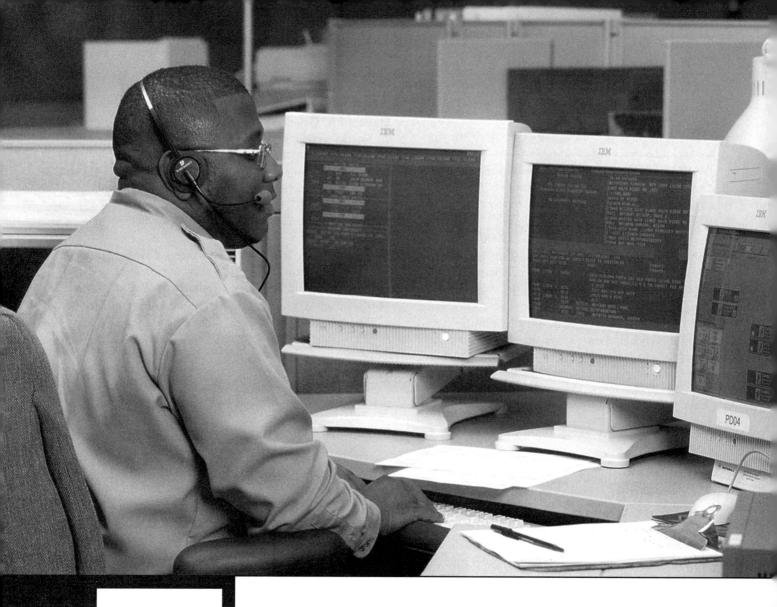

7 Administration, Management, and Operations

Richard Herrington
Gordon Bergh

Principles of This Chapter

After reading this chapter, you should be able to:

- Explain the different EMS system models and crew and response configurations.
- Describe the integrated process of field response.
- Recall the aspects of field clinical response.
- Explain the integration of the EMS system with community groups and citizens, the medical community, hospitals, public health, and public safety.
- Describe the infrastructure and support services functions.

THERE IS PERHAPS NO MORE MYSTERIOUS COMPONENT OF EMS to a medical director than the administrative and operational aspects of the system. It is helpful to think of an EMS system as a practice of medicine. The system exists to provide quality medical care to ill and injured patients. How that care is delivered has a significant impact on the quality and consistency of appropriate clinical care. The unique nature of an EMS system requires sophisticated, integrated approaches to care delivery. Although a medical director might believe that components of the system such as hiring requirements or fleet services have absolutely no place in the discussion of medical care, a poorly managed operation will ultimately result in poor medical care. Similarly, a well-coordinated operation enhances the opportunity to consistently provide clinically sophisticated care.

Although it is not the medical director's responsibility to run the entire EMS system (just as it is not an emergency physician's responsibility to run the entire hospital), it is beneficial to have a clear understanding of the essential elements of the entire system. Working in partnership with those responsible for making things happen not only expands a medical director's ability to facilitate important change but also allows the organization to benefit from the medical director's clinical expertise.

The purpose of this chapter is to introduce the EMS medical director (EMSMD) to the many facets of EMS administration and operations, with an emphasis on the interface with medical oversight.

System Design and Configuration

System design refers to the way an EMS system is structured and how medical care is delivered. Unlike most fire and police system design models, there is not a uniform standard that applies to EMS systems. Most fire and police departments are considered to be the backbone of the local public safety function and are usually publicly funded, especially in urban areas. This is often not the case with EMS systems. They will be private, hospital based, public (municipal), volunteer, or a hybrid. To add to the complexity, each of these different models varies in configuration throughout the country. One expert estimates that, combining the first response and transport categories, there are more than 80 different system configurations for providing patient care.[1] Some services employ only EMTs; others only paramedics; many both; and others paramedics and nurses. Many systems, especially in smaller, rural communities, provide BLS-level patient care. These areas often rely heavily on volunteer personnel to staff their ambulances. But in larger cities, ALS care is the norm.

In 2000, the predominant organization types in urban areas were **private** (44.5%), **fire department** (39%), and **third services** (12%).[2] Recently, several partnerships that combine fire and private services into a unified system have been established. The San Diego Medical Services Enterprise is an example that involves the San Diego Fire Department and Rural/ Metro Medical Services. Many systems provide both emergency and nonemergency services to their communities.

Within each of these ALS service organizations, the crew configuration varies. A widely used configuration is to have two paramedics on each ambulance. However, many systems use one paramedic and either an EMT-Basic or EMT-Intermediate per unit. Some communities use the **"tiered system" concept** of having both BLS units and a smaller number of ALS units available for response. Nationally, only 38.6% of patients require ALS intervention,[3] so the tiered system model is an attempt to reduce the higher costs of delivering ALS care to patients who require only BLS care. The Houston Fire Department is an example of a system that uses the tiered model. Although there are advantages and disadvantages to both models, there is considerable debate about whether BLS providers can consistently and safely determine which patients require ALS care and whether an all-ALS system can maintain paramedic skill proficiency. Studies do not provide a clear consensus.

The system design a community ultimately establishes is based on many factors, including but not limited to local regulations, elected official preferences, public opinion and will, economic circumstances, the medical community's influence, and level of satisfaction with the previous (or current) ambulance transport provider. Thus, a system that is best for one community might be unacceptable to another. Each of these organization types will be discussed briefly.

Fire EMS Provider

Fire-based systems are the most common public EMS systems in the country. They have evolved since the early 1970s when EMS as we know it was in its infancy. In many communities, there was a natural progression to expand the role and responsibilities of the fire departments as EMS came of age. Most fire-based EMS systems use firefighters who have been trained to the paramedic level (cross-trained) and spend time with the ambulance service. Some systems have separate medical and fire suppression divisions and no crossover of responsibilities. Most fire-based EMS systems provide both first response and transport.

One configuration within fire-based EMS systems, especially in the western United States, combines components of both the public and private sectors. In these systems, the fire department responds with ALS-trained personnel on non–transport-capable fire apparatus. If transport is required, a contracted private ambulance service transports the patient. The fire paramedic, depending on system configuration, will either accompany the patient or transfer responsibility for patient care to the transporting medics.

Third-Service EMS Provider

Third-service providers are government agencies separate from fire or police departments. They can be a distinct city department such as Austin-Travis County EMS, a health authority such as Denver EMS, or a function of county government such as Wake County (South Carolina) EMS. Compared to fire systems, which focus their resources on fire suppression as well as EMS, third-service models direct their resources to out-of-hospital medical rescue and patient care activities.

Private Contractor EMS Provider

Many communities have elected not to implement a public EMS system and rely on private contractors to provide EMS service. This usually results in either no taxation or a reduced tax subsidy to provide the services. Within larger urban areas, these services are usually awarded based on a competitive, performance-based exclusive contract. First response, either BLS or ALS, is usually provided by the local fire department. One advantage of this model is that the vendor is obligated to meet certain performance standards and could face penalties if it is not in compliance with those standards.

There are advantages and disadvantages for each of the models. Each community must determine what is the best model and configuration that meets its unique requirements.

Practice of Medicine

Again, think of an EMS system as a practice of medicine. Patients access the system with an expectation that they will be evaluated by competent practitioners, and that care will be initiated by a competent individual, in the appropriate time frame, with the right tools. The difference between the physician office or facility practice of medicine and an EMS system is in the methods used to carry out the process.

Clinical Care Administration

EMS continues to evolve as a serious participant in the emergency health care community. The days of the ambulance driver who had little more than basic first aid training have long gone, and a profession with skilled and educated out-of-hospital health care providers has taken its place. The depth of knowledge now present has led to a level of assessment and skill that was once unimaginable. Clinical skills once considered the domain only of physicians, such as tracheal intubation and 12-lead ECG interpretation, have become the norm for modern paramedics.

Many factors have influenced this development. Recently, more can be attributed to an increased emphasis on evidence-based standards of care, cooperative communication between EMS services and the medical community, targeted education programs, and sound quality improvement efforts. Each has a place in a sound practice of medicine that strives for high-quality care and focuses on positive results for those it serves.

In addition to changes in the level of clinical care, there have been new administrative challenges that are directly related to that care. Changes in the **Medicare Ambulance Fee Schedule** by the Centers for Medicare and Medicaid Services (CMS, formerly known as the Health Care Financing Administration, or HCFA) and increased privacy requirements brought about by the **Health Insurance Portability and Accountability Act (HIPAA)** bring about new challenges in the administrative practices that accompany out-of-hospital clinical services.

In order to meet these challenges, the medical director must be not only a skilled clinician and educator but also a competent administrator and a forward-thinking leader. Only then can the clinical administration of an EMS system thrive and move forward into the next generation of a rapidly evolving industry.

Medical Oversight

Medical oversight is a key component of an EMS system and a cornerstone to the management of its clinical operations. The EMSMD not only acts as the clinical manager of the system but also must mesh with the overall administrative management team. This allows the system to maintain a clear focus on the clinical aspects while recognizing that they are inseparable from those of operational consideration. It is important to be functionally cognizant of the role that the operational component has in ensuring the delivery of clinical care.

Many EMS systems have multiple medical directors. This is often due to multiple entities operating within one jurisdiction, such as a separate fire department and an ambulance provider. Coordination among the various medical directors and entities is paramount in ensuring a fluid system with consistent clinical care. Often it is beneficial to establish a committee within the system that includes all of the medical directors to facilitate coordination and consistency.

Some systems have transitioned to one EMS system medical director. This person coordinates clinical activities and ensures that the system is providing effective out-of-hospital clinical care in accordance with treatment standards approved among the several

agencies within the system. The complexity of clinical components has led many systems to add deputy or assistant medical directors to assist with the multitude of responsibilities. This allows expanded oversight, enabling each physician to focus attention on a piece of the overall clinical practice.

The EMSMD is essential in every facet of clinical operations. This includes providing direction and remaining in tune with the status of the system to facilitate the appropriate clinical support. Every step of the clinical process is affected by the medical director's involvement, including the structure for developing clinical standards of care, credentialing providers, continuing education, and quality management.

In addition to the leadership the EMSMD provides at the front end of clinical care, there is also a direct medical oversight element (directly available to the field provider) during the course of out-of-hospital care. Many systems use emergency physicians "online" when confronted with challenging clinical presentations to make sure that the system provides the most appropriate treatment. Using emergency physicians in this manner helps ensure appropriate care and supports providers as they actively treat patients in the field.

Protocols or Standards of Care for Field Clinical Practice

Every EMS system must have standard guidelines (treatment protocols, standard operating procedures, and so on) for the evaluation and treatment of patients. The exact manner in which these standards are created and used varies among states and regions. All providers must have an established standard of care that is consistent with accepted medical practice and approved by the physician who provides medical oversight. In addition, it is advisable to include the local medical community in the development and approval process of those standards to provide a cohesive continuum of care.

The creation and revision of a system's protocols or standards is an important process for both the EMS system and the medical director. These documents are the benchmark of out-of-hospital clinical care in the community and are the patient care script for the field providers. In order to provide the best opportunity for sound development of these documents, the development process should be a group effort. A protocol or standards development committee that is chaired by the medical director and includes representative clinical and education coordinators, field training officers, field providers, and members of the medical community is usually the most beneficial platform.

This group should regularly evaluate the effectiveness of the clinical standards and update them to ensure currency and appropriateness. An involved medical director must stay abreast of the current medical literature that supports the protocols or standards, as well as review data that provide direction for future enhancement. Evidence-based standards of care allow providers to provide the most up-to-date out-of-hospital care and contribute to new benchmarks in EMS for the future.

Orientation and Credentialing

Providers are certified by the state regulatory agency or National Registry of EMTs at a minimum competency level of clinical knowledge and skill proficiency. This assessment is usually determined through standardized written and practical examinations. After initial certification, a provider is usually required to complete a certain number of continuing education hours as part of the recertification process. Some states also require repeat competency testing.

It is the individual EMS medical director's prerogative (and some would argue responsibility) to further evaluate providers within the system to determine whether they meet defined system standards. This process is most appropriately termed credentialing. Although specifics vary among medical directors, most include some type of orientation process (or academy) and a field evaluation period in conjunction with other established competency assessment tools.

The orientation process is meant to expose the new provider to the clinical and operational standards of the practice in an educational classroom setting. Through a defined curriculum, this concept establishes a foundation from which the provider can build once in the field. This phase also allows an opportunity for the new practitioner to be exposed to the expectations and culture of the system.

During orientation, it is beneficial to introduce the provider to the field environment under the tutelage of a qualified evaluator, educator, and mentor, often called a **field training officer** or **field preceptor**. The field evaluation period brings classroom material to a real-life application and allows the field training officer to observe the ability of new field providers to complete predetermined skill competency modules while providing real-time feedback and enabling them to progress toward independent practice.

In addition to introductory education and field evaluation, it is also commonly required that providers pass local protocol or standards of care, written and scenario exams, or oral exams. Written exams test a core knowledge set, and oral exams attempt to simulate real-life patient encounters to evaluate the provider's understanding of the basic principles and his or her clinical decision-making.

Other aspects of the roles and responsibilities of the EMS medical director are covered in Chapter 6, "Medical Oversight and Accountability."

Provider Continuing Education

Continuing education is an important part of the field provider's ongoing development. It can be provided in-house by a system's internal clinical staff, outsourced to an EMS education firm, or obtained through regional programs and state and national conferences. Regardless of the source, it is usually necessary for all providers to maintain their credentials and is obviously important for the maintenance of clinical knowledge and skill proficiency.

EMS clinical administrators should be knowledgeable in individual state requirements for recertification. It is critical that the medical director be actively involved in all stages of the system's continuing education program. Continuing education requirements are often focused on specific clinical areas. Evaluation of these requirements makes it possible to ensure that certifications are met and providers are exposed to a wide range of targeted clinical information.

Many EMS systems are now expanding education beyond the limitations of the classroom through the use of technology. Education can be brought to the provider through the use of videotape presentations, audio programs, and Internet-based platforms. This technology has the potential to greatly enhance an EMS system's ability to provide high-quality, innovative education.

Research

During the early years of the EMS industry, little scientific study was present to support or refute the care that was being provided in the streets. Many of the early standards of care were implemented based on inhospital studies, but few evaluated the efficacy of out-of-hospital care. There is a growing trend of EMS systems designing and implementing targeted studies in the out-of-hospital environment. EMS systems might participate in outcomes trials or could provide an environment to field test new products prior to release in the EMS market. In addition to the significant benefit of critically evaluating the impact of care in the field environment, there are other advantages to participating in out-of-hospital research trials or demonstration projects. Research brings positive attention to the system, allows field providers to feel a sense of contribution to the industry, and enhances the system's ability to capture and evaluate data.

Research activities are discussed in more detail in Chapter 22, "Research."

Infection Control

Many EMS providers began their careers in a period when exposure to infectious disease was of little concern. Latex gloves, disposable gowns, protective eye shields, and HEPA masks were not in common use, nor were immunizations considered important. In today's environment, with the resurgence of tuberculosis and increased occupational exposure to infectious diseases, the administration of a comprehensive infectious disease program is not just appropriate; many components are required by law.

The details of a thorough and effective infection control program rely heavily on solid clinical guidance provided by a knowledgeable physician. Providing direction to the designated infection control officer regarding the education, immunization, postexposure prophylaxis, and followup care for an EMS system helps decrease morbidity (as well as anxiety) about this particular occupational risk.

Ideally, infection control programs should include an initial orientation at the start of employment (or when a volunteer joins the service) and should be reviewed and enhanced regularly. In addition, every provider and the occupants of every emergency vehicle and administrative office should have easy access to appropriate protective equipment and know when and how to use it. Even the best-prepared providers are still at risk for exposure due to the nature of the work environment. An infection control officer who can respond to accidental exposures and help providers obtain the appropriate immediate medical attention (including timely postexposure prophylaxis if necessary) should be designated.

More detailed information on infection control issues is outlined in Chapter 25, "Occupational Health Issues."

Emergency Response

Although most calls to an EMS system are not true emergencies, the EMS system must be designed to rapidly deploy the right resources with initial information regarding the nature of the illness or injury that suggests a reasonable probability that a potentially serious condition exists. Thus, in addition to the need for a clinically sophisticated system, the response must also be structured to get to the patient's side (wherever that patient might be) rapidly. Indeed, in the initial phases of acute illness or injury, the most prevalent public expectation is that help will arrive quickly.

Emergency response is more involved than the commonly held public view that EMS is simply an ambulance showing up and transporting someone to a hospital. For the purpose of this discussion, emergency response includes the spectrum of public education, 911 (or emergency) access, emergency communications/dispatch, first response, ambulance response, field clinical practice, and the local network of community and regional hospitals. This integrated process closely parallels the American Heart Association "Chain of Survival." The goal of the EMSMD within this context is to ensure that clinically appropriate care is delivered in an operationally appropriate manner.

Public Education

Public education is important to an EMS system's emergency response for two reasons. First, it provides opportunities to target localized problem areas such as lack of seat belt use or drowning. Second, it is the EMS system's how-to "user's manual" for the public. Effective public education should include information on the services the EMS system provides to the community, the various EMS participants (ie, Why does a red fire truck always show up when someone calls for an ambulance?) and the roles each agency has within the response system, how to access emergency medical services (ie, 911, 311, or other), and information/training programs on signs and symptoms of heart attack, stroke recognition, and lifesaving procedures such as CPR.

Public Access to EMS

Access to the EMS system begins with a call to 911 (or designated emergency number in communities not covered by 911). Although often neglected or unrealized, the 911 system and the EMS communications center are at the very core of a well-functioning EMS system. The 911 system primary **public safety answering point (PSAP)** is most commonly operated by law enforcement, either by county sheriff's offices or by the police department in most medium-to-large municipalities. Thanks in large part to improvements in technology, there is a trend toward consolidating smaller PSAPs to cover large service areas (multiple counties or cities). Although there are many operational models for primary PSAPs, the PSAP might be responsible for the entire process of call-taking and dispatching for law enforcement, fire, and EMS or any variation of that for single or multiple agencies. In a growing number of medium-to-large EMS systems, the actual call triage and ambulance dispatch function is performed by a secondary PSAP. Regardless of the structure, the EMSMD must understand specific processes and determine the medical standards for call processes, dispatch response levels, prearrival instructions, and related functions.

The EMSMD should also be aware of the proliferation of 311 or alternative public safety call systems. The 311 system was created to alleviate call volume loads on the 911 system for nonemergency calls. Most of these calls deal with law enforcement matters that usually do not require the dispatch of a law enforcement officer; however, many cities are also structuring their 311 systems to deal with all aspects of public interaction with local government. A large number of EMS 911 callers do not believe that their medical problems are true emergencies and might opt instead to call 311. It is important to develop guidelines for transferring these callers to the 911 center.

Emergency Dispatch and Prearrival Instructions

Obtaining correct information from callers requires a consistently applied approach to caller interrogation. Subsequent decisions regarding dispatch of resources and prearrival instructions are based on the ability to gather accurate information quickly. The questioning sequence might be part of a commercially available program, or it might be locally developed. Medical directors should have active roles in the initial program selection (or development) process, implementation, and ongoing performance assessment.

The 911 system and an EMS communications center should enable what Medical Priority™ has termed "zero-minute response times." With the implementation and use of a medical triage and dispatch protocol, 911 call-takers are able to provide appropriate medical instructions to callers over the phone (Figure 7-1). This can vary from an intervention as simple

as bleeding control and seizure support to truly lifesaving measures such as CPR. The implementation of concepts such as **dispatch life support** have significant potential to decrease morbidity and mortality as well as provide 911 callers with calm, reassuring support while they wait. These medical triage and dispatch systems also provide a structure for consistent caller triage and online medical support and provide a basis for targeted quality review and improvement.

Most EMS communications centers rely heavily on technology. **Computer-aided dispatch (CAD) systems** are used to enter and track calls for service. CAD systems use tools such as **automatic vehicle location (AVL)** to track and recommend the closest resources to an incident and facilitate interaction with mobile data systems for messaging and real-time status tracking of those resources. Many EMS systems interact with multiple agencies for first response. These agencies might use different radio systems that are characterized by the frequency on which they operate (VHF/UHF/800 MHz/Trunked 800/900 MHz systems). The communications center often has the responsibility for coordinating these multiple radio systems during incident response.

Other communications and dispatch considerations are covered in Chapters 9 and 10.

First Response

First response, usually due to strategic position and availability, provides initial on-scene emergency medical care until the arrival of the EMS transport ambulance. The first response component in any given community can include BLS or ALS providers (firefighters, police officers, or others) or other re-

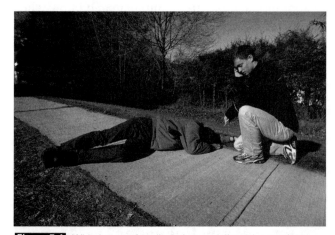

Figure 7-1 With the use of medical triage and dispatch control, 911 call-takers are able to provide appropriate medical instructions to callers over the phone.

sponders such as a school nurse, a security guard, or a corporate employee who volunteers as an emergency responder for her or his company. One of the most important aspects of first responder care is the ability to initiate immediate lifesaving measures, such as early defibrillation of a cardiac arrest patient.

Ambulance Response

Ambulance response involves the continuation of medical care from the on-scene first response team and during the EMS ambulance transport to the receiving medical facility. Care provided in an ambulance depends not only on the assessment and treatment capabilities of the provider but also on the availability of resources, both personnel and equipment. Additionally, there are unique challenges involved in providing medical care in the back of a moving vehicle that can have an impact on interventions, ability to assess, or priorities of management. Specific protocols should be developed to address when and how additional care providers should be used to join the providers in the ambulance en route to the hospital.

Field Practice of Medicine

Field clinical practice encompasses the very heart and soul of medicine — direct patient care by EMS providers (ie, first responders and ambulance medics). Support of the field practice of medicine is the bulk of an EMSMD's duties. Because the physician is not on the scene of every patient encounter, the delegated practice concept requires the development of protocols or standards for EMS providers to use. There are three common practices that delegate medical care to field providers: indirect (offline) medical oversight, direct (online) medical oversight, and a combination of both direct and indirect oversight.

Indirect (Offline) Medical Oversight

Indirect medical oversight involves the development of standing orders or protocols so that medics can treat patients without having to contact a physician directly.

Direct (Online) Medical Oversight

Direct medical oversight requires the medics to contact a physician (or designee such as a base station nurse or medic) with an assessment and treatment plan. The receiving base station then provides specific treatment orders. In some areas of the country, law or regulation requires direct medical oversight.

Combination of Direct and Indirect Medical Oversight

Most EMS systems have some combination of offline and online activities. This practice allows medics to perform specific designated treatment without contacting online resources. As the medics continue to manage the patient or the patient's condition becomes more complicated, the medics are required to contact online medical resources for additional patient care orders.

How much of what the medics do clinically offline versus online is a decision the EMSMD makes based on EMS system specifics, including the medical director's perceived competence of EMS providers. The trend of most EMS systems has been a migration toward more offline use of protocols for patient management.

This is only one aspect of a complex field clinical environment. The EMSMD must understand several other important aspects of field clinical operations, including the following:

- Scene authority for patient care
- Rescue
- Aeromedical transport integration
- Hazardous materials
- Special operations
- Weapons of mass destruction (WMD)
- Criteria for multicasualty incident management
- Transport destination requirements
- Legal issues

Scene Authority for Patient Care

This aspect concerns who has authority to make the final decision regarding how a patient is managed at the scene.

Rescue

Many EMS systems view rescue as a separate and distinct operation from field medicine. In reality, every step of a patient rescue operation has clinical implications, and those who respond must ensure that the rescue operation is patient centered.

Aeromedical Transport Integration

Some EMS systems have an aviation component among their system resources. Others have a hospital-based aviation program operating in the area. Directors must consider whether air resources are routinely dispatched as "first-in" units, and, if not, when the EMS system uses them.

Hazardous Materials

The EMS system's role at the scene of a hazardous materials (HazMat) event is the management of patients. The EMSMD must ask himself or herself: When and how? Are they part of a HazMat team? What type of specialized medical surveillance equipment is required? How does the EMS system provide preventive, rehab, and postexposure treatment of HazMat team members?

Special Operations

The EMSMD must determine what the role of EMS personnel is in such situations as confined space rescue or tactical law enforcement operations (see Chapter 20, "Operational EMS.").

Weapons of Mass Destruction

The EMS system must integrate the WMD role between its public safety and public health missions. The director must be aware of the roles of the other WMD participants (first responders, EMS transport agencies, hospitals, public health authorities, law enforcement). This is addressed in Chapter 19, "EMS Response to Terrorist Incidents and Weapons of Mass Destruction."

Criteria for Multicasualty Incident Management

The EMS director must know how the EMS system defines a multicasualty incident (MCI), as well as how the response system is activated, and by whom. Other factors to consider include whether it incorporates the principles of incident command; how patients are triaged; what the on-scene expectation for the EMS system medical director is; what triage protocol is used; how patients are distributed to area hospitals; whether the EMS system has an emergency operations center; whether EMS response units carry MCI equipment; and whether the system practices the MCI plan regularly.

Transport Destination Requirements

Other considerations for the EMSMD include whether the EMS system participates in a trauma system with patient categorization, how the EMS system integrates into the local/regional hospital trauma network, and whether there are specific designated cardiac, stroke, or pediatric receiving centers.

Legal Issues

The EMSMD must also consider legal factors, such as:

- Refusal of care process and requirements. This includes how EMS providers manage the patient refusal, whether it requires online consultation, what documentation is required, and what information the patient is given.
- Definition of a patient versus a nonpatient
- Definition of a minor (state statutes and local guidelines might be in conflict)
- Criteria for hospital diversion. The director must know how the EMS system integrates into the area hospital plan for diverting EMS patients from a hospital on diversion status. He or she must also know whether EMS manages the diversion process and whether it can override hospital diversion under certain conditions, as well as whether a designated trauma center can close to EMS trauma patients.
- Do not resuscitate (state statutes and local guidelines might be in conflict)
- Criteria for managing patients who are dead on scene (DOS). The director must know whether EMS providers can obtain field declarations of death with or without online consultation; what category of patient qualifies for a DOS; what state statutes require; and how the EMS system and medical examiner's office coordinate the DOS patient.

See Chapter 26, "Medical-Legal Concerns in EMS."

System Integration

EMS, no matter the method or model of delivery, is the newest member of the public safety triad. As such, the leadership of an EMS system must take special care to build partnerships, alliances, and effective methods of integration with other organizations to effectively deliver exceptional out-of-hospital care to the community.

This process of building relationships, both personal and organizational, is termed system integration. The effective EMSMD will work closely with the administration and management team of the EMS organization and EMS system participants to develop an effective system of routine communications and partnership development with a broad range of entities that represent various interested sections of the community. Examples of these organizations are community groups, elected officials, the medical community, hospitals and other health care facilities, the public health community, and the partner public safety organizations.

Community Groups and Citizens

EMS organizations, to be effective, need the support of the public they serve. The development of this relationship requires EMS to reach out to the community through such venues as neighborhood associations, philanthropic and service organizations, and general community participation and presence. This interaction provides a valuable venue for public education about the use and capabilities of EMS within their community, and it establishes a foundation of support that can be important when attempting to place new EMS stations, route emergency vehicle response paths, or develop support for additional funding or enhanced capabilities. Although a positive public image and presence can substantially benefit an EMS organization and contribute to its success, a poor public image can devastate a system's effectiveness. Careful maintenance of this relationship should be a critical priority of the leadership team, including the medical director.

Medical Community

It is clear that EMS represents a shared practice of medicine between the EMSMD and the community physicians whose patients use system services. The development of a strong relationship among the EMSMD, EMS operational leadership, and the medical community is key to ensuring that the EMS system has the support of the medical community, arguably the single most powerful and vocal stakeholder in the EMS system.

The maintenance of this relationship is largely the purview of the EMSMD and should be accomplished through formal (the local medical society) and informal (individual) relationships developed by the medical director. It is important to remember that these relationships are not limited to the physicians within the emergency medicine practice at local hospitals, but extend into a broad range of specialties and subspecialties that are affected by the performance of the EMS system.

Hospitals

Many EMS systems seem to ignore or, worse, assume an adversarial relationship with local hospitals. There is perhaps no relationship in EMS that can either be more symbiotic or pathologic than that between EMS providers and hospital staff. The effective management of this relationship is a substantial time commitment and requires aggressive response to concerns expressed by either side. When relationships are well maintained and successful, the benefits are enormous. Research, patient outcome data, quality management, continuing education, and public education are only a few of the areas that are positively affected when the EMS system and the hospital community are partners.

The current strains on hospital systems, especially in the area of personnel, are making this relationship more difficult to establish and maintain. The EMSMD is in a unique position to share a hospital perspective with EMS field providers while, in turn, sharing an out-of-hospital perspective with emergency department personnel.

Public Health

The terrorist attacks of September 11, 2001, and the subsequent biological pathogen deaths in Florida, Washington, DC, New York, and Connecticut forever changed the relationship between EMS and the public health community. In recent years, EMS has tried to explore the more proactive side of its nature, but public health has largely been ignored by EMS, and the reverse is equally true. Although it is clear that this relationship is necessary to successfully respond to the threat posed by a range of biological pathogens, the benefits of the relationship are far broader.

Community health initiatives, immunization programs, research and injury reduction programs, community outreach, and public education are only a few of the areas to which public health practitioners bring valuable experience. And while public health is frequently challenged by an effective means of moving in the community and delivering services door to door, EMS has an effective and well-developed mobile capability that in many systems has enough down time to offer opportunities for exciting partnerships. Additionally, most public health organizations have effective grant-writing and research staffs, two areas sorely lacking in almost all EMS organizations.

See Chapter 21, "EMS and Public Health."

Public Safety

EMS simply cannot safely and effectively deliver services without a strong relationship with the other public safety organizations. The maintenance of these relationships, both at the street and leadership level, is a daily task that must be approached with a high level of effort. The combination of strong emotions and strong personalities results in frequent misunderstandings that, if left unresolved, can result in problematic scene interactions and decreased effectiveness of patient care and decreased responder safety.

The leadership members of the EMS organization should maintain personal relationships with their public safety colleagues. Medical directors could also have the unique freedom to transcend typical hierarchical structures and communicate throughout the organization. This can be an effective tool for identifying challenges, or it can be problematic if information is shared at inappropriate times or in inappropriate venues. Although effective, this approach warrants caution. Domestic preparedness planning activities also allow EMS further opportunities to interact with other public safety agencies in a cooperative manner.

Supervision and Administrative Oversight

A broad range of factors will dictate the specific structure of supervision and administrative oversight within an individual EMS organization. In one form or another, two areas exist in most organizations: **operational supervision** and **clinical supervision** (often referred to as quality improvement). Although portions of clinical supervision must be segregated in order to be protected by state medical practice acts, clinical and operational management must work as a management team.

Operational Supervision

Many EMS organizations have some type of on-the-street supervision. In addition to the operational role of responding to and coordinating major incidents (a very small percentage of their time), these field supervisors typically perform a broad range of administrative tasks that are critical to the daily operation of the system. This can include employee scheduling; station, vehicle, and equipment inspections; incident investigations; and a full range of personnel management tasks. Operations supervisors are also in the ideal position to handle customer service issues. Their familiarity with the out-of-hospital environment and its employees, combined with the authority to solve the customer's problem, creates the

perfect combination to resolve issues, many times the moment one is reported.

The methods of deploying these personnel vary. Smaller organizations use supervisors who are also members of an ambulance crew. Larger organizations deploy one or more supervisors per shift in vehicles that allow them to respond to incidents as well as to travel throughout the system as they perform their duties. Supervisors are the front-line management of the organization and can usually provide a valuable perspective to the EMSMD regarding the actual functioning of the system and the performance of individual providers. The supervisors can also serve as an extension of the EMSMD, addressing clinical questions and issues with field personnel.

The most commonly neglected component of EMS supervision is the education provided to new EMS supervisors when they are promoted from the field. Most systems would never consider advancing a provider from a basic to an advanced level of practice without training, testing, and clinical internships — but that is almost the standard when promoting within the operational structure. The common practice has been to find the best paramedic and assume that he or she will make an excellent supervisor. In many cases, the candidate is provided an orientation to the disciplinary process, given new shirts and collar insignia, and sent off in a vehicle to supervise.

An effective leadership team will have a well-developed leadership/supervisory development program that includes education, projects, internships, testing, and frequent performance feedback. These build the foundation and provide the necessary tool set so that the supervisor can handle the daily personnel issues and truly understand the system's goals. This allows the supervisors to work as part of the management team to lead the system through challenges. It is a sad but true fact that the very skills that make paramedics effective, if not tempered with education and experiential learning, frequently result in their failure as supervisors. In these situations, the failure does not belong to the employee, but to the organization's leadership team.

Clinical Supervision

A less common but increasingly popular component of EMS system supervision is the clinical supervisor. Typically, these personnel provide an avenue for real-time collection of quality improvement data through observation, as well as providing immediate feedback and education to field personnel. To be effective, these positions require routine, interactive learning sessions with the medical director, access to advanced clinical opportunities, and a high level of trust within the medical community. The financial cost of this type of position is often a challenge in most systems, as it is viewed as redundant if effective education is not provided to organizational leadership.

System Performance Improvement

Measuring system performance has become an important medical, political, and financial tool in EMS. Measurement of patient outcomes is essential not only for individual EMS systems but also for the profession as a whole.

The EMSMD must have significant involvement in every aspect of performance improvement of the clinical elements of the EMS system. Measuring performance is the ultimate indicator of effectiveness of the infrastructure created to care for patients. A healthy EMS system thrives on quality improvement data to fuel programs in other clinical areas.

Usually occurring in the clinical QI program, the broader mission of performance assessment and improvement is to examine important aspects of the EMS organization's performance and develop methods for improving them. Although this sounds simple to EMS providers who really appreciate the "find-a-problem, fix-a-problem" approach to life, the actual execution of this type of program is complex and methodical.

To be effective, the EMSMD must have a significant role in establishing measurable standards that accurately reflect the goals of the EMS system, medical community, and consumers. Common performance issues are cardiac arrest survival rate, response times, customer satisfaction, critical vehicle failures, and emergency vehicle crashes.

Although objective measures are popular, largely because they tend to be easier to use and interpret, many of the things that people believe are important are subjective and do not lend themselves to counting. Effective performance assessment and improvement programs identify a mixture of objective performance criteria and subjective performance assessments that, when aggregated, can provide a useful view of performance and identify opportunities for improvement.

The system should be prepared to respond quickly to questions it might not typically answer. In today's world of 24-hour media, if an issue (such as diversion) becomes a major story in another part of the country, directors should anticipate that they will get at least one local media outlet that will want to put a local spin on the story. For example, local reporters might ask how often local hospitals are on diversion, and whether ambulances are aimlessly wandering the streets with patients.

Infrastructure and Support Services Functions

There are many components of an EMS system that might not be considered clinical in the purest sense but that still have a profound impact on patient care. For example, an EMS system with a high ambulance breakdown rate could have significantly delayed response intervals that have an impact on morbidity and mortality rates. Medical equipment failures during patient care can have similar catastrophic effects on patient outcome. A procurement process that emphasizes cost can result in the EMS system purchasing equipment that does not meet the performance requirements for effective clinical care. There might be a substantial financial or administrative impact associated with a new protocol that requires the purchase of an expensive, highly regulated medication or extensive time for in-service training of field personnel.

It is obviously not appropriate, nor should it be the intent, for the EMSMD to run all aspects of an EMS system. It is, however, important that the director consider all the components of an EMS system that might have an impact on patient care.

Critical Failures and Sentinel Events

Two keys areas of real-time operation performance within any EMS system that require exceptional levels of medical director involvement are critical failures and sentinel events. Generally, these areas are similar in that they identify key incidents that have the potential to have a negative impact on the morbidity or mortality of EMS system patients.

Critical failures generally refer to the failure, during any phase of response, of a piece of equipment or vehicle that in some way delays, impedes, or hinders the ability of the EMS system to respond to, manage, or transport a patient. Examples include the failure of a vehicle while responding to a call, the failure of the pacing function of a cardiac monitor, the failure of the balloon on an ET tube, and a flat tire while transporting the patient to a hospital. The EMSMD should be advised of and involved in the review and designation of critical failures and should make an assessment, either directly or through clinical staff, of the potential patient impact of any failure. Additionally, if the failure involves regulated medical equipment, specific reporting requirements must be met in compliance with US Food and Drug Administration regulations.

Sentinel events are more typically key events, errors, or omissions that require 100% review of the incident by either clinical and/or operations staff. Examples are new medication administrations, advanced airway management skills, unrecognized esophageal intubations, or any other patient type or procedure/medication that the medical director believes warrants a detailed review. Operations staff will also frequently use this type of process to examine vehicle crashes, rescue incidents, MCIs, or other high-risk, infrequent events. The medical director has a key role in determining specific sentinel events as well as the process by which they are examined and trended.

The value of either critical failure or sentinel event analysis is realized only if the information obtained is effectively used to improve organizational performance.

Procurement

Procurement is the process of buying goods and services to allow the EMS system to function. Purchases of ambulances, four-by-fours, or stretcher maintenance services are all handled through the procurement or purchasing system. The process used by an EMS organization to procure supplies and services is frequently a function of the organization's structure. It is critical that all leadership team members, including the medical director, have a working knowledge of the procurement process so that appropriate planning can be completed, especially when new equipment or supplies are being added to a system.

Typically, systems have various sets of rules for procurement based on the cost and/or life expectancy of the item to be purchased. As an example, purchasing $25,000 worth of medications is completed under a different set of rules than a single $25,000 cardiac monitor. The purchasing process in most large organizations, whether government or private, is frequently very structured, strictly monitored, and slow.

EMS personnel should understand the process for emergency purchases within the organization. EMS systems are frequently confronted with unexpected situations that must be solved by purchasing a specific piece of equipment or service in an emergent or urgent manner. Most organizations have a process for this type of purchase, but the time to investigate it is before it is needed.

Finance

Apart from the actual financial support structure of the entire EMS system, which is discussed in great detail in Chapter 8, "System Financing," the most important aspect of finance is the budget development process. It is critical that the EMSMD understand this structure and process. Most organizations operate on a fiscal year that does not coincide with the calendar year. To understand budget development, the EMSMD must understand the fiscal year. For example, as quantitative end-tidal CO_2 monitoring becomes an accepted standard, the acquisition of these monitors for all EMS units that provide advanced airway management becomes a priority. In most situations, EMS organizations will not have sufficient funds to make a major equipment investment that was not budgeted. In this situation, implementation of the new technology might have to wait for the next budget year, which could still be several months away.

Within government and other large organizations, it is not unusual to begin budget development and complete budget submission by April for an October fiscal year. This type of structure requires effective long-term planning and a well-developed clinical strategic plan.

Management Information Systems

Effective management of data of all types is critical for an effective and efficient EMS organization. These systems could include computer-aided dispatch, patient charting, billing, purchasing, employee performance, and system performance information collection, warehousing, and analysis tools. A common trend within all types of organizations is to move toward a comprehensive record management system so that a broad range of variables can be assessed against information historically thought to be unrelated. A secondary trend among organizations is to move away from customized software solutions and use off-the-shelf solutions to manage cost and allow for quicker implementation times of new information technology.

The management information system component will be key within an organization if it is used to implement the evolving technologies for electronic data collection, wireless information access, real-time information sharing, and other developing information technologies.

No matter which method is eventually used to collect patient and quality management data, a key consideration is confidentiality. The ongoing implementation of federal HIPAA regulations has mandated drastic increases in the protection afforded to patient information and care records. It is critical that the EMSMD investigate the organization's approach to ensuring confidentiality of all types of patient and medical information, whether electronic or paper. The protection of this data and the patient's rights under HIPAA must be carefully weighed against the need for patient information to be analyzed for quality improvement activities. In general, the access to patient information and medical records must be strictly limited to those personnel within the organization who have a direct and demonstrated need to access the data. This is further emphasized by the need to obtain a specific authorization for release and use of patient information. The structure of an individual organization's confidentiality program should be clearly outlined in policy and be a major component of the organization's Medicare compliance plan.

Summary

EMS is a practice of medicine. The role the EMSMD has in the management, administration, and operations of an EMS system is perhaps the least understood, often most uncomfortable, and unquestionably the most underemphasized. The role is not a separate entity or responsibility of some administrator type but an integral part of the medical director's everyday practice. EMSMDs who are capable of being good managers have the opportunity to become good leaders and influence patient care through previously uncharted channels. Additionally, the administration-savvy EMSMD has the ability to develop consensus among the many EMS stakeholders and is able to focus on the big picture of the EMS system.

Understanding the various diverse administrative elements of an EMS system maximizes the opportunity for any medical director to more effectively make his or her clinical mark on an EMS system. In addition, a knowledgeable physician partner is an extraordinarily valuable asset for any EMS system.

References

1. Ludwig G. How many different ways can you perform EMS? *Firehouse.* May 2001.
2. Cady G, Lindberg D. 200-city survey. *J Emerg Med Serv.* 2001;26:36–41.
3. Mayfield T, Lindstrom A. 200-city survey. *J Emerg Med Serv.* 2000;25:65.

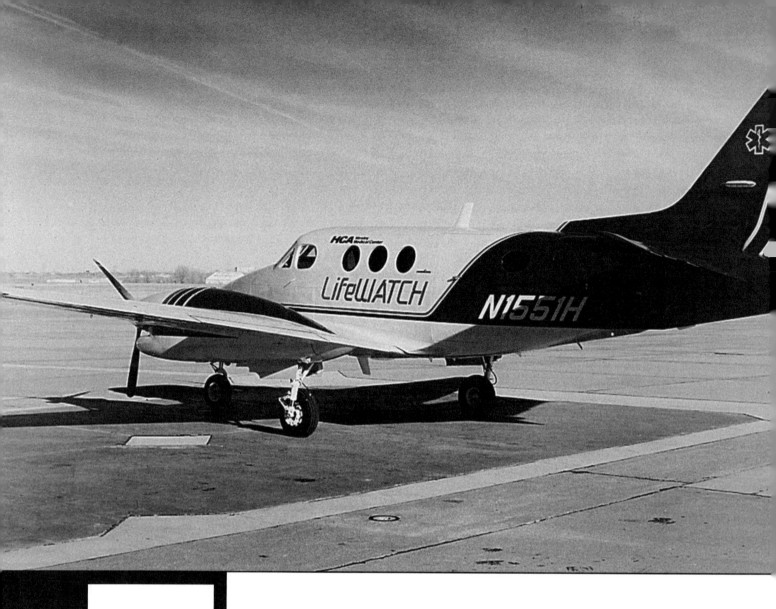

8 System Financing

Robert R. Bass, MD, FACEP

Principles of This Chapter

After reading this chapter, you should be able to:

- Discuss the major factors that affect the cost of providing EMS services, such as personnel, call volume, total time on call, level of service, quality of service, and response times.
- Explain cost versus outcome.
- Describe the various funding sources, including public, fee-for-service, and nongovernment contracts.

IN THE UNITED STATES, EMS DEVELOPED PRECIPITOUSLY in the early 1970s with significant federal grant support and guidance that defined essential system components. The guidance, however, did not include a national organizational model for providing local EMS services. That decision was left to local communities,[1] and thus, in contrast with many other countries, local EMS systems in the United States vary considerably in how they are organized and financed.[2] Depending on the community, EMS services are provided by private for-profit corporations, nonprofit organizations, government agencies, hospitals, and frequently combinations thereof. EMS providers might be salaried or might volunteer their services. This lack of uniformity has been and remains a major challenge to efforts to improve both the financing and the quality of EMS services.

Regardless of structure, all local EMS systems have expenses associated with providing service. The sources and amount of expenses vary considerably depending on the organizational model and other factors, but in any model, expenses must be covered by revenue. An EMS medical director will frequently need to advocate for improved funding or justify the cost of a medical intervention, an operational approach, or a system configuration that has an impact on patient care. Medical directors might be required to help establish processes to improve billing reimbursement or argue against a denial by a third-party payer. Thus, medical directors must have an understanding of factors that affect the cost of providing EMS services, as well as the methods for financing them.

Sometimes a medical director will be asked to render an expert opinion that more fundamentally addresses the organizational structure of the system. Such opinions are usually requested in the context of a communitywide process that is invoked to address a particular challenge in funding, patient care, or the social-political realm. A medical director who is familiar with the cost and financing implications associated with the various organizational models of EMS is more likely to be a resource to the community, ensure continued quality patient care, and perhaps survive the experience.

In many ways, providing emergency medical services can be regarded as a multistage production process, and a failure or even a delay in any step of the process can result in a poor outcome. Therefore, when the cost and funding of the overall EMS system are addressed, all components should be considered, including state and regional EMS programs, 911 access and dispatch, first responders, transport providers, receiving facilities, and rehabilitation services. Additionally, many EMS systems today have essential roles in injury prevention and supporting wellness in their communities, and these components also should be considered when funding requirements are addressed.[3]

It is highly doubtful that a single entity will have the overall fiscal responsibility for all these components. However, if the EMS system is to be maximally effective, all components must function effectively, which requires, among other things, that each is adequately funded. Sometimes the leadership of an EMS medical director serves to functionally link these components together with a focus on patient care. Similarly, it could be the EMS medical director who is called on to support funding for any of these components when such funding is necessary to improve the EMS system and ultimately patient outcomes.

Major Factors That Affect the Costs of Providing EMS Services

The cost of providing EMS services varies considerably among EMS systems, and it has been historically difficult and even politically challenging to document and characterize those differences. During the negotiated rule-making for the ambulance fee schedule in 1999, attempts by the Project Hope Foundation to study the cost of providing EMS services were frustrated by a limited access to data, difficulties in defining marginal, direct, and indirect costs, the significant variations in the organization and funding of EMS systems, and other factors.[4] Although we might not be able to accurately characterize the relative cost by system type (volunteer, career, fire, private, public utility), we are able to describe the various factors that influence the cost of care provided by an EMS system.

Personnel

Personnel costs can be a significant percentage of the overall cost of providing EMS, and they vary considerably depending on the type of service. Government services such as fire departments tend to have higher personnel costs than private services. There are regional variations in the costs of labor, with costs tending to be somewhat higher in urban areas.[5] Personnel costs also increase with the level of service provided, especially at the specialty care level. The cost of a medical director is a small but important factor in systems that pay or otherwise reimburse this person.

Volunteer systems generally have lower personnel costs than career systems, but there can be costs associated with recruitment and retention, which are quite challenging. Also, volunteers might receive certain benefits, including Worker's Compensation, tax credits, scholarships, training, and others. Frequently, volunteer EMS organizations are combination systems with career providers on duty during certain times of the day or week and volunteers at other times.

Personnel costs associated with training can be significant, especially in career systems that provide the initial and continuing education training for EMS providers.

Supplies

Supplies and equipment are generally not as significant a cost factor for EMS services as that of personnel. The cost of supplies and equipment varies significantly depending on the level of service provided. There are somewhat less regional variations in the costs of supplies and equipment than with personnel. Protocols can have significant impact on the cost of medications or medical equipment. Bulk or cooperative strategies for purchasing can reduce costs.

Call Volume

The volume of calls for EMS services varies considerably based on population and demographics. Total operating expenses go up as patient volume increases; however, the actual cost of service per patient is greater in low-volume services because insufficient numbers of patients consume the fixed costs of providing service.[6] In Maryland and other states, there is a bimodal increase in demand by age, with a slight increase in demand between ages 15 and 25 and a sharp increase in demand after age 65. Communities with older populations can have higher utilization rates.[7] Urban communities also experience higher utilization rates than suburban or rural communities.[8]

Call Time

The average time spent on a call can affect the cost. Situations that increase the time required to access, treat, or transport patients all contribute to increasing the average time on a call. In rural areas, geographic barriers and long distances can have a significant impact. In urban areas, heavy traffic, high-rise buildings, and crowds are factors. Emergency department crowding that prevents EMS providers from unloading patients or causes them to seek alternative destinations can have an impact on both urban and rural EMS systems.

Quality

EMS systems vary considerably in the level and quality of the services they provide to their communities. Generally speaking, quality EMS comes at a cost. This is not intended to imply that cost is the only factor that has an impact on the quality of care. Certainly, many EMS systems have improved the quality of care without increasing costs through vigorous quality management processes and improved efficiency. However, providing ALS service is more expensive than providing BLS service only. More ambulances and/or the use of first responders might be necessary to achieve acceptable response times. In systems with large geographic areas to cover, air medical transport services might be needed, adding significant costs. Communities and their EMS systems must balance the cost of providing quality EMS with the resources available and the demands for service. This is frequently a difficult task in which the medical director should have a central role. In particular, the medical director must be prepared to explain the cost and benefit of various options under consideration.

Negative and Positive Cost-Affecting Factors

Just as EMS systems vary in their configurations, they also vary considerably in their ability to provide an equivalent service at a given cost.[2] The inherent efficiency of a given EMS system can be affected both positively and negatively by a variety of factors. Some of these factors are fixed characteristics of the system or community, while others are affected by efforts to improve efficiency.

Organizational Configuration

The organizational configuration of the service can have a major impact on costs. Volunteer systems reduce the cost of labor, and in many communities in the United States they provide efficient and reliable, quality EMS services. Volunteer services, however, are not without other characteristics that negatively affect performance. Volunteerism tends to be cyclic, and there are times when it is not possible to maintain enough volunteers to adequately respond to calls for service. Volunteer systems also begin to have increasing difficulty recruiting and maintaining personnel when call volumes begin to place excessive demands on the volunteers, or when economic downturns require volunteers to seek supplemental employment. In communities that have the resources, career EMS providers might be employed to supplement the volunteers. In these combination systems, the community still benefits from lower labor costs while maintaining a level of service acceptable to the community.

Fire Departments

Fire departments provide EMS services in many communities, and some have a role in one or more of the components of the EMS system. Typically, fire departments are able to provide timely first responder service, benefiting the community in several ways. Most fire departments have a significant standing capacity in place to rapidly respond to fires, but fires have been on the decline over the past several decades. In many communities, this fire response capacity has been redirected to EMS without having a significant impact on the response times for fires. Additionally, since fire departments already have an existing capacity for responding to fires, using firefighters to respond to EMS calls is a marginal cost. Fire first responders can reduce the cost of maintaining the number of transport ambulances required to achieve an equivalent initial response time using ambulances. By carefully analyzing the resources available and the costs of various options, communities can design systems that provide excellent care in a cost-efficient manner. It is essential that medical directors be actively involved in such planning.

Matching Resources to Demand

Low-volume systems are inherently inefficient and more costly, but in rural communities that factor cannot be changed.[6] In urban communities, too many providers will result in a lower volume of patients per service and a higher overall cost of providing care per patient. This has led some communities to award an exclusive franchise to one service, to limit the number of services, or to group adjacent low-population areas into a multijurisdictional system. In some cases, local government will require that the local 911 service provide both interfacility and 911 responses on the premise that such a structure establishes an economy of scale that reduces the overall cost of the system.[2] In such situations, revenues from more profitable interfacility transports are used to offset the cost of 911 services, which typically have higher rates of underinsured or uninsured patients. Typically in the exclusive franchise model, the provider (either the government or a private entity) offering the best service at the lowest cost is awarded the contract. These principles are often incorporated into so-called high-performance systems with the goal of improving services while reducing costs. A number of additional cost-efficiency strategies can be used to achieve this goal, including system status management.[9]

System Status Management
System status management (SSM) is a strategy of matching resources to demand. Demand for EMS services is fairly predictable based on time of day, day of week, month of year, and location within the

service area. When these patterns are known, staffing and placement of units can be matched to demand for services. When successfully implemented, SSM results in maximal performance for the investment. On the negative side, some have argued that SSM creates excessive stress for providers because personnel typically have little idle time and might have no fixed base to which they can return.[10]

Tiered-Response Systems

Other strategies have been used with varied success in attempts to increase EMS system efficiency. Some systems have deviated from trends toward a specialized production model (which typically has a tiered response with ALS and BLS units) and have moved toward a single production model with ALS only.[11] The argument for tiered-response systems is that the need to provide a rapid ALS response can be reduced by deploying more readily available BLS units that can respond more quickly and can handle most transports. Others have argued that tiered systems are inherently inefficient because specialized units reduce the flexibility of system managers to match resources to demand and commonly require two ALS providers on each ALS unit.

Protocol Development

Although many of these approaches to reduce costs require the implementation of moderately sophisticated strategies, there are less onerous approaches that also yield cost savings. Some of these approaches involve development of medical and dispatch protocols that guide the appropriate use of resources such as first responders and air medical transport. Protocols might also be useful in reducing the routine use of interventions that are likely to have little or no benefit to the patient. The stocking of expensive medications that will have a low frequency of use and that will not result in any improvement in outcome in a particular community is one such example.[12] In such cases, the participation of a knowledgeable medical director who has good system and patient data is essential to safely ensure that the community gets the best outcome for the least cost. By using a public health approach, a medical director can balance resource availability with community needs to achieve the best outcomes.[2]

Cost Versus Outcome

When considering variables that have an impact on the cost of providing service, the impact on outcome of

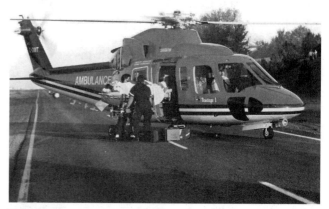

Figure 8-1 In a study of the effectiveness of helicopter transport of trauma patients, the magnitude of survival benefit was the most important factor in determining cost-effectiveness.

those variables must be considered. **Cost-effectiveness** can be measured as a ratio of total cost to outcome benefit. This model, in theory, can be used to compare the cost-effectiveness of one EMS system to another or a particular EMS intervention to other medical interventions. Unfortunately, EMS has been and remains challenged in measuring both the cost and the outcome of EMS systems and interventions.[13]

The importance of outcome cannot be overstated. In a study of the effectiveness of helicopter transport of trauma patients, the magnitude of survival benefit was the most important factor in determining cost-effectiveness[14] (**Figure 8-1**). However, relatively few EMS systems have good data on patient outcomes; overall, relatively little evidence has been published as to the overall clinical effectiveness of EMS or its effectiveness in treating specific clinical conditions.[15,16] Additionally, many of the studies have conflicting conclusions, likely confounded by the myriad of variables that exist in complex EMS systems. These factors make it difficult for EMS system managers and medical directors to make decisions regarding which clinical interventions a system should implement, curtail, or eliminate. One project funded by the National Highway Traffic Safety Administration (NHTSA) has published a list of outcomes referred to as the **five D's (death, disability, discomfort, destitution, and dissatisfaction)** in an attempt to standardize future research efforts to measure the effectiveness of EMS.[17]

There are little published data on the impact of system components and configuration on outcome.

One study has suggested that two-tiered systems have reduced response times and have resulted in better outcomes with out-of-hospital cardiac arrests.[18,19] On the other hand, the relative benefit of two-tiered versus all-ALS response remains unclear and could depend on the characteristics and resources of the community.[11]

Studies have looked at the outcomes for specific EMS interventions, such as endotracheal intubation. In one study of trauma patients, out-of-hospital endotracheal intubation was associated with a favorable impact on survival with good neurologic outcome.[20] In another study, endotracheal intubation of children was not associated with an improvement in outcome.[21]

Despite the limitations, there have been studies that have attempted to compare EMS interventions to other traditional health care interventions. In Tucson, Arizona, the cost-effectiveness of EMS treatment of out-of-hospital cardiac arrest was greater than heart, liver, and bone marrow transplants, as well as curative chemotherapy for acute leukemia.[22] In Ontario, a study of the cost-effectiveness of rural first responder defibrillation demonstrated a higher cost per life saved than in urban areas, but it was still economical when compared to other common treatments for life-threatening illnesses.[23]

What is clear is that more research is required.[24]

Funding EMS Systems

There are two major categories of funding for EMS systems: **public funding** and **fee-for-service reimbursement** (which includes nongovernment contracts for service). There is, however, significant variation in the type of public funding and in the relative contribution of each category used to support EMS systems. Generally speaking, the organization configuration of the EMS system is a significant factor in determining how EMS services will be funded. Although private providers have traditionally relied more on fee-for-service reimbursement and government providers have relied more on public funding, those differences have lessened over the past several decades, especially in regard to responding to 911 calls. Increasingly, government and volunteer providers are billing for services, and private ambulance companies that provide 911 responses are increasingly dependent on some form of public funding. Even when the local EMS service provider is entirely funded by fees for service, certain components of the EMS system are likely to be publicly funded, such as the 911 center and fire-based first response. The exception to this rule might be the private ambulance companies providing convalescent transport services and not responding to 911 calls. Although technically part of the overall EMS system, they do not have the expenses associated with maintaining the capacity to respond immediately to most requests for service. Many of these private ambulance companies get by on fee-for-service reimbursement alone.

The significant variation in methodologies to fund EMS systems is indicative of the relative newness of EMS and the unresolved debate as to whether EMS is an essential public safety service, a health care provider, or part of the public health system. In truth, EMS is all of these and therefore is unlikely to be funded by fees for service alone. In particular, third-party payers are not particularly interested in paying for standby time, rescue services, public safety infrastructure such as 911 centers and communications systems, and maintaining the capacity to respond to mass casualty situations or acts of terrorism. Even the federally funded Medicare program is currently reimbursing below the cost of providing services and will pay only if the beneficiary is transported.

Public Funding

Government-based EMS services, including fire departments and third-service providers, are usually funded through local tax-based general appropriations. In some cases, government EMS services receive funding through special funds, such as vehicle registration surcharges or fines on moving motor vehicle violations. Special funds can provide an entire agency's funding but usually provide supplemental funding, frequently through a grant program. One particular advantage of special funds is that they are less affected by variations in the economy than are tax revenues.

Volunteer EMS services traditionally have relied on donations from the community. Fundraising is a significant challenge for many volunteer systems, especially since volunteers are increasingly difficult to recruit and retain and have many other demands on their time, particularly continuing medical education. Donations, like tax revenue, typically decrease during economic downturns. Volunteer services sometimes contract with businesses that do the fundraising for them; however, the cost of this service can take a significant percentage of the funds that are raised. This has caused many volunteer systems to seek government assistance in the form of subsidies, grants, or salary support for paid personnel. The downside of government funding from the standpoint of volunteer services is that the government will typically expect something in return and a greater measure of control over the service.

Private EMS providers who respond to 911 calls are frequently supported by public funding. This support usually comes in the form of a subsidy associated with a contract for services. In the **public utility model,** a private provider is contracted by a government entity to manage EMS services in a defined geographic area, usually with defined performance standards. The private provider is paid for contracted services and penalized for not meeting performance standards. In some cases, the local government might own the vehicles and equipment, while the private provider manages the service and hires personnel. Public utility systems also derive funding through fees for service. **High-performance systems** are typically public utility models that are contracted to provide EMS services under tightly defined performance standards using strategies such as system status management.

Federal and State Grant Programs

Federal grant programs for EMS began with the Highway Safety Act of 1966 (PL 89-564). This was a matching grant program that provided funding for equipment and personnel, as well as demonstration projects and studies. In 1973, Congress passed the Emergency Medical Services Systems Act, which established a federal EMS program that provided guidance and significant funding for EMS systems until 1981. These grants required grantees to address 15 components but otherwise afforded EMS systems significant flexibility to meet local needs. In 1981, the federal EMS program was eliminated, and federal grants for EMS were made available through the preventive health block grant program that gave the states discretion to decide how to spend the grants. EMS had to compete with other traditional and underfunded public health programs, and as a result, grants for EMS dramatically declined. Section 402 of the Highway Safety Act currently provides some funding for state and local EMS systems through the state offices of highway safety.

Currently, there are several federal programs that provide EMS funding, mostly for national projects. These include NHTSA, the Health Resources and Services Administration (HRSA) in the Department of Health and Human Services, and the Centers for Disease Control and Prevention. NHTSA has traditionally supported the development of the **national standard curricula** for EMS providers and provided consultative evaluations of state EMS systems. NHTSA has also sponsored many innovative processes, such as the "EMS Agenda for the Future," the EMS Research Agenda, the EMS Managed Care Forum, and others. HRSA has several programs that provide funding for EMS, including the EMS for Children program that supports activities and funds national projects, and the Trauma and EMS Program that, in turn, funds state trauma systems development.

State EMS functions are typically funded through state general funds, although some states have innovative special funds, such as the one in Maryland that is based on a surcharge on vehicle registrations. This special fund supports the state EMS agency, including a statewide EMS communications system, a statewide fire and EMS training program, and a statewide air medical program. It also provides funding to trauma centers and trauma surgeons, local jurisdictions, and the state volunteer association. Most states are not as fortunate as Maryland. Other states derive special funds from vehicle registrations, driver's licenses, moving violations, or special taxes. Unfortunately, in too many states, the state EMS offices are underfunded and grant support for local EMS services is minimal.[25]

Fee-for-Service Reimbursement

Although private EMS providers have traditionally billed for services as a principal source of revenue, other types of EMS providers are increasingly billing to reduce the need for government funding and to improve the quality of services. Even volunteer services are increasingly billing for services as a significant source of revenue. This trend, which began in the late 1980s, has not gone without notice. Federal Medicare spending for ambulance services, even though accounting for only 2% of the Medicare budget, was one of the fastest-growing categories of expenditures. In 1997, Congress required the Health Care Financing Administration (HCFA, now the Centers for Medicare and Medicaid Services, known as CMS) to develop a national fee schedule for ambulance services that included a provision to address cost containment.[26] During the 1990s, health maintenance organizations (HMOs) were aware of the growth in ambulance reimbursement, and the industry anticipated that measures would be initiated to address it;

however, these initiatives never achieved widespread implementation.[27] Medicare, especially through its intermediaries, has been far more active in attempts to control costs by implementing review processes that sometimes deny reimbursement for services not deemed to be medically necessary. In 2000, CMS published new rules to more clearly define, and perhaps more narrowly define, when transport of a patient by ambulance was medically necessary.[28]

Billing for services has not turned out to be a panacea for declining government support or volunteer donations. Third-party payers typically reimburse only if the patient is transported. The additional requirements for documentation and the billing process add significantly to the complexity and cost of providing EMS service. This was initially problematic for government and volunteer services, but many are now billing routinely. The billing process can be difficult and has associated expenses, for it is not uncommon for services to hire a contractor to do the billing. Even with a good billing process, reimbursement can be relatively low, particularly in urban areas where many patients are uninsured, have Medicaid (which provides little or no reimbursement), or lack ambulance services as a benefit. Some urban EMS services receive less than 20% reimbursement for what they bill.[29] Despite these difficulties and shortcomings, many EMS systems have benefited from the new source of revenue.

Some EMS services contract with nongovernment parties, such as the sponsor of a special event, one or more hospitals, a residential community, an industrial facility, or another entity with a need for onsite or rapid access to emergency medical services. EMS services have also entered into contracts with HMOs, such as Kaiser Permanente. A subscription service is a form of contract with individuals in a community who typically pay a fee for access to the services of an EMS provider at no additional charge or at a significant discount.

Medicare Reimbursement for Ambulance Transports

For many services, especially those doing private transports, half or more of patients transported are Medicare beneficiaries. Medicare ambulance benefits, by law, cover only transportation and the services that are provided during transport. They are further restricted to situations in which transport by other means is contraindicated by the patient's medical condition. Additionally, the beneficiary must be transported to the closest facility that can provide the medically necessary test or intervention. Facilities are strictly defined as a hospital, a skilled nursing facility, a renal dialysis center, and home.[28]

As previously mentioned, in 1997, HCFA was instructed by Congress to develop a **national fee schedule** for ambulance services that included measures to address rising Medicare expenditures for such services. The fee schedule was developed through a negotiated rule-making process that brought together representatives from the industry and the medical community. The rule-making was narrowly focused on the fee schedule. Efforts to engage HCFA in dialogue on broader issues such as reimbursement for care without transport did not succeed. HCFA did allow a discussion of developing a list of condition codes that would supplement or replace ICD-9 diagnostic codes and more accurately communicate to Medicare carriers and intermediaries the medical condition that necessitated the patient being transported. HCFA, now CMS, continues to express interest in the condition codes that are widely anticipated to improve the Medicare billing process.

The fee schedule reimburses ambulance providers based on the level of service provided during transport and the miles traveled. The levels of service include BLS, ALS 1 (routine), ALS 2 (more complex), and specialty care transport (care beyond the scope of a traditional paramedic). These levels of care are more thoroughly defined in the Medicare regulations.[30] The fee schedule provides for an adjustment for rural providers to compensate for their higher costs per patient because of lower volumes and longer transports.

The fee schedule is phased in over 5 years and will provide a uniform level of reimbursement nationwide with slight adjustments in high- and low-cost areas.

One particular problem with the new fee schedule is that the reimbursement levels were not based on the cost of providing service. Rather, they were calculated to be budget-neutral with respect to the total amount of Medicare ambulance reimbursement in 1999. Based on recent studies, Medicare ambulance reimbursement will be significantly below the cost of providing ambulance services, especially with respect to private ambulance companies. This situation could force many EMS providers to improve efficiency or cut services, shift costs to other patients, or seek higher government subsidies. There is concern that many EMS providers without these options will be forced to stop providing care.[26]

Summary

Medical directors must be familiar with the financing of all components of the EMS system. Several factors affect the cost of providing EMS service, including personnel, supplies, equipment, call volume, time on call, level of service, quality of service, and response times. Factors that could mitigate the cost of providing service include the organizational configuration and efficiency of the service, as well as using a public health approach in protocol development. Major funding sources for EMS systems include both government sources and fee-for-service reimbursement. The organizational configuration of the system frequently determines how the system will be funded, although that difference has been diminishing over the past decade. Third-party billing for EMS services is not a panacea for financing quality EMS, and Medicare and Medicaid reimbursements, in particular, are frequently below the cost of providing service.

References

1. Boyd DR. The history of emergency medical services in the United States of America. In: Boyd DR, Edlich RF, Micik S, eds. *Systems Approach to Emergency Medical Care.* Norwalk, Conn: Appleton-Century-Crofts; 1983.

2. Overton J, Stout J. System design. In: National Association of EMS Physicians, eds. *Prehospital Systems and Medical Oversight.* Dubuque, Iowa: Kendall/Hunt; 2002.

3. Garrison HG, Foltin GL, Becker LR, et al. The role of emergency medical services in primary injury prevention. Consensus workshop. Arlington, Virginia, August 25–26, 1995. *Ann Emerg Med.* 1997;30:84–91.

4. Scott T. American Ambulance Association meeting summary of the negotiated rule making advisory committee on the Medicare ambulance fee schedule (minutes). December 6–8, 1999; McClean, Va.

5. Discussion on history of the Physician Geographic Practice Cost Index and the proposed changes for 2001-2002. Excerpted from: The notice of proposed rule making physician fee schedule for 2001 as published in 65 *Federal Register* 44175-44224 (2000). Available at: http://www.jems.com/insider/gpsi.html. Accessed February 4, 2005.

6. Mohr PE, Cheng CM, Mueller CD. Establishing a fair Medicare reimbursement for low-volume rural ambulance providers. *Policy Anal Brief W. Ser.* 2001;4:1–4.

7. Meador SA. Age related utilization of advanced life support. *Prehospital Disaster Med.* 1991;6:9–14.

8. Billittier AJ, Moscati R, Janicke D, et al. A multisite survey of factors contributing to medically unnecessary ambulance transports. *Acad Emerg Med.* 1996; 3:1046–1052.

9. Stout JL. System status management. The strategy of ambulance placement. *J Emerg Med Serv JEMS.* 1983; 8:22–32.

10. Morneau PM, Stothart JP. My aching back: the effects of system status management and ambulance design on EMS personnel. *J Emerg Med Serv JEMS.* 1999;24:36–40, 43–44, 47–48 passim.

11. Stout J, Pepe PE, Mosesso VN. All-advanced life support vs tiered-response ambulance systems. *Prehospital Emerg Care.* 2000;4:1–6.

12. Pazdral TE, Burton JH, Strout TD, et al. Amiodarone and rural emergency medical services cardiac arrest patients: a cost analysis. *Prehospital Emerg Care.* 2002;6:291–294.

13. Moore L. Measuring quality and effectiveness of prehospital EMS. *Prehospital Emerg Care.* 1999;3:325–331.

14. Gearhart PA, Wuerz R, Localio AR. Cost-effectiveness analysis of helicopter EMS for trauma patients. *Ann Emerg Med.* 1997;30:500–506.

15. Callaham M. Quantifying the scanty science of prehospital emergency care. *Ann Emerg Med.* 1997; 30:785–790.

16. Demetriades D, Chan L, Cornwell E, et al. Paramedic vs private transportation of trauma patients: effect on outcome. *Arch Surg.* 1996;131:133–338.

17. Maio RF, Garrison HG, Spaite DW, et al. Emergency medical services outcomes project I (EMSOP I): prioritizing conditions for outcomes research. *Ann Emerg Med.* 1999;33:423–432.

18. Nichol G, Detsky AS, Stiell IG, et al. Effectiveness of emergency medical services for victims of out-of-hospital cardiac arrest: a metaanalysis. *Ann Emerg Med.* 1996;27:700–710.

19. Nichol G, Laupacis A, Stiell IG, et al. Cost-effectiveness analysis of potential improvements to emergency medical services for victims of out-of-hospital cardiac arrest. *Ann Emerg Med.* 1996;27:711–720.

20. Frankel H, Rozycki G, Champion H, et al. The use of TRISS methodology to validate prehospital intubation by urban EMS providers. *Am J Emerg Med.* 1997; 15:630–632.

21. Gausche M, Lewis RJ, Stratton SJ, et al. Effect of out-of-hospital pediatric endotracheal intubation on survival and neurological outcome: a controlled clinical trial. *JAMA.* 2000;283:783–790.

22. Valenzuela TD, Criss EA, Spaite D, et al. Cost-effectiveness analysis of paramedic emergency med-

ical services in the treatment of prehospital cardiopulmonary arrest. *Ann Emerg Med.* 1990;19:1407–1411.

23. Jermyn BD. Cost-effectiveness analysis of a rural/urban first-responder defibrillation program. *Prehospital Emerg Care.* 2000;4:43–47.

24. Sayre MR, White LJ, Brown LH, et al. National EMS research agenda. *Prehospital Emerg Care.* 2002;6(3 suppl): S1–S43.

25. Wilson EM. State EMS offices in trouble. *J Emerg Nurs.* 1996;22:600–601.

26. Overton J. Reimbursement in emergency medical services: how to adapt in a changing environment. *Prehospital Emerg Care.* 2002;6:137–140.

27. National Highway Traffic Safety Administration. EMS and managed care final bulletin. Fall 1999. [NHTSA Web site]. Available at: http://www.nhtsa.dot.gov/people/injury/ems/emsbulletin/index.asp. Accessed February 4, 2005.

28. Garza MA. Medicare tightens rules for ambulance reimbursement. *J Emerg Med Serv JEMS.* 1999;24:16–17.

29. Hill J. *Revenue Recovery: Emergency Medical Services.* Washington, DC: International Association of Fire Fighters; 1997.

30. Centers for Medicare and Medicaid Services. Medicare program: fee schedule for payment of ambulance services and revisions to the physician certification requirements for coverage of nonemergency ambulance services. Final rule with comment period. 67 *Federal Register* 9099–9135 (2002).

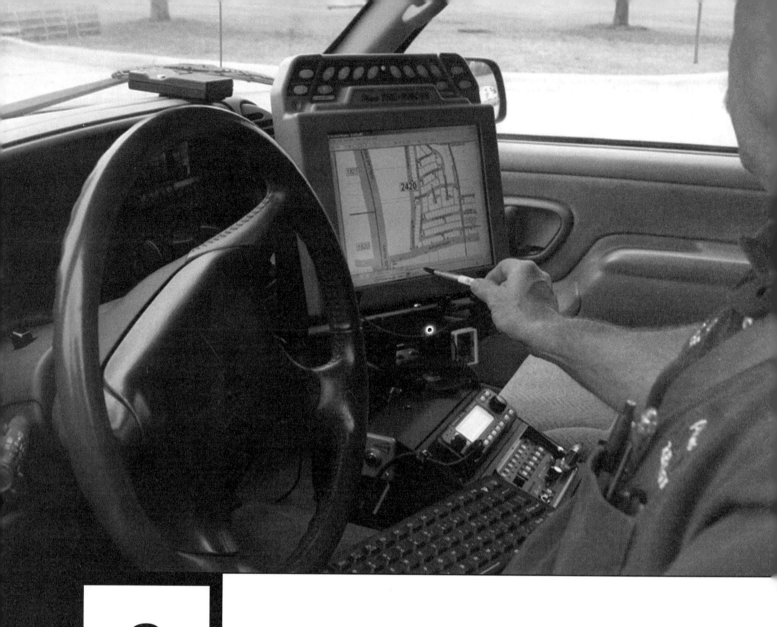

9 Communications

Robert E. Suter, DO, MHA, FACEP
Hon. Ricardo Martinez, MD, FACEP

Principles of This Chapter

After reading this chapter, you should be able to:

- Recall the components of a communications plan.
- Describe the various means of communication in an EMS system.
- Discuss the importance and role of offline and online communications.
- Describe the technology and equipment that have become the foundation for EMS communications.

COMMUNICATION AND THE TOOLS WITH WHICH IT IS AC-complished lie at the foundation of every EMS system. No matter what other resources and assets an EMS system possesses, if it has poorly coordinated communications arrangements, its performance will be mediocre at best.

EMS communications are dependent on the specific technologies needed to effect a transfer of information. The categories of communications operations are:

- Public access to the EMS system
- Operations control
- Medical direction
- Intra-agency communications
- Interagency/facility communications
- Information management
- Technology and equipment

Traditionally, each of the above operational areas has been considered a separate phase of the overall function of an EMS system. In many systems, the communications methods and modes for each opera-tional phase evolved independently from the others rather than being collectively planned. This often re-sulted in replication of resources or in establishment of conflicting communications structures.

Recently, EMS system managers have begun to appreciate the need for more coordinated and seam-less overall communications systems to improve the effectiveness and efficiency of their programs. EMS medical directors must have a clear understanding of the overall EMS communications system and how each phase interacts and influences the others. In this chapter, we will consider the various operational divisions of communication within an EMS system and the tools by which communications are accom-plished. We will look at specific technologies that are in use and will consider the strengths and weak-nesses of each. Finally, we will take a look at the new technologies being developed for future use in EMS systems. It should be clear that optimizing success in any EMS operation depends on a carefully planned and integrated communications system.

EMS Communication Theory and Practice

Communication is about transmitting information. If information is not successfully transmitted, with the correct meaning conveyed, then communication has failed. At its most basic level, a system for communi-cation consists of two people who send and receive messages and the medium through which a message is carried between them. In addition, there is noise. Noise is anything that might interfere with the clear transmission of a message. That could include physi-cal interference, actual noise, radio interference, or other adverse physical conditions. It could also be subjective noise, which includes differences in cul-ture, education background, life experience, and world view. Noise of this second kind is the most in-sidious obstacle to good communication because most people are not truly aware that it is there.

Public Access to the EMS System

An EMS system is of no use if the public cannot let re-sponders know when and where to respond. Early in the history of EMS, the primary tool the public had for contacting EMS was the telephone. This meant re-membering several 7-digit telephone numbers: one for fire, one for police, and maybe more than one for the ambulance. If an ambulance was needed on the road, the only recourse was a pay phone, *if* the right coin and the right number were available. That all changed in the late 1960s with the advent of the almost universal emergency number, 911. In addition, there are other means by which emergency responders can be summoned if needed, such as commercially available emergency response jewelry.

The 911 system is now the primary means of public access to emergency services for more than 93% of the US population. In the simple form of this system, dialing the number connects the caller with a **public safety answering point (PSAP)** operator who must decide which emergency services are required and then relay the call to dispatchers for the appropriate responders. In the case of fixed telephones, the caller's area code and exchange numbers are used to automatically route the call to the correct PSAP. The success of this form of 911 service is totally dependent on the quality of information the caller can provide to the PSAP operator. Over the years since the inauguration of the 911 service, telephone technology has advanced to the point where additional modes of information exchange automatically function when the PSAP is contacted. These advanced systems are referred to as enhanced 911 systems.

Enhanced 911 Systems

Enhanced 911 (E911) systems currently cover 95% of the population that has any form of 911 service and about 96% of the geographic United States. Assuming that a traditional telephone is used, these systems automatically transmit the location from which a call originates in the form of a street address, the call-back phone number, and the identity of the owner of the phone service at that location. Once the contact is made, this information is transmitted to the PSAP operator and is relayed to a dispatcher's computer screen even if the caller cannot speak. Theoretically, this allows help to reach a caller even if he or she cannot explain what is wrong or describe where responders should go.

When E911 systems were first brought online, cellular telephones were in their infancy and were extremely expensive. E911 systems were not designed to work with cellular technology, nor were they able to receive enhanced location or ownership information from cell phones. Currently, about 25% to 30% of the 911 calls in the United States originate from cellular telephones, negating much of the advantage of an E911 system. In 1990, the Federal Communications Commission (FCC) began pushing manufacturers of cellular telephones to develop the means for location and identification information to

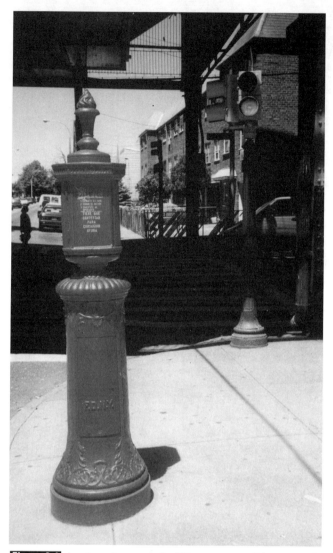

Figure 9-1 In a few urban areas, the 911 system can still be accessed by street corner fire alarm boxes.

be transmitted when a cell phone is used to access 911. Efforts to accomplish this have been delayed by many technical, political, and financial issues. Recently, the FCC established regulations setting deadline dates by which cell phone systems must be able to function as part of the E911 system.

In addition to standard and cellular telephones, public access to the emergency services system occurs by other means. Highway emergency call boxes, originally developed in the early 1970s, are becoming more common as a means of accessing the 911 system. In some areas, especially rural regions, citizens band radio channel 9 is still monitored by emergency services personnel, although this radio service has lost much of its former popularity. In a few urban areas, the 911 system can still be accessed by street corner fire alarm boxes (**Figure 9-1**). Although relatively uncommon, some systems are able to receive calls for help over the Internet from both fixed-location and wireless Internet sources. Finally, a growing number of patients with potentially serious chronic medical conditions equip their homes with special monitoring devices that can automatically dial 911 and request help when a panic switch is activated.

Operations Control

The day-to-day activities of emergency response organizations such as EMS agencies depend on carefully constructed and regulated operations communications systems. Such a system must have a substantial degree of redundancy for primary communications channels as well as multiple auxiliary channels for maintaining communication between the central coordinating center and field units. It must operate under a set of procedural protocols familiar to everyone in the system, while having sufficient flexibility to cope with unforeseen events and circumstances. In most EMS systems, operations control responsibilities have been vested in the communications and dispatching center, and these have become virtually synonymous terms.

EMS operations control centers take almost as many forms as do EMS organizations. They run the gamut from centers in tiny basement offices equipped with a single-channel very high-frequency (VHF) radio station and staffed by one dispatcher/operations controller, to highly sophisticated, state-of-the-art communications and operations centers with multiple communications consoles and data terminals, highly trained emergency medical dispatchers, and several communications modes and channels. In some systems, the processes of operations control and dispatch are combined, or at least are located in the same facility. In others, the two are separated completely. Some EMS systems depend on dispatching services from other public safety agencies, such as the county sheriff's office or local fire department, while others control their own resources and employ trained EMS dispatchers. Despite these many variations in resources and arrangements, all EMS operations control systems have a common basic purpose.

EMS Communications Center

Regardless of its size and sophistication, the principal purpose of an EMS communications center is to act as a central coordinating nexus for communications necessary to support EMS operations. The information about emergencies provided through the public access network is fed into the response system there. The PSAP could be a separate operation in a separate location and might receive information from the public through multiple communications channels, but received information is not put to use until it reaches the dispatchers, who determine the allocation of resources to respond to a given emergency. This can be done solely by rule of thumb and a good knowledge of the response area, or it can be accomplished with the help of sophisticated **computer-aided dispatching (CAD)** tools that assist in tracking the EMS system's assets and provide guidance about what units to respond. Initially, and possibly throughout the duration of a response, dispatchers can act as central coordinators for communication between agencies participating in a response. Dispatchers and controllers have a critical role in gathering information that becomes a permanent part of the operations record for the EMS service. Such records have a role in quality, financial, and resource management for the organization. The primary tools used by communications centers and dispatchers to provide coordinated communications are telephone links and radio systems. Computer networks and Internet connections increasingly supplement these more traditional links. Details regarding the technologies and hardware behind these devices are discussed in more detail later in this chapter. The effectiveness and flexibility of a communications control center are determined by the hardware and technologies available and the skill and insight used by dispatchers or controllers. Multiple telephone networks provide dispatchers instantaneous access to citizens calling the PSAP for assistance and can immediately provide them with all the transmitted data of an enhanced 911 system. This allows them to begin marshaling the necessary response resources while they are gathering more information about the emergency. Telephone networks can also automatically relay the information to other responders such as police and fire departments, allowing all needed personnel to respond together. Direct telephone tie-ins can link EMS dispatchers with dispatchers from these other services, or they might all be sitting at adjacent consoles in one communications/operations center. Telephones often are the most direct link between dispatchers and area emergency departments. In a growing number of systems, the use of cellular phones has become an important part of the overall communications network for responders, including notification, coordination, and hospital interaction.

Two-Way Radio
In most EMS services, the primary link between an operations or communications center and EMS

personnel in the field is currently the two-way radio. There has been substantial development of radio systems for use by EMS and other public safety agencies in the past 30 years. Radio systems might be as simple as a single-channel, low-band VHF system or as complex as computer-controlled, 800-MHz, truncated radio systems that provide tremendous flexibility in setting up communications networks. The most advanced systems also might provide special telemetry downlinks to transmit routing and location information. Communications centers could be linked to mobile units directly, transceiver to transceiver, depending strictly on the raw transmission power of the radios to effect a link. In more sophisticated systems, basic radio equipment could be supplemented by repeater systems or satellite downlinks. Details about the radio hardware available to EMS services and the potential capabilities of these technologies will be discussed later in this chapter.

Dispatchers and Operations Controllers

In addition to the primary role of coordinating communications during active operations, dispatchers and operations controllers have several secondary roles. When an emergency dispatcher receives a call from a citizen accessing the 911 system, he or she might provide over-the-phone medical instructions that the caller can implement until responders arrive. A growing number of EMS services employ dispatching personnel who are certified as emergency medical dispatchers in order to better provide this service. There are numerous documented cases where these prearrival instructions have positively affected the outcome of an EMS response. The EMS medical director should take an active role in oversight and protocol development of these programs.

In many medium-to-large systems, the operations control element of the communications center and the dispatchers extends to more than just active response operations. In many systems, dispatch personnel are designated system status managers, or controllers are empowered to both make operational decisions concerning policy and to issue binding directives to field personnel, such as hospital destination decisions. This authority seldom extends to medical care decisions, but it might extend to every other aspect of an on-duty crew's workflow. As part of this expanded operations control, dispatchers/controllers in many systems use a variety of methods to monitor the overall readiness status of service resources. These methods range from simply keeping paper notes and logs indicating the location and status of units, to using sophisticated systems that auto-matically update unit readiness status and locations by means of data obtained via global positioning technology that is transmitted to the communications center over dedicated telemetry channels. Regardless of the system used to maintain an updated picture of the readiness status of the system, modern dispatchers or controllers are often called on to continually alter the locations of EMS units. This is done as the system requirements change to ensure the optimal ability of available assets to respond. This process of actively managing system resources according to system status is commonly referred to as **system status management (SSM)**. Dispatchers might make the necessary decisions by best guess, and/or written standard operating guidelines, and/or the help of full-featured CAD decision-making systems.

Medical Direction

A well-designed multichannel communications link among medical directors, EMS managers, and field personnel is essential to effective medical operations in the EMS system. When people think of communications for medical direction, they tend to think exclusively of online communications, those conducted in real time between paramedics in the field and physicians in the emergency department. This is still a very important component of communications for medical direction, but not in the same way it once was. Equally important is the establishment of multiple routes of offline communication between EMS crews and medical direction. Offline medical oversight includes both prospective and retrospective communications, such as protocols, meetings, education, and quality management.

In modern EMS systems, online medical direction should rarely be required for EMS providers to perform procedures or administer medications defined by their standard protocols. A growing number of systems have redefined online medical direction as an expert resource for paramedics to consult when faced with perplexing or unusual cases beyond the scope of their protocols. (The "consult" concept is a good one to reinforce.) A few medical directors have dispensed with provisions for online medical direction completely, having provided their paramedics with a complete set of standing orders and the authority to flexibly interpret them to fit variable situations. This paradigm shift is a result of more sophisticated training provided for paramedics coupled with a higher level of confidence in the paramedics by physicians. This approach requires extensive offline education of out-of-hospital and physician providers. When a medical director is in the process of designing or revamping communications protocols for online medical direction, he or she must take stock of the communications modes available and must design the system to make the most effective use of available resources. In some cases, the medical director might be able to influence acquisition of communications equipment to provide a better online system. However, the secret to an effective online system lies in establishing a set of conditions under which communication and information exchange consistently occur. The medical director should provide paramedics with a clear understanding of the type and priority order of information they should relay. This will prompt them to be concise and not overburden the online providers with unnecessary information or commentary.

In some systems, paramedics are directed to contact the hospital that will receive the patient if online consult is needed. In this situation, there is a risk that paramedics will end up consulting with a physician who is not familiar with their protocols or their abilities. The medical director must provide clear guidance to out-of-hospital providers on how to proceed in these situations. When the number of emergency departments designated as online medical direction sites is limited, the smaller number of emergency physicians makes the online management responsibilities of the medical director easier. All persons providing online direction must be familiar with the EMS system resources and abilities and how to provide appropriate online direction; it is also the responsibility of the medical director to make sure that those personnel are appropriately educated.

Online Medical Direction Technology

There is no specific technology that must be used for online medical direction. In many EMS systems, EMS personnel contact online direction through a dedicated, accessible telephone line. This makes it fairly easy for them to establish contact from a patient's residence or place of business. Since cell phones have become almost ubiquitous, EMS crews can reach those dedicated numbers from almost anywhere. Radio communications systems are also still quite common. Many EMS services and hospitals have general communication radios and/or specialized ultra–high-frequency (UHF) biotelemetry radios. Recently, some medical directors, rather than assign online medical direction responsibilities to fellow physicians, have begun to manage the task themselves by using a dedicated cell phone or radio.

This idea is quite attractive to the medical director who likes to maintain direct involvement in the field activities of the medics but does not want to constantly monitor the radio. However, this can be quite invasive of the physician's time in a busy system. In a few systems, online medical direction can be provided with the added dimension of direct video links with the ambulance and crews. These out-of-hospital telemedicine systems have been in limited use for several years but are still extremely expensive and infrastructure intensive. Results so far call into question whether routine EMS telemedicine is worth the substantial costs and logistical problems it poses. Systems that allow the transmission of ECGs and other biotelemetry are also relatively expensive and seem to be of marginal benefit when physicians have a high comfort level with the paramedic's ability to interpret this information. Recently, with the advent of out-of-hospital 12-lead ECG, transmission of ECG telemetry has come back into practice. Some of the newest out-of-hospital ECG machines have available options to transmit a copy of the tracing to a fax machine in the emergency department via cellular telephone. The various technologies that are used to effect online medical direction communications will be discussed in more detail later in this chapter.

The Medical Director

Maintaining documentation of online contacts is important for quality assurance. Telephone contacts can easily be recorded using inexpensive equipment available at most electronics stores. These recordings can be useful as a quality improvement tool. Alternatively, a brief online contact log that details key information concerning each instance of a request for online medical direction is a very valuable tool for both quality management and legal reasons. The medical director should determine what core information he or she really believes is needed in a log, determine a suitable form, and work to establish policies for documentation at the emergency departments providing online medical direction.

Perhaps the best communication tool for medical direction is for the medical director to be active and visible in the EMS system. Some medical directors place themselves in the center of a large organizational structure from which they provide medical direction to many EMS services. In such systems, many of the day-to-day tasks and duties of the medical director are delegated to others, and the medical director is seldom, if ever, seen by the rank-and-file paramedics and rarely communicates with them as individuals. Physicians contemplating the role of medical director in any system must seek out ways to maintain direct contact and involvement with their paramedics. They need to see and be seen relatively often. This is a challenge for a busy physician to accomplish while managing a typical emergency practice. Therefore, it is probably best to place realistic limits on the number of EMS services and paramedics a medical director provides medical direction for, or to split medical direction responsibilities with other physicians. Medical directors must remain highly responsive to concerns of field personnel. Well-designed pathways and parameters for communication between the physician and the members of the EMS system he or she oversees are fundamental to the system's success. Prospective medical directors should consider communications issues carefully as they contemplate taking on the role. Where solid lines of communication are not in place, they should be established. Current medical directors should revisit the nature and effectiveness of their communications channels with EMS providers and should not hesitate to make needed changes. Successful communication does not depend simply on sophisticated technology and expensive infrastructure. It depends on establishing simple guidelines and procedures, making everyone familiar with them, and making sure they are followed.

Intra-Agency Communications

Communications among field EMS units within an emergency response agency are necessary for a variety of reasons. Units responding jointly to a call might need to coordinate their response, relay updated information, or interact with a special response unit. Regardless of the reason, it is important for an EMS communications system to provide an efficient means for this intra-agency communication.

In a growing number of systems, individual units are being provided with cellular telephones for medical direction communications. These phones provide an excellent means for interunit communications, although use might be limited by operational protocols and directives when no other resource is readily available. Many EMS system radio networks have provisions for multiple channels of radio communication that will allow intercommunication of responding units to occur on special operations frequencies. Services that use 800-MHz radio systems have even more flexibility for establishing lines of communication among EMS units, supervisory units, and special response units. Choices of radio and other communi-

cations hardware to be used for intra-agency communication should be based on the geographic features of the operating area, the typical operational profile for the service, and fiscal resources available for system development and maintenance.

Interagency/Facility Communications

An effective overall system for emergency communications must provide some practical method that allows communication among the different agencies involved in responses or patient management. This interagency communications capability should allow different responding agencies (police, fire, EMS, animal control) to exchange information. Another aspect of interagency communications is the link between EMS units in the field and receiving hospitals. In areas where there are multiple medical facilities, some practical means of direct communication between emergency departments is also essential. These capabilities are important in everyday EMS activities and become even more crucial in disasters and multiple-casualty incidents (**Figure 9-2**).

How communication occurs among different responding agencies is largely dependent on the sophistication and resources of the agencies involved. The optimum in efficiency and effectiveness occurs when responding units from different agencies can communicate directly rather than through a go-between. Unfortunately, in many areas, interagency communications must take place through the assistance of a dispatcher who is connected to counterparts in other agencies by special phone lines. Certain radio frequencies, notably those in the low VHF band, have been allocated for interagency communications at the countywide level and can be used to establish direct communications when all response organizations are equipped with them. Modern computer-controlled radio networks place all public safety organizations on the same set of frequencies. Dispatchers can arrange these frequency assignments as necessary to allow different agencies involved in the same response to communicate directly.

Communication between hospitals and EMS units is often tied to the function of online medical direction. The communication and medical direction are combined when each receiving hospital provides online direction for patients being transported to its facility. Contact with EMS units in these systems might be just to advise of a patient's status and impending arrival, or could involve a request for online

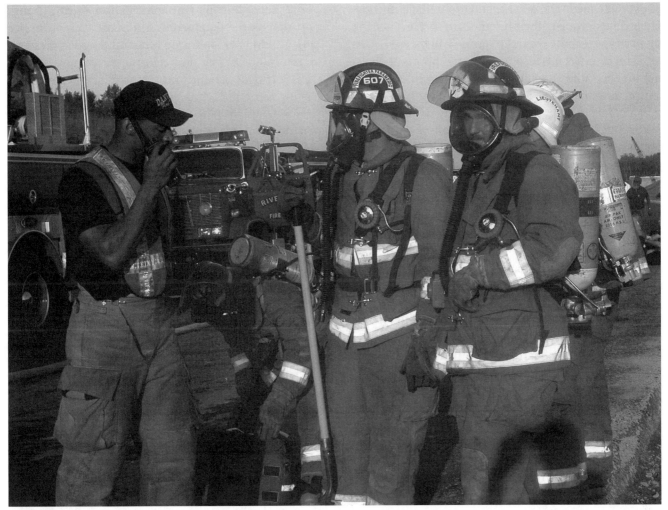

Figure 9-2 The ability for field responders to communicate with hospitals and response agencies becomes even more important in disasters and multiple-casualty incidents.

consultation. In other systems, only designated base facilities provide medical direction functions. In these systems, the task of notifying a receiving hospital might be undertaken by the online medical direction provider, or it could be accomplished by the EMS unit using a separate communications channel.

During the establishment of EMS communications systems in the 1970s, certain radio frequencies in the high VHF and UHF bands were designated specifically for medical communications of this type. Many of these radio networks are still in use today as either the primary communications link or as a backup system to phone links. Many hospitals also provide dedicated phone lines EMS units use to request online direction or notify of an impending patient arrival using a cellular phone.

The need to arrange rapid movement of patients from outlying hospitals to special care facilities such as trauma or cardiac centers highlights the need for formal hospital-to-hospital communications links.

The nature of such links is dependent on the number of hospitals in the area, the political relationships among medical facilities, and the available resources. In some areas, the only means of contact between facilities is by telephone through a hospital switchboard or to a general emergency department number. Where there are only two or three facilities, hospital emergency departments could be linked together by ring-down phone systems (explained later in the chapter) or a phone line reserved specifically for communication with other emergency departments. The VHF radio systems established for medical communications in the 1970s, known as the **HEAR (Hospital Emergency Administrative Radio) system,** are used effectively in some areas to link hospitals. Interhospital communications are especially important in the event of disasters or large mass-casualty incidents. The need for backup systems was underscored by the September 11, 2001, disaster, during which some cell phone networks were disabled or overwhelmed. The quicker and more efficiently hospitals can coordinate their resources in such events, the more successful the overall response will be.

The Internet has also become an important channel for the rapid transmission of certain information concerning the status of hospitals, EMS services, and aeromedical resources. Commercially available and custom-designed regional Web sites allow participating hospitals and response organizations to see at a glance the status of area hospitals regarding diversion or other operational issues. These Web sites also provide triage and transport officers a much more effective and rapid system for determining patient assignments to hospitals in disasters and mass-casualty incidents.

The ability for different agencies and hospitals involved in the rescue and treatment of emergency victims to communicate can directly affect patient outcome. The more inclusive and streamlined the arrangements provided for interagency communication, the more effective and efficient the overall response. Over the years, as different regions have improved their resources, and as new technologies have become available, the standards for interagency communications have evolved. These communications networks are important for day-to-day EMS operations but are *essential* for effectively dealing with masses of patients from disasters and mass-casualty incidents.

Information Management

Many aspects of EMS communications systems evolved independently and have traditionally been considered apart from one another. Information is gathered from numerous sources and might be filed in different reports kept in different locations. As new technologies designed to facilitate information-gathering have become available, a growing number of EMS services have taken steps to improve and streamline their information management strategies.

Run Report

EMS operations generate several types of primary records or data blocks. Perhaps the most fundamental is the patient chart, often referred to as a run report. This record is both a medical record and a legal document, just as a patient chart generated in the emergency department is. It usually is the primary source of billing information for services rendered to the patient.

Various problems are associated with these re-

ports. Recording patient information during transport diverts the paramedic's attention away from the patient. EMS personnel are often under great pressure to return to service and relocate very quickly after transporting a patient to the emergency department, leaving very little time for chart completion. EMS personnel might perceive that emergency department personnel do not consider their charting information of particular importance, which discourages them from preparing proper EMS medical charts. Another problem with the traditional EMS run report is its fragility. Medics might need to hand-prepare multiple copies of run reports in order to leave one at the emergency department, or they could depend on the availability of a copying machine. Many EMS services use NCR forms so that multiple copies can be distributed within the system. But because the original "top copy" is usually earmarked for EMS billing and general EMS record-keeping, the emergency department staff and QA director might receive copies that are partially or completely illegible. Some EMS services use charts that rely on check boxes and less narrative information. Such charts are similar to specialized charting instruments used by some emergency departments. Unlike those specialized charting systems, however, EMS charts do not provide different sheets for different types of chief complaints or diagnoses. Finally, some emergency departments do not seem to consider EMS chart copies to be of great importance or part of the patient's medical record. They might discard these reports, sometimes without review, rather than include them in the patient's hospital chart. Some EMS managers have adopted policies forbidding field personnel from leaving a copy of a run report at the emergency department, mistakenly believing that it will reduce legal exposure. The EMS medical director must assume a strong leadership role in establishing parameters for the preparation and management of these important documents.

Primary and Secondary Records

Other records routinely generated during EMS operations include dispatch/911 contact logs and individualized run reports. These reports record important information provided by 911 callers, as well as the times at which key events in the course of a response occurred. They can document the identities of additional responding organizations and personnel, as well as the weather and road conditions at the time of a particular response. All of these data could be important for quality management, discipline, and legal reasons. In many cases, such written records are complemented by audiotapes of 911 calls and related radio traffic. Although such recordings are not always retained for long periods, they might be of importance in verifying information recorded in other media. Other records include online medical contact logs generated by base hospitals. Participating EMS crews often generate special incident reports when there is something unusual about a case that might place it at high risk for later medical or legal review. These reports could be supplemented by additional information generated by an investigating supervisor or the EMS medical director.

Records that are secondary to the daily flow of EMS operations but equally important include daily vehicle inspection and inventory reports, controlled substance inventory and security reports, and reports generated during quality assurance review. All of these primary and secondary records contain pieces of the overall picture of an EMS service's operations and performance. The design of data forms and the policies adopted to regulate information-gathering and recording dictate the completeness and clarity of the resulting records. It is important for the medical director to have a clear understanding of the types of reports that are generated throughout the EMS system, the typical contents of each, and how to access that information.

In recent years, there has been much development toward paperless charting systems, both for in-hospital and out-of-hospital care. Such systems offer many advantages and, if they live up to their potential, could ameliorate many of the problems associated with the gathering of medical and other information. Depending on the sophistication of available paperless systems, information gathered in one phase of operations for an EMS case might be automatically shared across the entire EMS system. This could reduce the need for the same information to be independently gathered by multiple persons and could allow consolidation of all information into a single case or run record from which multiple special-purpose reports can be generated. More detail about these systems will be provided later in this chapter.

Technology and Equipment

EMS communication is dependent on a long list of technologies and devices, many of which have been in service for years. New technologies are being added to the list regularly. Although it is unlikely that an EMS system will use all available communications tools and instruments, it is important for the

EMS medical director to have a working familiarity with the plethora of devices and communications modes available. When decisions about new communications equipment or procedures are to be made, a knowledgeable medical director can influence decisions in a positive way.

Wire-Based Telephones

Despite the amazing developments in communications technology over the past 30 years, the telephone remains a mainstay of EMS communications. It is the primary communications tool for public access to the EMS system and a major component of the operational and intra-agency communications system. In many EMS systems, EMS providers still contact online medical direction by using telephones from the homes of their patients. Operational coordination among different EMS and public safety agencies and among these agencies and medical facilities is often achieved by telephone. Information management could also be assisted by use of standard telephone connections through which patient data and other information are transmitted to and from the field.

The telephone is the classic example of a **duplex communications device**. There are two functioning channels that allow both persons to hear and speak at the same time. Except under extraordinary circumstances, such as a disaster that damages or destroys its support infrastructure, the telephone system is the most dependable of all communications devices. It is also economical. Telephones are useful for much more than voice communication. The conversion of electronic data into modulated sounds makes it possible to transmit biomedical data, written documents, still pictures, and even low-resolution video information through telephone hookups if coding and decoding equipment is available at both ends of the call. When telemetry equipment uses sound frequencies outside the range of the human ear, transmission can even occur at the same time that voice communications are taking place.

Some variations of standard telephone equipment have applications in EMS communication. One of these is the dedicated telephone line or **ring-down phone**. This is a direct link between two or more locations that does not require the dialing of a number for access: just picking up the phone on one end causes the telephone at the other end to ring. These systems can be designed so that access to multiple points from the central control location can be effected at one time. The most common uses for ring-down phones are emergency communications with EMS stations, communications among operations control centers and medical facilities, and interagency communications among organizations that frequently participate in joint operations. Many emergency call boxes are nothing more than standard ring-down telephones tied to a specific emergency communications center based on their location. Newer wireless, digital, and satellite technologies have expanded the functionality of the traditional ring-down telephone to provide even more flexibility.

Another variation is the **radio tie line (RTL) system.** In this hybrid system, information transmitted through the telephone is fed into a radio transmission system for broadcast, or vice versa. The most common example of this technology is the telephone-accessed pager by which both digital and alphanumeric information can be transmitted. These systems are heavily used for operational communications in many EMS services and could also have a role in the medical direction system. Although less common since the advent of cellular phones, RTL systems that allow radio transmissions from EMS units in the field to link into the telephone system for online medical direction are also available. Another variation of the RTL is often used to provide emergency linkages between response agencies and regional disaster operations centers.

Radios

Radio systems have been an important component of emergency communications throughout the United States. The rapidly escalating demand for access to radio frequencies by commercial and government users has made it difficult for EMS and other public safety entities to obtain the radio channels and bandwidth needed for growing operational demands. Much of the new technology in recent years has been radio equipment operating on higher frequency bands. The International Telecommunications Union manages the entire usable electromagnetic spectrum worldwide, including radio waves. In the United States, two agencies oversee the allocation and use of radio frequencies. The **Interagency Radio Advisory Committee** focuses on radio use by the federal government, and the **Federal Communications Commission (FCC)** oversees all nonfederal usage.

All radio systems work by attaching meaningful information to light waves in the radio wavelength range of the light spectrum, a process called **modulation.** The most basic radio device operates using one discrete frequency, allowing only one person at a time to actively send a message. These devices re-

Table 9-1	Radio wave spectrum and specific band designations.

Spectrum	Band designation
30 KHz	Very Low Frequency (VLF)
30 to 300 KHz	Low Frequency (LF)
300 to 3,000 KHz	Medium Frequency (MF)
3 to 30 MHz	High Frequency (HF)
30 to 300 MHz	Very High Frequency (VHF)
300 to 3,000 MHz	Ultra High Frequency (UHF)
3 to 30 GHz	Super High Frequency (SHF)
30 to 300 GHz	Extremely High Frequency (EHF)

quire persons trying to communicate to take turns in transmitting or responding to messages. Various rules of radio procedure and etiquette have become standard to ensure that messages are not garbled or lost. Most radios used for EMS operational, intraagency, and interagency communications are of this basic type. More advanced radio systems use two or more frequencies within the same band. These systems allow conversation in a more natural and simultaneous manner and are less likely to cause communication problems. When such radio systems allow for two channels, one sending and one receiving, the system is referred to as a **duplex system.** Systems that allow more than two discrete channels to operate simultaneously are referred to as **multiplex systems.** The classic example of a multiplex radio is the now-obsolete Biophone biomedical radio. These provided two channels for voice communication and one or more additional channels through which biotelemetry information could be relayed simultaneously. A cellular telephone system is actually an example of a multichannel radio device.

The radio portion of the electromagnetic spectrum encompasses hundreds of thousands of frequencies that have been grouped together into discrete bands according to their properties (**Table 9-1**). Each band has unique properties, advantages, and disadvantages, and any discussion of radio systems must be based on the frequencies in which they operate. As radio technology has evolved, the trend has been toward development of radio systems operating on everhigher frequencies. It is entirely likely that radios for emergency service use in the "super high frequency" or even the "extremely high frequency" bands will be available, or at least on the drawing board.

VHF Low-Band Radios

Very high frequency (VHF) radio systems have been a mainstay of EMS communications for many decades. The VHF band is divided into three subbands, of which the lowest and highest have frequencies allocated for EMS use. The low-band portion of the VHF frequencies extends from 30 to 54 MHz. Within this heavily used band are scattered many frequencies allocated to public safety functions.

Radio waves in this frequency band are reflected by the upper atmosphere and are therefore able to follow the curvature of the earth. As a result, transmissions on these frequencies can travel for long distances without the need for a repeater or RTL. Unfortunately, these frequencies have some serious disadvantages that have caused them to become less desirable for emergency radio traffic. Natural problems with low-band VHF include interference by atmospheric conditions, weather, and electrical equipment. In addition, radio waves in this band do not penetrate static structures such as buildings and topographic features very well. VHF low-band transmissions are therefore prone to interruptions and dead areas, especially in urban areas or regions of rough terrain. In addition, the tendency of these radio waves to bounce or skip off the upper atmosphere can cause transmissions from far away to disrupt emergency traffic. For example, EMS services in the Dallas-Fort Worth area have occasionally experienced severe radio disruptions from shrimp boats operating in the Gulf of Mexico. At times, this skip traffic has rendered the EMS VHF low-band radio system all but useless. Added to these problems is the increasing assignment of adjacent frequencies to common short-range functions, such as pagers, wireless microphones, and business communications. For all these reasons, low-band VHF has become a poor choice for EMS communications. Some systems keep them as a backup radio system or for routine communications with hospital emergency departments. EMS services in major population centers now use VHF low-band radios only for communications during joint operations for interservice communications during disaster or mass-casualty incident operations. In more rural areas, these radio systems are also being replaced but are still commonly used for daily operations, especially in poorly funded volunteer organizations. VHF low-band radios are used only for voice communications. They cannot be used for telemetry of biomedical data.

Low-band VHF radios operate in a simplex mode with the same frequency used for both transmission and reception of information. As a result, only one of these functions can occur at a time. Radios are typically designed both to transmit and to receive signals, with transmission activated by pushing a button on the side of the microphone. Only one transmitter in an operational area can send at a time. All others must wait until that transmission is finished to respond. If two or more units attempt to transmit at once, the most powerful unit will override the others or the signals might interact to produce a completely unreadable signal. To avoid garbled communications, strict radio etiquette must be observed. In addition, personnel must be taught to fully push the transmit button before beginning to speak to avoid having the first part of a message cut off.

VHF High-Band Radios

Although not as common as in years past, VHF high-band radio systems remain an important part of the overall EMS communications system for many agencies. High-band VHF frequencies for public safety services are scattered from 150 to 174 MHz and differ in several important ways from those in the low-band VHF range. High-band VHF radio waves operate on line of sight. They travel in a straight line and are not prone to bounce off the atmosphere or follow the curvature of the earth. Unless augmented by a repeater system, the range of such radio systems is limited to the distance of the horizon. This reduces the possibility of interference from radio systems located in distant areas. Large buildings and dense terrain features such as hills can block VHF high-band transmissions, which makes high-band VHF radios less desirable in dense urban areas or in areas with hilly topography. Like frequencies in the low-band VHF range, high-band VHF frequencies are heavily allocated and are in great demand. Consequently, there can be a scarcity of available frequencies for EMS.

High-band VHF radios generally operate in a simplex mode and require correct use of radio etiquette to be effective. They are most often used for dispatching, interambulance, and unit-to-hospital communications. Care must be exercised in placement of base station radio antennae, and extensive use of repeaters might be necessary to prevent dead zones. For example, the high-band VHF radio system once used by EMS services on the San Francisco Bay peninsula, with its many hills and steep canyons, required a series of ganged repeaters placed on multiple mountain tops to provide acceptable radio communications. Even then, many areas contained dead zones from which radio transmissions could not be made or received. In many areas, high-band VHF radio systems are being replaced by systems operating in the UHF and 800-MHz ranges.

UHF Radios

Most EMS services in the United States use **ultra–high-band** radio systems. The UHF band extends from 300 to 3,000 MHz. Primary ranges of EMS radio frequencies include those between 450 and 470 MHz, those in the 800-MHz subband, and frequencies near the upper limits of the band, around 2,500 MHz, which are used for telemedicine applications.

UHF radio systems have several advantages over VHF. They operate strictly on line of sight, which means there is little likelihood of interference between radio systems operating in adjoining service areas (although it also makes the use of repeaters necessary for large geographic regions). Unlike VHF radio signals, UHF will easily penetrate most man-made structures. However, dense natural features such as hills, valleys, and large rock formations block them. These properties make UHF radio systems very useful in urban and suburban areas but limit their usefulness in rural areas and areas with rugged terrain features. Of the available radio systems for EMS use, those in the UHF band are the least susceptible to skipping or interference from atmospheric phenomena.

The early uses for UHF radios in EMS were for operational or medical communications. UHF radios allowed the transmission of simultaneous voice and biotelemetry. They were a standard fixture for online medical direction before the advent of cellular telephones. For this purpose, in the 1970s the FCC allocated several sets of paired frequencies that allowed duplex or multiplex operations. These 10 pairs of frequencies are known as the **Med Channels.** There are specific limitations placed on the use of each of the 10 channels. Additional paired and single frequencies have since been made available for use by public safety and EMS services, but these are still the most commonly used. In some areas, UHF radio systems were coupled with RTL systems to further enhance the flexibility and broaden access to multiple emergency departments and resources such as regional poison centers.

Recent developments in EMS-related telemedicine also make use of frequencies within the UHF band, as do special "trunked" or cycled-frequency radio network systems. These systems have the same general properties of the UHF band, along with unique capabilities inherent in the equipment designed to use the frequencies.

800-MHz Radio Systems

Public safety service radios operating in the 800-MHz range technically operate on the UHF band, but they have unique features. The FCC first made frequencies in the 800-MHz sub band available to emergency services in 1974. Originally, 70 channels

representing a pair of frequencies in the range between 809.9 and 860.9 MHz were allocated for public safety use. At the same time, additional channels in that range were allocated for use by businesses and for cellular communications systems. Because actual use by other entities did not occur immediately, EMS and other emergency services had this portion of the UHF band to themselves. In 1986, additional portions of the 800-MHz subband were allocated to emergency services, giving emergency services nationwide a total of 240 two-frequency channels. Each public safety entity or local group of entities is assigned a set of these channels distinct from adjacent users. They also have access to specially designated channels that all public safety entities using 800-MHz systems share. Like other UHF radio systems, 800-MHz systems are capable of using repeater systems and can be associated with satellite uplink systems. The most unique and useful aspect of 800-MHz systems to emergency services is its trunking capability.

The 800-MHz subband has become virtually synonymous with **trunked radio technology.** This technology, which is similar to that used in cellular telephone systems, allows a small range of channels to be used with great efficiency by a large service or group of services. Trunked radio systems use a central computer to manage frequency use. The controlling computer is programmed to place each group of users in a **talk group.** Talk groups are users who typically need to communicate with each other or with a shared control center. When the transmit button on a radio in the system is pressed, it sends a split-second digital signal to the central processor, identifying which talk group it belongs to. The computer rapidly assesses the system's status, determines which channels are currently unused, and switches all radios in that talk group to an unused frequency. Special protocols avoid switching any units within that talk group that are already transmitting on a different frequency. This all happens without human intervention and in a fraction of a second, so the technology is transparent to end users.

The primary advantage of trunked 800-MHz systems is that they provide tremendous flexibility and efficiency at a time when the radio spectrum is becoming more and more crowded. Another advantage is the ability for dispatchers or controllers to quickly create new talk groups for special multiple-agency responses. For example, in the event of a mass-casualty incident, all the police, fire, and EMS personnel actively involved in the response can be reassigned to a single temporary talk group, allowing them to communicate during the response without affecting other activities of the involved agencies. When two or more units in a single agency need secure communications, they can be temporarily assigned to a special talk group.

Originally, it was believed that this type of radio system would have the additional advantage of being impossible to monitor with a scanner, allowing more secure and discreet operations. The rapid and continuous channel reuse and switching provided by the controlling computer system was expected to prevent eavesdropping. Even though there is scanner equipment available that defeats the switching function, the erroneous idea that 800-MHz radio systems are unscannable persists. Therefore, great care must be taken during EMS operations not to transmit sensitive patient information over these or any other radios.

Theory and early experience also suggested that trunked 800-MHz radios would not be subject to interference by similar neighboring radio systems. As time passed and the commercial aspects of the technology began to be fully exploited, it was discovered that these expectations were too optimistic. Especially in high-density population areas, public safety communications systems using 800-MHz radios operate side by side with trunked business radio systems and digital cellular phone networks that use channels interwoven with those designated for emergency service. There have been increasing problems with these commercial and cellular communications systems interfering with public safety communications systems. In April 2000, the FCC brought together stakeholders from the public safety services, cellular service carriers, and commercial mobile radio services to discuss the problems of interference and seek positive courses of action. It was quickly verified that no one was causing the problems through operating license violations. The problem did not manifest earlier because, for many years, only public safety agencies were actively using the system. A work group consisting of representatives from Motorola, the Association of Public-Safety Communications Officials, Nextel Communications, the Cellular Telecommunications and Internet Association, and the Public Safety Wireless Network was formed to study the problem, pool knowledge, and develop a best practices guide to assist agencies experiencing interference.

The 800-MHz trunked radio systems represent one of the most important and effective developments in EMS and other public safety communications in many years. The inherent advantages of the UHF band, coupled with the digital computer control and frequency-allocation capability of the trunking

system, make these radios an excellent tool for EMS operations and multiple-agency responses. In addition, the development of trunking technology offers the chance to greatly extend the versatility of other radio systems in the future.

Microwave Systems

In many parts of the country, the long-distance links that bind local phone service providers into a nationwide communications network involve the use of microwave systems. Microwave transmission systems are also being used more commonly for certain aspects of EMS system communications.

By definition, **microwaves** are radio signals of a frequency between 1 and 300 gigahertz (GHz). Radio signals in this frequency range can be focused into tight beams that can be directed at receiving antennae as far as 60 miles from the origin point. This makes it difficult to intercept and monitor transmissions made in the microwave frequencies. Microwaves are also capable of carrying a tremendous amount of analog or digital information along a single radio beam. These properties make microwave transmission and relay systems ideal for relaying large numbers of individual phone messages from region to region.

For emergency services, microwave transmission systems have been used to establish a backup connection into the national phone communications network. Such systems can be brought online in the event that a large-scale natural disaster knocks out all or a portion of the local telephone system infrastructure. By using such systems, vital telephone communications can be maintained. Microwave communications systems might be used by EMS services covering very large geographic areas or areas that have unusual terrain features that make more traditional radio transmission systems ineffective.

A typical system of this type involves a central microwave transmission and receiving antennae array that beams and receives signals from a series of strategically placed microwave towers throughout the service area. Signals beamed to these towers are then converted into the standard operational frequencies used by mobile units and are rebroadcast by slave transmitters similar to traditional repeaters. Similarly, transmissions from mobile units are received by the nearest of the towers, converted into microwave signals, and beamed to the central communications tower. The benefits of such systems include clearer and more reliable coverage of large or rough-terrain service areas. Vulnerability to disruption from tower damage again emphasizes the need for backup communications systems. Such systems have the potential for being used to establish secondary closed-circuit communications systems among all participants in the emergency system. This includes transmission of voice, video, telemetry, and digital computer data, all in one beam to any facility equipped with the necessary antennae array and converter hardware. By using this technology, all hospitals, EMS services, and other responder organizations can maintain reliable interagency coordination and communication under adverse conditions.

Satellite Communications Systems

Some remote areas of the United States have no telephone or fixed radio communications linkage. Unfortunately, many of these areas are inhabited or have recreational attractions, and EMS units must be prepared to go there and communicate from there. In addition, certain EMS communications technologies such as telemedicine are hindered from reaching full potential because they are tied to a wire-based communications infrastructure. One technology that offers a possible solution is satellite communication.

Satellites have been used to carry international telephone and other communications traffic for several decades. What is relatively new is the availability of portable satellite communications gear that can be hand carried or mounted within an ambulance. In 1978, Acadian Ambulance achieved fame when it participated in a pilot program to use portable satellite communications units to support EMS operations. That experimental program focused on linking offshore oil drilling rigs serviced by the company to medical direction using a NASA communications satellite. The success of the program proved the potential of the technology. Recently, the Federal Emergency Management Agency and a variety of national organizations concerned with provision of vital services to rural and frontier areas have taken official positions in favor of federal support for the widespread development of satellite communications systems.

Satellite communications devices are similar to microwave systems in that they use tightly beamed radio signals in the microwave frequencies to send and receive information. Like microwave systems, such radio transmissions are difficult to intercept. They are also able to carry tremendous amounts of information, especially when first encoded into a digital format. A single beam can carry voice, telemetry, video, and other digital information all at once. Where these systems differ is in the nature of the relay. Instead of towers, these systems work by beaming information to satellites placed in geosynchronous orbit approximately 24,000 miles above the earth. Each satellite holds line of sight over one third of the earth's total surface, offering the ability for properly equipped persons located in the most remote areas to communicate effectively over large distances.

Satellite systems differ by orbit height. The ones for GPS and early communications were geosynchronous, ie, they take 24 hours to do one revolution, so essentially they do not move. They required, at least for uplinking, fairly powerful phones in a suitcase or attached to a vehicle. Receiving could be accomplished with much smaller antennae.

On the other hand, LEO, or low-earth orbit, systems are not geosynchronous and continuously move across the earth's surface. This requires more satellites (approximately seven), and each satellite is more like a cell tower, handing off the call. The good news is that much less power is required to reach the LEO satellite, allowing smaller, less powerful phones. More LEO satellites are going up all the time.

Currently, satellite communications systems suitable for use in daily EMS operations are very expensive and are not 100% reliable. Setbacks to practical use of satellite technology for routine EMS include the failure of at least one major satellite communications provider and failures of communications satellites themselves. Nevertheless, there is hope that, in the near future, such systems will become more widely available, cost-effective, and flexible enough to solve a variety of serious communication problems. Another development still in an early stage is a satellite communications downlink for EMS telemedicine applications that will allow freedom from current infrastructure requirements and access to this technology for rural EMS providers. It is unclear when, and to what degree, portable satellite communications systems will become a substantial component of the overall EMS communications system in the United States.

Repeaters

A repeater is nothing more than a slaved radio receiver and transmitter array that is designed to re-broadcast received signals while amplifying the signal strength and range. Repeaters can be fixed installations, placed at points of high elevation, or they can be mobile devices installed in an ambulance or other emergency response vehicle.

Repeaters are used by EMS systems for one of three reasons. First, services in areas with highly irregular terrain features have numerous locations from which radio signals cannot directly reach the communications center or medical direction facilities. Repeaters in these systems are generally placed at strategically selected high elevation points where they can receive local traffic and relay it throughout the radio network. Second, some EMS services have to operate over distances that extend beyond the horizon. These services use repeaters placed throughout their operating region to ensure no radio unit is beyond the range of the rest of the system. Finally, some services use a mobile repeater network installed in ambulances. These repeaters boost the signal of handheld units with too little power to reach directly to a central communications center or fixed repeater tower. Repeaters can be useful in both rural and urban settings.

Repeaters can be designed to receive signals on one frequency or in one band and retransmit the signal at another frequency or on another band. In fact, RTL systems, which feed received radio transmissions into the standard telephone system, can be considered a form of repeater.

Call Boxes

Once relatively uncommon, roadside emergency call boxes are becoming more readily available and offer yet another way to access the EMS system. As mentioned earlier, many call box systems use dedicated ring-down landline phone linkages. Other call box systems depend on cellular or RTL technologies to establish contact with emergency operators. Some of these call box systems automatically identify to the

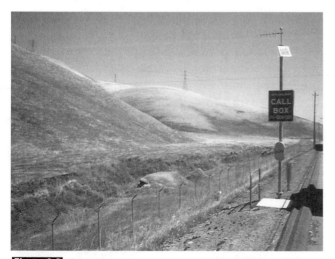

Figure 9-3 Once relatively uncommon, roadside emergency call boxes are becoming more readily available and offer yet another way to access the EMS system.

emergency operator exactly which box a caller is using, while others require the caller to identify the call box location by a reference number or code on the box. Such call box systems are most often placed along more isolated stretches of interstate highways where help would otherwise be difficult to obtain (**Figure 9-3**).

Cellular Communications Systems

In 2000, it was estimated that between 25% and 30% of all calls to 911 centers originated from cell phones. As discussed earlier, there are substantial problems with the use of cell phones as a means of public access to EMS. Beyond the use of cell phones by citizens for 911 access, cellular technology has become important to EMS services in operational, intra-service, interservice/facility, and data management applications.

Analog and Digital Systems

Cellular telephones are UHF radio systems that operate on a system of frequency cycling and reuse similar to, but far more elaborate than, that used by 800-MHz trunking systems. Depending on the type of service, cellular telephones can operate in the 400, 800, or 1,800 to 1,900 MHz portions of the UHF band. A given service area is divided into communications zones or cells, each served by one tower. Cells are generally placed so there is some degree of overlap to avoid or reduce dead areas. Cellular systems are computer controlled so that once a call begins, the call is routed through the cell tower that picks up the strongest signal from the phone. In the event the cellular telephone is moving and passes from one cell to another, the system is supposed to automatically switch the call to the dominant tower.

Cellular telephones can be either analog or digital depending on whether they are designed to send and receive messages as standard modulated radio signals (analog) or as digital encoded signals that are encoded and decoded by computer algorithms similar to those used by CD players and computer modems. Different equipment is required for the two types of cellular telephones, and not all areas with cellular coverage offer support for digital units. Digital cellular telephones offer better noise reduction and are especially useful for transmission of telemetry and wireless Internet connections. Some digital cell phone systems offer a variety of ancillary services in which the cellular telephone can act as a pager, a voice-mail system, or even an Internet access device. These types of cellular telephone systems are referred to as **personal communications service** systems. Cellular carriers are rapidly moving from analog to digital signals for two reasons. First, an analog channel can carry only one call at a time (similar to simplex radios), while a digital channel can carry many calls. Second, digital allows better, faster transmission of data, the fastest-growing segment of wireless transmission. The FCC has also dropped its mandate that carriers support analog.

Cell Phone Location Technology

Cell phone location technology is available but not widely used. The FCC issued guidelines requiring wireless communications carriers and manufacturers to integrate location technology into their products and systems in two phases, with the primary objective of assisting E911 centers. In Phase I of this development, carriers are required to provide a means for PSAPs to localize a call from a cell phone to the region covered by a specific cell tower. Not only will this allow the call to automatically be routed to the correct PSAP, but it will localize the caller's position to a single cell in the phone system. Phase II of the wireless E911 program requires that PSAPs receive both identification information for the registered owner of the cellular telephone and latitude/longitude information that will pinpoint the caller's location to within 400 feet. This is referred to as **automatic location identification (ALI)**. Efforts to accomplish this have been delayed by many technical, political, and financial issues. Recently, new FCC deadlines have been established by which cellular telephone systems must be able to function fully as part of the E911 system. In the 911 systems that have access to Phase I, the technology has already proved its value. At this time, some Phase II systems are online, and the FCC deadline for the completion of Phase II implementation is now December 31, 2005.

Originally, it was assumed the technologies necessary to allow cellular telephones to function with E911 systems would be carrier based, located at central reception and switching locations. Rapid developments in the technologies used in individual cellular telephones have made it more appropriate for the necessary enhancement to be built into the handsets themselves. To allow more time for phone manufacturers to perfect these technologies and begin tooling up for production, the FCC pushed back the deadlines for implementing the wireless E911 system.

For more information on wireless E911 implementation, requirements, and deadlines, go to www.fcc.gov/911/enhanced.

Benefits of Cell Phones in EMS

The applications for cellular telephone systems in EMS are limited only by the imagination of the personnel involved in operations. Cellular telephones have become so inexpensive that many EMS services include a cellular telephone as part of the standard equipment of each ambulance. These can be used for backup communications during normal operations or even to link multiple units or even multiple agencies together through a conference link established at the communications center. Cellular telephones are increasingly equipped with slimline headsets, making hands-free operation simple. In many EMS services, cellular telephones have totally replaced radios for online communications with medical directors. Special cellular phones equipped to link with portable monitor-defibrillators or other biomedical instruments transmit vital patient information to receiving hospitals at the same time that physicians and paramedics are consulting by voice communication. In some small-to medium-sized EMS systems, all online medical direction is handled personally by the medical director, who carries a cell phone at all times for just that purpose.

Weaknesses of Cell Phones in EMS

As with all other communications tools, cellular telephones have weaknesses. Most portable cellular telephones use batteries with a limited reserve of power. Multiple batteries must be available for such units, or an onboard system for charging the telephone must be provided. The limited useful life inherent in many types of cellular telephone batteries, coupled with heavy, daily use of cellular telephones, results in wearing out expensive batteries. Cellular telephones often lose contact with the network as they are moved from one cell to another. Analog systems might suffer from severe static or signal attenuation as the borders between cells are neared or in areas with unusual terrain features. Digital cellular telephones will simply drop a call without warning if the signal strength drops below a cutoff point. Despite careful planning, many cellular systems have dead zones in which phones will not operate. Services that cover large regions with both urban and rural areas might find that some parts of their operating area only support the analog system or do not have cellular access at all. Such weaknesses must be taken into account before cellular devices are formally incorporated into the communications plans and strategies for an EMS service.

The full evolution of the cellular communications system has yet to be realized. Many developments with the potential to affect or even revolutionize how EMS services operate are just over the horizon. It is clear that cellular communications will have an increasing role in EMS communications.

Global Positioning/Locator Devices

Global positioning system (GPS) technology has revolutionized EMS in several ways and offers still-greater benefits in the future. The modern GPS is a satellite-based technology that had its inception in 1973 with a design approval by the Department of Defense. The launch of the first component satellite took place in 1978, and the system was declared fully operational in 1995. This system was primarily developed for use by the US military, but its great potential benefit for civilian applications was soon recognized. In order to preserve national security and to avoid enemies of the United States from using the GPS against us, the system includes two separate systems in one, with access controlled by special digital encryption codes. Civilian users have access to what is termed **standard positioning service,** which is accurate to approximately 400 feet. US military forces alone have access to **precision positioning service,** the accuracy of which has not been published. In very basic terms, GPS works by measuring the time it takes for a signal from the remote GPS system to reach one of the several dedicated satellites and the angle at which this signal is received. The signal is timed by use of extremely accurate atomic clocks aboard each satellite. Computer programs use the time and angle data to calculate the user's position in terms of latitude and longitude.

One of the ways in which GPS has benefited EMS has been in regard to navigation. Coupled with special computer software called a geographical information system, GPS units in ambulances can be used to assist responders in reaching an emergency scene, creating a map on an LCD screen for them to follow. Similar systems allow emergency planners to accurately estimate the response times to reach various locations under different conditions. This allows better placing of EMS resources. Aeromedical services, especially those that commonly make scene responses, now rely heavily on latitude and longitude coordinates provided by first responders and their own GPS navigation systems to go directly to the site of an emergency, reducing the need to fly a search grid to find a critical patient.

Although not the only technology available for this purpose, GPS units connected to ambulance-mounted transponders are the most effective way of continually updating the position of an ambulance for dispatchers. When tied to the same type of GIS mentioned above, these systems allow dispatchers to pinpoint the location of each ambulance in the system with great accuracy. This improves the process of choosing the ambulance in the best position to make a given response. Automobiles equipped with the current generation of crash notification systems incorporate a GPS that allows service operators to locate them by latitude and longitude. They then relay this information to the EMS service, where these coordinates can be programmed into the responding unit's own GPS navigation system. At present, only some of the newer high-end model cars are equipped with these systems, but efforts are underway to make these systems more widely available and even more sophisticated.

GPS also improves efforts to incorporate cellular phones into the E911 system. New cell phone designs involve some form of GPS unit enclosed within the cellular telephone to establish the caller's location, within the accuracy available to civilian users of GPS.

The **geographical information system (GIS)** is an increasingly important tool for EMS operations. These systems consist of a large database of geographic information for a given area that is detailed in depth and scope. Subprograms associated with the database allow the information to be used for a variety of purposes across many disciplines. Emergency services GISs can be used to display detailed electronic maps in operations control centers and on view screens in mobile units. These can include detailed terrain features and street location and are useful for navigation to emergency scenes and medical facilities. For example, an ambulance crew responding to a particular location can enter the address into the terminal in their ambulance and rapidly obtain a street map showing the location. When interfaced with a GPS, such GIS programs can actually calculate and recommend routing to responders, possibly reducing response times. As discussed previously, GISs are often an integral part of the more sophisticated CAD systems and often this navigational function is controlled through the communications/operations center. This type of program augments and enhances communication of emergency scene locations and helps personnel get there in the most expedient manner.

GIS programs also aid EMS services in other ways. The program can be provided various parameters that allow for practice simulation exercises. This function makes it possible for emergency planners and operations managers to estimate typical response times to various locations within the operating area under a variety of conditions. This can be of immense value to the processes of system improvement, operational guideline development, and emergency management planning. The process by which the GIS database for a given area is developed is very complex and painstaking. Trained professionals under contract or from commercial sources develop a database. Once the database is assembled, EMS personnel can use the system with minimal training.

The final story regarding the full impact of GPS on EMS services and operations is yet to be told. The technology is not fully mature and, as it reaches full development, it is very possible that new EMS-related applications will continue to improve the safety and effectiveness of EMS responders.

Automatic Crash Notification Systems

Automatic crash notification (ACN) systems are a relatively new component of the emergency communications system, which, with further development, offer great potential to reduce mortality and morbidity from motor vehicle crashes. ACN systems are a melding of several separate technologies, including automated vehicle sensing systems, GPS, and wireless telephone/telemetry systems.

The current generation of ACNs is fairly simple. Occupants of the vehicle can push a button to activate an emergency call, or the vehicle might call automatically. The vehicle senses that an airbag or other restraint system has been activated and automatically connects with a centralized communications center. The GPS location of the vehicle, expressed in latitude and longitude coordinates, is transmitted at the time a communications link is established to the vehicle. Currently such communications centers belong to private **telematics service providers (TSP)** services, such as OnStar or ATX Technologies. TSPs can speak with the occupants of the vehicle to obtain more information about a crash and about occupant injuries and provide information and updates to the occupants. These services then relay information about a crash to the appropriate PSAP by using a 10-digit phone number culled from a database. The crash information is relayed to the PSAP either verbally or via fax. While these systems improve discovery and response times, these calls from TSPs to PSAPs do not go through dedicated 911 lines and therefore do not have the priority nor automated information of other local 911 calls. In addition, 10-digit numbers cannot access many PSAPs.

The real benefit of this developing technology is in its potential for expansion and solving some of the most basic problems in the operation of trauma systems, namely, timely discovery and notification of crash victims. Since 1993, an average of 7.5% of fatal urban auto crash victims and 30% of fatal rural crash victims took longer than 1 hour to reach a medical facility. In thousands of cases nationwide, it took longer than 10 minutes for emergency services to receive notice that an injury crash had occurred. In both urban and rural areas, the response time of rescuers to a scene was extended because of difficulties in locating the crash site. It has been estimated that just reducing the average crash notification time in rural areas from the current average of 9 minutes to 1 minute could save 600 to 1,200 lives per year. Further time reductions could be realized by more accurate, timely, and reliable location data on crash scenes. Coupled with appropriate EMS trauma management protocols to limit scene times, reduced crash notification and response times provided by advanced ACN systems could make a major impact on auto crash-related mortality in the United States.

Efforts are underway to integrate the data of emerging ACN technologies into the existing EMS communications systems, providing a rapid, nationwide means of identifying the location and severity of automobile crashes. The ACN system will eliminate the current delay in notifying emergency services that a crash has occurred and will provide highly accurate location data. It will result in better allocation of resources by helping to differentiate between a fender bender and a crash that likely produced injuries.

In a pilot program from 1995 to 2000, the National Highway Traffic Safety Administration, in cooperation with Cellular One, Veridian Engineering, and the Erie County, New York, Medical Center, installed an advanced ACN system using an URGENCY sensor/software system in approximately 300 vehicles in the Buffalo, New York, area. Using multiple accelerometers, this system activated with any type of crash, whether the air bag had deployed or not. The URGENCY software took information from the sensor system and used it to calculate the probability that the crash had produced injuries. This probability, along with the location of the crash, the precrash vehicle speed, direction of travel, and vehicle identification information was transmitted to the Cellular One communications center and relayed to appropriate emergency responders and the medical center. This pilot program was able to show that advanced ACN technology works, reduces EMS notification times (44 seconds), and can send information directly to a PSAP in a format that provides location, crash severity, and probability of injury. Limitations of this field test included the small number of crashes, failures to send information due to equipment problems and gaps in cellular coverage, and the fact that the number dialed from the car was a centralized 10-digit number rather than a direct call to the local 911 system.

As mentioned earlier, the FCC requirement for cellular phones to provide location information to PSAPs has created new approaches for transmission of GPS information to 911 using existing infrastructure. As use of in-vehicle telematics systems grows, the ability to transmit vehicle crash information increases, providing a firm foundation for rapid deployment of ACN systems in the years ahead.

Computer Software

EMS communications have been improved over the years not only by advances in hardware and other equipment, but also by advances in computer software. As it stands, the computer is a relative newcomer to the arsenal of tools available to EMS services for operations applications, but, as has been the case in other fields, these devices have become almost indispensable very quickly. The evolution of EMS-related software has occurred very rapidly.

Computer-Aided Dispatching

For communications applications, the most common EMS software tools are computer-aided dispatching (CAD) programs. Early CAD programs were custom written for a particular service or department and were usually based on a command-line interface, an arrangement where the program operates as the result of the user entering any one of several, often obscure, one- or two-word commands. In many of these older systems, the user had to enter almost as much information as he or she got back. The learning curve was steep and resulted in dispatchers bypassing the system in favor of traditional methods. Modern CAD programs vary in their specific features and setup but share some important features.

The typical EMS dispatcher or 911 operator working for a medium-to-large service today makes use of CAD almost without thinking about it. Available programs typically offer a graphical user interface, completely familiar to users of Windows-based and Macintosh computers (**Figure 9-4**).

Many of these programs tie a variety of separate functions together into one terminal, making all critical operational information available at the click of a mouse. Some programs directly link with the information transmitted by the E911 system's autolocation function, allowing the minimal information needed for a response to be automatically entered into the system. Along with this basic ability, some CAD programs fully integrate the call-taking function and provide a variety of tools to facilitate obtaining and preserving necessary information. A growing number of these programs incorporate a GIS that maps out the service area and, at the very least, displays the physical location of a dispatch-pending call on an on-screen map. More sophisticated programs are able to tie data streams from GPS or other location transponder equipment in each ambulance to the GIS and display the relative location of available ambulances to the location of an emergency call. This ability can partially or fully automate the process of primary resource management and emergency dispatching. Most programs also offer a rapid-access database and linkage system for other resources that might be needed by the EMS service. An additional valuable function that is available through many CAD programs is integrated records management. This function automatically extracts and records data from other call reception and dispatching programs for inclusion in permanent dispatching records. This reduces the possibility that important information will be logged incorrectly during peak activity periods.

Many of these programs can be linked by telemetry to display terminals installed in each ambulance and can automatically relay critical information and routing displays to crews responding to a call. Because such linkages can be two-way and can be tied to onboard GPS systems, it is possible for dispatchers to maintain continual monitoring of the system status automatically.

Many such systems even provide field medics with a way to alert dispatch that they are in trouble at the touch of a single button on the display console or on a handheld radio. This helps to protect personnel in this era of increasing risks and violence.

Of course, CAD systems incorporating all of these features require substantial technological infrastructure to operate. For this reason, the most sophisticated versions of these systems are normally seen only in larger cities and metropolitan areas and are used to provide dispatching for all emergency services in the service area. Most available CAD programs are designed in a modular format that allows for combinations of desirable features to be incorporated in customized implementations for a given EMS service. Many offer the option of upgrading and

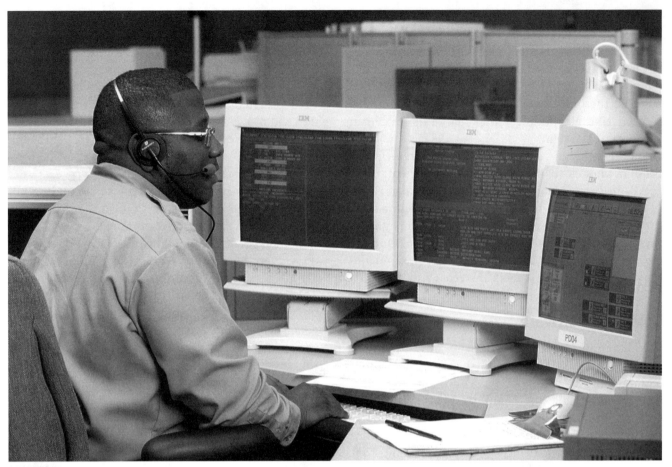

Figure 9-4 Available CAD programs today typically offer a graphical user interface, completely familiar to users of Windows-based and Macintosh computers.

adding additional features as needed and as resources allow. Overall, the ultimate outcome of these specialized communications control programs is the improvement of efficiency in dispatching/operations control activities and an increased effectiveness as evidenced by reduced response times.

Electronic Data Entry

The electronic data entry program, or paperless charting system, is another type of computer program related to communications now gaining increased importance within the EMS community. These programs, installed in a laptop or handheld computer, allow medics to enter data concerning EMS runs using a keyboard or stylus. When coupled with electronic run report forms and the appropriate computer hardware, these programs allow EMS crews to input data more quickly than would otherwise be possible. Such programs can save EMS services money normally used to print NCR run report forms and allow forms to be updated much more often and with far less expense than paper forms. It is even

possible to provide EMS providers with customized charting forms for a variety of commonly encountered chief complaints similar to some emergency departments. Such systems can be interfaced with a wireless data transfer system, allowing completed reports to be immediately filed in a central database. Using these programs, it is also possible to provide receiving hospitals with initial information on the patient's arrival in the emergency department, with a more complete report later by electronic transfer. This provides hospital personnel with immediate information about the patient and lets the medics go back into service as quickly as possible. Data input is either typed on a keyboard to begin with or is converted from handwriting to a typed format by algorithms associated with the palmtop computer supporting the charting program since these programs eliminate the problem of unreadable run reports. Paperless charting programs are not yet in widespread use, although several are commercially available. Due to the substantial advantage of solving several common operations problems, it is likely they will become prevalent even in small, rural EMS services as hardware prices fall.

To be sure, there are growing numbers of specially designed computer programs intended to support one phase or another of the overall operations of EMS and other emergency services. Those with limited budgets should be aware that commercially available computer programs can often be inexpensively adapted to do many of the same things the expensive custom programs can do.

For example, paperless charting can be accomplished by EMS services on a budget by use of specific software made for this purpose. This program, available for Windows, Macintosh, Unix, and some palmtop computer formats, allows the creation of blank forms that can then be filled in via keyboard or stylus in a manner exactly like the commercial paperless charting programs. Individual forms can even be linked to other documents after the same fashion as the different pages in a Web site. A primary form can be designed in house along with specialized auxiliary forms that can be called up by a single action for each common chief complaint. Completed forms can be printed, stored in a retrieval system, and transmitted by wireless or modem-based data transfer systems. This software also allows conversion of virtually any printed document, even large books, into an electronic file that can be read just like a book, page by page. Use of this program makes it possible for medical directors to provide an electronic copy of protocols and medical policies to each unit equipped with a laptop computer. Such electronic documents can be updated often without the problems and expense of having to reprint and distribute multiple paper copies. Such revisions can be distributed by e-mail. This is only one example of a commonly available computer program that can be adapted to the benefit of an EMS service and its medical director.

Summary

Whether using radio, telephone, computer programs, Internet-based applications, or old-fashioned face-to-face conversation, communication is essential to any EMS system. It is the cornerstone of medical direction and operations management. An effective communications network and plan are essential for a high-performing EMS system.

Bibliography

Augustine J, Paris P, Pappas G. Emergency medical services communications: In: Kuehl AE, ed. *EMS Medical Directors' Handbook.* St Louis, Mo: CV Mosby Publishing Co; 1989.

Cayten C, Oler J, Walker K, et al. The effect of telemetry on urban prehospital cardiac care. *Ann Emerg Med.* 1985;14:976–981.

Cross M, Maniscalco P. Cellular technology: an EMS overview. *Emerg Med Serv.* 1989;18(7):33–35.

FCC to give EMS new radio frequencies. *EMS Insider.* 1993;20(3):4.

Federal Communications Commission. Table of frequencies, allocations, and special requirements in international agreements and treaties. *FCC Rules and Regulations, Part 2.* Washington, DC: US Government Printing Office; 1985.

Gault ES. Scene communications pitfalls. *Emerg Med Serv.* 1992;21(8):23–25.

Guidelines for Developing an Emergency Medical Services Communications Plan. Washington, DC: HEW Division of Emergency Medical Services; March 1977. HSA 77-2036.

Lumpe D. Calling 911: who will answer? *Emerg Med News.* April 1993.

Mayron R, Long R, Ruiz E. The 911 emergency telephone number: impact on emergency medical systems access in a metropolitan area. *Am J Emerg Med.* 1984; 2:491–493.

McCorkle JE, Nagel EL, Penterman DG, et al. *Basic Telecommunications for Emergency Medical Services.* Cambridge, Mass: Ballinger; 1978.

Munn B. Cellular phones and 911. *Emerg Med Serv.* 1987; 16(8):12–14.

Nakata L. Microwave/satellite relays. *Emerg Med Serv.* 1990;9:30–31,56.

National Association of Emergency Medical Services Physicians. Position paper: Emergency medical dispatching. *Prehospital Disaster Med.* 1989;4:163–166.

Roush WR, Paris PM. EMS communications. In: Roush WR, ed. *Principles of EMS Systems.* Dallas, Tex: American College of Emergency Physicians; 1989.

Stewart C. Communications with emergency medical services providers. *Emerg Med Clin North Am.* 1990; 8:103–117.

Suter RE. Who's calling the shots? A theoretical analysis of EMS operations control. *Prehospital Disaster Med.* 1992;7:396–399.

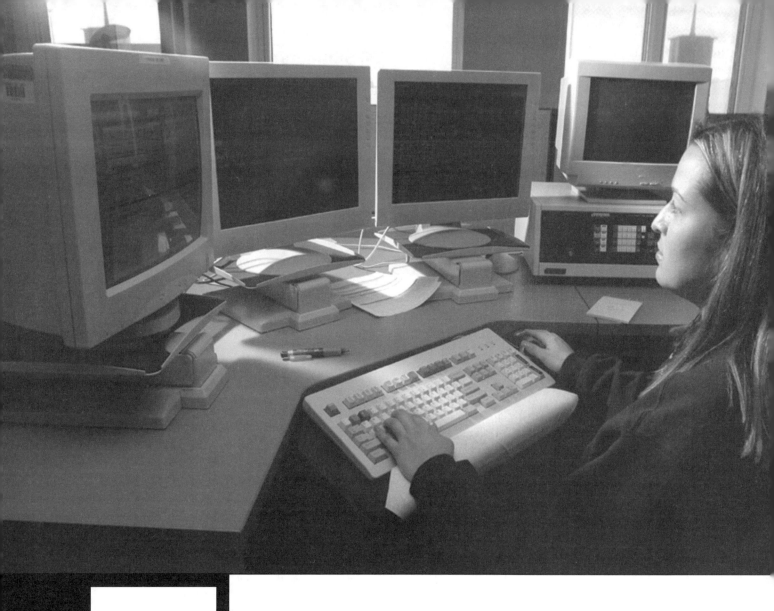

10 Emergency Medical Dispatch

Victoria A. Maguire, EMT-P, EMD-I
James N. Pruden, MD, FACEP

Principles of This Chapter

After reading this chapter, you should be able to:

- Explain the history of EMS dispatch.
- Describe the basic configuration of an EMS communications system.
- Recall the components of an emergency medical dispatch program.
- Discuss the enhancements of communications systems, such as ANI, ALI, and AVL.

THE EMS COMMUNICATIONS CENTER IS ONE OF THE MOST important links in the overall EMS system, and it is sometimes the most overlooked with regard to medical oversight. The communications center is the central nervous system of any EMS system; without a strong and stable central nervous system, the overall system will fail. The EMS communications center is the first link in the chain of survival of those patients who need access to emergency medical care. The objective of this chapter is to provide an understanding of how the EMS communications center functions, with emphasis on personnel selection, emergency medical dispatching, system components, terminology, technology, and other considerations that have an impact on the effectiveness of this vital function. It is impossible to describe the ideal EMS communications center or system because so many factors affect the process, including telephone access numbers, locations and types of response vehicles (fire apparatus, ambulances, helicopters), coverage areas (urban versus rural), and other considerations.

The History of EMS Dispatch

The history of the development of EMS dispatch is entirely different from the history of EMS in general. To say that dispatch took a backseat to the advancements that the field saw initially would be an understatement.

When EMS was first put under the US Department of Transportation (DOT) in the late 1960s, little or no thought was given to dispatch. Most dispatch rooms or "alarm rooms" were hidden away in dark and cramped spaces, typically in basements of fire or police departments. Personnel who staffed these dispatch rooms were police and fire dispatchers or lay personnel, secretaries or clerks, who were given additional responsibilities of dispatching. There was no special training provided to perform the duties. The perception of what a dispatcher did was to answer a telephone and then relay the information to the field providers who were responding. Secretaries and clerks already knew how to answer the telephone, and relaying information on a radio to field personnel was the same thing as talking on a telephone. The theory was that police and fire department personnel did not need any additional training because they were already dispatching police units and fire apparatus. The motto of the day was probably something like, "You call, we haul."

In the 1970s things began to change in the field, as well as in dispatch. In dispatch the first documented case of the use of prearrival instructions occurred in 1974 in Phoenix. A baby fell into a pool, and, when the family called the Phoenix Fire Department for help, a paramedic was put on the telephone with the family and successfully provided CPR instructions while EMS resources were being dispatched. As word of this event spread, fire departments attempted to staff the dispatch rooms with medical personnel whenever possible to provide self-help instructions over the telephone until EMS could arrive on the scene. In 1976, the DOT released the first guidelines for curriculum for emergency medical dispatching. Other dispatching programs soon developed. In 1978 the first edition of the **Medical Priority Dispatching System (MPDS)™** was released. The MPDS is a protocol-driven system that was first used by the fire department in Salt Lake City, Utah. In 1981, the cities of Aurora, Colorado, and Seattle, Washington, introduced scripted treatment sequence protocols to be used by dispatching personnel. In the early 1980s, the Dallas Fire Department experimented with a nurse call screening program in an attempt to identify situations in which ambulances might not need to be dispatched. Unfortunately, an individual nurse call screener did not follow the policies and procedures of the center and refused to send EMS to 65-year-old woman who was having difficulty breathing. This one event ended the call screening program and was a catalyst for identifying possible problems in many other dispatch programs. In the late 1980s and early 1990s, other commercial dispatch programs were developed.

Prior to 1989 there were no national standards for emergency medical dispatching. That year, the American College of Emergency Physicians (ACEP) approved guidelines for EMS, including recognizing emergency medical dispatchers as a critical part of EMS. Subsequently, the National Association of EMS Physicians (NAEMSP) presented a position paper on the need for medical control in emergency medical dispatching, which stated that, "EMS physicians are responsible for the provision of education, training, protocols, critiques, leadership, testing, certification, decertification, standards, advice, and quality control through the official authoritative position within the prehospital system."[1] The American Society for Testing and Materials (ASTM) released "Standard Practice for Emergency Medical Dispatch Management" in 1994, and in 1995 revised that document to further support the involvement of medical control in the oversight of the dispatching centers. The current version was published in 2001.[2]

Another big milestone for emergency medical dispatch occurred in 1992, when the American Heart Association recognized dispatch life support (DLS) in its 1992 "Guidelines for CPR and Emergency Cardiac Care," which was published in the *Journal of the American Medical Association*.[3] This publication recognized the critical role of the emergency medical dispatcher in providing CPR instructions over the telephone to callers reporting a patient in cardiac arrest. The decade of the 1990s brought much-needed attention to the area of dispatch. Telecommunications technology was in full bloom, with advancements in computer science happening every day. In many cases, the communications center was becoming the showcase of many public safety agencies. More attention was being paid to the hiring and training of new personnel, and no longer were dispatchers "out of sight, out of mind." In fact, many agency managers say that the dispatcher is the ultimate "minute-by-minute manager" of all agency resources.

Configuration

The basic configuration of an EMS communications system includes the following:

- An access telephone number
- A dispatcher
- A response crew with a vehicle

As simple as this design looks, its implementation is very complex. The question of the access number is sometimes related to politics and resources. There are some jurisdictions for which "home rule" is a critical consideration. In these areas, there might not be 911 access, but a local 7-digit number that a person must call for assistance. Sometimes that local number is the same for police, fire, and medical emergencies, and sometimes there are different telephone numbers for all three services.

In some systems, calls go through a **public safety answering point (PSAP),** which answers the incoming 911 calls and might or might not be responsible for dispatching resources. Some PSAPs act as a central answering point for all incoming 911 calls, and personnel interrogate callers to find out if they have a police, fire, or medical emergency need and then transfer them to the correct agency for actual dispatch. In some cases, the PSAP is a **central dispatch authority,** which not only acts as the primary call-taker for police, fire, and medical calls but also is responsible for dispatching the appropriate resources. Depending on its size, the PSAP might have one person or several persons on duty. If there is one dispatcher for all three services (police, fire, and EMS), that dispatcher must prioritize which call will go out first. Using an example of motor vehicle crash with a fire or an entrapment, consider the options that might go through the dispatcher's decision-making process. If the system uses a volunteer ambulance service, the dispatcher might put the ambulance call out first because it might have the longest response time. But if the crash occurred on a heavily traveled route where traffic control is an immediate and intense concern, the police might be dispatched first. But, if the car went down an embankment into a residential area and an ensuing fire put sleeping residents or property at risk, the first call might go out to the fire department. Training, protocols, and computer systems designed to consider these factors have a significant role. The role of the dispatcher is another issue that is more complex than it looks. At many PSAPs, there are separate dispatchers for each of the three services. The call-taker who receives the initial call at the PSAP routes the call to the appropriate dispatcher. There could be one, two, or several dispatchers for each service. It is not uncommon for one EMS dispatcher to receive the call and collect appropriate data while another dispatcher alerts a response crew.

Determining the appropriate response to a call requires some structure. The response options include redirecting the call to another agency (eg, the poison center), giving first aid (prearrival) instruction, dispatching a responder to evaluate the situation, dispatching a BLS crew, or dispatching an ALS crew. Not all communications centers have the resources to access all of these options. It is a critical function of the medical director to become involved with the response configuration of EMS calls. The response to EMS calls should be a well-thought-out, preplanned process. The medical director should meet with the appropriate agency (police, fire, EMS) heads to discuss the response configuration for the service area. Response times, geographic boundaries, medical first response (including use of police officers or firefighters with AEDs), level of out-of-hospital care (BLS versus ALS), trauma center location, air medical support, local hospital standard of care, and patient outcome statistics based on chief complaint types are just a few factors that must be considered when making decisions about response configurations. These configuration considerations include what resources to send (eg, first response and transporting services, or transporting services only) and the response manner (eg, emergency or nonemergency) for those vehicles. Every EMS system is different and needs local attention and physician participation in the development of specifics.

Prearrival Instructions

Since their first recorded use in 1974, prearrival instructions have undergone an interesting evolutionary process. Prearrival instructions began as instructions that were provided by dispatching personnel or medical personnel who would step in to help callers who needed immediate lifesaving instructions. The prearrival instructions were typically given for patients believed to be experiencing cardiac or respiratory arrest, choking, severe hemorrhage, or childbirth. Typically, these instructions were given off the cuff by dispatching personnel trying to assist the caller. The problem with doing prearrival instructions in this manner was that the personnel giving the instructions often used terminology or examples of how to do certain procedures that confused the nonmedically trained caller. It was also awkward for trained

medical personnel to give these instructions in the dispatching environment because they were out of their clinical element. To provide instructions over the telephone in a nonvisual environment is very difficult for medical personnel who are used to hands-on patient care. When scripted prearrival instructions were made available, such as those in the MPDS, it was found that the scripted prearrival instructions that were written for a layperson without medical training were much easier for the caller to understand and to follow. It also proved that prearrival instructions could be given to a nonmedically trained caller by a emergency medical dispatcher who had the appropriate training and certification and had the appropriate prearrival instructions to read. One of the initial concerns from a number of agencies was that prearrival instructions were dangerous and could result in liability for the agency that provided them. Many agencies initially refused to let their personnel provide prearrival instructions in the late 1970s and early 1980s because of this concern. What these agencies found out was that their concerns were completely unfounded. In fact, what happened was that agencies that did not provide prearrival instructions were the ones facing liability.

A popular television show in the 1980s called "Rescue 911" captured the value of well-thought-out instructions being given to patients as they awaited the arrival of EMS personnel. Although the show portrayed only those circumstances in which the victim survived, it did serve a purpose in demonstrating that this kind of service could be effective. This television show educated the general public on what to expect when calling 911 with a medical emergency. Because of the show's popularity, the expectation of the general public helped prearrival instructions become a national standard. Unfortunately, well-thought-out, consistent prearrival instructions were the exception rather than the rule. Even today, a fair proportion of the PSAPs are not in a position to provide prearrival instructions effectively. A recent ruling by the Federal Communications Commission mandated that PSAPs be prepared to provide prearrival instructions. Unfortunately, the implementation of that rule has been postponed.

Even though prearrival instructions are a national standard, there are still many agencies that do not provide them. In many small systems, the only dispatcher available is responsible for the dispatch of police and fire response, as well as EMS. When the call involves only a medical situation and there are no other calls coming up, it is possible to provide instructions. But when a more generalized response (as in a building fire) is needed, the need to coordinate the dispatch of police and fire resources will likely take precedence over the lone dispatcher's ability to provide patient management instructions.

Unfortunately, the setup of many of the PSAPs has the caller talking to someone other than the **emergency medical dispatcher (EMD)** at first. The call is received by the central call-taker (who in many cases is not trained as an EMD) and is then transferred to the EMS dispatcher who might or might not be in a position to provide prearrival instructions. The opportunity to have direct communication with the caller is lost. Additionally, the volume of calls received at a dispatch center might limit the amount of time the EMS dispatcher has to commit to one call.

In other systems, there is a central police dispatcher who forwards information about calls to either the fire department or the EMS dispatcher. This frees up the central dispatcher and allows the appropriate service to dispatch its own resources. In this configuration, the EMS dispatcher gets only basic information about the call and does not get a chance to speak to the caller.

There are several different proprietary programs that provide guidelines and scripts for call-taking questions, dispatch priority determination, and prearrival instructions. They include the MPDS™ and the APCO guide cards from the Association of Public-Safety Communications Officials, among others. These cards generally categorize the nature of the complaint with simple headings — "Animal Bite," "Chest Pain," and "Trouble Breathing." The dispatcher asks specific questions on the card, such as, "Is the patient choking?" "Can the patient talk?" "Is the patient turning blue?" The answers to the questions then determine the level of response (**Figure 10-1**), as well as lead to the prearrival instructions that the dispatcher gives to the caller (**Figure 10-2**). Some jurisdictions have chosen to develop their own guide cards.

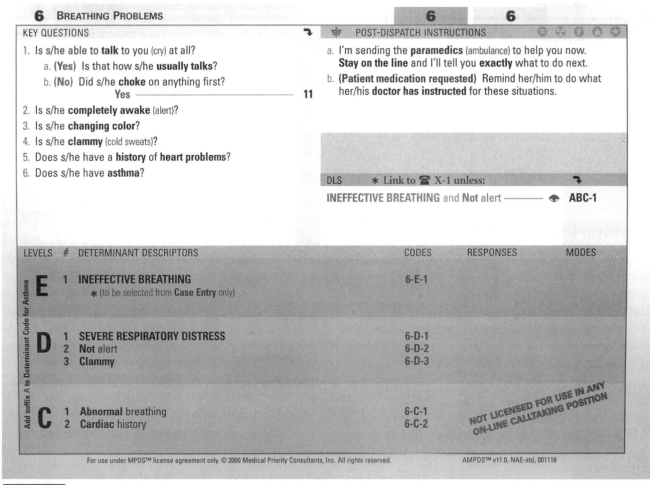

Figure 10-1 As a first step in providing prearrival instructions, the dispatcher will need to get more information from the caller. This sample from the MPDS™ system lists the questions to ask at the top of the card; the caller's answers then determine the level of response, as indicated at the bottom of the card. (Copyright 2000, Medical Priority Consultants, Inc. Reprinted with permission. http://www.prioritydispatch.net/)

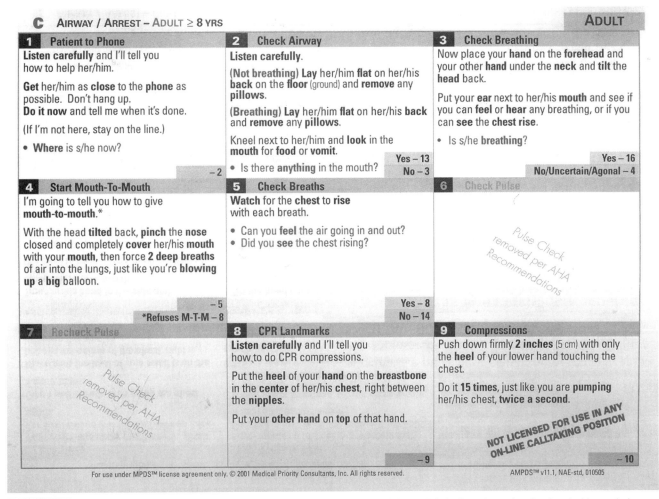

Figure 10-2 Sample prearrival instructions from the MPDS™ system. (Copyright 2001, Medical Priority Consultants, Inc. Reprinted with permission. http://www.prioritydispatch.net/)

In many systems, call prioritization and prearrival instructions are supplemented by computer-aided dispatch (CAD), which exists as a software package in many EMS dispatch systems (**Figure 10-3**).

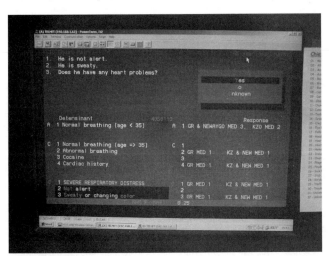

Figure 10-3 Computer-aided dispatch programs are used to supplement call prioritization and prearrival instructions in many EMS systems.

Caller Information

With few exceptions, the most important piece of information for a call-taker to obtain is the physical location of where the help is needed. Without an address and call-back telephone information, it is difficult to send help. Once the location is known, then moving on to specific problem-type information is appropriate.

One of the most important things to realize when gathering information on a chief complaint or problem type is that this information will result in the prioritization of the call, the resources that are sent, the prearrival instructions that are provided, and responder information, as well as taking care of scene safety implications. Therefore it is critical that a system of protocols is in place to make sure that the interrogation of the caller is uniform and consistent no matter which call-taker is handling the call. Using established, proven protocol systems provides for everything mentioned earlier and allows for local medical oversight.

Information about the nature of the call is important for determining the behavior of the responders and the kinds of resources to send. For example, a dispatcher receives a call about someone with trouble breathing, so questions might include, "Is the patient breathing?" "Is the patient awake?" "Does the patient have any known medical conditions (asthma, heart disease)?" "Does the patient use any medications for this condition, and if so, has he or she taken it? Does he or she have access to it?" In a response to a victim of a gunshot wound, the police should also be dispatched. Other questions include whether there is still shooting going on, if the wound was self-inflicted, if the gun is still at the scene, and so on (**Figure 10-4**).

Additional Dispatch Center Functions

There are other functions that dispatch centers perform beyond that of sending emergency resources to people in need. Some centers collect and disseminate information regarding the diversion status of local health care facilities. In times of mass-casualty incidents, the dispatch centers are frequently critical in coordinating the movement of resources to the scene, alerting receiving hospitals of the potential for incoming patients, and ascertaining the capabilities of these hospitals to take injured patients.

Quality Improvement

In order for the emergency medical dispatch division of the communications center to be successful, there must be a quality assurance/quality improvement (QI) program in place. Quality review is a critical function in any emergency dispatch system, and it is typically overlooked or is a very low priority. One of the first things that should be discussed with the agency administration as well as the line personnel is that QI is not a punitive process. They have to be reassured that QI is a positive improvement tool. There are three basic phases of the QI process, as outlined

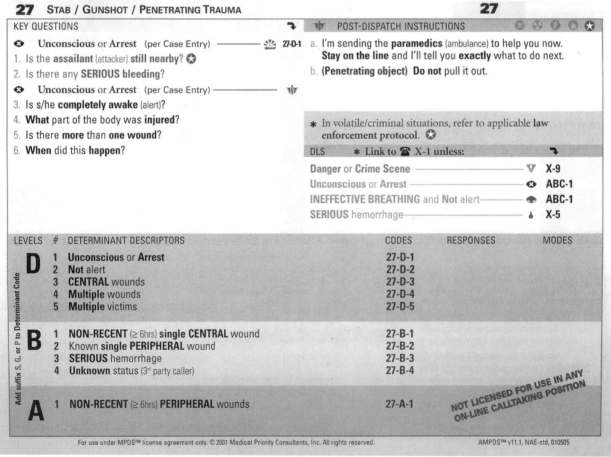

Figure 10-4 Sample questions and responses for a call related to a shooting or stabbing. (Copyright 2001, Medical Priority Consultants, Inc. Reprinted with permission. http://www.prioritydispatch.net/)

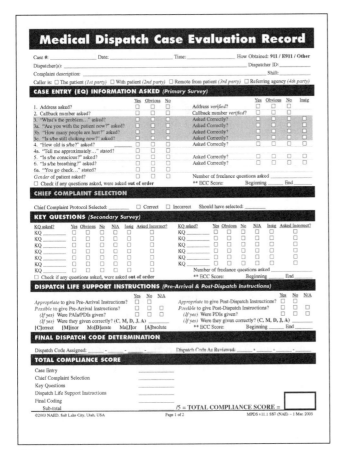

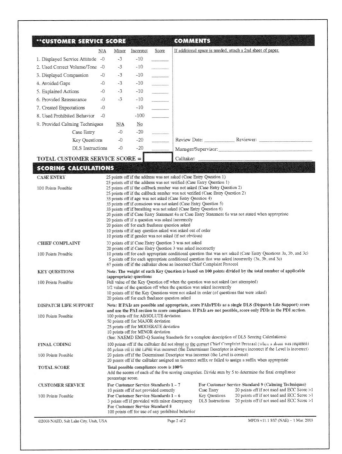

Figure 10-5 Sample check-off form that can be used to facilitate retrospective review of the calls handled by an EMD. (The National Academies of Emergency Dispatch. Available at: http://www.naemd.org/framesetR.html.)

here and described in Chapter 6, "Medical Oversight and Accountability."

Prospective Phase

The prospective phase includes the criteria for employment. This includes the hiring process and the initial orientation, training, and certification of the new employee. It also includes the selection and implementation of policies, procedures, and protocols (both administrative and EMD) that will be used in the communications center.

Concurrent Phase

The concurrent phase begins when the EMD starts taking emergency calls. It includes medical oversight, remedial education, and continuing education as needed. Direct observation is a standard way of providing feedback in the concurrent phase of QI. Besides seeing how effective the dispatchers are, direct observation allows a supervisor to assess ergonomic considerations (how many times the dispatcher has to roll from one area to another, flip

through screens, or collect or record information that is already collected or recorded elsewhere) and protocol compliance.

Retrospective Phase

The retrospective phase is the review of calls that have been handled by the EMD. Tape review is one of the best ways to accomplish this. The dispatch supervisor, medical director, or some other designee reviews a certain percentage of the calls to the dispatcher. These calls can be reviewed on the basis of particular worker, particular shift, or some other parameter. A predetermined check-off sheet should be developed to facilitate the review. This sheet can include time taken to handle the call, appropriateness of the resources dispatched, adequacy and completeness of the information recorded, appropriateness in selection and provision of prearrival instructions, clarity of communication, and so on (**Figure 10-5**).

There are commercially available quality assurance programs. Two of the most sophisticated and popular quality assurance tools for emergency medical dispatch are ProQA®, which is a computerized version of the MPDS protocols, and AQUA®. Both are distributed by Medical Priority Consultants Inc. No matter what tool is used, the reviews must be consistent in feedback and timely and constructive, not destructive.

Software and Hardware

Over the past 20 years, software and hardware advances have provided many essential tools to dispatching personnel. With many modern dispatch systems, the job of the dispatcher is greatly facilitated with these advancements. New technology such as ANI (automatic number identification), ALI (automatic location identification), and/or enhanced 911 (E911) give information about the call's point of origin. This is helpful if the call is interrupted, the caller is incoherent or incapacitated, or if the caller speaks a language not known to the EMD.

There are services that help with language barrier problems. For example, telephone companies and translation services provide a subscription language line program. When a caller is speaking a foreign language, the dispatcher calls the translation service, they briefly discuss the problem, and then an interpreter is added to the line.

Computer technology helps the dispatcher identify which resource is closest to the location of the request by using mapping, global positioning, or automatic vehicle locator (AVL) programs.

Communications System Issues

In establishing an effective and efficient communications system, one of the first things that should be accomplished is to set essential and obtainable goals. These goals should include but not be limited to the following:

- Communications center personnel hiring, orientation, and education practices
- Selection of the correct protocol or guide-card system that provides prioritization of EMS calls and prearrival instructions, followed by the implementation of that system
- Appropriate response times for the service area covered by local EMS, as they relate to the priority of the call
- Assorted policies and procedures that address daily operations of the communications center, including a communications center disaster plan

It is also important to achieve consistency in the EMD's communications with the public. The EMD must be trained in how to deal with callers who are emotionally distraught or verbally abusive. The EMD must understand the need for customer service and how to defuse an emotionally charged caller. Special training in dealing with callers in crisis is strongly recommended. The EMD must realize that he or she is the first contact with the 911 community and, as such, can set the tone of the entire encounter within the first few seconds.

The EMD must also be trained to interact with other agencies, public officials, and the media in a positive and professional manner. Developing good working relationships with all of these contacts will reduce the potential for negative press and liability. Additionally, education of the public through community education programs and public service announcements on how to use the 911 system correctly can also help alleviate some of the mystery and even abuse that sometimes surrounds the use of a 911 system.

Another issue for a communications system is that of the politics surrounding the day-to-day operations of the communications center. In many areas, the 911 communications center has control of the resources of many different departments and agencies. It is not uncommon to see a struggle for control over deployment of resources. This is especially seen in multi-jurisdictional communications centers where the center is responsible for dispatching multiple police, fire, and EMS agencies. These centers often have challenges meeting every police, fire, and EMS chief's specific requirements for deployment for their service areas. Many times these requirements are not universal, but are very specific to each jurisdiction and differ from scenario to scenario. An example of this is a call for a traffic accident with injuries. The jurisdiction where the accident occurs will dictate how the police department responds and with how many officers. The fire department in that same jurisdiction might or might not respond depending on whether it is a paid, full-time service or a volunteer service or if it has medical training or extrication equipment. The EMS service for that jurisdiction might or might not be the fire department. If it is not, then who responds and how will depend on whether it is a basic life support, intermediate life support, or advanced life support agency, or a combination thereof. What the communications center is required to do in a very short period of time is to decide who goes, how they go, how many of them go, and when they go — no small task. That, along with the number of different types of calls that come into the communications center, indicates the deployment challenges these centers deal with every day. The medical director must understand how these issues affect the day-to-day operation of the communications center, as well as the politics involved in working with each of the different agencies. This is a critical area of involvement for the medical director if he or she is to be successful in discharging the duties of medical oversight of dispatch activities. One of the most effective ways to deal with this challenge is to have a very active task force or committee made up of agency heads that meets regularly to discuss issues and solve problems. Standard operating policies and procedures that deal with daily operation are also a must for any communications center — no matter how large or small.

Personnel

An agency might have a multimillion-dollar communications system and communications center, but the most important piece of the communications system is the personnel who staff it. Even though the EMD position is critical, filling that position with sophisticated personnel has not always been a high priority of many agencies. The pay has also been historically low. In the past, it might have been filled by personnel who defaulted into the dispatching position. In fact, this happened so frequently in the past that dispatch became known as the "dumping ground" for personnel who were no longer able to function as field providers — for example, a police officer, firefighter, or paramedic who was physically injured while on duty and could no longer physically perform his or her duties in the field. There were also cases in which field providers were incompetent in the field and were put into dispatch. Finally, it was not uncommon to see dispatch used as a disciplinary tool for field personnel who were in a corrective action situation. Needless to say, personnel who were "dumped" into dispatch did not necessarily have the skills or aptitude to do the job, nor did they want to be there — which potentially affected the quality of the job they were performing. Unfortunately, this can still be seen in isolated cases today. Dr. Jeff Clawson, a longtime proponent of emergency medical dispatch, believes that there is positive movement toward changing the dumping ground mentality that has plagued dispatch staffing in the past. In his book, *Principles of Emergency Medical Dispatch,* he states,

> In response to the growing acceptance of priority dispatch, the standards of acceptable system design for communication centers have been redefined. No longer is it tolerable for the dispatch office to be the receptacle of marginal or disciplined field

providers. Once viewed as a good location for organizational dumping of sick or injured personnel, the up-to-date communication center now enjoys increased levels of respect and professionalism.[4]

The qualifications and requirements for personnel in dispatch positions must be carefully defined. Dispatchers ultimately are responsible for the minute-by-minute management of all the resources in the EMS system and must have the correct background, personality, education, and problem-solving skills to do the job correctly. Medical oversight, supervisory oversight, and the correct tools (ie, telecommunications equipment, maps, cross-reference material, policies, and procedures) must also be considered when planning for a successful communications center operation. Training of personnel once they are employed by the communications center is another critical area. In the past, the training frequently consisted of sitting with a senior dispatcher and doing what the senior dispatcher did for a specified period of time. Even though the trainer might have been an excellent dispatcher, the new dispatcher would only be trained in the calls that came across during that apprenticeship period.

Fortunately for many dispatch centers, there are more stringent training requirements in place. In Newark, New Jersey, the training module consists of a 40-hour basic telecommunications course, 32 hours of emergency medical dispatch training, 8 hours of CPR training, and extensive on-the-job training with a seasoned dispatcher. In addition, the dispatchers are trained in the use of a set of programmed question and answer cards that guide the collection of information.

Medical Oversight

The medical oversight of EMS dispatch is inherently an offline activity. In some major dispatch centers, there is a physician to deal with situations not covered by EMS protocols and prearrival instructions, but that is a luxury most systems do not have.

This could change as it becomes more of a standard to consider other options besides only transporting patients to hospitals. One only has to consider the 911 call for a diabetic patient who is hypoglycemic. The paramedics typically arrive and treat the patient to the point of full recovery. In many systems today, that patient would end up still being transported to the hospital. It might be more appropriate to have someone coordinate followup with that patient's primary caregiver than it is to go to the hospital. It would be critical in this kind of system for the medical director to establish parameters for release of the patient, parameters for dealing with patient refusal (including the consideration of direct physician contact when the refusal seems medically unwise), and so on.

Among the things that the medical director should consider in an EMS dispatch system are:

- Parameters for release against medical advice
- The selection/choice of using medical dispatch protocols or guide cards
- The appropriateness of prearrival instructions through direct observation or tape review (QI activities), especially for situations that do not fall directly into the algorithms of the guide cards
- Certifications and training of the dispatchers
- Response time compliance
- Turnaround times

Anyone with experience in the delivery of emergency care is intimately familiar with the importance placed on turnaround times. This certainly holds true in EMS dispatch. The turnaround times include the time from receipt of the call to the dispatch of a resource, which is generally accepted to be 30 to 45 seconds. Other times include:

- En route time (the time it takes the crew to depart from the time of dispatch)
- Arrival at scene time (this might also consider the interval from arrival at the scene to the time of patient contact, which is an issue in difficult access areas like high-rise buildings, buildings without an elevator, or where weather, entrapment, or wide-open spaces make immediate patient contact problematic)
- Depart scene time
- Hospital arrival
- Availability — the time the crew is available to take the next call or assignment

These times are then used to calculate the system response intervals.

FCC Rulings

The Federal Communications Commission (FCC) has many standard operating procedures and policies regarding communication and equipment practices.

The FCC is also responsible for the licensing of radio frequencies and radio equipment (www.fcc.gov).

Global Positioning System

Global positioning system (GPS) satellites are used by sophisticated communications systems to track the real-time location of their field resources. With GPS, dispatchers do not need to poll the field units' locations in order to give a call to the closest unit, which decreases the amount of time it takes to dispatch a call. It also provides for a security function when coupled with silent radio alarms for crews who might be involved in unsafe scene calls.

Cellular Telephones

Cellular telephones have become a widely used backup system to sometimes overloaded and congested radio frequencies. Many systems use cellular telephones for communication ranging from nonessential to critical, sensitive information. Some EMS systems use cellular technology to transmit 12-lead ECGs from the field to the hospital. Cellular telephones also create a challenge for the communications center when used by people calling 911. Unlike landline telephones, most cellular telephones are not capable of providing ANI and ALI information. Additionally, the possibility of the cellular telephone's signal being switched from one tower site to another increases the difficulty of the caller even getting in touch with the correct 911 center. New technology implemented in the early 2000s allows cellular phones to transmit location information based on GPS technology.

Summary

The communications system and communications center make up the central nervous system of any EMS system. Without an effective and efficient communications system, the EMS system will fail to function at an optimal level. It is important for the medical director to understand the vital role and function of the communications system and communications centers in the overall "health" of the EMS system.

References

1. National Association of Emergency Medical Services Physicians. Position paper: emergency medical dispatching. *Prehospital Disaster Med.* 1989;4:163–166.

2. American Society for Testing and Materials. F1258-95 (2001) Standard practice for emergency medical dispatch. *Annual Book of ASTM Standards.* West Conshohocken, Penn: ASTM; 2001.

3. American Heart Association Emergency Cardiac Committee and Subcommittees. Guidelines for cardiopulmonary resuscitation and emergency cardiac care, II: adult basic life support. *JAMA.* 1992;268: 2184–2198.

4. Clawson JJ, Dernocoeur KB. *Principles of Emergency Medical Dispatch.* 3rd ed. Salt Lake City, Utah: Liberty Press; 2000.

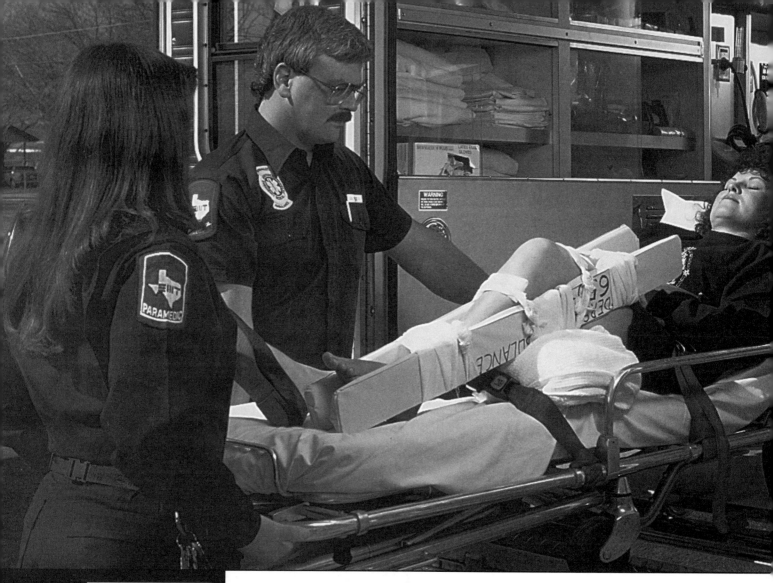

11

Medical Record Documentation and EMS Information Systems

Greg D. Mears, MD, FACEP

Principles of This Chapter

After reading this chapter, you should be able to:

- Explain the methods and components of EMS record documentation and information systems.
- Describe the two keys to quality documentation.
- Discuss the aspects of quality management and documents, as well as legal and security matters.

SINCE THE EARLY DAYS OF OUT-OF-HOSPITAL CARE, PROVIDERS have been less than enthusiastic concerning documentation. Examples of comments include:

- "I don't want to waste my time writing. I'm here to take care of patients."
- "This paperwork is killing me! I've just got too many other things to do, and the next call is stacked."
- "I always fill out these forms, and no one ever reads them when I leave them at the hospital."

These lamentations are understandable, and they often come from all levels of personnel and administration. But while the time spent preparing a comprehensive summary of patient care during an EMS run is both time-consuming and tedious, the run report itself is not a form of punishment for the out-of-hospital provider. Rather, it is necessary legal documentation of the EMS services provided and an integral part of patient care that is central to the maintenance, design, and improvement of an EMS system. The formal integration of data and/or documentation from several sources within an EMS system is called an **EMS information system.**

Historical Perspective

Emergency medical services are, in theory, no different from the rest of the health care field, although with respect to documentation and business structure, they are far behind. Federal and state legislation have mandated hospitals, clinics, physicians, and other health care providers to provide extensive documentation for several years. This documentation is typically associated with medical, legal, business modeling, or reimbursement needs. EMS in many areas grew from either a volunteer or tax-based approach. Although these funding streams are greatly different, both required less detail with respect to documentation because few bills were generated, and EMS was historically much less likely to be implicated in medical liability cases.

As the population grows, so does the demand for services, and there is competition with other public health and community needs. EMS is no longer isolated as an expensive source of transportation to the hospital. It is held accountable for its response times, the quality of its service, and the medical care it provides and for its cost or value to the customer. It is held to the standards of other medical specialties to prove its effect on patient outcome as a justification for its existence. Finally, as part of the health care system, EMS is required to interact with the rest of the system at the local hospital and regional, state, and federal levels through the exchange of information.

Several documents have been developed nationally either from legislative initiatives or national consensus projects and have become the models for documentation of EMS services and patient care. Several events have defined the EMS information system.

1973 EMS Enactment

In 1973, the Department of Health, Education, and Welfare defined the components of an EMS system (see Chapter 1, "History of EMS: Foundations of a System"). Although an information system was not listed as one of the 15 components, each component was shaped or defined as a piece to a puzzle. The completed puzzle required a significant amount of data to interact and monitor each of the pieces or components. Even more importantly, federal funding was provided to agencies that modeled their systems after these components. This was the first legislation for EMS, which required data or documentation of services through a coordinated patient record and a formal review and evaluation process (now referred to as quality management). These components were revised with the 1996 "EMS Agenda for the Future."

1991 Utstein

In 1991, the American Heart Association published "Recommended Guidelines for Uniform Reporting of Data from Out-of-Hospital Cardiac Arrest: The Utstein Style." This was the first major document to specifically address EMS systems and their performance with respect to patient outcome. Other documents had addressed patient outcome as an end point, but the Utstein Criteria comprised a standard data set with standard definitions for measuring cardiac arrest survival across systems. The Utstein Criteria required the exchange of information among the 911 dispatch center, the EMS system, and the hospital.

1993 Uniform Prehospital Dataset

In 1993, the National Highway Traffic Safety Administration (NHTSA) developed a consensus document that defined 81 elements important to an EMS information system. Of the 81 elements, 49 were considered essential and 32 were considered desirable. These elements were created in an effort to allow an EMS system to compare itself with respect to the service, patient care, personnel performance, patient outcome, and data linkage to other organizations or larger data sets. Perhaps even more important than the elements themselves is the creation of a standard definition for each element, which is critical for any information system.

1996 EMS Agenda for the Future

In 1996, NHTSA published "EMS Agenda for the Future." This is the most important modern EMS document to date in that it addresses EMS as a community-based health management system, fully integrated with the overall health care system. Included in this document were recommendations on the development of 14 distinct attributes of EMS (**Figure 11-1**). The goal of the document was to improve the quality of community health to achieve more appropriate use of acute health care resources, and yet allow EMS to remain as the public's emergency medical safety net. One of the 14 components addressed in the document was information systems.

Five recommendations for information systems were issued from the "EMS Agenda for the Future":

Figure 11-1 Attributes of EMS as a community-based health management system, from "EMS Agenda for the Future."

Integration of health services
EMS research
Legislation and regulation
System finance
Human resources
Medical direction
Education systems
Public education
Prevention
Public access
Communications systems
Clinical care
Information systems
Evaluation

- EMS must adopt a uniform set of data elements and definitions to facilitate multisystem evaluations and collaborative research.
- EMS must develop mechanisms to generate and transmit data that are valid, reliable, and accurate.
- EMS must develop and refine information systems that describe the entire EMS event so that patient outcomes and cost-effective issues can be determined.
- EMS should collaborate with other health care providers and community resources to develop integrated information systems.
- Information system users must provide feedback to those who generate data in the form of research results, quality improvement programs, and evaluations.

1998 EMS Agenda Implementation Guide

Finally, in 1998, NHTSA produced a followup document entitled, "The EMS Agenda for the Future Implementation Guide." This document took the 14 components of the original agenda and outlined suggestions or approaches to their development. This document reinforces the need for a standardized information system for every one of the essential EMS components identified. The information system, in fact, is the backbone for the development of these components. The future of EMS will be based on information systems.

2003 NHTSA Uniform Prehospital Dataset

In 2003, the NHTSA Uniform Prehospital Dataset was revised to Version 2 (**Figure 11-2**). Version 2 attempts to standardize data elements and definitions from a much

EMS Dataset
- Record Information
  - Patient care report number
- Unit/Agency Information
  - EMS agency number
  - Type of service requested
  - Primary role of the unit
  - Type of dispatch delay
  - Type of response delay
  - Type of scene delay
  - Type of transport delay
  - Type of turnaround delay
  - EMS unit call sign (radio number)
  - Response mode to scene
- Unit/Call Information
  - Complaint reported by dispatch
  - EMD performed
- Times
  - PSAP call date/time
  - Unit notified by dispatch date/time
  - Unit en route date/time
  - Unit arrived on scene date/time
  - Arrived at patient date/time
  - Unit left scene date/time
  - Patient arrived at destination date/time
  - Unit back in service date/time
  - Unit back at home location date/time

- Patient
  - Patient's home ZIP
  - Gender
  - Race
  - Ethnicity
  - Age
  - Age units
- Billing
  - Primary method of payment
  - CMS service level
  - Condition code number
- Scene
  - Number of patients at scene
  - Mass casualty incident
  - Incident location type
  - Incident ZIP code
- Situation
  - Prior aid
  - Prior aid performed by
  - Outcome of the prior aid
  - Injury present
  - Complaint anatomic location
  - Complaint organ agency
  - Primary symptom
  - Other associated symptoms
  - Provider's primary impression
  - Provider's secondary impression

- Situation/Trauma
  - Cause of injury
- Situation/CPR
  - Cardiac arrest
  - Cardiac arrest etiology
  - Resuscitation attempted
- Medical History
  - Barriers to patient care
  - Alcohol/drug use indicators
- Intervention/Medication
  - Medication given
  - Medication complication
- Intervention/Procedure
  - Procedure
  - Number of procedure attempts
  - Procedure successful
  - Procedure complication
- Disposition
  - Destination ZIP code
  - Incident/patient disposition
  - Transport mode from scene
  - Reason for choosing destination
  - Type of destination
- Outcome and Linkage
  - Emergency department disposition
  - Hospital disposition

Demographic Dataset
- Agency — General Information
  - EMS agency number
  - EMS agency state
  - EMS agency county
  - Level of service
  - Organizational type
  - Organization status

- Total service area size
- Total service area population
- 911 call volume/year
- EMS dispatch volume/year
- EMS transport volume/year
- EMS patient contact volume/year

- Agency — Contact Information
  - Agency contact ZIP code
- Agency — Vehicle Information
  - Unit call sign

larger perspective. This version defines EMS data elements as either associated with an EMS event or demographic data elements that describe an EMS system. Version 2 recommends a total of 64 EMS data elements and 14 demographic data elements to be collected nationally and more than 300 additional data elements for use by state and local EMS systems based on data need. The **National EMS Information System (NEMSIS) project** calls for the funding and development of a national EMS database that would collect, maintain, and provide reports on the national data elements. The national EMS database would receive data from each state and territorial EMS office, which would, in turn, receive data from local EMS systems. Reports from the national EMS database would provide descriptive in-

formation on EMS service and patient care delivery nationally to drive policy, resources, education, and funding. The NEMSIS project also calls for a data system to be implemented and maintained in every state EMS office. Reports from each state system would help to support each state's EMS initiatives. Information on the NEMSIS project and the NEMSIS data set can be found at www.nemsis.org.

Methods and Components

Although EMS systems across the country use many different methods of documentation, the overall goals and strategies are similar. A complete system must

Figure 11-3 EMS system documentation components.

Dispatch Center Data
- 911 call
- Computer-aided dispatch (CAD)
- Emergency medical dispatch
- Dispatch
- Prearrival instructions

Communications Data
- Dispatch and EMS
- EMS
- Hospital and EMS

Nonmedical Data
- Personnel records
- Scheduling
- Resources
- Vehicle maintenance
- Education
- Administrative policy and procedure
- Safety (OSHA, exposures, immunizations, etc.)
- Performance statistics
- Finance
- Grant funding
- Quality management
- History
- HIPAA
- Data use, maintenance, and linkage

Medical Care Information
- Dispatch
- Personnel
- Unit (vehicle)
- Incident
- Patient
- Past medical history
- Situation
- Assessment
- Intervention
- Disposition
- Medical direction
- Facility

Quality Management
- System
- Personnel
- Patient
- Peer review
- Outcomes
- Research

Financial
- Billing
- Reimbursement
- Grants
- Budget justification

Legal
- Legal requirements for documentation
- Record maintenance
- Liability
- Defense

maintain data that describe both system and patient care parameters, including dispatch, communications, nonpatient care issues, patient care issues, quality management, finance, and legal needs (**Figure 11-3**). This information is maintained manually or by computer with controlled access to authorized personnel.

Dispatch Center Data

The dispatch center can be a single entity, or it can be a **public safety answering point (PSAP)** that initially answers each 911 call and routes the call to the appropriate dispatch center. Regardless of the configuration, documentation of EMS service and patient care begins in the dispatch center. Information obtained from the 911 system documents a caller's phone number, and, if enhanced 911 (E911) service is available, the location of the land-based phone will be automatically provided to the dispatcher. This information is typically sent to the **computer-aided dispatch (CAD)** system, where it is stored with caller information and other system-specific data regarding the incident type and location. Emergency medical dispatch can assign a response priority to an EMS call based on a series of interactive questions between the caller and the dispatcher. This response priority can dictate the type and level of response among multiple agencies. Once an EMS response has been initiated, dispatch personnel can provide lifesaving prearrival instructions to the caller over the phone while EMS is en route. This is considered patient care and requires documentation. Several times are documented by the dispatch center and are important for documenting system response and performance. These times include: when the 911 call was received and answered; when the EMS response was initiated; and when the EMS unit was en route, arrived at the scene, left the scene, arrived at the hospital, left the hospital, returned to service, and was back in the service area. The times can also be recorded on the patient care report.

Communications Data

Documentation of all communication among dispatch, EMS, medical direction, and the hospital is required. Typically, the dispatch center records all voice communications with the 911 caller and the EMS responders. Additional communication occurs among EMS responders, online medical direction, and the hospital. The times and decisions associated with this communication must be documented with, or in addition to, the patient care report. These recordings should be monitored for the quality management of the system and for review of protocol compliance with respect to medical care.

Nonmedical Data

Extensive nonmedical documentation is created, maintained, archived, and analyzed with an EMS system. This includes individual personnel records that document hiring, firing, disciplinary actions, promotions, education accomplishments, certifications, contact information, and so on. This information should be connected to system data so that system performance and quality management issues identified through the performance improvement program can target personnel for improvement as needed. EMS systems have very complex vehicle maintenance and equipment allocation and distribution programs. Documentation of vehicle and personnel scheduling patterns is important for both day-to-day operations and as a component of disaster management, in which rapid mobilization of equipment and personnel is essential.

Several state and federal regulations address employee safety associated with the workplace and patient care. An Occupational Safety and Health Administration requirement associated with exposure to bloodborne pathogens is an example that requires detailed documentation and tracking. This requires specific policies and procedures related to operations and patient care, as well as mandatory continuing education for EMS personnel.

Each EMS system must document and maintain extensive operations and medical care protocols, policies, and procedures. An example of an operations policy is for the use of lights and sirens. An example of a medical care policy is for the use of air medical services. Many EMS systems have contractual requirements that are based on performance measures or statistics. This requires documentation and analysis of statistical and financial data generated from any point of the EMS event. Examples include response time parameters and service level requirements.

All EMS systems must document and maintain detailed statistics related to the cost of service. This includes *all* costs associated with providing EMS services. Included in this cost analysis are the costs of personnel, vehicles, equipment, reimbursement, bad debt, education, facility cost, tax subsidy, volunteer services, and any other cost associated with providing service. This information is useful for the detailed analysis of system cost and performance, as well as justification for improvements and to obtain grant funding.

As a component of the health care system, the EMS system should obtain and provide information to other health care entities. The ability to link EMS data with hospital, crash, trauma, medical examiner, and other registries provides additional information that can be used for performance improvement, outcomes measurement, research, and injury prevention initiatives. The threat of bioterrorism is a great example of the need for EMS information to be linked with public health initiatives as a component of a comprehensive bioterrorism surveillance system.

Medical Care Information

The documentation of an EMS encounter typically concentrates on patient care and expands beyond the actual patient contact to include dispatch and system information. A **patient care report (PCR)** includes dispatch information and the type of EMS response; the EMS personnel associated with the patient encounter; the EMS vehicle type and equipment; and the location of the incident. It also includes information about the patient, including the patient's name, gender, age, and address; the patient's medical history, including current medications and allergies; the situation that describes the need for EMS services, including the chief complaint; the assessment of the patient, including vital signs; any procedures or medications administered to the patient during the encounter; and the disposition of the patient. Finally, it includes information outlining any contact with medical direction and the facility associated with the disposition. The North Carolina PreHospital Medical Information System (PreMIS) paper form is an example of a documentation template for this information (**Figure 11-4**). The PCR should be standardized as much as possible for each state or region. This promotes improved documentation and standardization of care.

Quality Management

Quality management and performance improvement are critical components of an EMS system. EMS service and patient care must be evaluated from three different perspectives: the system, the personnel, and the patient. The EMS system must be evaluated and monitored based on providing a service, the level of that service, and the outcomes delivered to the community and the patient. Personnel must be evaluated for their performance in delivering quality care, following operational and patient care protocols, their success in skill performance, and the outcomes delivered to the community and the patient. The patient care should be evaluated based on the level of care provided, the

Figure 11-4 The North Carolina Prehospital Medical Information System form.

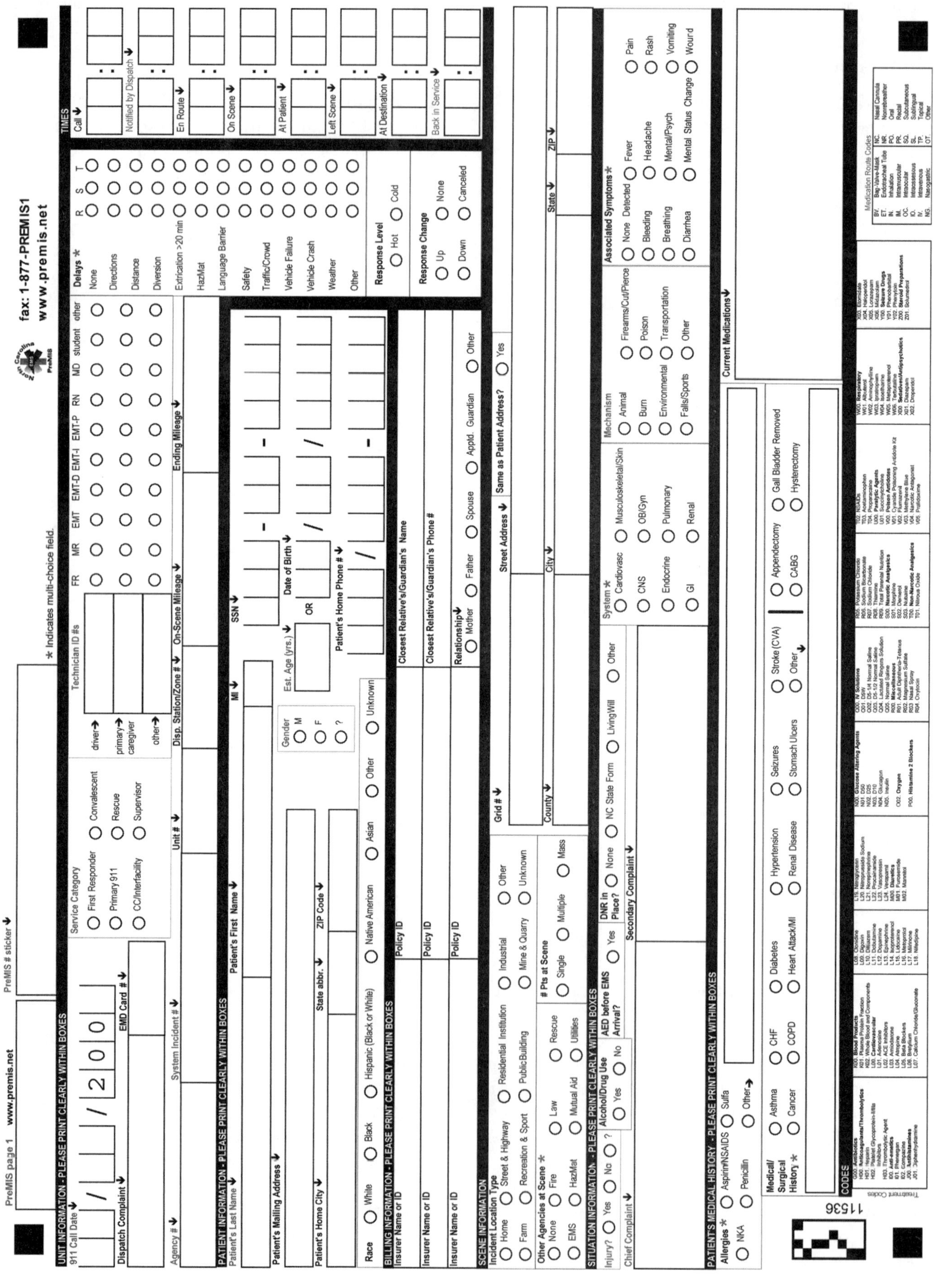

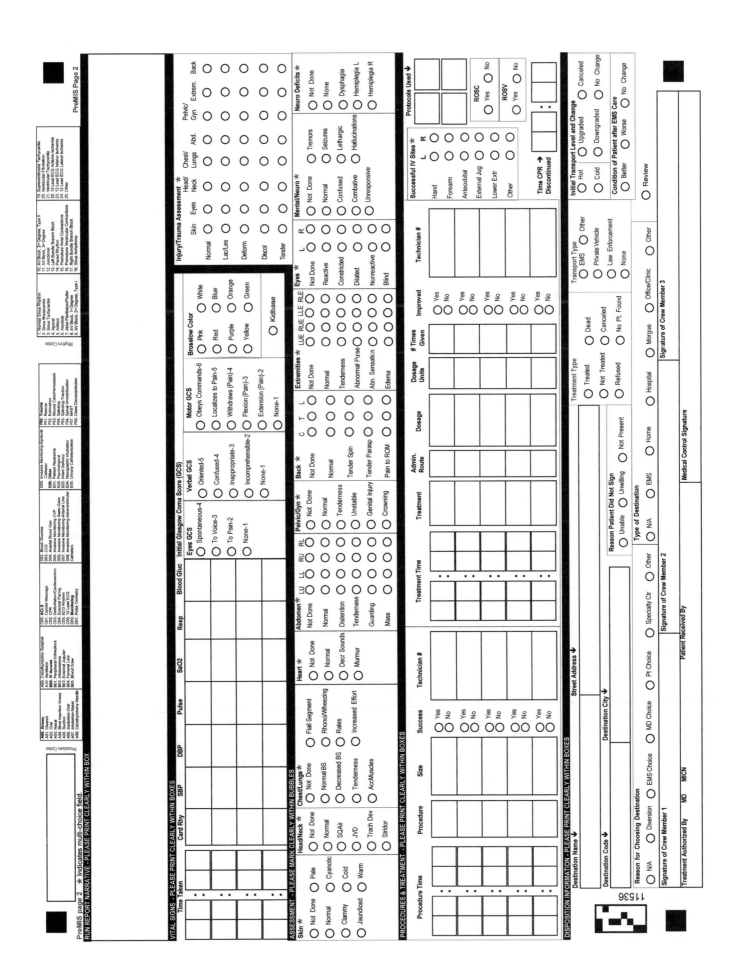

skills and service provided, and the outcomes delivered to the community and the patient.

Peer review is an important component of any quality management program. The discussion and evaluation of EMS encounters and patient care within a peer review structure are important for a system to evaluate and improve. Documentation of these peer review cases should be maintained according to the peer review laws of the state to protect the EMS system from legal discovery and the associated liability. Peer review should always end by identifying issues that need improvement and a plan for how to positively address them. Quality management is the evaluation of a component of service with the identification of any negative or positive issues associated with the event; the recommendation for interventions to correct negative concerns and promote positive findings; feedback to implement the interventions; and finally, reevaluation to make sure that the issue has been resolved.

Health care is migrating to an outcomes-based industry. Outcomes are typically defined in broad categories known as the six *D*s. These include:

- Death
- Disability
- Disease
- Discomfort
- Dissatisfaction
- Destitution

EMS systems should attempt to identify a specific outcome for each component of its service delivery and patient care. EMS must grasp outcomes and apply research principles to its service delivery and clinical care models. Documentation provides the data that drive research, and research should help define which data should be documented.

Legal Issues

Medical-legal issues must be considered when implementing a documentation or information system. Concerns fall into two major categories: legal requirements for data collection imposed by a federal or state agency, and potential defense in civil or criminal litigation. The EMS run report and dispatch records are integral parts of the patient's legal medical record because emergency medical intervention is considered to have started when someone tries to access the EMS system.

Legal risk associated with EMS services and clinical care can potentially involve the EMS system, the EMS personnel associated with the event, the medical director, or the political municipality. Criminal charges of assault and battery or illegal detention can be brought against EMS providers who attempt to treat and transport individuals against their will. Most individuals involved in EMS recognize that criminal charges are rarely a problem. On the other hand, the number of civil malpractice lawsuits is increasing. The potential for this problem was recognized during the early development of EMS-enabling legislation, and many states specifically enacted statutes to protect out-of-hospital providers from legal action. The original intent, apparently, was to protect EMS volunteers or Good Samaritans because they were providing care in emergency situations without expectation of reimbursement. In Ohio, for example, the law states that "no EMT or paramedic shall be liable in civil damages for administering emergency care or treatment outside of a hospital or doctor's office . . . unless the care, treatment . . . or assistance is provided in a manner constituting willful or wanton misconduct."

As EMS has moved away from volunteer organizations, out-of-hospital providers are more commonly full-time professionals. Because of this change, the courts — and to a lesser extent, civil law — now attempt to hold out-of-hospital providers to a higher standard. When tested in court, plaintiff's counsel will allege that, because the out-of-hospital provider is trained and certified, the conduct leading to poor patient outcome was willful (the provider knew what he or she was doing) and wanton (he or she did it anyway). These allegations, if accepted by a court, negate the out-of-hospital provider's statutory protection and place the provider and the EMS system at ever-increasing risk of litigation. Rather than depend on statutory protection, the system and the providers must depend on quality care and good documentation. The PCR is a key document and often a focal point in these claims. When a medical record is submitted in defense of civil litigation, the court generally assumes that anything not recorded was not performed. An objective, accurate, consistent, and complete PCR is pivotal to a strong defense.

These PCRs must be maintained by EMS systems for a period of time defined by the statute of limitations for each state. Typically, the statute of limitations is 3 years from the time of the event, but in the case of minors, it might extend to 3 years beyond the patient's 18th birthday. EMS systems should consult a local attorney to define the length of time records should be maintained.

Quality Documentation

There are two keys to good documentation: a functional form (paper or electronic) following the work flow of an EMS patient encounter, and its satisfactory completion. When designing a run report, it is useful to allow as much information as possible to be recorded by a simple check mark or filled-in box. There will be higher compliance with a chart requiring limited writing. Computerized forms allow predefined lists to be created and provide integrated logic and error-checking capabilities that can improve data accuracy and efficiency and speed.

Complete and proper documentation enhances the safe and orderly transfer of responsibility for medical care from the out-of-hospital provider to the physician in the emergency department. Vital information about the patient prior to arrival at the hospital can be lost if it is not precisely documented by the out-of-hospital provider. A rapid deterioration in the patient's condition might not be recognized without reference to baseline field data recorded on the run report. Paperwork should never interfere with patient care, but the PCR must be completed before EMS personnel leave the hospital.

To be useful, a PCR must be legible. Clear and accurate documentation also allows for more accurate quality management to evaluate system performance and clinical care.

EMS systems should incorporate time for the completion of the PCR into their operational structure. Documentation is most efficient and accurate if it is performed immediately after the encounter by the same EMS personnel who provided the care. Computerized systems can increase the speed and efficiency of documentation. All data that can be captured electronically should be transferred into the PCR electronically. Systems should strive to avoid dual entry of any data that can be provided electronically. With the computerization of health care, the expansion of the Internet, and the proliferation of handheld computing devices, EMS documentation is experiencing a paradigm shift.

Any successful documentation system must be well supported and have detailed instruction and user manuals. The data set must be well defined and documented.

Security

Security of an EMS information system is critical and can be split into the security and confidentiality of the patient's information and the security and confidentiality of the EMS system's information.

EMS system security is important for many reasons. EMS is a political entity and is subject to public and private scrutiny. EMS is also a component of the health care system that comes with a significant amount of medical-legal risk. EMS is many times in a competitive market where details of operational and system issues, if made available outside of the agency, could place a competitor at an unfair advantage. Finally, as a part of the health care system, EMS is responsible for quality management and benchmarking. This process provides a continuing analysis of patient care and system operations in an ongoing manner for improving service delivery and care.

An EMS information system should be designed from the ground up to provide top-level security to the EMS system and its personnel. Policies and procedures that define access and use of the system should be developed, complete with appropriate disciplinary actions to ensure their compliance.

Any information system that aggregates data from multiple EMS systems should have adequate policies and procedures in place to prevent the identity of EMS systems from being disclosed to any outside agencies or the public without the consent of that EMS agency.

Patient security is also critically important to an EMS information system. Policies and procedures to provide appropriate access to EMS personnel in need of patient data should be developed and implemented, but they should protect patients from undue or unnecessary exposure.

In 2000, the US Department of Health and Human Services released regulations to enforce the law that protects patients and health care data that are transmitted electronically. These regulations have significant implications for all of health care, including EMS. The law is known as **HIPAA,** or the **Health Insurance Portability and Accountability Act.** The regulations provide detailed requirements related to health care information that is collected by any health care entity. The rules address electronic transactions with respect to Medicare reimbursement, but there are significant sections on patient confidentiality and security. Definitions of what data are identifiable, when they may be released, what requires patient consent prior to release, and what punishment can occur when the regulations are not followed are included in the document.

From an EMS information system perspective, HIPAA basically divides security and confidentiality into four major components:

- Patient privacy and confidentiality
- User policy and procedure
- Physical security
- Software security

Any health care data or information system must have detailed policies and procedures describing who, when, where, how, and why any personnel can access the system. This includes user rules and disciplinary policy. The system must meet the physical security requirements of HIPAA, which include issues such as locked access, controlled access, entry logs, and so on. Finally, any health care information that is transmitted electronically must meet the HIPAA requirements. This includes issues such as user authentication and data encryption.

At the time of this publication, the implementation of HIPAA is in its early stages. For that reason, much of the detail within each of these components is still being interpreted.

Current Status

Two major forces are driving EMS computerized documentation systems at this time. First is the requirement for electronic transactions for billing and reimbursement. Most EMS systems are paper based, but with the implementation of the new EMS reimbursement program and HIPAA, there is a strong movement toward electronic documentation. Second, there is also a significant movement by the states to collect and use EMS data for statewide system planning, finance, and development.

There are still significant barriers preventing the proliferation of electronic documentation systems. These include cost, varying computer skills among EMS personnel, and general need for acceptance of electronic documentation systems within the day-to-day operations of an EMS system.

National EMS Information System

Since the early 1970s, various publications and legislation have contributed to the development of EMS information systems and databases. EMS systems vary in their ability to collect patient and systems data and to put these data to use. There is currently no way to easily link disparate EMS databases to allow analysis locally, statewide, and nationally. For this reason, the National Association of State EMS Directors is working with its federal partners at NHTSA and the Trauma and EMS program of the Health Resources and Services Administration Maternal and Child Health Bureau to develop a national EMS database. Such a database would be useful in developing nationwide EMS training curricula, evaluating patient and EMS system outcomes, facilitating research efforts, determining national fee schedules and reimbursement rates, addressing resources for disaster and domestic preparedness, and providing valuable information on other issues or areas related to EMS care.

The NEMSIS grant is ongoing. Current NEMSIS activity and project details can be found at www.nemsis.org. NEMSIS-related projects that have been completed as of July 2004 include:

- NHTSA Version 2 Uniform Prehospital Dataset
- NHTSA Version 2 XML Standard for Data Exchange
- A physical database schema that can be used locally, statewide, or nationally to receive, store, and use EMS data electronically submitted using the XML standard
- A 3-year NEMSIS business implementation plan, which calls for federal funding for the establishment of local, state, and national EMS information systems

Summary

EMS records are vital information links in the chain of patient care from the onset of the emergency to hospital discharge. A clear, well-written PCR is required to document the patient's medical problems and the need for out-of-hospital intervention. A complete, well-documented out-of-hospital record makes it easier for the emergency physician to receive and properly care for the EMS patient. Although most practitioners believe they will never be called on in a court of law to justify the care they provide to a patient, we live in an increasingly litigious society where protection for the out-of-hospital provider is limited and disappearing rapidly. A legible, high-quality EMS record will enhance the probability of a successful defense if the out-of-hospital provider, squad, municipality, or medical director is ever sued.

Medical and legal needs and reimbursement and system performance depend on data. Data must be documented. Documentation requires effort. A belief must exist within EMS administrators, medical directors, and personnel that data will drive the system. Information is the key to the future of EMS.

Bibliography

Braun O. EMS system performance: the use of cardiac arrest timelines. *Ann Emerg Med.* 1993;22:52–61.

Cone DC, Jaslow DS, Brabson TA. Now that we have the Utstein style, are we using it? *Acad Emerg Med.* 1999;6(9):923–928.

Cummins R. Why are researchers and emergency medical services managers not using the Utstein guidelines? *Acad Emerg Med.* 1999;6(9):871–875.

Cummins RO. The Utstein style for uniform reporting of data from out-of-hospital cardiac arrest. *Ann Emerg Med.* 1993;22:37–40.

Durch JS, Lohr KN, eds. *Emergency Medical Services for Children.* Washington, DC: National Academies Press; 1993.

Emergency Medical Services Systems Act of 1973: Pub L No 93-154, Title XII of the Public Health Services Act.

Garrison HG, Foltin G, Becker L, et al. Consensus statement: The role of out-of-hospital emergency medical services in primary injury prevention. In: Consensus Workshop on the Role of EMS in Injury Prevention; August 25–26, 1995; Arlington, Va. Final report.

Joyce SM, Brown DE. An optically scanned EMS reporting form and analysis system for statewide use: development and five years' experience. *Ann Emerg Med.* 1991;20:1325–1330.

Meislin HW, Spaite DW, Conroy C, et al. Development of an electronic emergency medical services patient care record. *Prehospital Emerg Care.* 1999;3:54–59.

Nagai M, Yamamoto M, Numata T. Current assessment and proposed improvement to emergency medical information systems in Japan. *Med Inform.* 1994;19:21–36.

National Academy of Sciences, National Research Council. *Accidental Death and Disability: The Neglected Disease of Modern Society.* Washington, DC: National Academy Press; 1966.

National Center for Injury Prevention and Control. *Data Elements for Emergency Department Systems: Release 1.0.* Atlanta, Ga: Centers for Disease Control and Prevention; 1997.

National Highway Traffic Safety Administration. *Emergency Medical Services: Agenda for the Future.* Washington, DC: National Highway Traffic Safety Administration; 1996.

National Highway Traffic Safety Administration. *Emergency Medical Services: Agenda for the Future: Implementation Guide.* Washington, DC: National Highway Traffic Safety Administration; 1999.

National Highway Traffic Safety Administration. EMS outcomes evaluation: key issues and future directions. In: proceedings from the NHTSA Workshop on Methodologies for Measuring Morbidity Outcomes in EMS. April 11-12, 1994; Washington, DC.

National Highway Traffic Safety Administration. Uniform Pre-Hospital Emergency Medical Services (EMS) Data Conference; 1994; Washington, DC. Final report.

North Carolina Prehospital Medical Information System. Available at: www.premis.net. Accessed January 18, 2005.

Peters J, Hall GB. Assessment of ambulance response performance using a geographic information system. *Soc Sci Med.* 1999;49:1551–1566.

Shahein H, Zaky MM. ESMIS — a computer-based emergency medical services management information system. Part 1: design procedure. *Int J Bio-Medical Computing.* 1983;14:451–462.

Shahein H, Zaky MM. ESMIS — a computer-based emergency medical services management information system. Part 2: database design. *Int J Bio-Medical Computing.* 1984;15:9–22.

Siscovick DS. Challenges in cardiac arrest research: data collection to assess outcomes. *Ann Emerg Med.* 1993; 22:92–98.

Spaite DW, Criss EA, Valenzuela TD, et al. Emergency medical services systems research: problems of the past, challenges of the future. *Ann Emerg Med.* 1995; 26:146–152.

Spaite DW, Valenzuela TD, Meislin HW. Barriers to EMS system evaluation — problems associated with field data collection. *Prehospital Disaster Med.* 1993;8:S35–S40.

Svenson JE, Spurlock CW, Calhoun R. The Kentucky emergency medical services information system: current progress and future goals. *KMA J.* 1997;95:509–513.

Swor RA. Out of hospital cardiac arrest and the Utstein style: meeting the customer's needs? *Acad Emerg Med.* 1999;6(9):875–877.

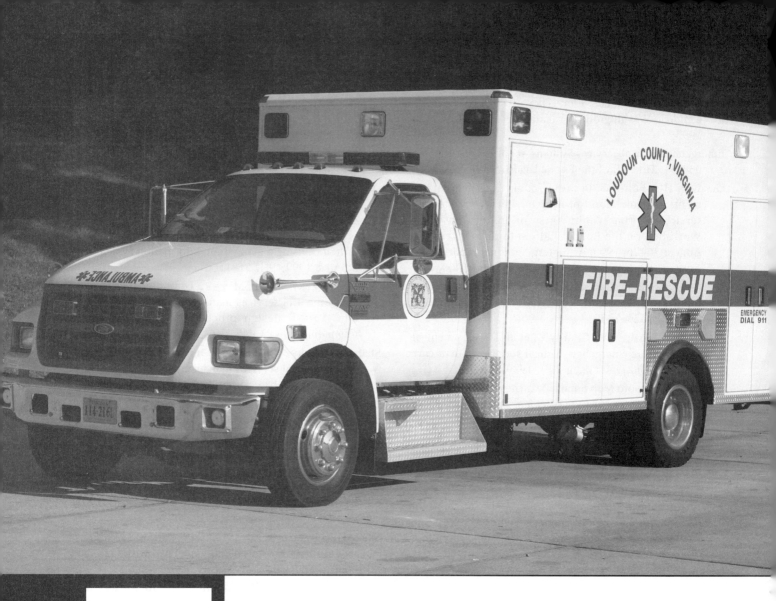

12

Ground Transport: Ambulances

Franklin D. Pratt, MD, FACEP
Jerry Overton, MPA

After reading this chapter, you should be able to:

- Describe the history and development of the ambulance and the evolution of the ambulance industry.
- Discuss the development of EMS training and equipment.
- Explain the use of response times and system status management to improve system operation.

THE AMBULANCE IS A SYMBOL OF OUR SOCIETY'S COMMITment to care for people in their time of most significant need: when they are ill or injured. Ground transportation of the ill and injured is a part of the EMS system that we take for granted. However, this has not always been the case. The ambulance is a relatively new entity in the history of medicine. In today's everchanging health care environment, the ambulance has medical, emotional, political, and financial implications. This chapter will review the history of the ambulance, discuss the diversity and maturation of the ground transport component of the EMS system, and identify future challenges for the ambulance in a post–domestic terrorism United States.

History of the Ambulance

The first reported use of a transportation device was during the 11th century, when an injured soldier was carried on the back of another to obtain help. The transporting person was sometimes paid a small fee for this work. During the Crusades in the 11th century, the Knights of St. John provided medical care after receiving first aid training from doctors on the battlefield. One must assume the injured soldiers were somehow taken to something that could be called aid stations. In 1487, the Queen of Spain supported the use of a cart to move wounded soldiers during the Siege of Malaga, and her son, Charles V, continued that tradition during the Siege of Metz in 1553. The next step in the formal use of a wheeled device to move patients was in the late 1700s, when Baron Dominique-Jean Larrey was appointed by Napoleon Bonaparte to develop a method for removing injured soldiers from the battlefield. Larrey created a system that took medical personnel to the injured soldier and brought the injured soldier away from the front lines to a location where medical care could be continued.[1] He also developed the "flying ambulance," a horse-drawn carriage that took trained medical personnel to injured soldiers and then took them back to a medical facility while providing care en route.

Just before the Civil War began, a five-member US Army board recommended the use of a two-wheeled cart to carry casualties from the battle lines.[2] The two-wheeled device was uncomfortable and possibly made the patients more ill during their movement to first aid. A four-wheeled design by Brigadier General Charles S. Tripler replaced the uncomfortable two-wheeled design and can be considered the forerunner of today's ambulance. Simultaneously, a civilian ambulance service was started in Cincinnati, Ohio. Shortly after the end of the Civil War, many civilian hospitals had ambulance services. Between the Civil War and World War I, the Red Cross used ambulances in the Crimean and Spanish-American wars. The invention of the automobile led to motorized ambulances, which were used by hospitals and the military. Motorized ambulances, dedicated to transportation without much additional care, then began to occupy the roadways. Although the French had experimented with fixed-wing aircraft modified for the movement of sick and wounded persons, the next most important development in ambulances was in the air — the use of helicopters in the Korean Conflict and Vietnam War.[3] Injured soldiers faced average evacuation times of 18 hours in World War I trenches, but those wounded in Korea and Vietnam were being seen by surgeons within an hour of being injured. Some young men who previously would have died instead survived.

Perhaps the most significant change in ground ambulance use was driven by the publication of the 1966 white paper *Accidental Death and Disability: The*

Neglected Disease of Modern Society.[4] This paper called attention to the need for care for victims of accidents and the parallel recognition of the benefit of early cardiac care by what were termed mobile intensive care units. Dr. J. Frank Pantridge, a physician at the Royal Victoria Hospital in Belfast, Northern Ireland, introduced the concept of bringing physicians with advanced life support procedures and equipment out of the hospital and to the patient.[5] Physicians in the United States attempted to replicate his system, but the cost of providing physicians and nurses in the out-of-hospital setting was prohibitive.

The Highway Safety Act of 1966 provided the first funding initiative for ambulance services at the federal level.[6] Federal funds were distributed as seed money in an attempt to establish EMS systems and address the concerns brought forward by the white paper. Advances in micromedical technology stimulated by NASA in the space program proved to have spillover benefits, as portable heart monitors/defibrillators and telemedical communications devices were developed and refined. Dr. Eugene Nagel of the University of Miami School of Medicine trained the first US paramedics, and soon paramedic training programs were established in Los Angeles, Seattle, and Columbus, Ohio.

The greatest cultural impact on out-of-hospital emergency services came in 1971. The paramedic service being developed in Los Angeles County caught the attention of an acclaimed television producer, and "Emergency!" was born.[7]

In 1972, federal funding was provided for EMS demonstration projects in five regions.[8] The Emergency Medical Services Systems Act of 1973 provided $185 million to establish EMS systems and created a template of 15 mandatory components for any EMS system seeking federal funding.[9] As the EMS system became a more accepted part of the community infrastructure, state and local governments recognized a responsibility to arrange access to EMS treatment and transport for its citizens, just as they provided for police and fire protection within their jurisdictions. The need for uniformity and minimum standards for ambulances, equipment, procedures, and personnel prompted the federal government, professional organizations, and the medical community to develop standards and guidelines to ensure the availability of safe, well-equipped, and well-staffed ambulances.[10] Minimal requirements (including those from OSHA) and laws regulating some aspects of EMS operations emerged, in part in an attempt to protect the public against unscrupulous and undependable providers of care and transport.

Ambulance Design

In the late 1960s and early 1970s, several documents developed and published by the federal government stimulated improvement in the design of ambulances. These articles defined an ambulance as:

> a vehicle for emergency care which provides a driver compartment and a patient compartment which can accommodate two emergency medical technicians and two litter patients so positioned that at least one patient can be given intensive life support during transit; which carries equipment and supplies for:
> (1) optimal emergency care at the scene as well as during transport
> (2) two-way radio communication
> (3) safeguarding personnel and patients under hazardous conditions
> (4) light rescue procedures and
> (5) which is designed and constructed to afford maximum safety and comfort and to avoid aggravation of the patient condition, exposure to complications, and threat to survival.[11,12]

Previously, many ambulances were modeled after hearses. In fact, in many communities the only suitable vehicle for transporting patients lying down *was* a hearse. Funeral directors provided patient transport services as a public service or a revenue stream, and funeral homes were the dominant provider of ground ambulance EMS through the 1960s.[13] In 1974, the federal government published "The Federal Emergency Medical Care Vehicle Specifications KKK-A-1822," or **KKK standards,** which provided engineering specifications that incorporated the general recommendations of the ambulance design criteria.[14] These standards detailed the construction and physical and safety requirements for ambulances.

At first, an attempt was made to have all ambulances built to conform to these federal specifications. Since then, however, only ambulances purchased using federal highway safety funds have been required to comply with these criteria. Still, this had a significant impact on the design of ambulances during the 1970s, when millions of federal dollars were spent to implement EMS systems. The KKK standards have been amended several times and remain the specifications by which federal agencies (and many other government entities) purchase ambulances.

A classification system was developed for the various configurations of these new mobile intensive care units. The Type I ambulance is a conventional truck

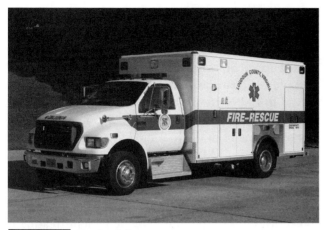

Figure 12-1 Type I ambulance.

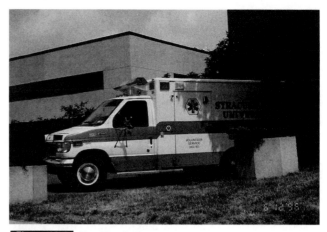

Figure 12-3 Type III ambulance.

cab chassis with a modular, usually transferable ambulance body mounted on it (**Figure 12-1**). A Type II ambulance is a conventional van, with the ambulance body conversion integrated into the rear spaces (**Figure 12-2**). The Type III ambulance is a specialty van with a cab-over-engine chassis, upon which a transferable modular ambulance body is mounted, or a specialty van with *unitized* cab and body (**Figure 12-3**). As a result of the KKK standards, the basic design of ambulances evolved from the modified hearse to the three types of vehicles commonly available today. Most ambulances provide space for two patient litters. One is usually on a wheeled-type stretcher that can be mounted in the center or on the left side of the vehicle. A center configuration allows room for rescue personnel on both sides of the stretcher (which is helpful during CPR), while the left-side configuration facilitates management of patients requiring transport on their left side to prevent aspiration. The second litter can be secured on the padded squad bench located on the right side of the patient compartment. The patient and driver

compartments are usually, but not always, connected. One basic floor plan with multiple options for placement of equipment and cabinets is standard, allowing for some customization to meet various needs and budgets. The most recent edition of the ambulance standards, KKK-1822-E, went into effect in June 2002.[15]

Equipment and Training

The American College of Surgeons Committee on Trauma first published a list of suggested ambulance equipment in 1970.[16] The American College of Emergency Physicians (ACEP) created a similar list. These lists were revised several times until 2001, when the two groups merged their lists and recommended a standardized regimen of ambulance equipment. The current document provides a suggested list for all ambulances that includes patient care supplies and equipment, radios and other communications equipment, and infection control and injury prevention equipment.[17] (See Figure 15-10 in Chapter 15, "EMS for Children.") In addition, the EMS for Children project collaborated with ACEP, the American Academy of Pediatrics, and others to develop a similar list of equipment appropriate for pediatric patients.[18]

National curricula were developed to define the professional, educational, and legal boundaries of those who would provide out-of-hospital emergency medical care.[19] Curricula were developed for the EMT-Basic,[20,21] the EMT-Intermediate, and the EMT-Paramedic.[22,23] These documents standardized the minimum medical background of the personnel staffing the ambulance and effectively defined a new allied health care professional.

Recognized professional organizations developed core curriculum textbooks[24] and specialty certification courses to further provide standardization and

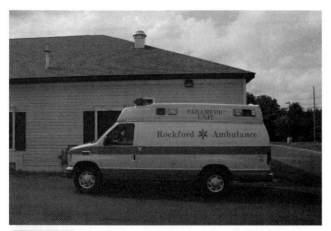

Figure 12-2 Type II ambulance.

focus in training, both in the field and in the hospital. Artificial ventilation and CPR courses were considered to be BLS training,[25] while specialty courses associated with advanced treatment interventions (intravenous therapy, drug therapy, intubation, and manual defibrillation) were known as ALS training.

The American Heart Association developed the ACLS (advanced cardiac life support) course in the mid 1970s[26] primarily for physicians who directed cardiac arrest resuscitation teams, but it soon became evident that this kind of training and this skill level were also needed at the scenes of out-of-hospital cardiac arrests. As a result, many paramedics and nurses were trained in cardiac arrest management, extending ALS care far beyond the hospital emergency department. Other organizations developed training in the areas of critical trauma, neonatal and pediatric emergency care, hazardous materials incidents, wilderness medicine, and, more recently, domestic preparedness and event management. As a result, more equipment, supplies, and medications were added to ambulances as physician expectations and state and local requirements for patient care activities increased.

The KKK standards, medical equipment lists, and personnel definitions provided the guideposts for the vehicles, equipment, and people they carried. Other critical issues related to system design, the actual placement/deployment of the ambulances, and funding of services became the next hurdles for optimal use of the ground ambulance.

Evolution of the Ambulance Industry

There have been major shifts in EMS delivery, system design, ambulance use, and patient transport funding during the past 10 to 15 years. The emergence of fire-based EMS brought ambulances into the realm of public safety. Corporate EMS also evolved as corporations began to invest in the ambulance industry, acquiring private EMS firms and attempting to develop economies of scale and reduce overhead. Many providers of EMS who had never billed for services before (fire departments, volunteer rescue squads) have now begun to try to recover some of the costs of providing ambulance service.

Fire departments have become more effective at fire suppression and prevention, and the volume of fires to be fought has decreased, but fire personnel and equipment levels must be maintained to meet fire threats. Pressures to justify staffing and budget levels and a focus on their mission of public safety led fire departments to increase their level of involvement in EMS substantially during the 1980s and 1990s. As their involvement increased, they took on more patient treatment and transportation responsibility. As a result, 85% of fire departments in North America are now involved in EMS, either providing first response or patient transport; and fire-based EMS is now the most common type of municipal EMS system.[27]

Fire service EMS has developed into several recognizable configurations. Some systems provide only an organized BLS response and depend on private or public ambulance providers for ALS treatment and transport. Other programs provide patient treatment and transport. Fire-based EMS offered an opportunity to blend existing public safety infrastructure with the patient's need for medical care and transport to a health care facility. Concepts integral to fire-based EMS programs include the following: existing facilities in strategic locations that can serve a dual purpose as EMS and fire stations; the availability of fire department personnel who can be cross-trained; dual-function emergency response (medical and fire suppression) providers; and the fire service's visibility in the community. Fire department-based systems usually did not and do not provide nonemergency transport or interfacility transfer services, creating a need for other ambulance entities within a community served by fire-based EMS response agencies. This duplication of services has raised questions by some about the cost-effectiveness of the fire-based EMS system.

As fire department-administered EMS systems evolved, some conflict has appeared within that structure. The problems of priorities when fire suppression is the department's primary role, and the personnel conflicts that can arise when firefighters are assigned a second function involving markedly different education and workloads have become apparent. As the composition of the fire service evolves, these problems are being resolved.

As the private EMS industry has become more sophisticated, it is applying business principles more carefully and producing managers with business and administrative experience. Many private ambulance firms are members of the American Ambulance Association (AAA), which has developed focused strategies of education and lobbying the government in support of EMS issues.

Other EMS entities such as the National Association of EMTs, the National Association of State EMS Directors, the National Association of EMS Physicians (NAEMSP), and ACEP have worked together to focus political pressure and to respond to state and national EMS issues. The AAA, the International Association of Fire Fighters, and the International Association of Fire Chiefs (as well as ACEP and NAEMSP) were integral participants in the negotiated rule-making process that is part of the Medicare Fee Schedule issue.

Another major event in the history of ambulance service development was the partial consolidation of the private ambulance industry. During the late 1980s and continuing into the 1990s, more than 200 smaller, privately owned ambulance companies were purchased by several larger corporations. Those larger organizations then consolidated into two even larger ambulance companies. The level of profit margin realized as a result of ambulance company acquisitions has apparently not been as great as anticipated, and those companies continue to seek a balance between adjustments in services and coverage provided. Independent, private EMS providers still exist and compete successfully within the industry.

EMS Transport Systems

The ambulance infrastructure described previously (vehicle, equipment carried, personnel levels) allows a very diverse operational, administrative, financial, and political environment for the delivery of ambulance transport services to a community. That infrastructure, combined with the delivery components, becomes the system design, and the resulting design significantly affects both operations and economic performance.

EMS response and transport systems use vehicles and personnel funded by fees for service (private ambulance companies and hospitals), by municipal taxes (fire, some public utility models, third service), by donations (volunteer), or by some combination of those sources. The response will be either single tiered or multitiered. In **single-tiered response systems,** all transport vehicles and personnel are capable of delivering essentially the same level of service, usually paramedic level (ALS). In **multitiered systems,** nontransport and transport vehicles and personnel of different capabilities respond according to a previously established systemwide dispatching plan; BLS transport units handle most calls, and ALS units can be summoned for more serious cases. In those systems, there sometimes is a delay if an ALS transport unit is needed when only a BLS transport unit is on the scene.

Private EMS Systems

Some EMS systems comprise one or more private companies located in the community or region delivering either emergency or nonemergency transport services, or both. Private EMS services can be broadly categorized

into commercial ambulance companies and hospital-based services. Each private entity owns the vehicles and equipment, employs all the personnel, and might be responsible for receiving patient access calls and dispatching the appropriate vehicles. Private companies then bill patients or insurance companies for the services provided, keeping in mind that income must equal expenses or the company will cease to exist.

Some hospitals have developed their own ambulance services to meet hospital and community needs for emergency response, interfacility transfers, and nonemergency transport. The ambulance service also provides the hospital with another product line to increase revenue and to capture a higher market share. These services are usually associated with the emergency department, and the personnel are hospital employees. The EMS personnel might also work in the emergency department when they are not on ambulance calls, which provides them a greater opportunity to observe and participate in patient care.

Municipalities can and should have some influence on the operation of all EMS agencies within their borders. This can be accomplished by ordinances that allocate market rights (franchises), license operators, set performance standards, monitor compliance through a medical advisory committee, and regulate rates.

As providers of the infrastructure for 911 emergency telephone systems, many municipalities have an obligation to ensure that equal access and rapid EMS response will be provided to citizens who use 911. Area physicians should have input into what constitutes the EMS standard of care for their communities. Municipal leaders should hold municipal and private EMS systems accountable for rates that have a basis in the cost to provide services, especially if they provide public money to help ensure an EMS response in their community.

Municipal EMS Systems

Municipal EMS systems are operated by the local government, which owns the vehicles and equipment, and the personnel are government employees. These systems can be based in the fire department, police department, or in a separate EMS department (sometimes referred to as a third service). The municipality might or might not bill for services, but most are now trying to capture this potential revenue.

Combined Services

Combined private and municipal services have emerged from these basic models and are usually referred to as ambulance or EMS trusts or public utility models. In the first model, the trust is responsible for providing all EMS out-of-hospital service, ensuring the quality of the service, and operating a billing and collection system. When operating as a trust, the service is responsible to a board of trustees rather than to the local government. This limits the intrusion of political influence on the operation of a multijurisdictional or regional system. Examples of cities with ambulance trusts are Reno, Nevada, and Little Rock, Arkansas.

With the **public utility model (PUM)**, one or more municipalities create a public trust or EMS authority for the purpose of providing EMS, which is usually governed by a board of directors appointed by the municipality.[28] The EMS authority then contracts with a private company to manage the EMS personnel and provide out-of-hospital care to the region for a predetermined cost, which would be fixed or tied to a formula based on transport volume. The authority establishes clinical performance and response time standards for the system and uses an independent physician organization for medical audit and quality improvement. The authority controls or owns all equipment used in the system, reducing the chances for an interruption of services if the service provider's contract is terminated. The authority usually bills users or insurance companies directly. The authority pays the service provider based on contracted fees. In the public/private partnership of a public utility model, the contractor is encouraged by incentives and disincentives to concentrate solely on providing rapid, appropriate EMS response, prioritized dispatch services, and quality patient care. Some areas using the public utility model include Richmond, Virginia; Kansas City, Missouri; Tulsa and Oklahoma City, Oklahoma; and Pinellas County, Florida.

Another combination of public and private delivery of EMS occurs when local governments or municipalities contract directly, rather than through a trust, with a private ambulance company, as in Syracuse, New York. This company is either contracted to respond only to emergency calls or to provide care and transport of all patients outside the hospital, including invalid transport and interfacility transports. If the contract is for response to emergencies only, other private ambulance companies can participate in nonemergency transport services and interfacility transports. Remuneration from the municipality to the ambulance service contractor will be a fixed amount for the service provided regardless of usage or a subsidy in excess of collectable billing provided to cover bad debt and indigent care.

Whether a community contracts for service or is directly responsible for the service, it should create an independent medical advisory panel to develop and monitor standards of performance. The municipality should also require full financial disclosure from either the municipal or private provider to determine the appropriate user rates and/or subsidies, and provision should be made for public ownership or control of the vehicles and equipment so that emergency service can be continued if there is a change of operators.

Response Times and System Status Management

Response Times

The most important factor in successfully resuscitating a patient in cardiac arrest is the speed of response. The survival rate from untreated ventricular fibrillation decreases up to 10% for every minute that passes and definitive care is not provided (**Figure 12-4**).[29] The American Heart Association, ACEP, and other respected organizations recommend that EMS vehicles should respond to deliver BLS skills within 3 to 4 minutes, with ALS skills available within 6 to 8 minutes. The ALS-within-8-minutes concept developed from research that showed the survival rate for cardiac arrest victims decreases significantly with each passing minute, and that optimal probabilities for survival increase when BLS has been provided within 4 minutes, followed by ALS within 8 minutes.[30,31]

Before a response time can be measured, it is important to determine the response interval that will be used. A **response interval** is defined as two points of the response for which there are starting-point and stopping-point times. For cardiac arrest, the Utstein style has provided many of these points.[32] Because times for several of the points cannot be accurately attained (such as the exact time of patient collapse or the exact time of arriving at the patient's side), it is important to measure the response interval with times that are readily available and captured accurately. The starting point could be the time when the telephone rings in the 911 dispatch center, or alternatively, the time the call is received by the EMS dispatcher. In all cases, the end point is the time the appropriate response vehicle arrives at the scene.

Historically, response times have been measured as an average. Using this method, all response times are added and divided by the number of responses. This often leads to a problem of inequity of service, because, by definition, 50% of the patients have re-

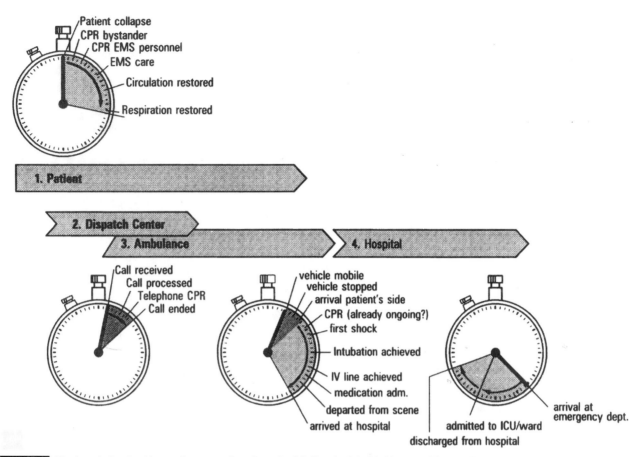

Figure 12-4 The four clocks of sudden cardiac arrest. From Cummins RO, Chamberlain DA, Abramson NS, et al. Recommended guidelines for uniform reporting of data from out-of-hospital cardiac arrest: the Utstein style. Task force of the American Heart Association, the European Resuscitation Council, the Heart and Stroke Foundation of Canada, and the Australian Resuscitation Council. *Ann Emerg Med.* 1991;20(8):862. Reprinted with permission from ACEP.

sponse times longer than the average response time goal.

To ensure a more equitable service to all areas of the community, **fractile response time** measurement was introduced and now is commonly used by EMS systems. To calculate a fractile response time, all applicable response times are placed, by minute, in ascending order. The number of calls within a predetermined minute are then calculated as a percentage of the total number of calls. This establishes a percentage of reliability that often must be met for patients needing an emergency response. The 90th percentile is most commonly used. **Figure 12-5** shows a sample fractile response time report from Richmond, Virginia.

System Status Management

To achieve acceptable response time goals, EMS systems must use ambulance deployment strategies, sometimes called **system status management,** or **SSM.** All providers of EMS services use SSM in some form.[33] SSM simply refers to the strategy used in placing and deploying ambulances to meet the demand for EMS services.

In a **static deployment system,** EMS vehicles are housed in fixed stations and are deployed from there as needed. In a dynamic or **flexible deployment system,** EMS vehicles are not station based, but are constantly positioned at predetermined points where the EMS demand can best be covered by the number of units available for deployment in the system at any moment. In a static system using flexible deployment, EMS vehicles are moved among their fixed stations to provide the best coverage for the number of units still available for deployment in the system. Of these strategies, the dynamic flexible deployment system is viewed by many as the most effective. Most fire service-based EMS is configured with a static deployment method. Of course, a progressive EMS system also requires that personnel are ready to respond at all times, that system status controllers (dispatchers) are well trained, and that ambulances use reasonable shift schedules (avoiding long hours).

Sophisticated, computerized methods to predict

1m Intervals	Count	System Interval %	Accum %
00:00–00:59	36	2.15%	2.15%
01:00–01:59	32	1.91%	4.06%
02:00–02:59	96	5.73%	9.80%
03:00–03:59	202	12.07%	21.86%
04:00–04:59	291	17.38%	39.25%
05:00–05:59	298	17.80%	57.05%
06:00–06:59	230	13.74%	70.79%
07:00–07:59	229	13.68%	84.47%
08:00–08:59	144	8.60%	93.07%
09:00–09:59	40	2.39%	95.46%
10:00–10:59	27	1.61%	97.07%
11:00–11:59	17	1.02%	98.09%
12:00–12:59	14	0.84%	98.92%
13:00–13:59	4	0.24%	99.16%
14:00–14:59	4	0.24%	99.40%
15:00+	10	0.60%	100.00%
Total Count	**1,674**		

Figure 12-5 Richmond, Virginia, ambulance authority fractile response times.

demand for EMS services are used to implement SSM. Based on historical demand patterns for each hour of each day, the computer can anticipate the most likely location and time of the next call for EMS assistance. Ambulance location and density can be adjusted to provide response times that are within the desired standard (eg, flexible deployment). Of course, no computer can always predict when or from where the next call will occur, but definite patterns of EMS demand can be documented. If managers use these tools properly, matching demand to resources, significant system performance and efficiencies are possible.

Staffing

Ambulances can be staffed by full-time career professionals or by part-time, paid staff who have other vocations. Most modern fire department-based systems are staffed by cross-trained and dual-role personnel who are firefighters and EMS personnel. One variation in staffing for fire department systems has been the employment of civilian (nonfirefighter) EMS personnel, while another makes use of volunteer or part-time personnel to staff the vehicles. Some systems deliver care with a combination of full-time and part-time paid personnel. Seventy percent of the EMS personnel in

this country are considered part-time, paid volunteers and provide a large part of the care given to the ill and injured in our country. The use of nonpaid or part-time personnel paid per call can be a significant cost savings, but it is becoming more difficult to recruit and retain those personnel.

Volunteer EMS personnel and firefighters have made a significant contribution to the public safety arena, particularly in rural areas. Faced with their own logistical problems, such as being unable to depend on a uniform response from a dispatch summons, volunteers often provide the only form of EMS within large geographic areas. They are often passionate about their desire to protect and serve their communities, and they might bring access to additional funding sources, creating a savings for the operation and the government. Despite the challenges, many suburban and rural EMS systems are staffed with well-trained, highly motivated, part-time, paid staff.

Summary

The ambulance embodies much of what we define as medical care and humanity in the out-of-hospital setting. This vehicle and all it symbolizes represent a significant component of the emergency medical care system. This common ideal can be served by a multitude of vehicle, equipment, personnel, deployment, and financing combinations. The local jurisdiction authority must decide the combination that serves its community most appropriately while maintaining the high medical standard that community expects.

Author's note: This chapter has been adapted from Weigand JV. Prehospital ground transport: system structure and function. In: Roush WR, ed. *Principles of EMS Systems.* 2nd ed. 1994.

References

1. Richardson GR. *Larrey, Surgeon to Napoleon's Imperial Guard.* London: John Murray; 1974.

2. Stewart MJ. *Moving the Wounded: Litters, Cacolets and Ambulance Wagons, US Army, 1776–1876.* Fort Collins, Colo: Old Army Press; 1979.

3. Dorland P. *Dust Off: Army Aeromedical Evacuation in Vietnam.* Washington, DC: Center of Military History, US Army; 1982.

4. *Accidental Death and Disability: The Neglected Disease of Modern Society.* Washington, DC: National Academy of Sciences, National Research Council; 1966.

5. Pantridge JF, Geddes JS. A mobile intensive care unit in the management of myocardial infarction. *Lancet.* 1967;2:271–273.

6. Highway Safety Act of 1966.

7. Page JO. *The Paramedics.* Morristown, NJ: Backdraft Publications; 1979.

8. Emergency Medical Services Act of 1972.

9. Emergency Medical Services Act of 1973. Pub L No 93-154.

10. Safar P, Esposito G, Benson DM. Ambulance design and equipment for mobile intensive care. *Arch Surg.* 1971;102(3):163–171.

11. *Ambulance Design Criteria.* Washington, DC: National Highway and Traffic Systems Administration (NHTSA); May 1971.

12. US Department of Public Health. *Medical Requirements for Ambulance Design and Equipment.* Washington, DC: US Government Printing Office; 1973. Publication No. (HSM), 73-2035.

13. Boyd DR. The history of emergency medical services systems in the United States of America. In: Boyd DR, Edlich RF, Micik S, eds. *Systems Approach to Emergency Medical Care.* Norwalk, Conn: Appleton-Century-Crofts; 1983.

14. US Department of Transportation. *The Federal Emergency Medical Care Vehicle Specifications.* Washington, DC: US Department of Transportation; 1974. KKK-A-1822.

15. US Department of Transportation: *The Federal Emergency Medical Care Vehicle Specifications.* Washington, DC: US Department of Transportation; 2001. KKK-A-1822-E.

16. Committee on Trauma, American College of Surgeons. Essential equipment for ambulances. *Am Coll Surg Bull.* 1970;55(5):7–13.

17. Committee on Trauma, American College of Surgeons and the American College of Emergency Physicians. *Equipment for Ambulances.* ACEP and ACSCOT; 2001. Available at: http://www.acep.org/library/pdf/ambulance_equip.pdf. Accessed December 30, 2004.

18. Committee on Ambulance Equipment and Supplies, National Emergency Medical Services for Children (EMSC) Resource Alliance. Guidelines for pediatric equipment and supplies for basic and advanced life support ambulances. *Pediatr Emerg Care.* 1996;12(6): 452–453.

19. Washington Committee on Emergency Medical Services, National Academy of Sciences. *Training of Ambulance Personnel and Others Responsible for Emergency Care of the Sick and Injured at the Scene During Transportation.* Washington, DC: National Research Council; 1968.

20. National Highway Traffic Safety Administration. *Basic Training Program for Emergency Medical Technicians — Ambulance.* Washington, DC: US Department of Transportation; 1971.

21. Division of Medical Sciences, Committee on Emergency Medical Services and the Subcommittee on Ambulance Services, National Academy of Sciences. *Advanced Training Program for Emergency Medical Technicians — Ambulance.* Washington, DC: National Research Council; 1970.

22. US Department of Transportation. *Emergency Medical Care: A Manual for the Paramedic in the Field.* Washington, DC: US Government Printing Office; 1979.

23. US Department of Transportation. *National Standard Curriculum: Emergency Medical Technician — Paramedic.* Washington, DC: US Government Printing Office; 1985.

24. American Academy of Orthopedic Surgeons. *Emergency Care and Transportation of the Sick and Injured.* Chicago, Ill: AAOS; 1969.

25. American Heart Association, National Research Council. Standards for cardiopulmonary resuscitation and emergency cardiac care. *JAMA.* 1974;227(suppl):833–868.

26. American Heart Association. *Textbook of Advanced Cardiac Life Support.* Dallas, Tex: American Heart Association; 1981.

27. Journal of Emergency Medical Services. Annual 200-city survey 2002. *JEMS.* 2002;12.

28. Stout JL. The public utility model revisited. *JEMS.* 1985;11:32–34.

29. Advanced Life Support Working Party of the European Resuscitation Council: Guidelines for adult advanced cardiac life support. *Resuscitation.* 1992;24:111–121.

30. Eisenberg MS, Bergner L, Hallstrom A. Paramedic programs and out of hospital arrest: factors associated with

successful resuscitation. *Am J Public Health.* 1979;
69:30–38.

31. Cobb LA, Conn RD, Samson WE. Prehospital coronary
care: the role of a rapid response mobile intensive/coro-
nary care system. *Circulation.* 1971;44(suppl 2):11–45.

32. Cummins RO, Chamberlain DA, Abramson NS, et al.
Recommended guidelines for uniform reporting of data
from out-of-hospital cardiac arrest: the Utstein style.
Ann Emerg Med. 1991;20:861–874.

33. Stout JL. System status management. *J Emerg Med Serv.*
1983;8:22–32.

Additional Reading

Kuehl AE. Perspectives on international EMS system development. *Emerg Med Serv.* 1989;3:37.

Kuehl AE and the National Association of EMS Physicians.
Prehospital Systems & Medical Oversight. 3rd ed. Mosby
Lifeline; 2002.

Lewis AJ, Ailshie G, Criley JM. Prehospital cardiac care in
a paramedical mobile intensive care unit. *Calif Med.*
1972;117:1–8.

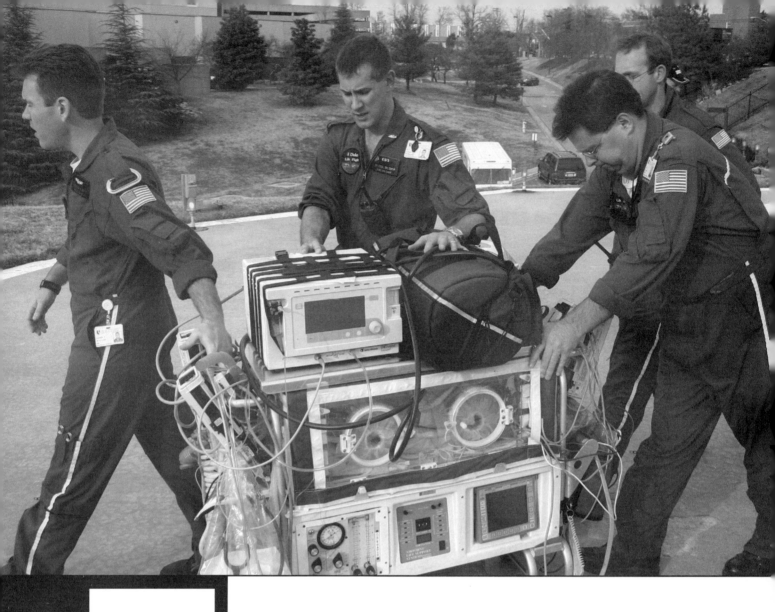

13

Ground Interfacility and Specialty Care Transfer

Robert M. Domeier, MD, FACEP

Principles of This Chapter

After reading this chapter, you should be able to:
- Explain why patients are transferred to other facilities.
- Describe the risks related to patient transfer, such as possible deterioration of a patient's condition.
- Discuss the logistics of patient transfer, including method of transfer, level of staffing required, communications, and medical oversight.

INTERFACILITY PATIENT TRANSFER IS A FUNDAMENTAL COMponent of any EMS system. The transfer of patients was originally identified as one of 15 essential components of EMS.[1] The regionalization of the health care system necessitates the transport of patients from one health care facility to another. This regionalization of medical care provides for the efficient use of resources and the concentration of specialty services, which results in making higher levels of care available to patients. Regionalization also allows the health care system to reduce the duplication of services that would be necessary if interfacility transfer were not routinely available.

Transfers occur with an expectation that patients will arrive at the receiving facility in a condition similar to that at the time they leave the sending facility. Despite this expectation, there are often potential complications that must be managed during the transport.[2] The interfacility transport system should have preestablished mechanisms to ensure safe transfer. These mechanisms must take into consideration the severity of illness and have contingencies for specialty needs.

The responsibility for interfacility transports is fragmented. The EMS medical director understands the system's capabilities, but not necessarily the patient's needs. Conversely, the sending physician understands the patient's needs, but not necessarily the system's capabilities. In some systems, as a result, patients might be transferred by personnel unprepared to handle potential complications and be unaware of the adverse effects that might be caused by treatments initiated at the sending facility.

The referring facility and physician bear the legal responsibility to ensure that the patient is transported in a safe and medically appropriate manner.[3] In order to make sure patients are transferred safely, all physicians who use the interfacility transport system must be aware of the capabilities of that system. Despite the responsibility of the sending facility, the interfacility transport system also has responsibility for the transfer and should have established safeguards to ensure that transfer vehicles have the necessary equipment and medications and are staffed by personnel able to appropriately manage the patient during that transfer.

Justification for Interfacility Transfer

The transfer of emergency patients to tertiary centers in order to access higher levels of care not available at primary care facilities is one of the most common uses of interfacility transport. Many primary care and urgent care facilities and rural, suburban, and urban emergency departments do not have the ability to provide definitive care for all patients. The types of emergency patients for whom transfer to a secondary or tertiary care facility might be necessary include those who have suffered cardiac problems, burns, trauma, or stroke, as well as pediatric, high-risk obstetrics, neonatal, and neurosurgery patients, and those experiencing other complex medical conditions. Improved outcome has been demonstrated for patients transferred to centers providing that higher level of specialty care. These benefits have been reported in both adult and pediatric trauma patents, patients transferred for coronary angioplasty, and for high-risk obstetric patients not in active labor.[4-7]

Nonemergent transfer to higher-level facilities might also be done to provide definitive care, evaluation by specialty physicians, or evaluation and treatment with procedures not available at the sending facility. Nonemergency patients are often transferred for diagnostic cardiac catheterization or specialty scanning such as MRI.

Additional reasons for transfer include continuity of care and patient preference. During a perceived emergency, patients might seek treatment at a facility other than that which usually provides their care. In order to avoid duplication of testing inherent to multiple-facility care, and to provide continuity and continued care by physicians familiar with the patient's condition and medical history, patient-requested transfer to a "home" facility might be beneficial.[8] Patients might also request transfer for nonmedical reasons. These include proximity of home and family, familiarity with a particular facility, and dissatisfaction with the care at the primary facility. They might also want to seek a second opinion.

Finally, in a managed care environment, interfacility transfer of patients from out-of-plan facilities to those that are part of the managed care organization allows reduction in costs to the managed care organization. Transfer of stable patients to in-plan facilities is an integral part of many managed care cost-containment plans.[9] When patients are treated at out-of-plan facilities for emergency conditions, the cost is often higher than it would be at in-plan facilities. Physicians and hospitals must be careful, however, to effect transfers in accordance with EMTALA. A patient's request for transfer must not be the result of economic coercion or a suggestion by someone associated with the hospital that the federally mandated medical screening examination and stabilizing treatment won't be covered by the patient's insurance.

See Chapter 27 for a more in-depth discussion of EMTALA.

Risks of Transport

The decision to transfer a patient must be preceded by an analysis of the potential benefits of the transfer measured against the potential risks. There are risks during transport not only to the patient but also to the transport personnel.[10] Whenever possible, the patient must be involved early in the transfer decision. If the patient's condition makes this involvement impractical, the family must be involved with the decision.[11-13]

The risk-benefit analysis should include a determination of the patient's current medical problems and the most suitable facility for management. In addition, the patient's likelihood for deterioration without transfer, the urgency of definitive management, and the availability of tertiary resources must be factored into the decision.

There is a significant risk of deterioration during the transfer of critically ill patients.[14-20] Prior to initiation of a transfer, the patient should be adequately monitored and stabilized for transfer. The extent to which this can be accomplished is dependent on the resources available at the transferring institution, the type of medical problem, and the age of the patient. In some cases, such as seriously ill pediatric and neonatal patients, the stabilization efforts might be best accomplished by a specialty transport team coming to the facility to pick up the patient.[21] To achieve stability in some patients (trauma patients, for example), interventions unavailable at the referring facility might be required.[21] Obstetric patients and women having labor contractions present special problems and considerations.[17] To avoid the potential complications of a delivery during transfer, women having labor contractions should generally deliver prior to transfer, even in the case of high-risk pregnancy.

The Logistics of Patient Transfer

Methods of Transport

Important considerations in choosing the mode of transport and level of care required during transfer include time and distance. For the unstable, critical patient, rapid interfacility transfer to a more comprehensive facility is required. In contrast, nonemergent interfacility transfer might not require speed or sophisticated transfer services. Interstate and international transfers require significantly more complex planning. Fixed-wing aircraft transport and anticipation of complications during transport requiring a higher level of care during the transport are important considerations for longer transports.

Most interfacility patient transfers are managed by ground ambulance personnel, whose primary responsibility is the provision of out-of-hospital emergency medical care.[22] These might be private, hospital-based, or municipal EMS services, depending on the role and availability of each type of service in the community. Additionally, air medical and specialty ground transport units participate in the transfer of patients with the need for specialty care during transport. The most commonly used ground vehicle is an ambulance, either in traditional form or with a specially modified patient care module designed for the needs of the specialty transport unit.

Responsibility for Interfacility Transports

Although fragmented, the responsibility for the patient during the traditional interfacility transfer resides primarily with the transferring physician and institution. Matching the medical needs of the patient, which the transferring physician should determine, with the appropriate level of care for the transfer is often difficult for the transferring physician. Reasons include a lack of clinical guidelines to assist in making level-of-care decisions and the frequent lack of knowledge of the capabilities of the local interfacility transport system.

The local EMS medical director or specialty transport unit medical director, who is most knowledgeable about the treatment capabilities of the transporting units and their personnel, might not be affiliated with the transferring facility. Consequently, the capabilities of the EMS system to provide interfacility transfers is not always universally known, and referring physicians are often not cognizant of the capability of the local providers. Additionally, the specialty transport systems that might be available for patient transport often originate from outside the local area. In many EMS systems, there is no provision for specialized transport using local resources.

Most patients are adequately cared for by the existing local BLS or ALS system. However, patients with a higher severity of illness or need for specialty care might not be adequately cared for by these local providers. The local EMS system and medical director should provide appropriate education to referring facilities as to the capabilities of the available interfacility transport resources. In addition, the EMS medical director should define a standard scope of practice consistent with the training of the personnel involved in the various segments of the EMS system. This scope of practice should be used to determine if the local system has the capability to provide interfacility transport for any patient. If the severity of illness or the medications used to stabilize the patient are beyond this scope of practice, the local EMS providers should have the authority to decline the transport and the sending physician must make alternative arrangements.

Alternative Practices

Alternatives to the local ground EMS providers for the provision of interfacility transfer depend largely on the resources available in the community. For much of the country, patients requiring care beyond the scope of practice of the local EMS system are transferred by ground ambulance with supplemental hospital staff to provide the required level of care.[22] Another alternative is to terminate nonessential treatments such as medication drips, which might be temporarily withheld without patient harm, in order to mold the patient to the scope of practice of the available system.

In most cases, this is not ideal. The sending facility might also decide to further stabilize the patient to a point that would allow for local EMS transport. Finally, in systems without safeguards to prevent transfer by inadequately trained personnel, a sending physician might believe that the only available method of transport of a critical patient is with inadequate providers. The sending physician might arrange such a transfer in order to deliver the patient to a facility more able to provide the needed care than the sending facility. This last alternative clearly puts the patient at risk during transport and would violate the obligations of the transferring physician and facility under EMTALA. (See Chapter 27, "EMTALA and EMS.") This is not advocated as a viable alternative.

Ground Specialty Transport Units

The types of specialty transport units vary, and some critical care transport units can fulfill multiple roles. Types of specialty units include those for coronary care, pediatrics, and neonatal transport and nonspecialized mobile intensive care units (MICUs) (**Figure 13-1**). Specialty missions performed by critical care transport units include the transport of patients receiving support with intra-aortic balloon pumps, a ventricular assist device, or extracorporeal membrane oxygenation.[23]

The first ground specialty transport units predated the widespread deployment of organized EMS systems and paramedics in this country. In 1966, Pantridge placed resuscitation equipment designed for use in the hospital on an ambulance, staffed it with physicians and nurses, and demonstrated the ability to perform cardiac care in an out-of-hospital setting.[24] Hospitals in the United States developed similar systems with variations in equipment and staffing. At the time, interfacility transfer for specialty cardiac care was rare, as the treatment modalities for cardiac patients were limited, and most patients could be cared for at home or in primary care facilities. As the EMS system in this country became more mature, paramedics demonstrated that they were proficient at managing acute coronary emergencies in both the emergency response and interfacility venues. Today, most cardiac patients who must be transferred for specialty care have been stabilized by the primary facility and can be transported within the scope of practice of the modern paramedic. For patients requiring care beyond that scope, hospital-based or ambulance-based MICUs, which do not emphasize a particular medical subspecialty, can be used to transport the more seriously ill or injured patients. These include ground and air medical units. The ground MICUs most often use conventional ambulances but

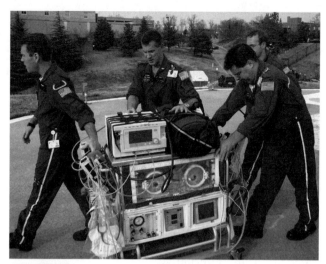

Figure 13-1 Neonatal transports are often conducted using specialty care units and transport teams.

are supplemented with additional equipment and staffed in such a manner as to be capable of managing a variety of medical and surgical conditions.[25,26]

Children's hospitals and large medical institutions that have neonatal and pediatric intensive care units frequently have specialty ground transport units with specialized personnel and equipment such as transport incubators. They also frequently carry special equipment to allow for airway management and intravenous therapies. Neonatal transport services have been well organized since the inception of modern EMS.[27,28]

MICUs often have the capability to manage high-risk obstetric patients. Those who are not at risk for imminent delivery might generally be safely transported to facilities specializing in managing high-risk pregnancies and the delivery and management of premature infants. Women having labor contractions, especially those for whom delivery is imminent, are best managed by delivery of the infant at the transferring facility and transport of mother and baby to specialty care units. Resources to care for mother and child at the referring facility are far superior to those available in a transporting unit. Once the baby is delivered, mother and child can be more safely transferred.

Unit Staffing

The medical team configuration should consist of the health care professionals best suited to the type of transfer being made by the specialty transport unit. The staffing of specialty and critical care transport units varies and provides for various levels of patient care capabilities. Specially trained critical care

paramedics and nurses provide most of the staffing for critically ill patients.[25,29-34] The need for physicians during transfers is probably limited to the most serious patients who require frequent or extensive interventions.[29,35-40] In some situations, a flexible staffing model is used, providing various levels of patient care providers for the transport depending on the severity of illness or injury.[34,41]

Although several organizations have published guidelines or position papers concerning interfacility transport,[41-46] there are no generally accepted standards describing specific staffing requirements for specialty care transports. The level of licensure required for providers of care during transport is dependent on the severity of illness of the patient, the complexity of the technology involved, and the level of training of the providers. A variety of functional transport unit models exists, providing appropriate care to patients within the defined scope of practice of the specialty unit.[25,34,40] Staffing, whether by physicians, nurses, respiratory therapists, paramedics, or EMTs, should be dictated by the needs of the service and individual patient.

Most routine patient care can be managed by one care provider in the patient compartment of the transport vehicle. However, at least two medical crew members should be available to manage patient care in case the patient's condition deteriorates and to provide for the routine lifting of the patient in and out of the transport vehicle. More seriously ill patients might require two or more providers in the patient compartment (**Figure 13-2**).

The transport team should have policies or protocols that define the staffing requirements.[45] Consultation with the transport agency's medical director should be available when staffing level questions arise. Whatever the team composition, adequate training should be available initially and regularly thereafter to ensure the provision of the highest level of care required and available.

Communications

The efficient operation of a specialty ground transport system requires a carefully planned dispatch and medical communications system. A full-time dispatcher to initiate and follow the progress of the transport is a valuable resource. The communications center generally performs several functions. It receives requests for service, dispatches the transport unit, and maintains constant communication with the transport unit and its medical crew. Additionally, the communications center could act as a full-service transfer center and

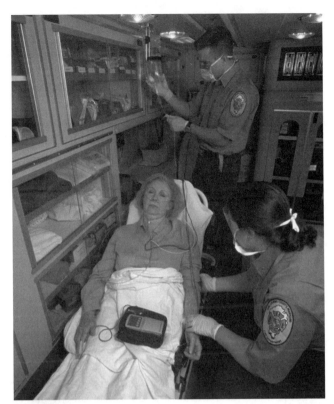

Figure 13-2 Seriously ill patients might require two or more providers in the patient compartment.

arrange for the acceptance of patients at receiving institutions. The communications center could also relay information when direct communication between the transporting unit and the receiving facility is not immediately possible.

A plan to ensure some form of medical communication with both the sending and receiving facilities should be in place for any specialty transport unit. This communication is important to accommodate for unexpected changes in patient condition, allowing the medical crew to consult with the referring physician, the receiving facility, or the medical director of the transport unit as needed. Although direct communication is best, information could also be relayed through the communications center. Because transports might involve great cross-country distances, radios might not be completely reliable as the sole way to provide medical direction. Cellular telephones have proved to be a valuable tool to enhance the ability of specialty transport units to maintain medical communications

throughout the transport. Specific protocols and standing orders must be developed to provide guidance for routine medical treatment and to cover those circumstances where direct communication is not possible.

Medical Oversight

Medical responsibility during the transfer should be arranged prior to patient transport. This might be done at the time of initial contact between the referring and receiving physicians. Transfer orders should be written by the referring physician after consultation between the sending and receiving physicians. Options for medical responsibility during the transport include:

- The sending physician assumes medical responsibility, or
- The receiving physician assumes medical responsibility, or
- The medical director of the transport unit assumes medical responsibility, or
- The physicians share a predefined responsibility, with a transfer of that responsibility en route when transport distances exceed communications capabilities.[46]
- The selection might be based on prearranged agreement, communications capability, or it might even be defined by statute.

A specialty transport unit should have a defined medical director who has responsibility for the medical operations of the unit. The medical director is responsible for establishing protocols and procedures for routine care and for management of expected and unexpected complications during transport. The medical director should be available or have a preestablished mechanism in place to allow for online consultation for the specialty unit. The specialty transport unit, similar to EMS units, must have the capability to contact online resources to assist in circumstances that are not anticipated by offline protocols.[46]

Summary

Ground interfacility and specialty transport is an important part of the EMS system. In order to be successful and be of maximum benefit to patients and the medical system, these units must have appropriate levels of training, a defined scope of practice, and sufficient planning for medical oversight and must provide the community with education about the unit's practice capabilities.

References

1. Boyd DR. The history of emergency medical services (EMS) systems. In: Boyd DR, Edlich RF, Micik SH, et al. eds. *Systems Approach to Emergency Medical Care.* Norwalk, Conn: Appleton-Century-Crofts; 1983:1–82.

2. Swor RA, Storer D, Domeier RM, et al. Medical direction of interfacility patient transfers. *ACEP-PREP.* January 1997.

3. Examination and treatment for emergency medical conditions and women in labor. 42 USC 1395dd, §1867 of the Social Security Act.

4. Baxt WG. The impact of a rotorcraft aeromedical emergency care service on trauma mortality. *JAMA.* 1983;249:3047–3051.

5. Macnab AJ, Wensley DF, Sun C. Cost-benefit of trained transport teams: estimates for head-injured children. *Prehospital Emerg Care.* 2001;5:1–5.

6. Straumann E, Yoon S, Naegeli B, et al. Hospital transfer for primary coronary angioplasty in high risk patients with acute myocardial infarction. *Heart.* 1999;82:415–419.

7. Towers CV, Bonebrake R, Padilla G, et al. The effect of transport on the rate of severe intraventricular hemorrhage in very low birth weight infants. *Obstet Gynecol.* 2000;95:291–295.

8. Thomas SH, Orf J, Peterson C, et al. Frequency and costs of laboratory and radiograph repetition in trauma patients undergoing interfacility transfer. *J Emerg Med.* 2000;18:156–158.

9. Selevan JS, Fields WW, Chen W, et al. Critical care transport: outcome evaluation after interfacility transfer and hospitalization. *Ann Emerg Med.* 1999;33:33–43.

10. Society of Critical Care Medicine. Guidelines for the transfer of critically ill patients. *Crit Care Med.* 1993;21:931–937.

11. Kellermann AL, Hackman BB. Emergency department patient 'dumping': an analysis of interhospital transfers to the regional medical center at Memphis, Tennessee. *Am J Public Health.* 1988;78:1287–1292.

12. American College of Emergency Physicians. Principles of appropriate patient transfer. *Ann Emerg Med.* 1990;19:337–338.

13. American College of Emergency Physicians. Appropriate interhospital patient transfer. *Ann Emerg Med.* 1997;30:365.

14. Olson CM, Jastremski MS, Vilogi JP. Stabilization of patients prior to interhospital transfer. *Am J Emerg Med.* 1986;5:33–39.

15. Braman SS, Dunn SM, Amico CA, et al. Complications of intrahospital transport in critically ill patients. *Ann Intern Med.* 1987;107:469.

16. Kanter R, Tompkins J. Adverse events during interhospital transport: physiologic deterioration associated with pretransport severity of illness. *Pediatrics.* 1989;84(1):43–48.

17. Katz V, Hansen A. Complications in the emergency transport of pregnant women. *South Med J.* 1990; 83(1):7–9.

18. Martin G, Cogbill T, Landercasper J, et al. Prospective analysis of rural interhospital transfer of injured patients to a referral trauma center. *J Trauma.* 1990;30:1014–1020.

19. Valenzuela T, Criss E, Copass M, et al. Critical care air transportation of the severely injured: does long distance transport adversely affect survival? *Ann Emerg Med.* 1990;19(2):169–172.

20. Himmelstein DU, Woolhandler S, Harnly M, et al. Patient transfers: medical practice as social triage. *Am J Public Health.* 1984;74:494–497.

21. Crippen D. Critical care transportation medicine; new concepts in pretransport stabilization of the critically ill patient. *Am J Emerg Med.* 1990;8:551–544.

22. Wuerz R, Meador S. Adverse events during interfacility transfer by ground advanced life support services. *Prehospital Disaster Med.* 1994;9(1):50–53.

23. McBride LR, Lowdermilk GA, Fiore AC, et al. Transfer of patients receiving advanced mechanical circulatory support. *J Thorac Cardiovasc Surg.* 2000;119:1015–1020.

24. Pantridge JF. Mobile coronary care. *Chest.* 1970; 58:229–234.

25. Domeier RM, Hill J. The development and evaluation of a paramedic-staffed mobile intensive care unit for interfacility patient transport. *Prehospital Disaster Med.* 1996;11(1):37–43.

26. Greco A. Development of an interfacility transport program for critically ill cardiovascular patients. *AACN Clin Issues Crit Care Nurs.* 1990;1(1):3–12.

27. Segal S. Transfer of a premature or other high risk newborn infants to a referral hospital. *Pediatr Clin North Am.* 1966;13:1195–1205.

28. Hackel A. A medical transport system for the neonate. *Anesthesiology.* 1975;43:258–267.

29. Macnab AJ. Optimal escort for interhospital transport of pediatric emergencies. *J Trauma.* 1991;31:205–209.

30. Pristas LR, Rausch T. Transport considerations for the critically ill child. *Crit Care Nurs Q.* 1997;20(1):72–80.

31. Johnson CM, Gonyea MT. Subspecialty clinics: pediatrics, transport of the critically ill child. *Mayo Clin Proc.* 1993;68:982–987.

32. Edge WE, Kanter RK, Weigle CG, et al. Reduction of morbidity in interhospital transport by specialized pediatric staff. *Crit Care Med.* 1994;22:1186–1191.

33. Pon S, Notterman DA. The organization of a pediatric critical care transport program. *Pediatr Clin North Am.* 1993;40(2):241–261.

34. Boyko SM. Interfacility transfer guidelines: an easy reference to help hospitals decide on appropriate

vehicles and staffing for transfers. *J Emerg Nurs.* 1994;20(1):18–23.

35. McCloskey K, King WL, Byron L. Pediatric critical care transport: is a physician always needed on the team? *Ann Emerg Med.* 1989;18(3):35–37.

36. Crippen D. Interhospital transport of critically ill patients: problems and pitfalls. *Int J Emerg Intensive Care Med.* 1997;1(4).

37. McCloskey KA. Emergency interhospital critical care transport for children. *Curr Opin Pediatr.* 1996;8(3):236–238.

38. Rubenstein JS, Gomez MA, Rybicki L, et al. Can the need for a physician as part of the pediatric transport team be predicted? *Crit Care Med.* 1992;20:1657–1660.

39. McCloskey KA, Johnston C. Critical care interhospital transports: predictability of the need for a pediatrician. *Pediatr Emerg Care.* 1990;6:89–92.

40. Gebremichael M, Borg U, Habashi N, et al. Interhospital transport of the extremely ill patient: the mobile intensive care unit. *Crit Care Med.* 2000;28:79–85.

41. Day S, McCloskey K, Orr R, et al. Pediatric interhospital critical care transport: consensus of a national leadership conference. *Pediatrics.* 1991;88:696–704.

42. Emergency Nurses Association. Care of the critically ill or injured patient during interfacility transfer [ENA Web site]. Available at: http://www.ena.org/about/position/CareCriticallyIll-INTER.asp. Accessed February 14, 2005.

43. Society of Critical Care Medicine. Guidelines for the transfer of critically ill patients. *Crit Care Med.* 1993;21:931–937.

44. American Academy of Pediatrics Task Force on Interhospital Transport. *Guidelines for Air and Ground Transport of Neonatal and Pediatric Patients.* 2nd ed. Elk Grove Village, Ill: American Academy of Pediatrics; 1999.

45. American College of Emergency Physicians. Medical direction of interfacility patient transfer. *Ann Emerg Med.* 1998;31:154.

46. Shelton SL, Swor RA, Domeier RM, et al. Position Paper; National Association of EMS Physicians: Medical direction of interfacility transports. *Prehospital Emerg Care.* 2000;4:361–364.

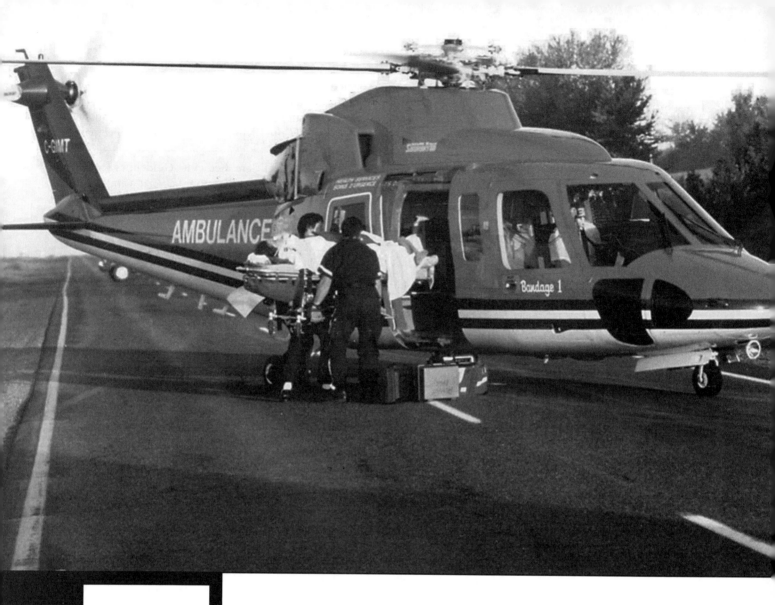

14 | Air Medical Transport

Kenneth A. Williams, MD, FACEP
Kenneth J. Robinson, MD, FACEP

AIR MEDICAL TRANSPORT IS THE USE OF AIRCRAFT IN THE care and movement of patients. It developed from the expediency of aircraft use in battle conditions, where geography, time, and hazards sometimes made air travel preferable over land travel. Similar logic, with some adaptations, applies for civilian and peacetime air medical systems. Proper use of air medical transport requires knowledge of system capabilities and limits. This chapter presents those capabilities and limits in three sections, with suggested topics of interest for physicians who might request air transport for their patients, for flight physicians who provide care in aircraft, and for air medical program medical directors.

Goals of Air Medical Transport

Enhance Patient Care by Expanding the Range of Time-Sensitive Care

A goal of air medical systems is to provide critical care medical transport that results in similar or better pa-

tient outcome over a larger geographic area than can be achieved by ground transport during the same elapsed time. In other words, patients with similar illness or injury can potentially receive sufficient care to have equal or better outcomes from more remote areas when air medical care is available. This is a reasonable goal, but it could be unrealistic to expect a better outcome for all patients. The appropriate use of air medical transport can markedly improve patient outcomes.

Comparison of interfacility helicopter transport times in one study suggests that a dedicated critical care air medical system has equal to or better than average transport times when compared with one-way ground transport.[1]

The round-trip disadvantage of the helicopter is offset by greater transport speed, ability to fly in a direct line, prompt response time, and efficient patient assessment at the referring institution. The ability to reach out further into the community more rapidly than ground transport has the potential to improve outcomes for individual patients, make specialty services (neonatal, cardiac, trauma, for example) available to a wider range of patients, and allow regionalization of tertiary care. This ability to enhance patient care by expanding the range of time-sensitive care is a realistic goal.

Decrease Out-of-Hospital Time for Critically Ill or Injured Patients

Patients are often transferred from an emergency department or critical care unit to a tertiary care facility for care that is not available at the referring facility. These critically ill or injured patients can suddenly become unstable en route. In the transport environment, there often are not as many resources available on the transporting vehicle as at the referring or receiving hospital. An unnecessarily prolonged out-of-hospital time can have adverse effects on a patient's condition. The increased speed of the air medical transport vehicle decreases the time that the patient is out of the hospital setting in most cases, and thereby can decrease the possibility that the patient's condition will deteriorate during transport.

Provide Access to Care From Remote Areas

Another benefit of air medical systems is access to care in remote areas. Remote could mean rural, with a distance of many miles to the nearest hospital or definitive care, an area inaccessible by ground vehicles (such as an island or mountaintop), or an area isolated by ground due to traffic patterns, bridges, tunnels, etc. In some cases, the remote nature of the requesting agency is constant and well known, such as an offshore oil rig or tourist island. In other cases, the requesting agency will ask for air medical assistance because of a transient condition such as icy roads, a natural disaster blocking highway access (including forest fire, flood, or hurricane), or episodic traffic (such as holiday or rush-hour congestion). Some programs use aircraft to deliver specialized staff such as cardiologists or gastroenterologists to remote areas for scheduled diagnostic testing or specialty care. Others are referenced in the regional disaster management plan as a resource for staff, supplies, reconnaissance, and communications, as well as patient transportation if a mass-casualty event occurs far from ground resources.

Promote Efficient Use of Advanced Critical Care Transport Teams

In order for patients to benefit from air medical transport, the critical care team aboard the aircraft must be trained and experienced in delivering a variety of advanced care interventions. The air medical systems must efficiently develop, maintain, and use the skills of a scarce resource, the clinical professionals who provide or support critical care medical transport through the use of aircraft. Although critically ill or injured patients can certainly become unstable and require advanced care, most remain stable during transport. This does not relieve the referring institution or agency from the responsibility of requesting a means of transport that maintains or improves the level of care available for the patient. In addition, it does not relieve the air medical transport system of the responsibility of making available a medical crew capable of providing both the care required and care that might become necessary if the patient's condition deteriorates.

The cost of training and experience necessary to manage critical care patients, along with the cost of personnel with advanced credentials, is a major expense for any critical care transport program. The use of aircraft allows more efficient use of a smaller number of such teams. Each helicopter ambulance, for example, can efficiently cover the same area as six ground ambulances. The cost of a single helicopter is more than offset by the cost of staff, training, equipment, and facility for six ground ambulance bases.[2]

Facilitate Regionalized Care Systems

Often stated indirectly, one goal of air medical transport systems is standardization and integration of local care within a specialty or regionalized tertiary care system. For example, a tertiary care hospital in a rural area might want to develop a neonatal intensive care program but does not have the patient volume within a reasonable driving time of the hospital. An air medical transport system might provide the ability to establish and support the program through its ability to safely transport patients from a larger geographic area and therefore a larger population base. This ability provides a standardized regional resource with training and role-model influences on EMS and hospital care. Although not typically stated as a goal of air medical transport, this ability provides a mechanism for bringing current care practices to a large referral area and for standardizing patient care in a beneficial way. In particular, these benefits are important where standardized care systems such as trauma systems involve a regional geography.

Rotor wing (helicopter) air medical programs are best integrated into local EMS and hospital care delivery systems through planning, adherence to standards for safe and high-quality care, and education. These mechanisms, including programs on safe landing zones, patient care and preparation for flight, communications/request/acceptance procedures, and patient followup have dual benefits. While directly improving the safety and care of individual patients, the dissemination of current best practice education indirectly aids the entire medical region.

In EMS systems with tiered response protocols, the inclusion of helicopter air medical transport can improve response times and care. Fixed-wing aircraft, which typically fly longer missions than helicopters, can have a similar effect through the dispatch of medical specialists or teams to remote sites.

Provide Research and Training Opportunities

The best clinical practices in critical care air and ground transport, EMS, and emergency medicine can be determined only through research. Air medical transport programs, through their ability to reach a broad distribution of providers with a relatively small number of professional crews, provide an excellent means to gather research data. In addition, many aircraft have the ability to carry observers and serve as an excellent training platform for EMS providers, other health care professionals, and others (media, administrators, politicians, or regulators, for example) with public interest in emergency care.

Provide Aviation Resources

Transport systems must provide an opportunity for the effective, proper, and safe use of rotor and fixed-wing aviation resources in support of civilian medical care objectives. They should do so in a way that is economically and socially viable and provides for professional and personal development of those involved.

Both helicopter and fixed-wing aircraft represent the commercial aviation industry in a variety of ways. Air medical transport programs, through use of aviation equipment, personnel, and support systems, support the aviation industry. Many commercial helicopter pilots employed in transient, seasonal, and/or temporary situations (eg, logging, construction, crop dusting, power line maintenance, sightseeing) are also air medical transport pilots. These pilots now have the benefit of both job and location security because air medical care systems provide steady, scheduled employment with aviation operations from a fixed base. Similarly, aviation support providers such as helicopter manufacturers, interior completion firms, vendors of helicopter equipment, services and personnel, maintenance professionals and their support network, fuel and hangar providers, and others involved in the aviation industry now have hundreds of relatively fixed sites of helicopter operation to rely on, whereas previous operations were typically airport based and transient. This allows both improved stability and reliability in both planning and operations. In addition, those directly involved in air medical care have an interest in safety, economic viability, and social support for their efforts. Advances in medicine and aviation should be accommodated in air medical transport programs in a way that facilitates professional development and challenge, as well as personal satisfaction and growth for those involved.

One goal of air medical programs is to provide safe and effective use of aircraft in support of patient care and transport, but there are risks involved with the use of any transport system or vehicle. Patient movement, even within the hospital, increases the risk of falls, inadvertent removal of lines and tubes and other medical devices, as well as unrecognized or untreated adverse events. The use of personnel and equipment chosen and trained for the transport of critically ill patients reduces this risk. Another risk is injury to the patient and transport staff if a transport vehicle crashes. Ground ambulances crash approximately 10 times

more often than air medical helicopters on a per-mile basis, but helicopter crashes are more likely to cause serious injury or death on a per-crash basis.[2] Air medical helicopter programs, in an effort to improve safety, often address issues such as pilot training and experience, crew resource management and teamwork training, interior design (ie, elimination or padding of objects in the head-strike zone, secure mounting for all equipment, load-absorbing seats, patient and crew restraints), and emergency exit and survival training.

Helicopter crashes, not surprisingly, are often related to unexpected bad weather, night operations, operations in unfamiliar terrain, and mechanical failure. Measures to reduce these factors include pilot training and familiarization; the use of predesignated landing sites, careful mission planning, including the best available weather information; cautious operational parameters for night and unfamiliar terrain operations; and rigorous mechanical inspection and maintenance programs. In some crashes, teamwork failures during a chain of errors lead to avoidable crashes. Efforts to improve teamwork coordination through training and use of team simulator sessions are measures that can improve safety.[3]

Physician Interface With Air Medical Care

Referring Physician

The referring physician will interface with air medical services through medical oversight of EMS care at the scene or by requesting transport from a hospital or other facility. In order to provide online medical direction or consultation via radio, cellular telephone, or other means for EMS services involved with or requesting air medical support, the emergency physician should understand basic air medical transport concepts and be familiar with the air medical service capabilities in the area.

Others requesting service, including intensivists, neonatologists, and surgeons, should be familiar with the best way to obtain service at their facilities and the type of care provided by local air medical services. The hospital emergency department and related EMS communications center, if any, should provide knowledge and resources to others in the hospital community seeking air medical transport.

Emergency physicians, and EMS medical directors in particular, requesting air medical services should have knowledge and information about the services in their areas, as follows:

- Services locally available
- Level of care provided by each service
- Typical response times and criteria
- The best way to request service
- Preferred patient care practices of the flight program
- Followup procedures

Services Locally Available

Emergency physicians should know how many air medical programs are in the service area and whether they provide services using helicopters, fixed-wing aircraft, ground vehicles, or a combination of vehicles. The physicians should know their operations parameters, such as hours of operation and number of aircraft or teams available. They should also be aware of the programs' weather capabilities, any restrictions on a patient's weight and size, and whether they can accommodate a patient's family.

Level of Care Provided by Each Local Service

Emergency physicians considering air transport must be aware of crew composition, equipment, size and type of vehicle, and what type of care can be provided by each service. They must also consider whether the transport vehicles are equipped with devices such as incubators or balloon pumps. The training levels of the medical care team and whether they vary with the mission should also be considered. Preferably, the requesting agency can discuss the level of care needed with the medical director or accepting physician prior to mission launch. Emergency physicians should know what medications and equipment for monitoring and treatment are aboard the aircraft. Physicians should consider whether there are any medical devices or situations that make the air medical option difficult or impossible (cervical traction devices, patients contaminated with hazardous materials, or uncontrolled patient agitation, for example), and what alternatives are available for these patients.

Typical Response Times and Criteria

There are many ways to discuss times involved in medical transport and many definitions. Two time parameters that are important to the requesting physician are the time from the initial request until the medical crew is at the patient's bedside, and the time from initial request until patient delivery at the definitive care site. Knowledge of these times in typical circumstances (aircraft ready and at base, weather acceptable, patient prepared as requested, patient accepted at receiving facility) allows the requesting physician to judge trans-

port options if there is a choice to be made. Similar times should be sought for ground transport and other options such as fixed-wing air transport and use of local 911 ambulance services so that the referring physician can choose the best option for each patient.

In addition to time, other operational criteria should be known. Requesting physicians must know whether the program flies at night. They must know if, and under what circumstances, the program takes multiple patients. Whether the flight program will find an accepting physician or hospital for the patient, or whether that effort is required prior to the request, should be understood. In some locations, the air transport programs require verification of payment before response. This is not unusual for fixed-wing programs and can apply to helicopter programs depending on local practice, licensing, and regulatory climate. Although a requesting physician might believe that the choice of patient destination is determined by the requesting and accepting physicians, the air medical program might have internal policies or parameters that create preferences or even absolute requirements for receiving hospitals (the presence of a helipad on the premises, for example). If there are requirements that seem unfair, improper, or a violation of good medical practice or EMTALA regulations, the referring physician should discuss them with the air medical program medical director in order to understand the basis for the requirements, and with other physicians if the situation still appears improper.

Best Way to Request Service

Most air medical programs require telephone or radio contact from medical professionals to accept a mission. The lay public, in most locations, cannot request helicopter ambulance service to their home or hospital bed. A direct request to the flight program communications system is the most efficient means to request service. Air medical programs should have a way to contact accepting physicians and provide awareness about available intensive care beds or other capabilities at receiving hospitals. This system of patient acceptance gives the referring facility an efficient means to transfer patients, without having to hunt for an accepting physician by calling the main hospital number. Most air medical programs use a form, either paper or computer based, to record the information necessary to accept a mission. Referring facilities should understand this process and explore options such as faxing the information simultaneously with a telephone call, sending secure information over the Internet, or even having copies of the relevant forms available to simplify the request conversation.

Preferred Patient Care Practices of the Flight Program

Some issues often arise when a critically ill or injured patient must be moved rapidly between facilities. They include air medical programs that prefer all patients to have two patent intravenous lines; those that have latex-safe or latex-free requirements in place for the flight program or the accepting facility; and instructions for securing and maintaining the airway. Also, the best way to handle concentrations and drip rates of intravenous medications should be determined. Requesting physicians should consult with the air medical program to determine whether thrombolytics should be completely administered before flight and how the spine is to be stabilized. Air medical programs have developed preferred ways to handle these and other issues. Requesting physicians and their respective facilities should be aware of these preferences, accommodate those that are reasonable, and resolve any issues prior to transport whenever possible. For example, if a referring hospital typically mixes a pressor at double the concentration of the flight program, a protocol or understanding of how that patient care issue should be resolved when that medication is in use can be developed among the involved staff long before it creates the potential for patient delay or harm.

Followup Procedures

Questions pertaining to the completion of the mission must also be answered. Some programs will ship or deliver EMS or hospital equipment that was used in transport; others ask that it be picked up at the destination hospital. Many programs provide maps and directions explaining their service and ways for the family to get information from the destination hospital or how to travel there. Requesting physicians should be aware of the procedures for obtaining information in patient followup, for reasons of medical knowledge or even personal health (in a body fluid exposure situation, for example). Confidentiality should be maintained. For example, followup letters bearing the patient's name should not be posted on bulletin boards in the referring hospital or EMS agency, but it might be acceptable to post letters referring to the "child with fever and seizures transported on May 11."

Flight Physician

Operations

In addition to the knowledge required for referring physicians, flight physicians (and other members of the medical care team) should have significantly greater understanding of the air medical program's operational capabilities. These topics should include:

- Air medical transport history, operations, associations, and research
  - History and development of air medical care
  - Indications for air medical transport
  - Air medical associations and their function, to include the Air Medical Physician Association (AMPA) and its handbook and positions, and the Commission on Accreditation of Medical Transport Systems and its standards
  - Air medical research
- Aviation operations and equipment (tables)
  - Master switch
  - Fuel shutoff valve
  - Rotor brake (where applicable)
  - Oxygen shutoff valve
  - Refueling
  - Aircraft maintenance
  - Aircraft startup and cool-down procedures
  - Aircraft egress, including emergency egress
  - Safety around the aircraft during all phases of operation
  - Basic concepts of aircraft spotting and reporting
  - Emergency fuel shutdown
  - Fire extinguisher location and use
  - ELT location and use
  - Safety briefing information
  - Maintenance requirement and schedule basics
  - Airframe safety basics
  - Navigation basics
  - Landing zone and approach procedures
  - Takeoff and landing procedures and checklists
  - Proper use of communication equipment
  - Securing patient and equipment in aircraft
  - Understanding of weight and balance limitations of aircraft
- Program operations
  - Staff shifts and scheduling
  - Charting procedures
  - Dispatch procedures
  - Medical equipment maintenance requirements
  - Aircraft stocking and cleaning
  - Policies and procedures
  - Communications equipment and procedures
  - Patient acceptance and transfer procedures
  - Safety training

- Flight briefing and debriefing
- Quality improvement process, medical and programwide
  ▪ Flight physiology
  - The pressure, volume, and temperature relationships of gases (Boyle, Henry, and Charles laws) and the expected effect of these laws on patients and patient care devices in the program service area
  - Basics of weather recognition and forecasting, including local weather patterns
  - The physical and physiologic effects of noise, vibration, and acceleration on flight crew and patient, with particular emphasis on motion sickness and patient monitoring capabilities
  ▪ EMS and mass-casualty response
  - Familiarity with disaster plans for the region, state, and hospital, with emphasis on the specific role of the EMS helicopter service
  - Applicable and acceptable systems for incident command, disaster response and staging, patient identification, decontamination, assessment, triage and care, and transport routing
  ▪ Search, rescue, and survival
  - Ground and marine, if applicable, search patterns and the local protocols for coordination of air and ground search and rescue teams
  - Wilderness survival techniques appropriate to the area served by the flight program, such as fire starting, signaling, the provision of food and shelter, and compass use and map-reading skills
  - Program policies and procedures regarding search and rescue missions, missing aircraft, aircraft incidents and accidents, and emergency egress in unusual situations such as water ditching
  ▪ Hazardous materials
  - The meaning of common transportation system placards
  - Basics of hazardous materials scene approach and response at the OSHA level appropriate for the program mission profile
  - Introduction to and basic understanding of the Department of Transportation *Emergency Response Guidebook*
  - Policies and procedures on the containment of commonly encountered hazardous materials and pathophysiology and medical management of victims of exposure

- Program policies and procedures regarding hazardous materials operations

Vehicles and Equipment

The flight physician should be intimately familiar with the aircraft and ground vehicles used by the flight program and with all medical equipment and procedures related to patient care aboard that aircraft or vehicle.

Because air medical teams are small, typically two providers only, the physician must be able to assist with and use equipment such as monitor-defibrillators, ventilators, intravenous pumps, intravenous pacemakers, radios, oxygen supplies, Doppler stethoscopes, and any other devices aboard the aircraft (**Figure 14-1**). The physician's knowledge must include more than observing the device in use; the flight physician should know how to change batteries, charge batteries, adjust the unit during operation, clean and pack the unit for next use, and troubleshoot common problems. The flight physician must be familiar with procedures such as mixing intravenous medications, obtaining intravenous access, and performing endotracheal intubation, tube thoracostomy, and so on, in three ways. First, the flight physician must be able to perform the procedure well and know how the air medial environment influences both performance of the procedure and patient monitoring thereafter. Second, the flight physician must know where to find the necessary equipment for performing the procedure aboard the aircraft. It is not enough to ask for a chest tube kit; the flight physician should be able to find the necessary supplies rapidly and confidently in the aircraft's medical bags or cabinets. Third, the flight physician must understand enough aerospace medicine to know if the procedure places the patient at additional risk with changes in altitude, vibration, and so on, and be able to monitor the patient for these effects and accommodate them.

Clinical Care in the Aviation Environment

Flight physicians providing care for critically ill or injured patients in the aviation environment must understand the relevant patient conditions and treatment in an EMS or hospital setting, as well as how the aviation environment influences both the medical condition and the treatment.[4] Flight physician training curriculum would include topics such as:
  ▪ Neurologic disorders
  - Increased intracranial pressure
  - Closed- and open-head injuries
  - Spinal cord injuries
  - Thrombotic, embolic, and hemorrhagic cerebrovascular events

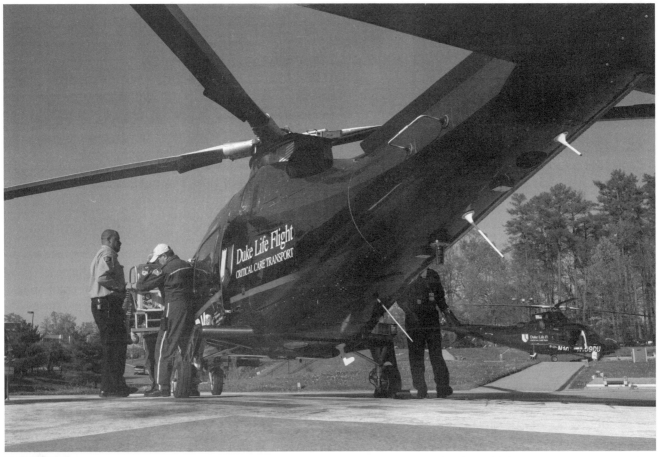

Figure 14-1 The flight physician must be able to assist with and use any of the medical equipment aboard the aircraft.

- Respiratory disorders
  - Respiratory arrest
  - Pulmonary edema
  - Pulmonary embolism
  - Bronchospastic and obstructive airway disease
  - Pneumothorax and hemothorax
  - Upper airway problems
  - Use of mechanical ventilation
  - Management of a difficult airway
  - Indications for hyperbaric oxygen
- Cardiovascular disorders
  - Acute myocardial infarction
  - Ventricular and supraventricular dysrhythmias
  - Left ventricular failure and shock
  - Malignant hypertension
  - Aortic dissections/aneurysms
  - Cardiopulmonary arrest
- Trauma
  - Splinting of fractures and spinal immobilization techniques
  - Airway management of the trauma victim
- Management of suspected hemothorax and pneumothorax
- Management of shock
- Management of neurologic trauma
- Assessment and management of abdominal injury
- Assessment and use of various scoring systems as used by regional EMS agencies and trauma centers
- Management of the burn victim
- The regional trauma plan (adult and pediatric)
- The regional burn plan
- High-risk obstetric and neonatal patients
  - Pre-eclampsia and eclampsia
  - Pregnancy-induced hypertension
  - Normal vaginal delivery
  - Preterm labor
  - Obstetric hemorrhage
  - Neonatal hypoglycemia
  - Respiratory distress syndrome
  - Meconium aspiration
  - Tracheoesophageal fistula

- Myelomeningocele
- Gastroschisis and omphalocele
- Cyanotic heart disease
- Apgar scoring system
  - Pediatric disorders
    - Croup and epiglottitis
    - Asthma/bronchiolitis
    - Child abuse and neglect
    - Infectious diseases common to childhood
    - Special considerations in pediatric trauma
    - Assessment of pediatric hemodynamics, respiratory and neurologic status
    - Seizures
    - Psychosocial development of infants, children, and adolescents
    - Vascular access
  - Policies and procedures
    - Relevant regional, state, local, hospital, and program laws, regulations, policies, and procedures related to aircraft, EMS, and air medical operations

Infection Control and Prevention

Because of the potential for transmission of infectious diseases during health care encounters, all flight physicians should use universal precautions. Procedures and policies for universal precautions, sharps safety, decontamination, biologic spills, and body fluid contact/exposure should be developed and demonstrated. Particular challenges in the air medical environment include the need to depart the scene of care (and perhaps leave body fluids or contaminated materials behind), the lack of handwashing facilities in the aircraft (often necessitating an exception in hospital handwashing policies and alternative cleansing solutions), and the need to perform procedures in the aircraft. Pathophysiology and communicability of potentially encountered infectious diseases should also be part of the training.

Air Medical Program Medical Director

Physician medical directors for air medical programs should have an understanding of all aspects of program operations, from aviation to business management. A knowledge focus on medical aspects of critical care transport, integration of the air medical program into the local EMS and health care system, and the local regulatory environment are paramount. As the program's leader and medical supervisor, the physician medical director should also understand issues that concern the program mechanics, pilots, communicators, and administrators, as well as flight nurses, paramedics, respiratory therapists, and physicians. Thus, the medical director should be familiar with all of the information expected for a referring physician and a flight physician, with the additional understanding necessary to lead the program wisely and safely. The medical director is the final arbiter of all medical care delivered by the program and of all operations from a medical standpoint. Requirements and qualifications for a medical director are noted below.[4-9]

Basic Requirements and Qualifications

The basic requirements/qualifications for a medical director in air medical transport are as follows:

- Appropriate professional medical credentials with the jurisdiction governing operations of the air medical system
- Knowledge and training in clinical care consistent with the mission profile
- Skill and training in the resuscitation and stabilization of the acutely ill and injured patient, including all age ranges appropriate to the program mission profile
- Capability to implement both initial and continuing medical education appropriate for air medical personnel
- Knowledge and/or training in unique aspects of air medical operations, including altitude physiology, occupational health, regulatory aspects, safety and survival techniques, vehicle and vehicle capabilities, and equipment requirements and performance, including general knowledge about air medical operations and detailed knowledge about the equipment and other operations used by the program
- Operational knowledge of communications equipment and procedures, including familiarity with various emergency communication and location systems used in the program service area or those likely to be used in the event of a program emergency
- Knowledge of issues in out-of-hospital and interhospital transport, both current and literature based as well as political and managerial
- Knowledge and/or training in medical command and control, including the development and use of protocols, standing orders, triage procedures, incident command, and the capabilities of patient care providers

- Skill at performing utilization reviews of flight program resources
- Working knowledge of disaster planning and mass-casualty incident management
- Working knowledge of quality improvement processes and programs
- Administrative skills and knowledge, including communication and negotiation skills, a basic understanding of fiscal and employment issues, interviewing and hiring skills, skill in stress recognition and treatment, and an understanding of principles of risk management and medical-legal issues, including transfer regulations
- Knowledge or training in the basic principles of research

Desirable Characteristics

The desirable characteristics of the medical director in air medical transport are as follows:

- Board certification in a specialty appropriate to the mission profile
- Prior experience as a member of an aviation or medical flight team
- Training in hazardous materials management
- Public relations skills
- Experience with online medical direction
- Knowledge of search and rescue techniques
- Knowledge of occupational health issues as they relate to the air medical environment
- Training or experience as an educator
- Knowledge of planning and implementation of outreach education and safety programs
- The capability to conceptualize, conduct, and report original research
- Knowledge of EMS system design and configuration

Summary

Physicians involved in air medical or other critical care transport should be knowledgeable about such operations in relation to their involvement. Physicians who request air medical services should have an understanding of the procedures and systems involved in arranging transport services for their patients. Flight physicians have additional responsibility to understand aspects of transport medicine that include clinical care of patients in the transport environment and the unique aspects of that environment, as well as the operational and safety requirements. Program medical directors should be familiar with the knowledge base of requesting and flight physicians, and in addition have the responsibility to understand managerial, financial, political, regulatory, and human resources aspects of directing a critical care transport system.

References

1. Salton G, Brozen R. A comparison of air and ground transport times. Poster presented at: Critical Care Transport Medicine Conference; April 9–11, 2001; San Antonio, Tex.
2. Bruhn J, Williams K, Aghababian R. True costs of air medical vs ground ambulance systems. *Air Med J.* 1993;12(8):262–268.
3. Williams K, Rose W, Simon R. Teamwork in emergency medical services. *Air Med J.* 1999;18:149–153.
4. Fromm RE Jr. Training of the air medical flight crew: practical applications. In: Blumen I, ed. *Air Medical Physician Handbook.* Salt Lake City, Utah: Air Medical Physician Association; 1995.
5. Alonso-Serra H, Blanton D, O'Connor RE. NAEMSP position paper: physician medical direction in EMS. *Prehospital Emerg Care.* 1998;2:153–157.
6. Carrubba C, Air Medical Physician Association Consensus Group. Role of the medical director in air medical transport. In: Rodenberg H, Blumen IJ, eds. *Air Medical Physician Handbook.* Salt Lake City, Utah: Air Medical Physician Association; 1999.
7. Eljaiek LF, Norton R, Carmona R. NAEMSP position paper: medical director for air medical transport programs. *Prehospital Disaster Med.* 1995;10(4):283–285.
8. Stone RM, Seaman KG, Bissell RA. A statewide study of EMS oversight: medical director characteristics and involvement compared with national guidelines. *Prehospital Emerg Care.* 2000;4:345–351.
9. Blumen I, ed. *Air Medical Physician Handbook.* Salt Lake City, Utah: Air Medical Physician Association; 1995.

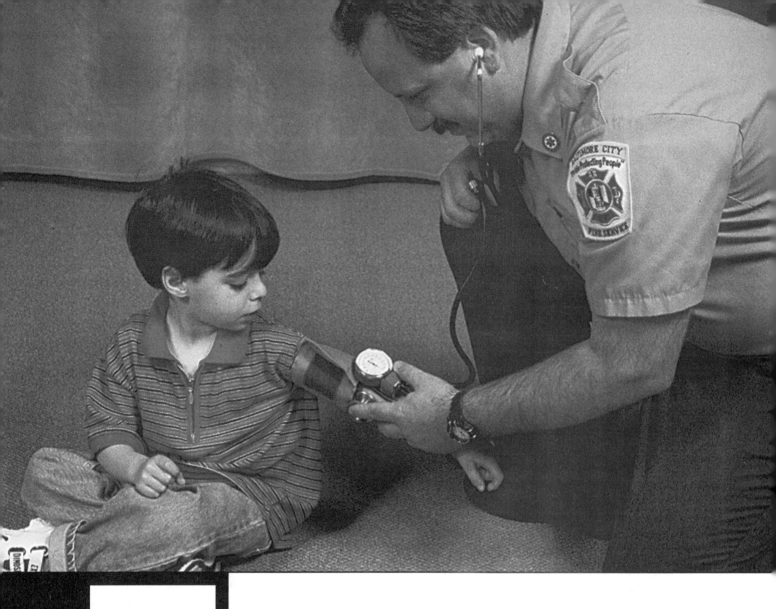

15

EMS for Children

Marianne Gausche-Hill, MD, FAAP, FACEP
John A. Brennan, MD, FAAP, FACEP
Robert K. Waddell II

Principles of This Chapter

After reading this chapter, you should be able to:

- Explain the impact of EMSC on the health and welfare of children in the United States.
- Describe the EMSC grants that have funded improvements in all 50 states and US territories.
- Discuss the resources and partnerships available to EMS administrators and medical directors, other health care professionals, and parents.

History of Emergency Medical Services for Children

THE EMERGENCY MEDICAL SERVICES FOR CHILDREN (EMSC) PROgram, a national initiative of the Health Resources and Services Administration (HRSA) Maternal and Child Health Bureau (MCHB) and the National Highway Traffic Safety Administration (NHTSA), was established in 1985 to help reduce childhood disability and death due to severe illness or injury.[1-3] This national initiative has had a tremendous impact on the health and welfare of children in the United States. It began with the recognition that EMS systems, which had originally focused on much-needed trauma and cardiac care for adults, were not meeting the needs of the children within that system.[4,5]

Dr. James Seidel and colleagues, in a series of articles in the early 1980s, outlined data on the epidemiology of out-of-hospital care for children and noted that children represent approximately 10% of the paramedic calls. They also found that trauma death rates were twice those of adults, and survival from cardiopulmonary arrest was poor.[4] In a survey of EMS training programs,[5] Seidel later found that little time was spent educating out-of-hospital providers in pediatric emergency care. He reported that 40% of the programs had less than 10 hours of pediatric didactic training, and 41% had less than 10 hours of clinical experience in pediatrics. EMS providers were also lacking in pediatric-sized equipment such as resuscitation masks (79% did not have all of the sizes of masks), pediatric manual resuscitators or bag-mask devices (20% did not carry appropriate sizes for pediatrics), pediatric backboards (52% carried only adult sizes), and infant and child blood pressure cuffs and IV catheters (20% to 32% were missing various sizes).[5]

These data and personal experiences with the emergency care system at that time prompted Senators Orrin Hatch (R-Utah), Lowell Weicker (R-Connecticut), and Daniel Inouye (D-Hawaii) to sponsor the first EMSC legislation, which established a national EMSC program.[2,6,7] This legislation (Public Law 98-555) made funding available through the Department of Health and Human Services, Bureau of Maternal and Child Health Resources Development, to improve care of children within EMS systems.[2,7] The goal of the EMSC program is to ensure that state-of-the-art, child-sized emergency equipment is available and that all EMTs and health care providers offer age-appropriate care, including rehabilitation. The first four states to receive funding were Alabama, California, Oregon, and New York in 1986.[2,6] By 1997, all 50 states and US territories had received funding to improve pediatric care.[6]

EMSC is continually being integrated into EMS at local, regional, state, and national levels. Components of EMSC within EMS systems are shown in **Figure 15-1**.[7,8] These components help to ensure an appropriate con-

Figure 15-1 EMSC components within EMS systems.

System planning and financing
Universal access to quality emergency care for all persons through a 911 system
Dispatch, including telephone triage and EMS prearrival instructions
Triage policies for EMS providers to transport to pediatric-capable facilities
Timely transport to definitive care with personnel and equipment to care for children
Emergency department preparedness for the care of children
Specialty facilities for children (pediatric critical care and pediatric trauma centers)
Interfacility transfer agreements between emergency departments and specialty centers
Public and professional education
Data collection and analysis to be used for pediatric performance improvement
Public health and safety agencies (eg, poison center, child protective services)
Clinical research in EMSC

Figure 15-2 EMSC continuum of care.

Prevention phase
Entry phase
- Systems of access (911 and enhanced 911)
- Dispatch
- Out-of-hospital care
Hospital phase
- Emergency departments
- Inpatient care
- Intensive care
Rehabilitation phase
Ongoing care phase
- Medical home/family-centered care
- Mental health services

tinuum of care. This continuum includes the prevention phase, entry phase, out-of-hospital phase, hospital phase, rehabilitation phase, and ongoing care phase (**Figure 15-2**).[1,8] Many of these components will be integrated by the primary care provider as part of a child's **medical home** (**Figure 15-3**).[9] Emergency physicians, EMS providers, and EMS administrators will continue to establish relationships with primary care providers, specialists, and public agencies to achieve injury and illness prevention and well-coordinated medical care for ill and injured children entering the EMS system.

The Institute of Medicine and EMSC

In 1993, the Institute of Medicine (IOM) published a report on EMSC in the United States.[10,11] Although the IOM panel recognized that pediatric emergency care had improved significantly over the previous decade, they suggested seven essential areas of EMS system responsibility (**Figure 15-4**).[10] They also recognized problems in communication, access to care, data collection, physician involvement, equipment, education of providers, research, and EMS system infrastructure (**Figure 15-5**).[2,11] The panel then made a series of recommendations in the following areas: education and training; putting essential tools in place; communication and 911 systems; planning, evaluation, and research; and federal and state agency funding (**Figure 15-6**).[2,11]

Since its beginnings, the EMSC program has sought feedback from out-of-hospital providers, physicians, nurses, administrators, parents, and legislators on the job being done by the program. Over the past 17 years, the EMSC program has responded to the perceived and documented needs of EMS systems, including those recommendations by the IOM panel.[1,6] As a result, several initiatives have evolved to address these needs, as described in the following sections.

Figure 15-4 IOM report: seven essential areas of EMS system responsibility for EMSC.

Identifying emergencies
Ensuring access to the services of the system (911 telephone service)
Providing appropriate out-of-hospital care
Transporting patients
Providing definitive medical care
Communicating among emergency care providers and with others, to include parents and primary care providers
Using information systems and feedback to assess and improve patient care, to enhance system performance, and to identify injury prevention needs

Figure 15-5 IOM: problems within EMS systems that affect children.

Many communities lack 911 and enhanced 911 capabilities.
Data sets are not uniform and lack outcome measures.
Physician involvement in EMS is lacking in many communities.
Some EMS systems lack proper equipment to care for patients of all sizes and ages.
Some systems lack protocols and education to care for infants and children.
EMS systems lack involvement of health care professionals with both pediatric and EMS expertise.
Research into optimal paradigms, approaches, and modalities to care for children in all phases of EMS is lacking.
Regionalization of care for critically ill and injured children is lacking.

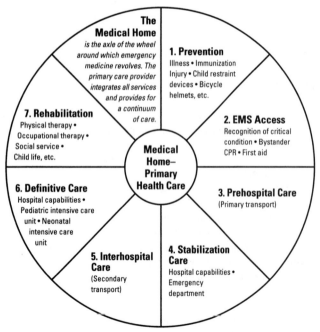

Figure 15-3 The medical home and integrated medical care for children. Reprinted with permission from Singer JS, Ludwig S, eds. *Emergency Medical Services for Children: The Role of the Primary Care Provider.* Elk Grove Village, Ill: American Academy of Pediatrics; 1992.

Figure 15-6 IOM report: recommendations of the Committee on Pediatric Emergency Medical Services.

Education and training
- States and localities develop and sustain programs to provide the general public of all ages with adequate and appropriate levels of education and training in the following areas:
  - Safety and prevention
  - First aid CPR
  - How to use the EMS system appropriately for children
- States and localities develop and maintain specific guidelines or criteria to ensure quality curricula in pediatric emergency care for EMT-Basic, EMT-Intermediate, and EMT-Paramedic providers, allied health care professionals, and nurse and physician graduate education programs.
  - Education to include pediatric basic and advanced life support (as appropriate), medical, developmental, and social needs of children, and children with special health care needs

Putting essential tools in place
- All state regulatory agencies with jurisdiction over hospital emergency departments and emergency response and transport vehicles have available and maintain equipment and supplies appropriate for emergency care for children.
- All state regulatory agencies in EMS address the issue of regionalization and categorization of pediatric care and oversee the integration of EMSC within EMS systems.

Communication and 911 systems
- All states ensure that 911 systems are implemented and, wherever possible, implement enhanced 911 systems.

Planning, evaluation, and research
- States adopt ICD-9-CN E codes for improved reporting of childhood injury.
- States implement a program for data collection and analysis based on a national uniform data set and report results on the nature of EMS provided for children.
- Develop methodology for linking data sets in emergency care from the field to rehabilitation.
- Expand research in EMSC and give priority to seven areas: clinical aspects of emergencies and emergency care; indices of severity of illness and injury; patient outcome and outcome measures; costs; system organization, configuration, and operation; effective approaches to education and training, including retraining and skill retention; and prevention.

Federal and state agencies and funding
- Congress directs the Secretary of the Department of Health and Human Services:
  - To establish a federal center or office to conduct, oversee, and coordinate activities related to planning, evaluation, research, and technical assistance in EMS for children
  - To establish a national advisory council for this center — members to include representatives of relevant federal agencies, local and state governments, the health care community, and the public at large
- States establish a lead agency to identify specific needs in EMS for children and to address mechanisms to support those needs.
  - Establish state advisory councils
- Congress appropriates $30 million each year for 5 years to support activities of the federal center and the state agencies related to EMS for children.

Adapted from Durch JS, Lohr KN, eds. *Emergency Medical Services for Children: Summary.* Washington, DC: National Academies Press; 1993.

◼ EMSC Initiatives

As part of its commitment to children, the EMSC program supports two resource centers: the **EMSC National Resource Center (EMSC NRC)** and the **National EMSC Data Analysis Resource Center (NEDARC).*** The NRC, located in Washington, DC, is dedicated to providing technical support, information dissemination, and

---

* For information, contact EMSC (202-884-4927 or www.ems-c.org), EMSC NRC (703-902-1203), or NEDARC (801-581-6410 or http://nedarc.med.utah.edu).

topic-specific expertise. NEDARC, located in Salt Lake City, Utah, is dedicated to providing data collection, analysis, and linkages. Both resource centers are accessible to EMSC coordinators, health care providers, parents, and the general public.

The EMSC program has 88 active grants (FY 2004). Other programs supported by the federal EMSC program are: the Clinical Practice Guidelines program; the Enhancing Pediatric Patient Safety demonstration project; the Emergency Medical Services for Children partnerships demonstration grants; the Network Development Demonstration Project cooperative agreement; EMSC research opportunities; Emergency Medical Services for Children regional symposium supplemental grants; and the Partnership for Children consortium.

Clinical Practice Guidelines

The purpose of the Clinical Practice Guidelines program (Public Health Service Act, Title XIX, Section 1910, 42 USC §300W-9) is to develop and to demonstrate the usefulness of a set of clinical practice guidelines applicable to all medical personnel who are responsible for treating children's emergency conditions (eg, pediatricians, family practitioners, nurse practitioners, emergency physicians, and physician assistants). These guidelines are intended to improve care for common problems treated in emergency departments and physician offices. They will be based on an assessment of published research and will be used to accumulate valid summary data for EMS.

Enhancing Pediatric Patient Safety

In November 1999, the IOM published *To Err is Human: Building a Safer Health System.*[12] This report generated significant concern and more articles and publications in both the medical literature and the lay press; however, several articles raising concern over medical errors were in print before the IOM report.[13-23]

The IOM report highlighted one critical aspect of health care quality — the ability of the system to render care to patients without causing injury in the process. The report synthesized the available evidence on patient safety and noted that medical errors are a leading cause of death and injury.[12]

The Enhancing Pediatric Safety initiative evolved from a growing recognition that children have unique needs in emergency situations — needs that often vary from those of adults due to the physiological, developmental, and psychological differences between children and adults. The purpose of this demonstration project is to support the assessment of an existing strategy or tool that has the potential to improve patient safety in pediatric emergency care delivery in multiple out-of-hospital and emergency department settings.

EMSC Partnerships Demonstration Grants

The purpose of these state partnership demonstration grants (Public Health Service Act, Section 1910, 42 USC §300W-9) is to provide a funding mechanism for activities that represent the next logical step or steps to take in order to institutionalize EMSC within EMS and to continue to improve and refine EMSC. Proposed activities should be consistent with documented needs in the state and should reflect a logical progression in enhancing pediatric capabilities. For example, funding might be used to: address problems identified in the course of a previous EMSC grant; increase the involvement of families in EMSC; improve linkages among local, regional, or state agencies; disseminate standards developed for one region of the state under previous funding to include the entire state; devise a plan for coordinating and funding poison centers; or ensure effective field triage of children in physical or emotional crisis to appropriate facilities and/or other resources.

Network Development Demonstration Project Cooperative Agreement

The goal of the Network Development Demonstration Project (NDDP) cooperative agreement is to demonstrate the value of an infrastructure for collaborative research in EMSC, as follows:

- A well-conceived and fully operational infrastructure can be put in place to conduct clinical trials and observational studies on EMSC using rigorous study designs and methodologies.
- A consensus-derived and well-informed research agenda can be developed and used to actively guide the network's activities.
- A research and development process can be instituted fully within the network to develop proposals, conduct pilot studies, and carry out full-blown investigations with support from MCHB or other federal agencies.
- A plan to study and encourage the transfer of network findings to EMSC practices can be designed and instituted.
- A collaboration of EMSC personnel, nurses, practitioners, and researchers can be fostered to provide opportunities for bidirectional education and exchange of ideas, information, and values between the treatment and academic communities.

EMSC Research Opportunities

HRSA and other Health and Human Services agencies have responded to children's unique emergency medical needs by issuing a first-time, multiagency program announcement highlighting research opportunities in the field.

A consensus group was convened using the Rand-UCLA consensus process to develop priorities for research in EMSC.[24-26] This group reviewed the priori-

Figure 15-7 Priorities for research in EMSC.

Major clinical entities, including shock, respiratory distress, asthma, brain injury, multiple-organ trauma, seizures, poisoning, behavioral disorders, burns, and fever
Development and validation of outcome measures
Injury prevention
Medical informatics
Effective ways to measure, improve, and upgrade the quality of EMS care and systems
Prevention and relief of physical and emotional pain
Effectiveness and cost of out-of-hospital interventions
Pediatric resuscitation
Costs of EMSC: direct, indirect, and marginal
Access to EMS for children
Development and validation of injury and illness scores
Educational issues such as training, retraining, and skill retention
Public education in injury prevention, basic emergency care skills, and the use of EMS systems
Triage in the out-of-hospital and emergency department settings
Children with special health care needs

ties for research as described in the IOM report. Fifteen topic areas from the 32 suggested by panelists were placed in the seven priority categories identified in the IOM report. Clinical aspects of emergency care, systems organization, configuration and operation, and injury prevention were given high-priority rankings. These priorities are listed in **Figure 15-7**.[24-26]

The Interagency Committee on EMSC Research joint program announcement identifies each agency's EMSC-related research programs, as well as eligibility and funding information. The committee is composed of representatives of HRSA, the Agency for Healthcare Research and Quality, the Centers for Disease Control and Prevention, and the National Institutes of Health. This federal collaboration resulted from a 1997 meeting of a multidisciplinary group of professional organizations that came together to establish research priorities in light of the IOM recommendations for increased EMSC research.

EMSC Regional Symposium Supplemental Grants

The purpose of the EMSC regional symposium supplemental grants (Public Health Service Act, Section 1910, 42 USC §300W-9) is to provide supplemental funds to existing state partnership grantees for regional roundtable meetings that are convened for the purpose of knowledge sharing. In collaboration with schools of medicine, regional consortia of state EMS programs meet annually to develop and evaluate improved procedures and protocols for treating children. Meetings involve coordinating, exchanging, and demonstrating innovative activities of common interest to participating states and provide a forum for knowledge transfer on EMSC-related issues between individual care providers and care-providing organizations.

Partnership for Children

The EMSC program has established strong collaborative relationships among national organizations dedicated to the safety and well-being of children. In 2003, the Partnership for Children Consortium became the **EMSC Partnership for Children Stakeholders**, and several organizations, grantees, and federal agencies were integrated into the group for the purpose of providing input into EMSC program goals and objectives. These organizations are listed in **Figure 15-8**.

As a result of these collaborative relationships, EMSC sponsors task forces to address issues such as research priorities (discussed earlier in this chapter), supplies for BLS and ALS ambulances, equipment and medication supplies for emergency departments, education needs for out-of-hospital providers, the development of an emergency information form for children

Figure 15-8 EMSC Partnership for Children Stakeholders.

Ambulatory Pediatric Association
American Academy of Family Physicians
American Academy of Pediatrics
American Association of Poison Control Centers
American College of Emergency Physicians
American College of Osteopathic Emergency Physicians
America's Health Insurance Plans
American Pediatric Surgical Association
American Trauma Society
CDC National Center for Injury Prevention and Control
Emergency Nurses Association
Family Voices
EMSC Grantees (state partnership, targeted issues, NEDARC, PECARN)
Indian Health Services
International Association of Fire Fighters
National Association of Children, Hospitals and Related Institutions
National Association of Emergency Medical Technicians
National Association of EMS Physicians
National Association of State EMS Directors
National Association of School Nurses
National Association of Social Workers
National Council of State EMS Training Coordinators
National Highway Traffic Safety Administration
National Safe Kids Campaign

with special health care needs, pediatric protocols for out-of-hospital providers, and guidelines for pediatric preparedness of emergency departments.

Emergency Information Form

Children with special health care needs create a challenge for EMS providers and emergency physicians. These children often have complex medical problems that require special knowledge of the interaction of their anatomy with childhood physiology. These children often are cared for by multiple specialists, and it can be difficult for emergency care providers to access information on all their care from one source. In 1996, members of the Pediatric Committee of the American College of Emergency Physicians (ACEP) suggested the development of a data set or information form to be available to emergency physicians who care for children with special health care needs.[27] This emergency information form (EIF) would contain a summary of the child's medical problems and important drug interaction information, as well as physician contact information. This effort led to the collaboration of the federal EMSC program with ACEP and the American Academy of Pediatrics (AAP), and ultimately to the establishment in 1998 of policy statements outlining an EIF that can be completed by a patient's physician and used by emergency physicians to obtain much-needed information on types of illness, allergies, medications, and reactions to certain emergency therapies (**Figure 15-9**).[28] This joint effort by ACEP and AAP was the first time that these organizations had collaborated on a policy to serve the mutual needs of patients cared for by members of both societies. The EIF has become a national initiative involving such organizations as ACEP, AAP, the Emergency Nurses Association (ENA), the National Association of School Nurses (NASN), the National Association of Children's Hospitals and Related Institutions (NACHRI), the National Association of EMS Physicians (NAEMSP), the National Association of Emergency Medical Technicians (NAEMT), and NHTSA.

The form can be downloaded from the ACEP Web site (http://www.acep.org/library/pdf/EIF.pdf).

Ambulance Equipment

In 1996, a multidisciplinary task force was assembled by the National EMSC Resource Alliance (NERA) as part of the EMSC program in order to develop guidelines for pediatric equipment to be carried by BLS and ALS ambulances. This multidisciplinary committee included representatives from the American Ambulance Association, ACEP, the American College of Surgeons (ACS), ENA, the International Association of Fire Chiefs,

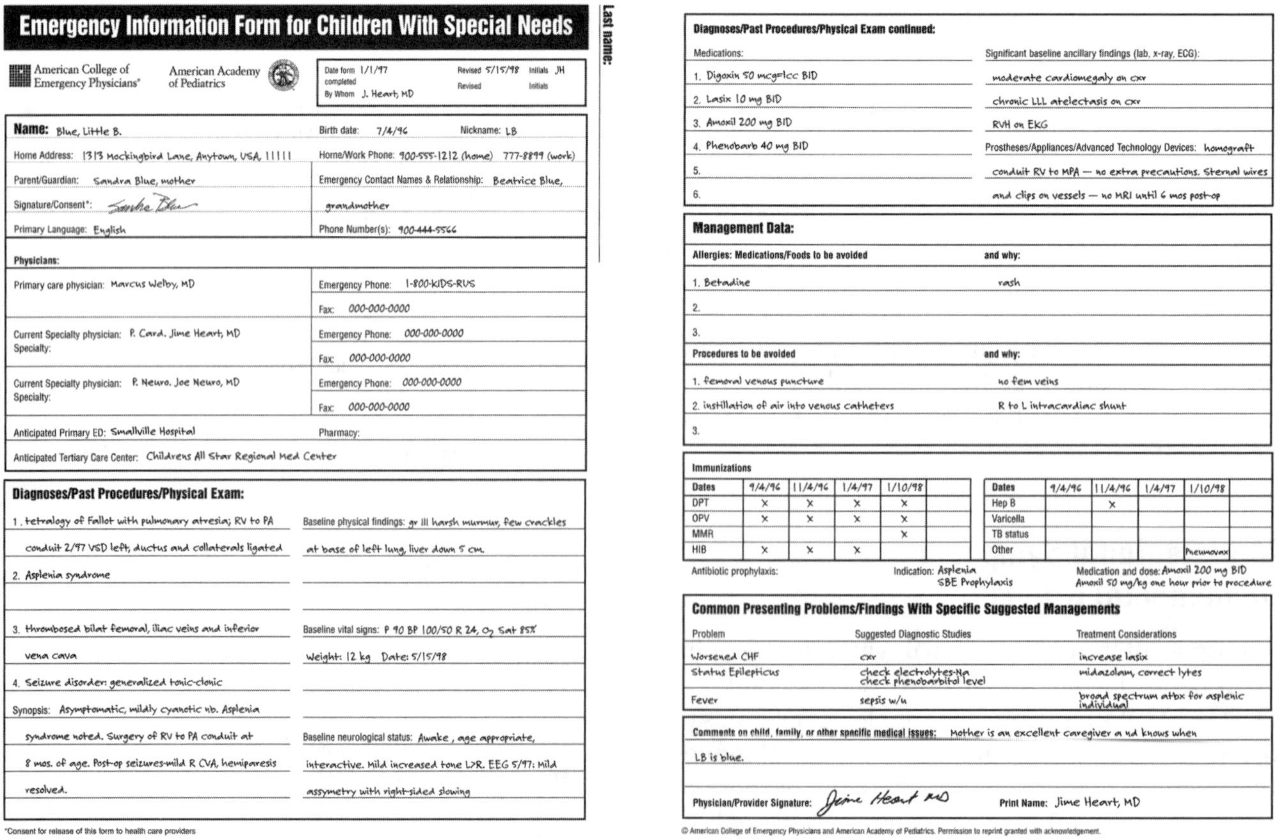

Emergency Information Form for Children With Special Needs

Last name:

American College of Emergency Physicians® — American Academy of Pediatrics

Date form completed: 1/1/97 — By Whom: J. Heart, MD — Revised: 5/15/98 — Initials: JH — Revised: — Initials:

Name: Blue, Little B. — Birth date: 7/4/96 — Nickname: LB

Home Address: 1313 Mockingbird Lane, Anytown, USA, 11111 — Home/Work Phone: 900-555-1212 (home) 777-8899 (work)

Parent/Guardian: Sandra Blue, mother — Emergency Contact Names & Relationship: Beatrice Blue, grandmother

Signature/Consent*: Sandra Blue

Primary Language: English — Phone Number(s): 900-444-5566

Physicians:

Primary care physician: Marcus Welby, MD — Emergency Phone: 1-800-KIDS-RUS — Fax: 000-000-0000

Current Specialty physician: P. Card. Jime Heart, MD — Specialty: — Emergency Phone: 000-000-0000 — Fax: 000-000-0000

Current Specialty physician: P. Neuro. Joe Neuro, MD — Specialty: — Emergency Phone: 000-000-0000 — Fax: 000-000-0000

Anticipated Primary ED: Smallville Hospital — Pharmacy:

Anticipated Tertiary Care Center: Childrens All Star Regional Med Center

Diagnoses/Past Procedures/Physical Exam:

1. tetralogy of Fallot with pulmonary atresia; RV to PA conduit 2/97 VSD left, ductus and collaterals ligated
2. Asplenia syndrome
3. thrombosed bilat femoral, iliac veins and inferior vena cava
4. Seizure disorder: generalized tonic-clonic

Synopsis: Asymptomatic, mildly cyanotic nb. Asplenia syndrome noted. Surgery of RV to PA conduit at 8 mos. of age. Post-op seizures-mild R CVA, hemiparesis resolved.

Baseline physical findings: gr III harsh murmur, few crackles at base of left lung, liver down 5 cm.

Baseline vital signs: P 90 BP 100/50 R 24, O_2 Sat 85% — Weight: 12 kg — Date: 5/15/98

Baseline neurological status: Awake, age appropriate, interactive. Mild increased tone L>R. EEG 5/97: Mild assymetry with right-sided slowing

*Consent for release of this form to health care providers

Diagnoses/Past Procedures/Physical Exam continued:

Medications:

1. Digoxin 50 mcg=1cc BID
2. Lasix 10 mg BID
3. Amoxil 200 mg BID
4. Phenobarb 40 mg BID
5.
6.

Significant baseline ancillary findings (lab, x-ray, ECG): moderate cardiomegaly on cxr; chronic LLL atelectasis on cxr; RVH on EKG

Prostheses/Appliances/Advanced Technology Devices: homograft conduit RV to MPA — no extra precautions. Sternal wires and clips on vessels — no MRI until 6 mos post-op

Management Data:

Allergies: Medications/Foods to be avoided	and why:
1. Betadine	rash
2.	
3.	

Procedures to be avoided	and why:
1. femoral venous puncture	no fem veins
2. instillation of air into venous catheters	R to L intracardiac shunt
3.	

Immunizations

Dates	9/4/96	11/4/96	1/4/97	1/10/98	
DPT	x	x	x	x	
OPV	x	x	x	x	
MMR				x	
HIB	x	x	x		

Dates	9/4/96	11/4/96	1/4/97	1/10/98	
Hep B		x			
Varicella					
TB status					
Other				Pneumovax	

Antibiotic prophylaxis: — Indication: Asplenia; SBE Prophylaxis — Medication and dose: Amoxil 200 mg BID; Amoxil 50 mg/kg one hour prior to procedure

Common Presenting Problems/Findings With Specific Suggested Managements

Problem	Suggested Diagnostic Studies	Treatment Considerations
Worsened CHF	cxr	increase lasix
Status Epilepticus	check electrolytes-Na check phenobarbitol level	midazolam, correct lytes
Fever	sepsis w/u	broad spectrum atbx for asplenic individual

Comments on child, family, or other specific medical issues: Mother is an excellent caregiver and knows when LB is blue.

Physician/Provider Signature: Jime Heart MD — Print Name: Jime Heart, MD

Figure 15-9 Sample completed Emergency Information Form.

Figure 15-10 Equipment for BLS and ALS ambulances.

Basic Level Providers

A. Ventilation and Airway Equipment

1. Portable and fixed suction apparatus
   - Wide-bore tubing, rigid pharyngeal curved suction tip; tonsillar and flexible suction catheters, 5F–14F
2. Portable and fixed oxygen equipment
   - Variable flow regulator
3. Oxygen administration equipment
   - Adequate length tubing; mask (adult, child, and infant sizes), transparent, non-rebreathing, Venturi, and valveless; nasal cannulas (adult, child, and infant sizes)
4. Pocket mask with one-way valve
5. Bag-valve mask
   - Hand-operated, self-reexpanding bag (adult and infant sizes), with oxygen reservoir/accumulator; clear mask (adult, child, infant, and neonate sizes); valve (clear, disposable, operable in cold weather)
6. Airways
   - Nasopharyngeal, oropharyngeal (adult, child, and infant sizes)

B. Monitoring and Defibrillation

Automatic external defibrillator is strongly recommended for systems that do not have immediate availability of an advanced life support service.

C. Immobilization Devices

1. Cervical collars
   - Rigid for children ages 2 years or older, infant, child, and adult sizes (small, medium, large, and other available sizes)
2. Head immobilization device (not sandbags)
   - Firm padding or commercial device
3. Lower extremity (femur) traction devices
   - Lower extremity, limb-support slings, padded ankle hitch, padded pelvic support, traction strap (adult and child sizes)
4. Upper and lower extremity immobilization devices
   - Joint-above and joint-below fracture (adult and child sizes), rigid-support appropriate material (cardboard, metal, pneumatic, vacuum, wood, or plastic)
5. Radiolucent backboards (long, short) and extrication device
   - Joint-above and joint-below fracture site (chin strap alone should not be used for head immobilization), adult and child sizes, with padding for children, hand holds for moving patients, short (extrication, head-to-pelvis length), long (transport, head to feet), with at least 3 appropriate restraint straps

D. Bandages

1. Burn pack
   - Standard package, clean burn sheets (or towels for children)
2. Triangular bandages
   - Minimum 2 safety pins each
3. Dressings
   - Sterile multitrauma dressings (various large and small sizes)
   - ABDs, 10"×12" or larger
   - 4"×4" gauze sponges
4. Gauze rolls
   - Sterile (various sizes)

5. Elastic bandages
   - Nonsterile (various sizes)
6. Occlusive dressing
   - Sterile, 3"×8" or larger
7. Adhesive tape
   - Various sizes (including 2" or 3") hypoallergenic
   - Various sizes (including 2" or 3") adhesive

E. Communication

- Two-way radio communication (UHF, VHF) between EMT, dispatcher, and medical direction (physician)
- Two-way disaster communication
- Cellular phone

F. Obstetrical

1. Kit (separate sterile kit)
   - Towels, 4"×4" dressing, umbilical tape, sterile scissors or other cutting utensil, bulb suction, clamps for cord, sterile gloves, blanket
2. Thermal absorbent blanket and head cover, aluminum foil roll, or appropriate heat-reflective material (enough to cover newborn)
3. Appropriate heat source for ambulance compartment

G. Miscellaneous

1. Sphygmomanometer (infant, pediatric, and adult regular and large, for example, thigh sizes)
2. Stethoscope (pediatric and adult)
3. Length/weight-based chart for pediatric equipment sizing
4. Thermometer with low temperature capability
5. Heavy bandage or paramedic scissors for cutting clothing, belts, and boots
6. Cold packs
7. Sterile saline solution for irrigation (1-liter bottles or bags)
8. Flashlights (2) with extra batteries and bulbs
9. Blankets
10. Sheets, linen, or paper (minimum 4), and pillows
11. Towels
12. Triage tags
13. Disposable emesis bags or basins
14. Disposable bedpan
15. Disposable urinal
16. Wheeled cot (properly secured patient transport system)
17. Folding stretcher
18. Stair chair or carry chair
19. Patient care charts/forms
20. Lubricating jelly (water soluble)

H. Infection Control*

*Latex-free equipment should be available.

1. Eye protection (full peripheral glasses or goggles, face shield)
2. Masks
3. Gloves, nonsterile
4. Jumpsuits or gowns
5. Shoe covers
6. Disinfectant hand wash, commercial antimicrobial (towelette, spray, liquid)
7. Disinfectant solution for cleaning equipment

(continued on next page)

Figure 15-10 Equipment for BLS and ALS ambulances (continued).

8. Standard sharps containers (EMT-Basic, -Intermediate, and -Paramedic)
9. Disposable trash bags (identifiable color, such as red)
10. HEPA mask

I. Injury Prevention Equipment

1. Appropriate restraints (seat belts, air bags) for patient, crew, and family members
2. Child safety restraints
3. Protective helmet and coat with reflective material (1 each per crew member)
4. Fire extinguisher
5. Hazardous material reference guide
6. Traffic signaling devices (reflective material triangles or other reflective, nonigniting devices)

J. Optional Basic Equipment

1. Pneumatic antishock garment (PASG)
   - Compartmentalized (legs and abdomen separate), control valves (closed/open), inflation pump, lower leg to lower rib cage (does not include chest)
2. Respirator
   - Volume-cycled valve, on/off operation, 100% oxygen, 40–50 psi pressure (child/infant capabilities)

Advanced Level Providers

For EMT-Paramedic, include all the equipment listed for the basic level provider plus the following additional equipment and supplies. For EMT-Intermediate (and other nonparamedic advanced levels), include all the equipment for the basic level provider and selected equipment and supplies from the following list, as appropriate.

A. Vascular Access

1. Intravenous administration equipment (fluid must be in bags, not bottles)
2. Crystalloid solutions, Ringer's lactate or normal saline solution (1,000-mL bags × 4), 5% dextrose in water (optional)
3. Antiseptic solution (alcohol wipes and povidone-iodine wipes preferred)
4. IV pole or roof hook
5. Intravenous catheters 14G–24G, 1" long
6. Intraosseous needles
7. Tourniquet, rubber bands
8. Syringes of various sizes, including tuberculin
9. Needles, sizes 19G–25G
10. Intravenous administration sets (microdrip and macrodrip), Burretrol, and in-line blood pump (as differentiated from intravenous tubing with an in-line blood filter)
11. Intravenous arm boards, adult and pediatric

B. Airway and Ventilation Equipment

1. Laryngoscope handle with extra batteries and bulbs, adult and pediatric
2. Laryngoscope blades, sizes 0, 1, and 2, straight; sizes 3 and 4, straight and curved

3. Endotracheal tubes, sizes 2.5–6.0 mm uncuffed and 6.5–8.0 mm cuffed (2 each), other sizes optional
4. Meconium aspirator
5. 10-mL non-Luerlock syringes
6. Stylettes for endotracheal tubes, adult and pediatric
7. Magill forceps, adult and pediatric
8. Lubricating jelly (water soluble)
9. Nasogastric tubes, pediatric sizes 5F and 8F, Salem sump sizes 14F, 16F, and 18F
10. End-tidal CO_2 detectors
    - Colorimetric or quantitative

C. Cardiac

1. Portable, battery-operated monitor/defibrillator
   - With tape write-out/recorder, defibrillator pads, quick-look paddles or hands-free patches, ECG leads, adult and pediatric chest attachment electrodes, adult and pediatric paddles, with capability to provide electrical discharge below 25 watt-seconds.
2. Transcutaneous cardiac pacemaker
   - Either stand-alone unit or integrated into monitor/defibrillator

D. Other Advanced Equipment

1. Nebulizer
2. Glucometer or blood glucose measuring device
   - With reagent strips
3. Pulse oximetry with pediatric and adult probes

E. Medications (pre-load when available)

Medications used on advanced level ambulances should be compatible with current standards as indicated by the American Heart Association's Emergency Cardiac Care Committee, as reflected in the Advanced Cardiac Life Support Course, or other such organizations and publications (ACEP, ACS, National Association of EMS Physicians, and so on). In general, medications should include:

- Cardiovascular medication, such as 1:10,000 epinephrine, atropine, lidocaine, bretylium tosylate, adenosine, diltiazem hydrochloride, propranolol, nitroglycerin tablets, aspirin, dopamine
- Cardiopulmonary/respiratory medications, such as albuterol (or other inhaled beta agonist), 1:1,000 epinephrine, furosemide
- 50% dextrose solution (and sterile diluent or 25% dextrose solution for pediatrics)
- Analgesics, such as morphine, meperidine hydrochloride, nitrous oxide
- Antiepileptic medications, such as diazepam or midazolam
- Activated charcoal, sodium bicarbonate, magnesium sulfate, glucagon, naloxone hydrochloride, flumazenil
- Bacteriostatic water and sodium chloride for injection

F. Optional Advanced Equipment

1. Portable automatic ventilators
2. Alternative airway devices (double lumen tube airways)
3. Umbilical vein catheters (sizes 3.5F and 5F)
4. Blood sample tubes, adult and pediatric
5. Automatic blood pressure device

(continued on next page)

Figure 15-10   Equipment for BLS and ALS ambulances (continued).

Extrication Equipment

Adequate extrication equipment must be readily available to the EMS responders, but is more often found on heavy rescue vehicles than on the primary responding ambulance.

In general, the devices or tools used for extrication fall into several broad categories: disassembly, spreading, cutting, pulling, protective, and patient-related.

The following is necessary equipment that should be available either on the primary response vehicle or on a heavy rescue vehicle.

Disassembly Tools

- Wrenches (adjustable)
- Screwdrivers (flat and Phillips head)
- Pliers
- Bolt cutter
- Tin snips
- Hammer
- Spring-loaded center punch
- Axes (pry, fire)
- Bars (wrecking, crow)
- Ram (4 ton)

Spreading Tools

- Hydraulic jack/spreader combination
- Boss tool with spreading device

Cutting Tools

- Saws (hacksaw, fire, windshield, pruning, reciprocating)
- Air-cutting gun kit

Pulling Tools/Devices

- Ropes/chains
- Come-along
- Hydraulic truck jack
- Air bags

Protective Devices

- Reflectors/flares
- Hard hats
- Safety goggles
- Fireproof blanket
- Leather gloves
- Jackets/coats/boots

Patient-Related Devices

- Swiss seat
- Stokes basket

Miscellaneous

- Shovel
- Lubricating oil
- Wood/wedges
- Generator
- Floodlights

Local extrication needs may necessitate additional equipment, that is, water, aerial, or mountain rescue.

American College of Emergency Physicians, American College of Surgeons. Equipment for ambulances [policy resource and education paper]. ACEP Web site. Available at: http://www.acep.org/library/pdf/ambulance_equip.pdf. Accessed January 11, 2005. Reprinted with permission.

the International Association of Fire Fighters, NAEMT, NAEMSP, the National Association of EMS State Directors, and NHTSA. These recommendations were published[29] and then served as a reference for the development of recommendations by ACS and ACEP (**Figure 15-10**).[30]

Education of Out-of-Hospital Providers

The EMSC program has made sponsorship of education efforts in pediatric emergency care for the public and health care professionals a priority. In the beginning of the EMSC program, education efforts for out-of-hospital providers in pediatric emergency care were fragmented and without a national focus. The EMSC program established a national Education of Out-of-Hospital Providers task force that met in August 1996 and November 1997 with the goal of evaluating current EMS curricula and making recommendations on curriculum design and topic areas to be included.[31,32] The task force reviewed previous efforts in provider education and concluded that many of the curricula were diagnosis based. The task force believed this

was not practical for emergency providers because they often do not establish a diagnosis in the field, relying instead on assessment findings (history, signs and symptoms) to guide their care. Several recommendations were made regarding curriculum design, including that the education be assessment focused and that there be well-defined objectives, a well-defined lesson plan, consistent materials used throughout, and a valid and reliable evaluation tool.[31,32] Controversies were also addressed, including the use of hyperventilation to reduce intracranial pressure, bag-mask ventilation techniques used to educate paramedics (tools such as "squeeze, release, release" and the EC-clamp were highlighted), other education tools such as the **Pediatric Assessment Triangle**, the scope of practice for paramedics in pediatric airway management, the need for vascular access in children in the out-of-hospital setting, the use of the pneumatic antishock garment, and the need for continuing education guidelines.[33-38] Topic areas to be covered in education curricula are listed in **Figure 15-11**; special emphasis was placed on using con-

Figure 15-11 Topics to be covered in out-of-hospital provider curricula in pediatric emergency care.

Patient assessment
Growth and development
EMSC
Illness and injury prevention
Respiratory emergencies (airway and breathing problems)
- Respiratory distress, respiratory failure, respiratory arrest
- Possible causes of respiratory emergencies:
  – Airway obstruction (upper and lower)
  – Fluid in the lungs
Cardiovascular/circulatory emergencies
- Shock (compensated and decompensated)
- Rate and rhythm disturbances, cardiopulmonary arrest
Altered mental status
- Possible causes:
  – Airway/breathing problems
  – Shock
  – Seizures
  – Poisoning
  – Metabolic problems
  – Occult trauma
  – Serious infection
Trauma
- Burns
Child abuse and neglect
Behavioral emergencies
- Suicide, aggressive behavior
Child-family communications
Critical incident stress management
Fever
Medical-legal issues
- Do-not-resuscitate (DNR) orders
- Consent
- Guardianship
- Refusal of care
Newborn emergencies
Near-drowning
Pain management
Poisoning
Sudden infant death syndrome (SIDS) and death in the field
Transport considerations
- Destination issues
- Methods for transport (safety seats and parental transport)
Infants and children with special health care needs
- Technically assisted children
  –Apnea monitors, central lines, chronic illness, gastrostomy tubes, home artificial ventilators, and shunts

Adapted from Gausche M, Henderson DP, Brownstein D, et al. The education of out-of-hospital medical personnel in pediatrics: report of a national task force. *Ann Emerg Med.* 1998;31(1):58–63, and Gausche M, Henderson DP, Brownstein D, et al. The education of out-of-hospital medical personnel in pediatrics: report of a national task force. *Prehospital Emerg Care.* 1998;2(1):56–61.

Figure 15-12 Recommendations for essential skills in the education of paramedics in pediatric emergency care.

Assessment of infants and children
Use of a length-based resuscitation tape
Airway management
- Mouth-to-mouth barrier devices
- Oropharyngeal airway
- Nasopharyngeal airway
- Oxygen delivery system
- Bag-mask ventilation
- Endotracheal intubation
  – Optional: Endotracheal placement confirmation devices (CO_2 detection), rapid-sequence induction
- Foreign body removal with Magill forceps
- Needle thoracostomy
- Nasogastric or orogastric tubes
- Suctioning
- Tracheostomy management
Monitoring
- Cardiorespiratory monitoring
- Pulse oximetry
- End-tidal CO_2 monitoring and/or CO_2 detection
Vascular access
- Intravenous line placement
- Intraosseous line placement
Fluid/medication administration
- Endotracheal
- Intramuscular
- Intravenous
- Nasogastric
- Nebulized
- Oral
- Rectal
- Subcutaneous
Cardioversion
Defibrillation
Drug dosing in infants and children
Immobilization/extrication
- Car seat extrication
- Spinal immobilization

Adapted from Gausche M, Henderson DP, Brownstein D, et al. The education of out-of-hospital medical personnel in pediatrics: report of a national task force. *Ann Emerg Med.* 1998;31(1):58-63, and Gausche M, Henderson DP, Brownstein D, et al. The education of out-of-hospital medical personnel in pediatrics: report of a national task force. *Prehospital Emerg Care.* 1998;2(1):56-61.

sistent terms. The task force also outlined essential pediatric skills for paramedic providers (**Figure 15-12**).

Several innovative programs in pediatric emergency care education have been established since the meeting of the task force. These include the Center for Pediatric Emergency Medicine *Teaching Resource for Instructors in Prehospital Pediatrics* (www.cpem.org)[34] and the first national course for pediatric education for out-of-hospital providers, the **Pediatric Education**

Figure 15-13 Topics for model pediatric protocols.

General patient care
Trauma
Burns
Foreign body obstruction
Respiratory distress, failure, or arrest
Bronchospasm
Newborn resuscitation
Bradycardia
Tachycardia
Nontraumatic cardiac arrest
Ventricular fibrillation or pulseless ventricular tachycardia
Asystole
Pulseless electrical activity
Altered mental status
Seizures
Nontraumatic hypoperfusion (shock)
Anaphylactic shock/allergic reaction
Toxic exposure
Near-drowning
Pain management
SIDS

for Prehospital Professionals (PEPP) course (www. PEPPsite.com) developed by AAP in collaboration with Jones and Bartlett Publishers.[38]

Pediatric Protocols

Model protocols for out-of-hospital care of children have been developed by NAEMSP.[39] Pediatric protocols from many EMS systems in the country were reviewed for content, and the existing literature was evaluated to identify those out-of-hospital interventions that are evidence based. **Figure 15-13** is a list of the pediatric emergency protocols that were developed; the protocols can be downloaded from the NAEMSP Web site (www.naemsp.org).

Pediatric Preparedness Guidelines for Emergency Departments

Some of the first efforts to develop guidelines for emergency departments that care for children began in California.[40,41] These guidelines address the reality that hospitals within an EMS system have varying pediatric capabilities and resources. Some EMS systems have opted for regionalization of pediatric care, and others have sought to improve the entire system's pediatric capability. Guidelines for pediatric preparedness of emergency departments have been subsequently developed by the American Medical Association (AMA), AAP, and ACEP, as well as various states and regions.[42-46]

Despite efforts to establish preparedness guidelines for emergency departments, none have received widespread use — even though data suggest that some

emergency departments are not fully prepared.[47,48] Therefore, in 1998, the EMSC program established a multidisciplinary task force of stakeholders in pediatric emergency care, led by representatives from ACEP and AAP, to develop guidelines for pediatric preparedness of emergency departments that would be national in scope and in implementation. These stakeholders included the following:

- American Association of Health Plans
- American College of Healthcare Executives
- American College of Surgeons
- American Hospital Association
- American Medical Association
- EMSC National Resource Center
- Joint Commission on Accreditation of Healthcare Organizations
- National Association of Children's Hospitals and Related Institutions
- National Association of State EMS Directors
- National Committee on Quality Assurance
- US Department of Health and Human Services, Health Resources and Services Administration Maternal and Child Health Bureau

These guidelines were published as a joint policy statement in the April 2001 issues of *Annals of Emergency Medicine* and *Pediatrics*.[49,50] They call for the establishment of a physician coordinator and nursing coordinator for pediatrics to oversee quality improvement, policy development, and staff education, as well as to serve as liaisons with other pediatric-related committees in the hospital and the community. The

Figure 15-14 List of policies and procedures as part of a quality or performance improvement plan.

Child maltreatment (physical and sexual abuse, sexual assault, and neglect)
Consent (including situations in which a parent is not immediately available)
Death in the emergency department
Do-not-resuscitate orders
Illness and injury triage
Sedation and analgesia
Immunization status
Mental health emergencies
Physical or chemical restraint of patients
Family issues, including:
• Education of the patient, family, and regular caregivers
• Discharge planning and instruction
• Family presence during care
Communication with patient's primary health care provider
Interfacility transfers (must be conducted in accordance with the screening, stabilization, and transfer requirements of EMTALA)

guidelines recommend that pediatric quality improvement plans be created and integrated into the overall emergency department plan. The guidelines also identify policies and procedures for children that should be addressed in the quality improvement plan (**Figure 15-14**). Interfacility transfer agreements should be established to ensure timely transfer and continuity of care. Equipment and supplies for the emergency department are also listed. Periodic updates of the policy and equipment lists will be posted on the ACEP and AAP Web sites (www.acep.org; www.aap.org).

Other EMSC Products

As of early 2005, EMSC had 198 products in 38 categories. They are too numerous to list here but can be found on the EMSC Web site, along with product descriptions and ordering information. To access the complete list, go to http://www.ems-c.org/products/frameproducts.htm and click on the product catalog link.

Summary

The EMSC program has done much to improve the care of children since its initiation. EMSC has been integrated into the EMS systems of all 50 states. The programs outlined in this chapter have served to establish standards in education, research, system development, and medical care for children along the EMSC continuum. The EMS medical director and EMS administrators have important roles in EMSC as advocates for the welfare of children served by EMS systems; they can implement effective EMSC programs, and they can educate parents and health care providers in EMSC issues.

There is a bright future for our nation's children with the establishment of public, government, and health care partnerships, and with the continued focus of the EMSC program on meeting the challenges of preserving health for children.

References

1. Seidel JS, Henderson DP, eds. *EMSC — Emergency Medical Services for Children: A Report to the Nation.* Washington, DC: National Center for Education in Maternal and Child Health; 1991.

2. Foltin GL, Tunik MC. Emergency medical services for children. In: Barkin RM, ed. *Pediatric Emergency Medicine: Concepts and Clinical Practice.* St Louis, Mo: Mosby-Year Book, Inc; 1997.

3. Seidel JS. History of EMS for children. In: Dieckmann RA, ed. *Pediatric Emergency Care Systems: Planning and Management.* Baltimore, Md: Williams & Wilkins; 1992.

4. Seidel JS, Hornbein M, Yoshiyama K, et al. Emergency medical services and the pediatric patient: are the needs being met? *Pediatrics.* 1984;73:769–772.

5. Seidel JS. Emergency medical services and the pediatric patient: are the needs being met? II: training and equipping EMS providers for pediatric emergencies. *Pediatrics.* 1986;78:808–812.

6. Gausche M, Seidel JS. Out-of-hospital care of pediatric patients. *Pediatr Clin North Am.* 1999;46:1305–1327.

7. Seidel JS. Emergency medical services for children. *Emerg Med Clin North Am.* 1995;13:255–266.

8. Dieckmann RA, Schafermeyer RW. EMS for children. In: Roush WR, ed. *Principles of EMS Systems.* 2nd ed. Dallas, Tex: American College of Emergency Physicians; 1994:51–82.

9. Singer J, Ludwig S, eds. *Emergency Medical Services for Children: The Role of the Primary Care Provider.* Elk Grove Village, Ill: American Academy of Pediatrics; 1992.

10. Durch JS, Lohr KN, eds. *Emergency Medical Services for Children.* Washington, DC: National Academies Press; 1993.

11. Durch JS, Lohr KN, eds. *Emergency Medical Services for Children: Summary.* Washington, DC: National Academies Press; 1993.

12. Kohn L, Corrigan J, Donaldson M, eds. *To Err is Human: Building a Safer Health System.* Washington, DC: National Academies Press; 1999.

13. Committee on Quality of Health Care in America, Institute of Medicine. *Crossing the Quality Chasm: A New Health System for the 21st Century.* Washington, DC: National Academies Press; 2001.

14. McDonald CJ, Weiner M, Hui SL. Deaths due to medical errors are exaggerated in Institute of Medicine report. *JAMA.* 2000;284:93.

15. Lesar TS, Briceland L, Stein DS. Factors related to errors in medication prescribing. *JAMA.* 1997;277:312–317.

16. Gausche M, Goodrich SM, McCollough MD, et al. Accuracy of epinephrine dosing in children in cardiac arrest by prehospital providers. *Acad Emerg Med.* 1996;3(5):404.

17. Leape LL, Bates DW, Cullen DJ, et al. Systems analysis of adverse drug events. *JAMA.* 1995;274:35–43.

18. Adams JG, Bohan JS. System contributions to error. *Acad Emerg Med.* 2000;7:1189–1193.

19. Leape LL. Error in medicine. *JAMA.* 1994;272:1851.

20. Selbst SM, Fein JA, Osterhoudt K, et al. Medication errors in a pediatric emergency department. *Pediatr Emerg Care.* 1999;15:1–4.

21. Cole T. Medical errors vs medical injuries: physicians seek to prevent both. *JAMA.* 2000;284:2175–2177.

22. Handler JA, Gillam M, Sanders AB, et al. Defining, identifying and measuring error in emergency medicine. *Acad Emerg Med.* 2000;7:1183–1188.

23. Brennan TA. The Institute of Medicine report on medical errors: could it do harm? *N Engl J Med.* 2000; 342:1123.

24. Seidel JS, Henderson DP, Tittle S, et al. Priorities for research in emergency medical services for children: results of a consensus conference. *Ann Emerg Med.* 1999;33(2):206–210.

25. Seidel JS, Henderson DP, Tittle S, et al. Priorities for research in emergency medical services for children: results of a consensus conference. *J Emerg Nursing.* 1999;25(1):12–16.

26. Seidel JS, Henderson DP, Tittle S, et al. Priorities for research in emergency medical services for children: results of a consensus conference. *Pediatr Emerg Care.* 1999;15(1):55–59.

27. Sacchetti A, Gerardi MJ, Barkin R, et al. Emergency data set for children with special needs. *Ann Emerg Med.* 1996;28:324–327.

28. American College of Emergency Physicians. Emergency information form for children with special health care needs. *Ann Emerg Med.* 1999;34:577–582.

29. Committee on Ambulance Equipment and Supplies, National EMSC Resource Alliance. Guidelines for pediatric equipment and supplies for basic and advanced life support ambulances. *Ann Emerg Med.* 1996;28:699–701.

30. American College of Emergency Physicians, American College of Surgeons. Equipment for ambulances [policy resource and education paper]. American College of Emergency Physicians Web site. Available at: http://www.acep.org/library/pdf/ambulance_equip.pdf. Accessed February 1, 2005.

31. Gausche M, Henderson DP, Brownstein D, et al. The education of out-of-hospital medical personnel in pediatrics: report of a national task force. *Ann Emerg Med.* 1998;31(1):58–63.

32. Gausche M, Henderson DP, Brownstein D, et al. The education of out-of-hospital medical personnel in pediatrics: report of a national task force. *Prehospital Emerg Care.* 1998;2(1):56–61.

33. Cooper A, Tunik M, Foltin G, et al. Teaching paramedics to ventilate infants: preliminary results of a new method. In: Chameides L, ed. *Proceedings of the International Conference on Pediatric Resuscitation.* Washington, DC: Washington National Center for Education in Maternal and Child Health; 1994:8.

34. Foltin GL, Tunik MC, Cooper A, et al, eds. *Teaching Resource for Instructors in Prehospital Pediatrics (EMT-Basic).* Rockville, Md: Maternal and Child Health Bureau; 1998.

35. Gausche M, Stratton SJ, Henderson FP, et al. Bag-valve-mask ventilation (BVM) for children in the prehospital setting. *Acad Emerg Med.* 1996;3:404–405.

36. Gausche M, Lewis RJ, Stratton SJ, et al. Effect of out-of-hospital pediatric endotracheal intubation on survival and neurological outcome: a controlled clinical trial. *JAMA.* 2000;283:783–790.

37. Gausche-Hill M, Lewis RJ, Gunter CS, et al. Design and implementation of a controlled trial of pediatric endotracheal intubation in the out-of-hospital setting. *Ann Emerg Med.* 2000;36:356–365.

38. Dieckmann RA, Brownstein D, Gausche-Hill M, eds. *Pediatric Education for Prehospital Professionals.* Sudbury, Mass: Jones and Bartlett Publishers; 2000.

39. EMSC Partnership for Children. National Association of EMS Physicians. Model pediatric protocols, 2003 revision [NAEMSP Web site]. Available at: http://www.naemsp.org/ModelPediatricProtocols.pdf. Accessed February 1, 2005.

40. Seidel JS, Gausche M. Standards for emergency departments. In: Dieckmann RA, ed. *Planning and Managing Systems for Pediatric Emergency Care.* Baltimore, Md: Williams and Wilkins; 1991.

41. McNeil M, Dieckmann RA, Westlake D, et al, for the Emergency Department Subcommittee. Administration, personnel and policy guidelines for the care of pediatric patients in the emergency department [California EMS Authority Web site]. Available at: http://www.emsa.gov/aboutemsa/emsa182.pdf. Accessed February 1, 2005.

42. Committee on Pediatric Equipment and Supplies for Emergency Departments. Guidelines for pediatric equipment and supplies for emergency departments. *Ann Emerg Med.* 1998;31:54–57.

43. American Medical Association Commission on Emergency Medical Services. Pediatric emergencies. An excerpt from "Guidelines for the Categorization of Hospital Emergency Capabilities." *Pediatrics.* 1990;85:879–887.

44. American College of Emergency Physicians. Emergency care guidelines. *Ann Emerg Med.* 1997;29:564–571.

45. American Academy of Pediatrics, Committee on Pediatric Emergency Medicine. Guidelines for pediatric emergency care facilities. *Pediatrics.* 1995;96:526–537.

46. American College of Emergency Physicians. Pediatric equipment guidelines. *Ann Emerg Med.* 1995;25:307–309.

47. Athey J, Dean JM, Ball J, et al. Ability of hospitals to care for pediatric emergency patients. *Pediatr Emerg Care.* 2001;17:170–174.

48. McGillivray D, Nijssen-Jordan C, Kramer MS, et al. Critical pediatric equipment availability in Canadian hospital emergency departments. *Ann Emerg Med.* 2001;37:371–376.

49. American Academy of Pediatrics, Committee on Pediatric Emergency Medicine, and American College of Emergency Physicians, Pediatric Committee. Care of children in the emergency department: guidelines for preparedness. *Ann Emerg Med.* 2001;37:423–427.

50. American Academy of Pediatrics, Committee on Pediatric Emergency Medicine, and American College of Emergency Physicians, Pediatric Committee. Care of children in the emergency department: guidelines for preparedness. *Pediatrics.* 2001;107:777–781.

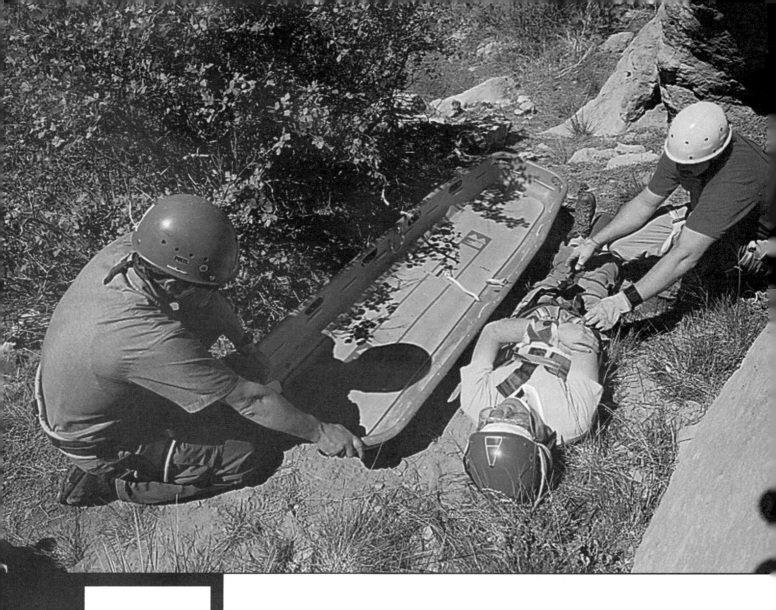

16 Rural EMS

Bob W. Bailey
Dan Manz

Principles of This Chapter

After reading this chapter, you should be able to:

- Describe the challenges affecting the rural EMS setting, such as limited personnel, equipment, and funding, as well as extended response and transport intervals, communications, and medical oversight.
- Explain how EMS acute care activities, prevention programs, and primary care activities are integrated with rural health systems.

THE CHALLENGES OF PROVIDING QUALITY EMS IN A RURAL setting are much the same as challenges faced by other rural health care providers. There are resource limitations on both personnel and equipment. Finances can be challenging. The experience level of EMS providers is sometimes low. Response times can be extended well beyond what would be acceptable in an urban setting. Communications can be challenging. Nonetheless, the public expects that the EMS system will provide a health care safety net for medical emergencies.

The term rural can mean many things. A very common definition is the federal Office of Management and Budget's designation of a **Metropolitan Statistical Area (MSA).** An MSA is an urbanized area with at least 50,000 people in a county or counties having a total population of at least 100,000.[1] Rural or non-MSA consists of everything else. Although this is a commonly used definition, the problem is that a town or community encompassed within an MSA might have attributes commonly associated with rural areas. The terms suburban, rural, and wilderness all form grada-tions of communities that at some level share the attributes of small populations, low population densities, and remoteness of location from a larger urban setting.

Challenges

Those attributes that make an area rural also tend to make it naturally difficult to serve with EMS. Small populations tend to generate fewer EMS calls than larger populations. This decreased frequency of EMS demand contributes to problems of skill retention by personnel and limited financial resources. Low population densities and remoteness of locations contribute to extended response times. Transport times to an initial receiving hospital will be longer than in most urban settings. Transport of patients directly from an emergency scene to tertiary care is often not a viable option, and interfacility transfers commonly involve complex logistics of time and distance.

Many EMS providers are volunteers with the task of acquiring and maintaining increasingly higher levels of EMS competency, while at the same time working in other full-time careers. The compensation of paid EMS providers is often not at a level sufficient to attract and retain the most qualified personnel in rural settings. The reasons vary, but the rapid turnover of both volunteer and career EMS personnel is a commonly mentioned problem in rural service delivery.

The technology available to support EMS in rural areas varies widely. The development of cellular telephone service has tended to follow population centers and transportation corridors, leaving many rural areas without cellular coverage or only sporadic coverage. Similarly, 911 emergency calling services have commonly first been provided in urban settings and later in rural areas, if at all. Radio communications systems to support EMS dispatch and medical direction are excellent in some rural areas and barely functional in others.

Rural EMS settings have often been best able to justify a need for high-level out-of-hospital care based on the likelihood of an extended out-of-hospital contact with a patient and, at the same time, being least able to provide it. The alternative argument can also be made, that life-threatening emergencies tend to be infrequent in rural areas, so the expense and difficulty associated with supplying and maintaining high-level EMS might not be considered worthwhile. There are no simple answers and no absolute rights or wrongs to the design of a rural EMS system. The dilemmas described frame the challenges associated with planning and building an EMS system to meet the needs of a rural area. The key to developing efficient rural EMS systems is balancing the demands for service with the ability to meet those demands.

Some rural hospitals that have been threatened with failure of survival due to financial problems, have received help from the **Critical Access Hospital (CAH)** program, which offers cost-based reimbursement to those facilities.[2] Congress recognized that community hospitals in rural settings are an essential community health resource. Leading the list of needs that community hospitals fill is access to emergency care. The potential failure and closure of a local community hospital creates overwhelming challenges to local EMS providers. The assistance that these hospitals receive from the CAH program has positive effects for the support of their local EMS systems as well.

On July 25, 2001, then Secretary of the US Department of Health and Human Services Tommy G. Thompson issued a press release to announce new initiatives for rural communities.[3] Thompson announced the ". . . creation of a HHS Rural Task Force that will conduct a department-wide examination of how HHS programs can be strengthened to better serve rural communities." One of the charges of the task force is "examining the use of Title XII of the Public Health Services Act, which gives HHS broad authority over EMS provider funds for training, recruitment, and retention grants. The HHS goal is to keep good EMT personnel on the job in rural America, where EMS systems are stretched thin."[3] This type of action by the federal government indicates that it understands that the delivery of rural health care and EMS services is in crisis and needs to be addressed.

There are many challenging issues facing rural EMS delivery systems. It is unlikely that rural communities will have the resources to independently resolve all these issues. But with local commitment and federal recognition of the need for resources to address the issues, they can be resolved.

Rural EMS Finance

The financing of EMS in rural areas is one of the most complex aspects of ensuring adequate delivery of out-of-hospital emergency care. The structure of an EMS organization's financing has often evolved over time in ways that reflect local culture. Third-party reimbursement, particularly Medicare and Medicaid payments, have also had significant roles in how EMS organizations secure the financial resources necessary to function. An understanding of EMS finance requires an examination of both costs and revenues.

Costs

Many of the cost components of delivering EMS are **fixed costs.** The costs of an ambulance vehicle, a crew to staff it, housing, insurance, training, communications, and medical oversight all must be incurred whether an organization responds to a small or large number of calls. Fixed costs are sometimes referred to as **readiness costs,** or the cost of being prepared or ready to respond at all times.

The **variable costs** of EMS delivery include items such as fuel, medical supplies, vehicle maintenance, and capital equipment. Variable costs tend to be lower than fixed costs.

The relationships between fixed and variable costs combine to give EMS operations a definite economy of scale. A study completed in 2000 by Project Hope indicated that the most cost-efficient size for an ambulance service is around 8,000 calls per year.[4] Generally, the lower the call volume of an EMS organization, the higher the readiness costs as a percentage of the overall cost of doing business. Rural EMS organizations normally have fewer responses than their urban counterparts and accordingly do not enjoy any real economy of scale and have high readiness costs.

Revenues

The revenues supporting any particular EMS organization vary widely. Often, **hidden revenues** tend to understate the actual cost of service delivery. One of the largest hidden revenues for many rural organizations is volunteer labor. Consider the following example of the minimum staffing necessary to provide personnel for one ambulance vehicle for a year:

- 24 hours/day × 365 days per year = 8,760 hours
- Two-person crew coverage requires 8,760 × 2 = 17,520 hours covered
- 17,520 hours × an hourly wage of only $8/hr would result in annual personnel costs of $140,160 (without fringe benefits)

Even with a modest per hour wage, the real cost of staffing one ambulance vehicle can run into hundreds of thousands of dollars per year (**Figure 16-1**). If volunteers staff the organization, this is the contributed value of their labor with no actual dollar outlay.

There are many other examples of hidden revenues that are sometimes not well understood or accounted for. A few examples include:

- The cost of medical oversight, which is sometimes absorbed by the medical director volunteering his or her time or by a hospital, the

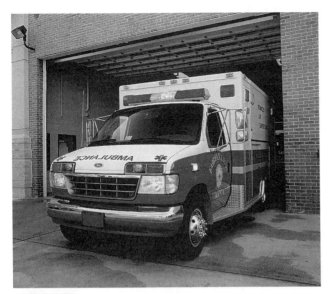

Figure 16-1 The cost of staffing one ambulance vehicle is sometimes hundreds of thousands of dollars per year.

physician organization, or some other institution supporting that time

- The cost of EMS housing, which might be provided by a fire station and absorbed in a budget other than that of the EMS organization
- The cost of dispatch and other communications (eg, 911 system or some radio systems) for EMS, which might be shared with several other emergency organizations

When someone other than the EMS provider organization pays for these expenses, it represents a revenue or subsidy to the real cost of EMS delivery in a community.

Revenues for EMS are generated through many different mechanisms. Commonly, EMS providers bill patients and attempt to recover costs through third-party reimbursement such as private insurance, Medicare, or Medicaid. However, there are still some volunteer EMS organizations that do not bill for services and rely on subsidies or contributions. Although some EMS providers are able to cover their costs through billing, many require additional public subsidies, generally through some form of local taxation. Depending on local circumstances, many rural EMS providers also rely on voluntary contributions, special fundraising campaigns, bake sales, dinners, raffles, subscription programs, grants, or other mechanisms to meet an annual budget. Each of these mechanisms has advantages and disadvantages, which are worth understanding.

Third-party reimbursement for EMS has followed a somewhat nontraditional pathway when compared to third-party reimbursement for other types of health care. Medicare payments typically represent the largest single source of third-party reimbursement for ambu-lance services, so Medicare policies have tended to drive the reimbursement practices of other insurers. Medicare is statutorily limited to payments for ambulance transportation. That limitation translates into a separation of how EMS is delivered in many communities and how it is reimbursed. Medicare will not pay for the costs of nontransporting first response or advanced life support. Medicare is not able to support any of the legitimate readiness costs of being prepared to have EMS in a community, except through reimbursement on a patient-by-patient transport basis. This practice by Medicare is in contrast to reimbursement mechanisms at the hospital level, where small rural hospitals have been able to receive cost-based reimbursement under the CAH program.

Historically, Medicare reimbursement for ambulance transport has been based on a profile of what services in the same area were charging. Medicare would set an allowable rate by examining all of the ambulance charges in an area and selecting the number at the 75th percentile. Services that billed at or above that number were reimbursed 80% of the allowable rate and were required to bill the patient for the remaining 20%. The profile system resulted in widely varying allowable rates in different parts of the country, largely driven by the billing practices of organizations in a particular area. One common problem was that many volunteer or heavily subsidized municipal/county services billed at rates well below the actual cost of service delivery. This practice drove the profile down in many areas, usually in rural settings. Because of the profiling process and the historical billing practices of many EMS organizations, the relationship between cost of service delivery and charge for service delivery has been eroded.

Beginning in the late 1990s, the Health Care Financing Administration (HCFA), now the Centers for Medicare and Medicaid Services (CMS), started on a course to level the reimbursement for ambulance services nationwide through the establishment of a common fee schedule. Congress placed certain requirements on HCFA efforts, including the use of a process called **negotiated rule-making.** In negotiated rule-making, HCFA included important outside parties with an interest in developing the fee schedule in exchange for a commitment that if the fee schedule could be developed by consensus, the outside groups would not oppose its adoption. Congress also imposed a requirement of cost neutrality in the establishment of the fee schedule. **Cost neutrality** means that, for a set volume of calls, the reimbursements under the fee schedule could not exceed the reimbursements provided under the profile system in a preselected base year.

HCFA completed negotiated rule-making discussions in February 2000. The formal announcement of the fee schedule and accompanying rules regarding adoption were published in *Federal Register* in September 2000. HCFA received significant negative commentary from ambulance providers around the country who would be reimbursed at levels lower than they were receiving in the profile system. The fee schedule announcement failed to include a proposed system for basing reimbursement on an EMS assessment of the patient's condition rather than an ICD-9 diagnosis. The fee schedule was subsequently adopted in early 2003.

As the transition to the fee schedule occurs, some fear that many private insurers will cap their level of reimbursement at the fee schedule rates. If this occurs, it will limit the opportunity for ambulance services to cost shift in favor of patients with private insurance. The adoption of the fee schedule could also include the mandatory acceptance of assignment by the EMS agency. When a service accepts assignment, it is prohibited from billing patients for any amount other than the difference between the allowed amount and the reimbursed amount (typically the 20% copayment). Additionally, when a service accepts assignment, it must bill the patient for the copayment that Medicare does not cover. This requirement has caused some concern for volunteer organizations that historically have not billed patients. This requirement represents another limitation on the ability of ambulance services to recover actual costs of service delivery that might be higher than the allowed amount.

Subsidies

When an EMS organization is unable to recover its costs of operation from patient-generated revenues, it commonly turns to its community for some form of subsidy. These subsidies vary widely. Some communities contract with private providers, and a predetermined sum of money is exchanged for ambulance service that meets some agreed-on specifications. In other situations, the ambulance service is owned or operated by the town, city, or county and has a specific line item in the municipality's budget. Often, some portions of EMS costs are included in the budget for the community's fire department. In other situations, the municipality makes an annual contribution to a community-based private volunteer EMS organization. Each of these subsidy mechanisms has greater or lesser strengths in terms of paying for and receiving EMS delivery.

Grants

Other support for EMS delivery costs comes from special grants or funds. Some states have established funds

from "sin taxes," such as safety belt violation fines, a portion of speeding ticket fines, or motor vehicle registration fees. These monies commonly support capital projects or local service operations, or they might be committed to the support of other EMS system infrastructure costs such as maintaining a statewide communications or training system.

Federal funds for programs such as EMS for Children or highway safety grants from the Department of Transportation (DOT) are commonly awarded to state government agencies. Some support the costs of EMS system improvements rather than provide a specific subsidy to any local EMS provider. Many of these grants have recently focused on the rural EMS community.

Funding Models

The subject of the optimal financing model has been widely debated in EMS management circles, and there is no clear consensus. From a medical oversight perspective, it is important to know that whatever financing model is in place must be sufficient to support the necessary and legitimate costs of service delivery. Some questions to answer include:

- Is the current EMS funding model survivable over time? For example, if a system is currently heavily dependent on volunteer labor, it might be important to ask what provisions have been made or can be made if it becomes necessary to supplement the volunteer labor pool with paid providers.
- Is there an understanding between EMS providers and the communities they serve regarding the costs and revenues in place to provide local EMS service delivery?
- Is there competition among local EMS providers that has financial implications?
- What, if any, economies of scale are present? Is there any possibility of improving economies of scale (eg, through group purchasing arrangements among several rural services)?
- How is the cost of medical oversight covered? Are enough resources committed to ensure adequate medical oversight of EMS to provide quality patient care?
- Are local EMS organizations doing everything possible to recover patient revenues (eg, billing at levels that reflect true cost, filing claims in a timely and appropriate manner)?

More information on finance issues can be found in Chapter 8, "System Financing."

Human Resource Issues

In rural America, maintaining a qualified EMS workforce is essential in ensuring adequate service delivery. Attracting, developing, and maintaining that qualified workforce is among the most significant challenges facing rural EMS systems. Recruitment and retention of EMS personnel are major concerns in most states. A survey of all state EMS offices conducted on behalf of the National Association of State EMS Directors identified recruitment and retention as the number one issue facing rural EMS.[5]

Historically, most of the EMS workforce in rural America has been volunteers. That is still true today. Inherent in the use of volunteers is the conflict of competing demands for time. Family, career, recreation, and other life interests all compete with the time any volunteer has to devote to EMS. Voluntary involvement with EMS takes many forms, including time to be on duty for calls, time to train, time for administrative meetings, and in some cases time for additional functions such as fundraising, vehicle maintenance, and so on.

The concept and definition of an EMS volunteer are continually evolving. Similarly, the sophistication of EMS organizations to attract volunteers is also evolving. Years ago, EMS volunteers might have been expected to commit time for being on duty, pay their own tuition for training, purchase their own uniforms, raise money to support the EMS organization, and so on. Today's volunteers might be offered immunizations before beginning EMS duties, be supplied with uniforms and personal protective equipment, have any tuitions for training paid or reimbursed, and in some cases receive a stipend for time spent on duty or responding to calls. Many volunteer organizations are now providing continuous recruitment programs aimed at keeping the ranks full. Some rural agencies are supplementing volunteers with paid administrative or daytime clinical staff who are charged with recruiting new volunteers and who provide coverage on nights and weekends.

Similarly, many organizations are recruiting non–EMS personnel to help with a variety of nonclinical duties. Involving persons from the community specifically to perform station and vehicle maintenance, fundraising, and even child care to free up on-duty EMS parents are all examples of how squads are changing in an attempt to better meet the needs of their members.

Recruitment and Retention of Personnel

Two strategies for establishing a more secure personnel base are first, recruit more persons into the organization, and second, keep the people in the organization

for longer periods of time. Establishing and maintaining long-term commitment by volunteers to EMS organizations require an understanding of why people leave their organizations. Some EMS organizations conduct exit interviews with personnel to identify their reasons for leaving. The reasons are multifaceted. A study conducted in 1999 of volunteers in the Old Dominion EMS Alliance region of Virginia found that the number one reason volunteers stopped volunteering was family demands. This was closely followed by conflict within the volunteer organization and burnout.[6] Another study published in the *Journal of Consumer Research* found that self-reporting allows for overestimating altruistic reasons and underreporting reasons such as personal development, career, and social recognition.[7] Yet another study published in the *Journal of Personality and Social Psychology* found that, in volunteers, most often self-centered motives dictate the length of service donated.[8]

In rural communities, EMS providers are more likely to know their patients and, consequently, more likely to be personally affected than providers in urban areas. Difficult or troubling cases can lead to the burnout or stress of personnel who have little experience dealing with similar cases. Critical incident stress management programs are aimed at keeping providers functional within the EMS system after exposure to stress-producing calls. Very low call volumes can be a factor in the loss of EMS providers who take significant amounts of training, invest hundreds of hours on duty, and then rarely encounter a critical patient who requires important EMS interventions.

Training

The training and continuing education of rural EMS personnel are other issues facing rural EMS delivery systems. Access to quality training is a factor commonly given as the reason persons choose to enter an EMS system. Initial training leading to the credentialing necessary to function in an EMS organization, as well as ongoing inservice continuing education, must be considered. Many states and localities are experimenting with distance learning technologies and other programs aimed at providing quality training to rural EMS personnel at convenient times and requiring minimal, if any, travel.

Physicians who provide medical oversight to EMS systems have important roles in building and supporting a qualified rural EMS workforce. EMS personnel, whether they are volunteer or paid, like any other professionals, need feedback about their performance. Ongoing organized programs of quality improvement invest providers in the betterment of the entire EMS system. EMS personnel view emergency physicians as the clinical experts who set the standard for how care should be provided. Physician involvement at all levels of EMS operations is important. This is especially true in rural EMS, as it provides rural EMS personnel with the opportunity to feel they are part of the overall health care team and have someone (the medical director) they can rely on.

Communications

The technology boom has created opportunities to improve EMS communications in rural areas, and at the same time has created pressure on existing systems. A functional EMS communications system must consider elements of system access, prearrival instructions, dispatch, medical oversight, and data management.

Many EMS communications systems in both rural and urban areas were initially built in the 1970s. The goals at that time were often no more complex than ensuring that EMS providers could be dispatched by radio and that ambulances could have voice contact with receiving hospitals. In some systems, especially in the most rural areas, this basic level of capacity remains fundamentally unaltered. In a few areas, even this basic level of communications capability is not well established, resulting in the inability to communicate with dispatch, hospitals, or even other ambulances due to geographic and distance factors. Another concern for rural EMS communications systems is that these 1970s-era communications systems are so old that the equipment routinely breaks down and manufacturers no longer provide service or parts.

According to a 2001 press release from the National Emergency Number Association (NENA), 97.8% of the US population has access to EMS by dialing 911. The press release goes on to say that

> . . . 231 counties, comprising almost 6% of the land in the US, do not have 9-1-1 support. These counties are generally rural areas with sparse population, high poverty levels, Native American lands, and military locations, and often do not have the funds needed to implement 9-1-1 infrastructures. . .[9]

This disparity represents the tendency to develop 911 systems in urban population centers before the technology reaches rural areas. Even rural areas that have 911 service today often have basic 911 capacity that cannot display a locatable address and call-back number (ie, enhanced 911). Wireless 911 now comprises 25% of national 911 calls, and the number is expected to double in the next few years, according to NENA. A significant issue regarding wireless 911 is that not all 911 centers can identify the location of wireless callers. This creates problems in emergency response for both rural and urban settings. The Federal Communications Commission (FCC) requires that this problem be solved by the end of 2005.

Once an emergency call has been received, it must be dispatched. Most rural systems have the capacity to reach their responders by radio, but the ability to accurately prioritize emergency calls and send the most appropriate resources in the most appropriate response mode varies widely. Having communications personnel trained to provide medical prearrival instructions to callers is another element of the communications system that is improving but not uniformly available today in rural areas.

The radio technology that is in place to support EMS dispatch, coordinate responses, and communicate with medical oversight also varies widely. The age of equipment, the design of what the system was initially intended for, the availability of frequencies, funding, and a host of other factors create whatever local communications system is in place. In rural areas, funding and the lack of communications technical expertise are serious barriers to providing effective communications systems. In addition, geographic barriers and distance make effective communications in rural settings more difficult.

In many parts of the country, EMS communications systems are evolving to take advantage of new technologies to improve capacity and efficiency in supporting the delivery of EMS. No specific equipment or technology is definitively superior. It is more important to consider whether the current or proposed communications technology adequately and efficiently supports the EMS system operations as they exist today and as they are envisioned for the future.

Although existing EMS radio systems function to one extent or another, there are some common problems identified with many systems. These include:

- Radio coverage problems or dead spots in certain areas. This could be the result of topography, technology, or system design problems.
- Frequency overcrowding. The number of frequencies set aside by the FCC for EMS purposes is limited. Technology changes in radio designs for the future hold the promise of expanding the number of available frequencies by narrowing the space needed between adjacent channels. Using this technology will require funding to replace entire communications systems.

- Lack of interagency operability. In many cases, it is not possible for fire, police, and EMS responders within a community to talk on a common radio frequency for coordination purposes. In some cases, not every ambulance within a specific jurisdiction can communicate with the others. These problems are exacerbated during large-scale operations such as a mass casualty incident or large fire emergency. One of the goals of post-9/11 domestic preparedness planning activities is to address this interoperability concern.
- Inability to upgrade existing systems. In some cases this is a funding problem. The infrastructure of many state and local communications systems was initially purchased with federal grant funds that are no longer available. In other cases, the current technology is functioning at the limits of its capability and must be replaced or upgraded to meet future demand.

For most communications problems, a solution can be found if there is enough time, money, and planning. Evolving technologies are bringing solutions to communications problems with increasing speed and in some cases for lower costs.

The ability to transmit information in a digital, rather than analog, format is increasing both the volume and the speed of information transfer. The ability to transmit and receive a 12-lead ECG via wireless or landline telephone is at least technologically possible in many systems today. Many two-way radios now support digital communications that can identify the status of a unit in the field without the need for a voice transmission.

The interface of traditional radio systems with the power of the Internet is offering a host of communications enhancements that only a few years ago seemed impossible. Some organizations are placing **geographic information system**, or **GIS**, mapping technologies on their ambulances to provide crews with instant access to the location of emergencies during responses. Mobile data terminals in vehicles are used to record patient information and provide it to hospitals, dispatchers, and EMS managers in real time. Personal digital assistants and other lightweight computers are being used to capture data on scenes and avoid data reentry after the call. The transmission of video imaging from EMS scenes to medical oversight is being explored in some areas. Satellite cellular phones are providing voice communications capability to very remote areas previously not served by traditional EMS communications. However, most of these technologies are not being used in the rural areas of the country. Most rural EMS organizations are still struggling with ways to fund and upgrade or replace basic, reliable voice communication systems.

Private automobile companies are pioneering **automatic crash notification (ACN)** programs. Many late-model automobiles are being equipped with automatic crash notification devices from a variety of vendors, such as OnStar. In addition to ACN, this capability allows drivers to push one button and contact someone to give directions, unlock doors remotely, and other activities. This technology has significant ramifications for the quick notification and response of emergency personnel to crashes. This is just one example of a broader long-range initiative of the DOT to make highways safer through the application of technology. It is important to include rural EMS systems in these technological advances as they become available.

More information on communications issues can be found in Chapter 9, "Communications."

◼ Medical Oversight

The medical oversight of rural EMS operations presents some significant and unique challenges to involved physicians. In some areas, medical oversight takes place at the individual organization level. In others, it is structured regionally. Medical oversight for EMS might be a primary duty for a physician, or it might be part of a much broader range of responsibilities. In recent years, there have been improvements in the opportunities for physicians to prepare themselves for assuming this role.

As we progress into the 21st century, the concept that EMS is an extension of a physician's practice into the out-of-hospital environment is increasingly well understood. EMS personnel look to physicians to provide leadership in identifying the relevant interventions for patient care and working with the system that delivers care to ensure and improve quality (**Figure 16-2**).

In the mid-1990s, the **national standard curricula** used to train EMS providers from the first responder through paramedic levels were revised, in part to reflect the legitimate role of medical oversight.[10] These curricula form the foundation of most EMS training programs and have extended the concept of medical oversight beyond the advanced life support realm and into the most basic aspects of EMS care. Although this step appropriately recognizes the need for physician involvement in all aspects of EMS and for all levels of EMS personnel, it has created demands on physicians that previously did not exist.

In many rural settings, medical oversight falls to the physicians practicing in a local hospital emergency

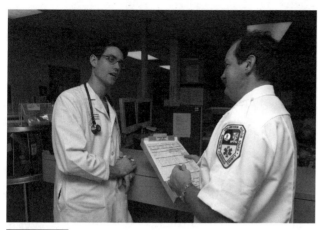

Figure 16-2 EMS personnel look to physicians to provide leadership in delivering appropriate and quality patient care.

department. These might or might not be physicians formally trained or board certified in emergency medicine. In rural areas where there are few hospitals, family physicians or other physicians having little formal emergency medicine training might provide medical oversight. Both of these models are common. Physicians practicing in the emergency department of a hospital are generally in the best position to see the work of EMS personnel. This exposure provides impressions about quality of care, training needs, adjustments to protocols, and other patient care issues.

Success as an EMS medical director in a rural area requires a range of skills. The physician must be thoroughly familiar with the operations of the EMS providers in his or her area. He or she must understand the realities of providing emergency care in the out-of-hospital environment and be able to help ensure that patients have the best care possible given the field settings encountered. A successful local medical director must be a good clinician and stay current in evolving EMS trends and technologies. He or she must have the personality to be accepted as part of the team by the field EMS personnel. The medical director must be an advocate for EMS and have the political awareness to bring about results. Sometimes the medical director must serve as peacemaker among various organizations. He or she needs an understanding of state requirements placed on EMS and must be a consensus-builder to bring about long-term change. The role of medical director is critical for the successful EMS system to meet the needs of the patients and community it serves.

Physicians serving or willing to serve as EMS medical directors must develop an understanding of several issues, including:

- Responsibilities of the medical director
- Scope and authority of the medical director
- Availability of medical director training
- Medical director compensation

Responsibilities of the Medical Director

A physician considering serving as a medical director should be able to answer the following questions: Is there a written job description? What level of involvement is there in the development or refinement of protocols for patient care activities? Does the position include offline functions such as oversight of training programs, review of patient care, and serving as a peacemaker among various organizations? What online expectations are there in the oversight of actual emergency cases in progress? What is expected of the medical director when representing the EMS system to other health care providers and the public? What resources are available to support the medical director in the performance of both online and offline duties?

Scope and Authority of the Medical Director

Prospective medical directors should also consider the following questions: Is one medical director responsible for the oversight of all EMS personnel and organizations in the jurisdiction? Is it clear that the medical director has the authority to limit the practice of EMS personnel and organizations, following appropriate due process activities, in cases where there are significant concerns about the provision of care? May the medical director amend care protocols? To whom is the medical director responsible within the structure of the EMS system?

Availability of Medical Director Training

In 2001, the American College of Emergency Physicians (ACEP) and the National Association of EMS Physicians cooperated in the development of national medical director's guidelines. These guidelines are available from the NHTSA Web site,[11] state EMS offices, ACEP chapters, and other sources. Educational programs based on these guidelines are offered at some EMS and emergency medicine conferences. In addition to national curriculum courses, there are state and local seminars, meetings of regional medical directors, and similar functions that provide education and training for EMS medical directors.

Medical Director Compensation

Financial compensation for medical oversight duties is an important consideration. It is also important to consider how liability insurance for medical oversight functions is provided. This coverage might be provided as part of the physician's clinical insurance or by the organization's insurance. The medical director should have the necessary financial resources, personnel, information, equipment, and other resources to ensure that the job description can be reasonably fulfilled.

More information on medical oversight can be found in Chapter 6, "Medical Oversight and Accountability."

Integration of EMS With Rural Health Systems

The following scenario is a vision from the "EMS Agenda for the Future": Ella is 78 years old, and she trips and falls in her living room. Although initially she is unable to get herself up, she summons EMS via a voice recognition habitat monitor. The EMS providers do not find serious injuries but suspect an ankle sprain. They schedule an appointment for Ella later that day with her primary care source via a palm-sized computer. They also are able to request transportation for her after consultation with the medical command center. While at Ella's, the EMS providers note that her home is oppressively hot due to a malfunctioning air conditioner, and that there are numerous risk factors for future falls. Using their computer, they arrange for social services to follow up; they notify her primary care provider and her building maintenance supervisor, and schedule an EMS return visit to check on her progress. Ella avoids an emergency department visit, is treated for her ankle sprain, and receives attention that reduces her numerous risk factors for future health problems.[12]

EMS systems exist within the broader continuum of health service delivery. How well the EMS system in any area is integrated with the other health care components remains an issue for many rural and urban areas. Traditionally, EMS has held the role of responding to acute emergency medical situations in an out-of-hospital setting. Today, there are many reasons to rethink whether EMS should continue solely with that mission of emergency response.

The fire service in the United States began with the mission of putting out fires. Over time, the fire service discovered that the most effective approach to reducing loss of life and property was through prevention rather than suppression. The fire service has successfully approached prevention through improved building codes, public education, technology (eg, smoke detectors), and other avenues. They have used fire-loss data to develop and document the effectiveness of fire-prevention strategies.

Most EMS systems are in their infancy in an evolving role of preventing acute injuries and illness as part of the overall health care system. Many providers see their role as limited to emergency response rather than maintaining the health and safety of the community. The ability to combine prevention education, engineering, enforcement, funding, and evaluation into a cohesive program is a challenge well beyond the capacity of most EMS systems. Although hard data to support the effectiveness of EMS involvement in injury prevention are scarce, many believe it is simply the right thing to do. For example, in 1996, NHTSA and the Maternal and Child Health Bureau of the Health Resources and Services Administration jointly sponsored a project to develop "Consensus Statement on the Role of EMS in Primary Injury Prevention."[13]

In rural areas in particular, there are many arguments in favor of integrating EMS with other elements of the health care system, including the following:

- EMS is visible and established in most communities.
- EMS has a workforce that might not be functioning at full capacity conducting only emergency responses.
- Prevention is likely to be more cost-effective than acute care.
- Some communities or elements of the health care system have gaps that EMS could fill.
- The use of EMS for functions other than emergency responses might contribute to the visibility and financial viability of maintaining EMS in the community.

When attempting to integrate EMS with the community's health care system, physician input is essential. By its nature, EMS is community based and has responsibility for the needs of a broad population. In that sense, EMS is truly public health care. An EMS medical director must balance the need to maintain a priority for prompt emergency response with other valuable but potentially competing agendas. Physicians must carefully consider the issues of training, equipment, oversight, finance, and quality while considering options for EMS and health care system integration issues.

Summary

The assumption that rural EMS systems are simpler or less complicated than urban EMS systems by virtue of their setting is erroneous. Rural EMS faces the challenge of providing quality patient care in an environment that often has limited provider resources, fewer facilities, less robust communications systems, and longer transport times. Specific issues facing rural systems include the development and maintenance of EMS personnel, appropriate integration of technology, and the ability to ensure a firm financial foundation for operations. There is an increasing recognition of the unique needs and challenges of rural systems by federal agencies involved in supporting or paying for EMS. Well-prepared physicians participating in medical oversight are essential to ensure that the elements of state and local EMS systems are logically and optimally configured to meet the legitimate needs of emergency patients.

References

1. 55 *Federal Register* 12154 (1990).
2. Office of Rural Health Policy, Health Resources and Services Administration. *Rural Hospital Flexibility Program: The Tracking Project, First Year Findings.* Washington, DC: Health Resources and Services Administration; 2001.
3. US Department of Health and Human Services. HHS Secretary Tommy G. Thompson announces new initiatives for rural communities [press release]. July 25, 2001. Available at: http://www.os.hhs.gov/news/press/2001pres/20010725b.html. Accessed January 4, 2005.
4. Mohr PE, Cheng CM, Mueller CD. *Establishing a Fair Medicare Reimbursement for Low-volume Rural Ambulance Providers.* National Opinion Research Center, Walsh Center for Rural Health Analysis. Policy Analysis Brief, July 2001; 4(2). W Series.
5. Bailey B. Challenges of rural emergency medical services: an opinion survey of state EMS directors [NASEMSD Web site]. Available at: http://www.nasemsd.org/rural_emergency_medical_servic.html. Accessed January 4, 2005.
6. Hughes J. EMS volunteers in the ODEMSA region: a study of demographics, attitudes and perceptions [Virginia Department of Health Web site]. Available at: http://www.vdh.virginia.gov/OEMS/Recruit/recruitr.asp. Accessed January 4, 2005.
7. Fisher R. The effects of recognition and group need on volunteerism: a social norm perspective. *J Consumer Res.* 1998;25:262–274.
8. Penner L. Dispositional and structural determinants of volunteerism. *J Pers Soc Psychol.* 1998;74(2):525–537.
9. National Emergency Number Association. Nation's first report card on 9-1-1 grades U.S. service as "B"; notes future of 9-1-1 as "threatened" [press release]. September 11, 2001. Available at: http://www.nena.org/initiatives/rcn/rcn%5Fpress%5Frelease.htm. Accessed January 4, 2005.
10. National Highway Traffic Safety Administration. National standard curricula [NHTSA Web site]. Available at: http://www.nhtsa.dot.gov/people/injury/ems/nsc.htm. Accessed January 4, 2005.
11. National Highway Traffic Safety Administration. 2001 guide for preparing medical directors [NHTSA Web site]. Available at: http://www.nhtsa.dot.gov/people/injury/ems/2001GuideMedical.pdf. Accessed January 4, 2005.
12. National Highway Traffic Safety Administration. EMS agenda for the future [NHTSA Web site]. Available at: http://www.nhtsa.dot.gov/people/injury/ems/agenda/emsman.html. Accessed January 4, 2005.
13. National Highway Traffic Safety Administration. *Consensus Statement on the Role of Emergency Medical Services in Primary Injury Prevention.* Washington, DC: National Highway Traffic Safety Administration; 1996.

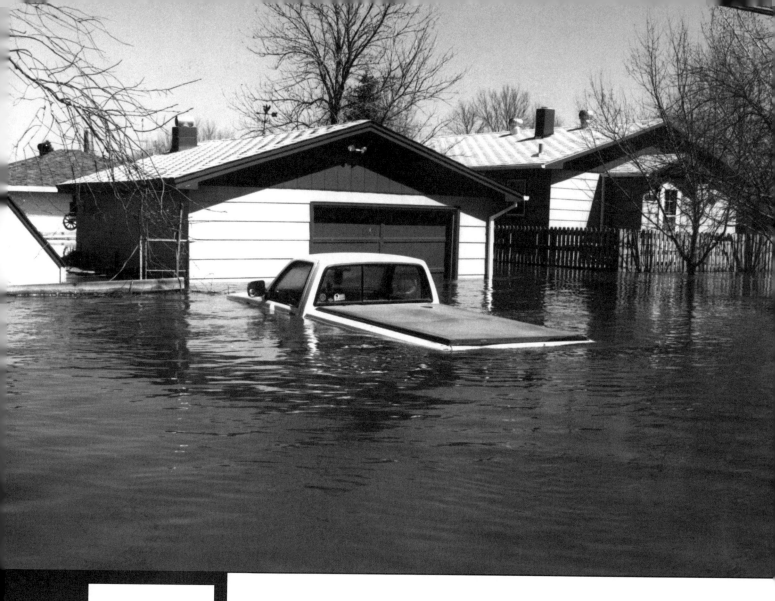

17 Disaster Response

Stuart B. Weiss, MD, FACEP, FAAP
Peter I. Dworsky, MPH, EMT-P
William A. Gluckman, DO, FACEP, EMT-P

Principles of This Chapter

After reading this chapter, you should be able to:

- Describe the differences between a disaster and a mass-casualty incident.
- List the different types and phases of a disaster.
- Discuss the role of triage in a disaster.
- Explain what is involved in the development of an EMS disaster plan.
- Recall the basic tenets of the incident command system.
- Explain the importance of communication in a disaster.

ALTHOUGH MOST PEOPLE CONSIDER DISASTERS TO BE RARE events in their lives, they actually are occurring every day throughout the year. In 2003, the American Red Cross responded to 72,000 events. On average over the past 5 years, the American Red Cross has responded to 67,000 events per year. According to personal communication with the Red Cross press office and various press releases, most of these events are fires at single-family homes, but more than 2,300 per year are disasters large enough to require national resources. That translates to more than six disasters requiring national resources every day. During the past 20 years, disasters have resulted in the deaths of more than 3.4 million people. In 2002, an estimated 600 million people worldwide were affected by floods or drought.[1] A search of the United Nations ReliefWeb for 2003-2004 shows 206 major disasters worldwide.[2] This figure is set to rise as continued urbanization in developing countries results in an increased density of population at risk for earthquakes, hurricanes, and floods. In addition, increasing global travel and commerce raise the risk of potential infectious disease disasters such as an influenza pandemic, avian flu, SARS, and more. In addition, the increased frequency of international acts of terrorism using chemical, biological, radiological, nuclear, or explosive/incendiary (CBRNE) devices will add to the at-risk population.

Since the World Trade Center disaster of September 11, 2001, many people have an increased awareness of the potential for disasters in their communities. In the United States, however, large mass-casualty events have been very rare. Only eight disasters in US history have resulted in more than 1,000 fatalities each, and seven of them occurred prior to 1936.[3] This low probability of large-scale human fatality-producing events has led to some complacency with regard to disaster planning as other problems take priority in the current fiscal environment. People continue to underestimate the impact a major disaster would have on our population, our lifestyle, and our economy. In addition, steps to mitigate disasters have often been overlooked. For example, hospitals and other critical resources have been built on fault lines; an increasing number of people live in flood plains; population centers have been built close to areas with potential volcanic activity; and large chemical plants have been constructed close to urban areas.

EMS, fire, and police departments are invariably the first to respond to or recognize a major event. The level of preparedness, planning, and coordination among these agencies and the actions taken in the first few minutes will dictate the level of success in mitigating the medical consequences of a disaster.[4]

This chapter addresses the underlying principles of EMS disaster management and the common pitfalls in disaster planning, and it can serve as a planning guide for EMS agencies. One important point to keep in mind: the *process* of developing a disaster preparedness plan and the resulting *relationships* can be just as important, if not more important, than the plan itself.

The Definition of Disaster

One of the most difficult aspects of discussing disasters is the lack of a common definition. The word **disaster** is used quite liberally to describe many types of events. The Center for Research on the Epidemiology of Disasters defines a disaster as: "Situation or event, which overwhelms local capacity, necessitating a request to national or international level for external assistance." One of the following four criteria is required for inclusion in the Center's database: 10 or more people killed, 100 people reported affected, a call for international assistance, or a declaration of a state of emergency. Other agencies have used other definitions. The American College of Emergency Physicians policy on disaster medical services states that "a medical disaster occurs when the destructive effects of natural or man-made forces overwhelm the ability of a given area or community to meet the demand for health care."[5]

To add to the confusion, events that have been routinely labeled as disasters, such as plane crashes, might not satisfy disaster criteria or definition, and events that should be classified as disasters, such as multicar pileups in rural areas, are not.

The key concept in accurately defining what is or is not a disaster is to look at how the event relates to the available response resources at the time of the event. If an event overwhelms local resources available at the time, then it meets the definition of a disaster. For example, a multicar crash with 10 trauma victims could easily be absorbed into a large, urban EMS system, but the same event in a rural environment would constitute a disaster — it might require activation of a disaster plan and, at a minimum, would require mutual aid. The same definition applies to hospitals and health care systems. A large city with multiple hospitals could handle a train crash with many trauma victims; the same event in a more rural environment would overwhelm the local resources and would clearly constitute a disaster.

A term that is often confused with a disaster is a **mass-casualty incident (MCI)**. An MCI is an event that creates a large number of victims. This event would meet the definition of a disaster if it overwhelms the local resources available at the time; however, an MCI does not necessarily constitute a disaster.

Types of Disasters

Disasters can be classified using several different schemes based on different aspects of the disaster. One way is to classify the disaster based on the degree of mutual aid required. Classically, a **type one disaster** had been defined as one in which local resources could handle the event. This is somewhat confusing: as described, a type one event does not even meet the definition of a disaster. A **type two disaster** is one in which local resources are overwhelmed and regional mutual aid is required. A **type three disaster** is a large event in which regional assets are overwhelmed and state and/ or federal resources are required.

Disasters can also be classified by causative agent. This is an especially useful concept when conducting an analysis of the hazards and threats in a community. There are four major types: natural, technological, civil, and special hazards. These often overlap; for example, a large natural disaster can create a technological disaster, and so on.

A **natural disaster** is one that occurs in nature and results in human casualties. Examples of this type of disaster include infectious disease outbreaks, coastal storms, cold weather events, hot weather events, high wind events, wild fires, earthquakes, droughts, floods, volcanic activity, and mudslides or avalanches.

Technological disasters are related to manmade structures and infrastructure. Examples of this type of disaster include hazardous material events or industrial accidents, structural failure events (building or bridge collapse, tunnel cave-in, dam failure), structural fires, utility interruption, communication disruption (loss of 911, dispatch, paging), and transportation events (plane crash, train derailment, ferry accident, major roadway event).

Civil disasters result from human activity. These disasters include labor events (strike, walkout, slowdown), criminal or terrorist events, civil disturbances (protest, demonstration, march), hostage events, planned large events (concert, VIP visit), armed conflicts, and wars.

The **special hazards** category includes types of disaster that disrupt services, leading to potential harm to patients. This category includes, for example, critical supply shortages, VIP visits that close roads and block EMS access, and treatment of a large number of persons under arrest.

Finally, hospitals and EMS systems based at hospitals tend to classify disasters as either internal to the facility or external. One type tends to fold into the other, as a large external disaster can create an internal disaster as systems fail, and vice versa.

Several authors have attempted to bring the different classification systems together. One such attempt is the **potential injury-creating event**, or **PICE**, nomenclature.[6,7] This system involves assigning several modifiers to each event (**Table 17-1**). These modifiers describe the potential for additional casualties (column A); indicate whether an overwhelmed system is disrupted and needs augmentation or is paralyzed and needs reconstitution (column B); classifies the extent of geographic involvement (column C); and assigns a staging number to describe the projected need for outside aid. Stage 0 means there is little chance that outside medical assistance will be needed; Stage I means there is a small chance; and Stage II means there is a moderate chance. Stage III means local resources are clearly overwhelmed. This system might be useful for

Table 17.1	Potential injury/illness-creating event (PICE) nomenclature.			
A	**B**	**C**		**PICE stage**
Static	Controlled	Local		0
Dynamic	Disruptive	Regional		I
	Paralytic	National		II
		International		III

academic research but too complex for use in EMS response.

Perhaps a more useful classification for EMS would be to use a scale that combines several disaster response aspects. Such a classification system could be based on type of event, current number of victims, potential number of victims, and potential duration. No widely used, standardized system is in place at this time. A recent Australian study highlighted the need for a standard system to be developed.[8] This survey of state and territory health service emergency management plans revealed that 13 different terms were being used to describe casualty-producing incidents, and that there were four different definitions for the word disaster, and eight for the word emergency.[8]

Role of EMS in a Disaster

As one of the initial responders to a disaster event, EMS has a critical role in determining how the event develops and how patient care is delivered. The initial steps that are taken and the information that is relayed back to the medical community can mean the difference between a well-run and coordinated response and true chaos. The ability to provide efficient patient triage, treatment, and transport depends on EMS organization and management. EMS must help bring order to the chaos surrounding a disaster response by using a well-rehearsed incident management system. One such system is the incident command system (ICS) discussed later in this chapter.

EMS must be the eyes and ears for the rest of the medical community and relay accurate and timely information back to dispatch centers for dissemination to local hospitals and other responders.

Even before an event occurs, EMS leaders must bring patient care knowledge to emergency management planning occurring in their communities. EMS representatives must be at the table when community disaster plans are drawn up to make sure that patient care issues are taken into account and that plans are operationally sound. EMS leadership should provide valuable input into state and federal ESF 8 plans and local/county/parish/state office of emergency management plans, and should be active members of local emergency planning committees.

Anatomy of a Disaster

When an event that ultimately becomes a disaster occurs, there is a chronology of events that routinely occurs. This sequence can vary slightly depending on disaster type (natural, technological, civil, or special hazards). In an explosive event, the actual event is short lived. In a large natural event such as an infectious disease outbreak, the disaster-creating event is more prolonged and might not be recognized for some time. In a coastal storm, the buildup to the event might be prolonged but the actual event short lived. In all cases, the sequence of events is similar, as depicted in **Figure 17-1**.

Recognition

Most disaster response begins with the recognition that an event has occurred. In most disasters, the actual event is obvious, for example, an earthquake, explosion, or hurricane. In some cases, however, the actual event is not as obvious and recognition comes only when the health care system is embroiled in the response. An example of this would be an infectious disease outbreak. In this case, the slow rise in EMS and emergency department volumes might go unnoticed initially. For intentional infectious disease outbreaks, there have been several initiatives put in place to augment early recognition. One such program is Biowatch, which routinely collects air samples in major US cities to monitor for any release of a bioterrorism agent.[9]

Activation

Once a disaster-creating event is recognized, the EMS system must be activated. This phase includes notifica-

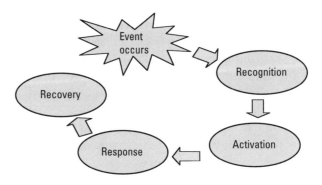

Figure 17-1 Sequence of events in a disaster.

tion of all relevant personnel, EMS agencies, and local hospitals. Health care facilities must be notified immediately of the potential disaster because, in many past events, large numbers of victims have evacuated themselves to the closest hospitals.[10,11] In the Oklahoma City bombing in 1995, the closest hospitals received most of the patients, as is consistent with most disasters. In this event, only 33% of patients arrived via EMS; 55% arrived via privately owned vehicle; 10% walked in; and 1% arrived via other mode.[11] In New York City, after the 2001 World Trade Center attack, the closest hospital received more than 350 patients, and the closest trauma center received more than 300 patients within the first 2 hours.[12]

Several states have developed notification systems for hospitals. In New Jersey, the 800-MHz Hospital Emergency Radio System is a stand-alone, fully redundant notification and communications system that links together all acute care hospitals, EMS dispatch centers, the New Jersey State Emergency Operations Center, and the Department of Health and Senior Services. This system is tested daily and allows for rapid notification of facilities across the state.

Notification is quickly followed by initial response to a specific location, if applicable. In events such as explosions or fires, there is such a place; in widespread events such as floods or hurricanes, there might not be.

A second and equally important aspect of activation is the organization of command structure and initial scene management. The initial steps taken to organize command structure and response will greatly affect the ability of responding units to provide the best level of patient care. Many disaster responses have been hindered by a lack of initial organization. One example of this is the 1990 Avianca Airlines plane crash off Long Island, New York. There was only one road into the crash area, and it was very quickly filled with boxed-in emergency response vehicles. As a result, responders had to hike up to 2 miles to reach the site.

The initial command structure must be consistent with an established incident management system, such as the fire service incident command system (ICS). Using a standard ICS brings several distinct advantages to command and control of a disaster response. First, an ICS incorporates a standard vocabulary for job titles and functions. By using an ICS, everyone involved in a response will understand who is doing what and what their titles are.

Second, by adopting ICS and training and exercising its use, an EMS agency will have people who are comfortable with a management system that will rapidly bring much-needed order to a chaotic situation. Third, ICS comes with predefined **job action sheets** that

clearly delineate the responsibilities of the individuals who step into the jobs within the ICS (**Figure 17-2**). Finally, ICS is an easily scalable management solution. It can be rapidly expanded to many positions for large or prolonged events and collapsed into a small system for small events.[13,14]

EMS disaster planners and EMS incident commanders must also remember that the need for routine EMS services will not disappear during a disaster. In fact, the demand for EMS services might actually increase as a community and its population are stressed by a local disaster.

Response

During this phase, the actual patient care activities begin, including patient extrication, search and rescue if needed, triage, stabilization, treatment, and finally transport. Additional resources for patient care are activated during this phase. As mentioned previously, many patients will self-triage and transport themselves to distant health care facilities by means other than EMS. According to the New Jersey Office of Emergency Management, after the 2001 World Trade Center attacks, patients were seen at health care facilities throughout the region, some more than 100 miles away from New York City.

The final aspect of this phase includes definitive scene management. If a disaster-creating event is confined to one area, scene control and containment are fairly straightforward. In evolving or slow-moving disasters, scene management can be more difficult, especially if the scene is spread over a large geographic area or if the search, rescue, and extrication phases are prolonged.

Recovery

This phase is often underemphasized in disaster planning, but it is critical to allow restoration of a sense of normalcy to an affected community. During this phase, response agencies stand down and release units and resources. Treatment and support are provided for responders, including initial counseling and referral for additional services. In some services, **critical incident stress debriefing (CISD)** is used, although there is a growing discussion as to the usefulness of classic CISD in many settings.

In this phase, the role of EMS changes from triage, treatment, and transport to support of response agencies.

Equally important during this phase is to perform an assessment of the response, develop a corrective

MEDICAL/HEALTH BRANCH DIRECTOR

Position Assigned To:	
You Report To:	

Mission: Organize and direct activities relating to the Medical/Health operations. Carry out directives of the EOC Director, local Health Officer, and EMS Agency Medical Director. Coordinate and supervise the medical and health resources within the operational area.

Immediate _____ **RECEIVE APPOINTMENT**
Receive appointment from the Operations Section Chief or EOC Director. Obtain packet containing Section's Job Action Sheet and forms.

_____ **REVIEW JOB SHEET**
Read this entire Job Action Sheet and review organizational chart.

_____ **OBTAIN BRIEFING**
Obtain briefing from the Operations Section Chief or EOC Director, which should include times of future briefings.

_____ **ESTABLISH EOC POST**
Establish a post in the operational area EOC as the Medical/Health Branch Director. Clearly mark your post and identify yourself (eg name badge).

_____ **APPOINT GROUP SUPERVISORS**
Appoint Group Supervisors as needed to obtain information and liaison with various components of the medical and health community (e.g. Medical Transport Services, Public Health Services, Inpatient Services, Outpatient Services, Ancillary Services, Animal Services, Specialty Services). Distribute Job Action Sheets and forms to Group Supervisors.

_____ **DEVELOP INITIAL ACTION PLAN**
Brief all Medical/Health Group Supervisors on current situation and develop the section's initial action plan (for the first 12-hour operational period). Designate time for next briefing.

_____ **INITIAL ASSESSMENT**
Perform an initial assessment of the medical/health needs and possible impact on resources (RIM Medical/Health Status Report form).

_____ **CONTACTS**
Review county and municipal emergency organizational charts to determine appropriate contacts and message routing. Coordinate with the Logistics and Finance Sections regarding the process of obtaining needed supplies.

_____ **RELAY STATUS REPORT**
Contact state Medical/Health Officials, EMSA and DHS. Provide a brief overview of the event and forward RIMS Medical/Health Situation report to state officials through the operational area EOC Planning Section.

_____ **RESOURCES NEEDS**
Establish communication with the Operational Area Disaster Medical/Health Coordinator (OADMHC) from within the EOC. Relay current status of medical and health resources and any resource needs to the OADMHC, using the RIMS Resource Request form.

(Continued on next page)

Figure 17-2 Sample job action sheet.[16]

<table>
<tr><td></td><td>_____</td><td>**PUBLIC INFORMATION**
Coordinate with the Public Information Officer to issue periodic public health & safety information.</td></tr>
<tr><td></td><td>_____</td><td>**DOCUMENT**
Assure that all communications and times are documented, as well as all actions and decisions.</td></tr>
<tr><td>_Intermediate_</td><td>_____</td><td>**STAFF/SUPPLY**
Ensure that each of the Group Supervisors has adequate staff for the next two operational periods (12-hour shifts) and adequate supplies. Relief staff should arrive 30 minutes early to allow for briefing prior to shift change.</td></tr>
<tr><td></td><td>_____</td><td>**BRIEFINGS/UPDATES**
Conduct briefings and updates with all Group Supervisors on a regular basis.</td></tr>
<tr><td></td><td>_____</td><td>**UPDATE ACTION PLAN**
Develop the Medical/Health Action Plan for the upcoming operational period.</td></tr>
<tr><td></td><td>_____</td><td>**COMMUNICATE UP**
Brief the Operations Section Chief routinely. Attend Planning Meetings as appropriate.</td></tr>
<tr><td></td><td>_____</td><td>**RESPOND TO PROBLEMS**
Respond to requests and complaints from incident personnel regarding inter-organization problems.</td></tr>
<tr><td>_Extended_</td><td>_____</td><td>**DOCUMENT**
Assure that a system for logging and organizing all documentation is established.</td></tr>
<tr><td></td><td>_____</td><td>**LONG-TERM STAFFING**
Ensure that adequate staffing is being considered for the projected duration of the incident. Observe all staff for signs of stress. Report concerns to the Operations Section Cheif. Provide for staff rest periods and relief.</td></tr>
<tr><td>_Recovery_</td><td>_____</td><td>**DISASTER RECOVERY**
Ensure that information for public health and safety are used during disaster recovery stage. Notify public of:
• safe drinking water requirements
• safe reoccupancy of damaged homes and buildings (structural integrity, gas leaks, etc.), appropriate personal protective clothing and equipment (gloves, masks, etc.)
• handling and disposal of foodstuffs, refuse, clothing, hazardous materials
• animal control</td></tr>
<tr><td></td><td>_____</td><td>**AFTER ACTION CRITIQUE**
Participate in critique of activated medical/health disaster response plans and overall county disaster response plans.</td></tr>
</table>

Figure 17-2 Sample job action sheet (continued).[16]

action plan, and then implement the corrective actions. No EMS agency should ever return to "normal" after a disaster response. There are always lessons to be learned, and these must be incorporated into EMS protocols to allow for an improved response the next time.

Developing an EMS Disaster Plan

There are five steps in the development of a disaster plan. All steps in this process are of equal importance. These steps include:

- Gathering information
- Developing the plan with partners
- Training using the plan
- Exercising the plan
- Evaluating the plan and making corrections

Gathering Information

Before beginning to write a plan, it is essential that planners take a moment to look around their communities for potential hazards and threats. This is the basis for performing a **hazard vulnerability analysis (HVA)**. The idea behind performing an HVA is to look at all the potential hazards and threats in your community and then assign a level of risk to each one. The list of potential hazards and threats can be developed by referring to the four disaster classes discussed earlier in this chapter. Data can be obtained from local offices of emergency management, local emergency planning committees, and from industry under the Superfund Amendment and Reauthorization Act of 1986. Additionally, data for communities in areas affected by natural disasters such as tornadoes, hurricanes, blizzards, floods, and mudslides can be obtained from government experts (National Oceanic and Atmospheric Administration, US Geologic Survey, National Weather Service, US Army Corps of Engineers). Finally, population figures, including density and special needs populations, must be obtained. Urban areas can be expected to have higher numbers of casualties as well as a higher number of bystanders. Both must be managed. Low-density rural areas might require a more extensive search and rescue component, and it can be difficult to set up triage, treatment, and transport points. Special needs considerations could include populations who do not speak English, large influx of seasonal visitors in resort areas, large elderly or nursing home populations, incarcerated persons, large military bases, large venues such as stadiums and arenas, and special facilities such as nuclear power plants.

The assignment of risk is related to how likely or probable (based on historical data) it is that the hazard or threat will generate a disaster and how vulnerable the community is to damage if this hazard or threat were to occur.

Last, the immediate impact on the system (people, equipment, supplies, economy) if the threat or hazard results in a disaster must be assessed.

Developing a grid that lists hazard or threat, probability, vulnerability, and impact is useful. Once this list of hazards and threats is created and a risk factor is assigned to each one, the items should be ranked: the highest-risk/largest-impact events should be planned for first.

The final step is to develop the grid into a matrix that lists hazard or threat, risk, and impact, as well as mitigation and consequences, as shown in **Table 17-2**. Mitigation activities are those that help reduce the medical consequences of a threat or hazard. Consequences are the long-term impact of the threat or hazard on a system.

After the HVA is completed, planners must look at the agency's assets and capabilities. This asset list must include personnel, equipment, supplies, and so on. Finally, a review of applicable laws, regulations, and mutual aid agreements must be completed.

Developing the Plan With Partners

No EMS agency can plan in a vacuum. All disaster responses will include a multitude of response agencies. One only has to recall any recent disaster to realize the magnitude of response in a large-scale event. Not only will local EMS be present, but responding agencies will include local police and fire; there might be county response, state response, and even federal response. This will include police, fire, health department, mutual aid agencies, office of emergency management, FEMA, FBI, military assets, EPA, ATF, utilities, NTSB, to name a few. It is imperative that initial EMS plans are created while planning how EMS will fit into the larger disaster response. Other local responders and then regional responders must be brought into the planning process early to ensure that realistic plans are created and that they translate into good operations in the field.

Plans must also be developed with the principles of comprehensive emergency management (CEM) in mind. CEM has four components: mitigation, planning, response, and recovery. Plans should also be developed as an all-hazards type of plan with special annexes to handle the hazards identified in the HVA. By creating an all-hazards type of plan, unforeseen and unpredicted disaster-creating events can be handled using the same plan.

Finally, the plan should allow individual responders to perform job actions they normally do. People do best what they do every day. A person who is asked to do something completely out of his or her job description during a disaster will often revert back to what he or she is comfortable with and will ad-lib and not follow the plan.

One of the key points in disaster planning is that the *process* of developing the plan is sometimes more important than the plan itself. During the process of disaster planning, relationships that can be used during a disaster response should develop. If the chief of EMS develops a good working relationship with the police and fire chiefs, then during a disaster response each one can pick up a telephone and speak to another and already have a relationship. This will greatly improve the seamless integration of different responding agencies.

As part of the planning process, a **threat-response matrix** should be developed. On this matrix, each hazard and each threat is listed, and next to each one an initial response should be planned. For example, if a chemical plant is identified as a high-risk/high-impact threat, then next to the chemical plant the matrix should list what resources should be sent to each call

Table 17.2	Sample hazard vulnerability analysis.

TYPE OF HAZARD/ THREAT[a]	Reported Events/Incidents PAST 10 YEARS[b]	RISK Probability (P) Vulnerability (V)[c]	IMPACT on System or Community[d]	MITIGATION Activities[e]	CONSEQUENCES[f]
Hurricane Cat. III or IV	8	P: Moderate V: High	High	Storm shutters upgraded. Alternative care sites planned, and supplies predeployed.	Widespread disruption of health care. Loss of communications system due to towers down. Drinking water contaminated. Hospital A in coastal flood zone.
Hazardous material incident	764	P: High V: Moderate	Low	EMS trained to use personal protective equipment. HazMat team upgraded to 24 × 7. Hospital decon. room completed.	Minimal in small events. Tanker gas release might require evacuation of north end of town (prevailing winds usually S→N).
Lightning strikes	545	P: High V: Moderate	Low	Lightning rod education program implemented for homeowners.	Local fires. Communications system failure if towers struck.

[a] Type: Disaster events that have historically occurred or those that are concerning.
[b] Reported Events/Incidents: From historical data.
[c] Risk: Probability = number of specified events per year/total events per year. Vulnerability = how susceptible the system is to damage if the event occurs.
[d] Impact: Impact of event on people, equipment, supplies, economics, and so on.
[e] Mitigation: Steps taken to lessen the impact of an event on the system.
[f] Consequences: What would happen to the system if the event occurs.

at that plant. The threat-response matrix should also list the preplanned resources staging area. For the chemical plant, for example, it should indicate that, for all responses, initial BLS and ALS units are sent, and they stage at the corner of First Street and Fifth Avenue and wait for fire department escorts into the area. A similar listing should be entered for each hazard and threat in the HVA.

Training Using the Plan

No plan is worth the paper it is written on if it is not trained on. A plan in a book on a shelf that is not pulled out until disaster strikes will not be useful. Therefore, once you have developed your emergency management plan, you must train your staff on using the plan. Start by giving people a broad overview of the plan. Then break it down into small, digestible chunks and train people in the individual smaller parts. Finally, after training on all the smaller parts, put it all together

and train people on how the plan fits together. While designing your training, it is important to keep two points in mind. First, make sure people are trained for jobs that are similar to the tasks they perform in their daily routines. Second, train several people for each job. Do not make the mistake of assuming that the one person trained to do a job will not be on vacation when the disaster occurs.

Exercising the Plan

Tabletop, functional, and full-scale exercises are commonly used. All three types of exercises serve different purposes, and all three should be used routinely.

Tabletop Exercises

Tabletop exercises are perhaps the most useful of the three. A tabletop is organized to have all responding agencies at one table. A scenario is presented, and the agency representatives talk through their response plans and capabilities. The scenario, in a compressed timeframe, should be allowed to play out as much as possible. During the interchange, ideas should be shared, deficiencies identified, relationships formed, and a summary document prepared. The summary document should outline corrective actions that should be incorporated into an updated plan. The tabletop exercise should focus on a small, carefully identified part of the plan. It should test specific aspects that need to be validated. No actions are taken during a tabletop exercise. The exercise is all done by talking through the problem. Tabletop exercises are the least expensive of the three types but have limitations, such as limited participation by personnel (ie, open to a limited number of invited participants) and lack of real-time operations.

Functional Exercises

A functional exercise builds on the results from the tabletop exercise. In a functional exercise, the participants actually make the calls and notifications required in their plans. No equipment is moved, but questions are asked about response capabilities. For example, during a functional exercise, EMS command would call the notification number listed in the plan and ask if the required resources are available, how long it would take to get the equipment and personnel, and so on. Functions of the disaster plan would be tested, but no resources would actually be moved. Functional exercises should also test specific parts of the plan. These parts should have already been tested through the tabletop exercise.

Full-Scale Exercises

A full-scale exercise is one in which resources are actually moved in accordance with the disaster plan. During a full-scale exercise, people, equipment, and supplies are mobilized and deployed. All participants who would normally respond to a disaster should participate. The more realistic the response, the more effective the exercise will be. However, safety must be built into the exercise scenario, and there must be controllers who watch for safety problems. For example, most responders limit the lights-and-siren response to an exercise by prepositioning assets close to the exercise site. These resources are then temporarily held back so that their time for response is the same as if they were responding from quarters. This allows for greater realism and maintains a higher level of exercise safety. It is critical for a successful full-scale exercise to have clearly established objectives and a scenario and playbook based on the objectives.

One of the most important parts of a full-scale ex-

ercise is the debriefing of participants and the development of an after-action report. The lessons learned and deficiencies identified in the after-action report must then be included in an updated disaster plan. This is often the missing link: lessons to be learned are *not* learned and are not incorporated into the disaster plan. The old adage that people who do not learn from their mistakes are doomed to repeat them is especially true in disaster planning.

There are several common problems with EMS exercises that should be avoided, as follows:

- EMS training only within the EMS organization. In disaster responses, multiple agencies will be involved. Exercises at all levels must involve other response agencies.
- No clear objectives are predefined. Unless clear objectives are established prior to running an exercise, there will be no means to measure success or failure of individual parts of the plan and make the necessary corrections.
- Disaster exercise planners jump right to full-scale exercises and bypass tabletop and functional exercises. Many EMS agencies plan initial exercises that involve the movement of people, equipment, and other resources. Because too many parts of the plan are being tested at the same time, people improvise to get the job done and incorrect behaviors are reinforced.
- Disaster scenarios are too complex or outlandish. Although it might be exciting to design a scenario involving a planeload of deaf paraplegic passengers that crashes into a school that happens to sit next to an oil refinery that catches on fire, this exaggerated sce-

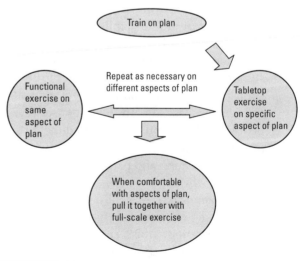

Figure 17-3 Sequence for training and exercising a disaster plan.

nario is too complex. When scenarios are this complex or unlikely, people get lost in the scenario and the exercise is ineffective. Planners should choose scenarios that are realistic and based on the community HVA. To further test the incident commander, throw in one or two realistic confounding factors only after there is a consistent level of confidence with the plan.

Overall, training and exercising should follow the sequence depicted in **Figure 17-3.**

Evaluating the Plan and Making Corrections

The final part of all planning, training, and exercising is the evaluation and correction phase. As mentioned earlier, incorporating corrections into response plans is how improvements are made and mistakes are redressed. Unfortunately, many response agencies discover problems with plans during exercises only to have the same problems recur in the next exercise because the deficiencies were not corrected.

Incident Management System

The **incident command system (ICS),** also referred to as the **incident management system (IMS),** provides a comprehensive method for managing people, resources, and operations during both emergency and nonemergency events. It is equally applicable to small-scale, daily operational activities and major mobilizations, both planned events and emergency responses. It is the preferred method of command and control used by almost all fire departments across the United States. IMS provides a useful and flexible instrument that is particularly adaptable to incidents involving multijurisdictional and/or multidisciplinary responses.

The basic tenets of IMS are as follows:

- **Management by objectives** — The objectives should be established at the outset of the response, and they should be agreed on by all of the agencies tasked with the response. The people in charge must understand the local policies, establish the incident objectives, select the strategies, and perform the operations to achieve the goal.
- **Chain of command** — Establishing and publishing the chain of command ensures that each person operating at the scene reports to only one person, and each person knows who reports to him or her. It also allows for informa-

tion to be disseminated in an orderly manner so no one is left out. This also implies that there is an orderly ranking of personnel and that each has the authority of that position. This is very important because personnel from one agency might be assigned to another agency for a specific task or function (**Figure 17-4**).

- **Span of control** — In the IMS plan, each person should have no more than seven people reporting to him or her. It is preferable, when possible, to limit this to no more than a 1:5 ratio. In a crisis situation, this limits the amount of information the individuals who are in critical decision-making areas need to process. It also assists management personnel in the provision of safety and accountability of the manpower and resources assigned to the event.
- **Common terminology** — The terms used to identify resources or communicate vary throughout regions. Some agencies use codes to identify events, and others use plain text or a combination. This is often problematic when EMS is responding to a mutual aid request. Agency A might call a building collapse a 10-54, and Agency B will use the same code for a motor vehicle crash. Imagine a person requesting on the radio that he needs a COW. To the uninitiated this might mean something that goes, "Moo," and to others it is a communications device (cell on wheels) provided by a local wireless provider. Thus, plain text communication is a hallmark of IMS. Another complication that is resolved through the implementation of the IMS is that of rank. When personnel are placed into the IMS structure, they adopt an IMS title, such as "incident commander" or "staging officer." The title or rank from the home agency does not transfer for the duration of the event. Thus, the police

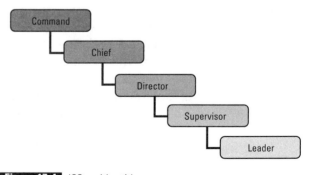

Figure 17-4 ICS position titles.

captain might be designated as the "north sector team leader."

- **Incident action plan** — This is a document that is prepared for the event. For small events, this might be no more than a summary page listing what happened. For large-scale incidents, it is more complex and serves as the blueprint that guides the responders. It has several sections that cover the statement of objectives, the organizational structure, all tasks and assignments, and supporting documentation. FEMA has developed several forms (ICS-201 through 209) to aid in the writing of this plan.[15] It is of utmost importance to have an incident action plan when an event involves multiple jurisdictions, crosses over shift changes or operational periods, or is very complex.

IMS is most notably known for its visual structure, that of an organization chart. IMS is broken down into five functional areas, as depicted in **Figure 17-5**, each with specific responsibilities. Each box represents a function or an activity. They are interrelated in that each supports the other. The functions of command, operations, planning, logistics, and finance are referred to as the **general staff positions**. When assigned, operations, planning, logistics, and finance report directly to the incident commander. Also reporting to the incident commander are four **command staff positions**.

As previously discussed, predefined job action sheets will help individuals perform their duties, especially if they are unfamiliar with the specific tasks associated with the job.[16]

General Staff Positions

Command
The function of the command position is to assume responsibility for the overall management of the incident. Command establishes the strategy and tactics for the incident and has the ultimate responsibility for the success of the incident activities. The person assigned to this role is the **incident commander.** The command position is established at every incident no matter how small or whether it involves only a single resource.

The major responsibilities of the incident commander are as follows:

- Organizing to meet the needs of the incident
- Establishing incident control objectives
- Setting priorities for work accomplishment
- Ensuring development of the incident action plans
- Approving resource requests
- Approving public information briefings
- Interacting and coordinating with public officials and other agencies

Operations
The function of the operations position is to implement and accomplish the objectives and strategy developed by the command position. The operations chief directs all the incident tactical operations and assists command in the development of the action plan. Operations people are the "doers" in the organization, where the work of incident management is accomplished. Operations is charged with carrying out command direction.

Responsibilities include:

- Achieving command objectives
- Directing tactical operations
- Participating in the planning process
- Providing intelligence to planning and command
- Maintaining discipline and accountability

Planning
The function of the planning position is to collect and evaluate information that is needed to help the incident commander make logical decisions. This position provides past, present, and future details regarding the events occurring at the incident. This information includes real-time resource and situation status.

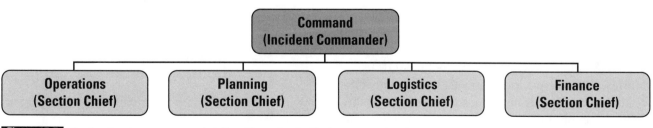

Figure 17-5 Five functional areas, or general staff positions, of an incident management system.

It is often easier to think of the planning function as future operations because one of its primary objectives is to plan for the next operational period, which might be 12 to 24 hours later.

Responsibilities include:

- Maintaining accurate resource status
- Gathering and analyzing situation data
- Providing displays of situation status
- Estimating future probabilities
- Preparing alternative strategies
- Conducting planning meetings
- Compiling and distributing approved action plans

The planning function incorporates positions for technical specialists and advisors. These positions are filled by qualified people who provide the planning section with expert information or technical data that are essential to managing the incident. In the case of a chemical spill, for example, a chemical engineer could advise in planning.

Logistics

The function of the logistics position can be described as the quartermaster's role for the incident. The logistics position provides the services and supplies that will support the functions being performed by operations. When operations needs tow trucks, a request goes up the chain of command through the operations chief to the incident commander, who passes the message to the logistics chief, who will obtain the trucks.

The logistics function has two missions. One is to focus on supporting the needs of the event (**support branch**) by providing the responders with the resources necessary to achieve the objectives that are set forth by the incident commander. This includes tools, lighting, additional manpower, and so on. The other mission is to provide for responders and their personal needs (**service branch**). This includes shelter, food, medical care, and so on.

It should be noted that, once logistics obtains the requested resources, it becomes a joint effort of operations and planning to use them.

Finance

The function of the finance position is to maintain all of the fiscal documentation and records that are produced as a result of the event. This includes payroll records, Worker's Compensation documentation for injuries, and receipts for contracts, goods, and services obtained. This is important if there is to be any chance of reimbursement. In many cases, damages can be assessed against a responsible party for the purpose of repayment.

Command Staff Positions

There are typically four command staff positions — public information officer, safety officer, liaison officer, and medical director. These positions are implemented to help the incident commander fulfill the responsibilities associated with managing the emergency. They handle essential activities that enable the incident commander to concentrate on managing the incident. The command staff positions are not considered part of the incident commander's span of control, although they report directly to the incident commander (**Figure 17-6**).

Public Information Officer

The public information officer, or PIO, is responsible for the development and release of information regarding the incident. This person serves as the point of contact for the media and other agencies requiring information. It is the responsibility of the PIO to establish an area for the media away from the command post and a safe distance from the incident. There the PIO will provide updates based on a predetermined schedule, answer questions, and if possible, arrange for photo opportunities of the incident. Each response agency might have its own PIO, who will respond with them; however, the incident commander will designate one to be the lead PIO, and the others will be deputy PIOs. The PIO will also be the incident representative at a joint information center if one is established.

Safety Officer

The safety officer is responsible for the safety and well-being of the responders. This person must monitor activities for unsafe practices or situations and notify the incident commander of unsafe acts and conditions. Because the size of the event can be widespread, deputy safety officers must be appointed; they have the full authority of the safety officer. The person designated

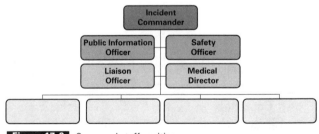

Figure 17-6 Command staff positions.

as safety officer must have the requisite knowledge of the task at hand. If the major event is fire related, it makes sense to have someone with detailed knowledge of the fire service serve as the safety officer. If the incident involves search and rescue activities at a building collapse, it is prudent for this person to have search and rescue and engineering or construction knowledge.

Although it is the duty of the safety officer to notify the incident commander of unsafe acts or conditions, it is the responsibility of the safety officer to take immediate corrective action to stop a dangerous practice (eg, using a cutting torch without proper protective eyewear, removing personnel from the threat of imminent danger, as in a collapse zone). Whenever this is done, the safety officer must advise the incident commander and line managers of the corrective action and the nature of the hazard as soon as possible. If the threat is not imminent, the safety officer should follow the normal chain of command to accomplish the corrective action.

Liaison Officer

A liaison officer might be required at an incident that involves multiple agencies. The liaison officer's responsibilities are to provide a point of contact for agencies not involved in the command function, such as the Red Cross. The liaison officer coordinates the efforts of the other agencies and reduces the risk of their operating independently.

Each agency that responds to an event should have a representative with whom the liaison officer can work. These relationships must be well established prior to any disaster response.

Medical Director

The medical director organizes, prioritizes, and assigns physicians to areas where medical care is being delivered (ie, treatment area) and should oversee the activities in this sector. This person advises the incident commander on issues related to the medical care of the victims and provides onsite medical oversight for EMS agencies. This person also coordinates with the transportation officer with regard to patient destination and oversees the establishment of field hospitals and rehabilitation sectors if needed.

EMS Within the IMS Structure

EMS normally operates an IMS structure at most small-scale events without even realizing it. Examining a two-car motor vehicle crash, the first unit on scene splits the tasks at hand: one team member assumes command and assesses the scene, chooses the plan of action, and obtains additional resources (police, fire, traffic control), while the other members begin triage and treatment.

The common IMS chart for EMS operations is depicted in **Figure 17-7**.

It is imperative for all EMS providers to realize that, at a large-scale event, they are not an island unto themselves; they are part of a larger plan. The entire structure of the EMS IMS plan can be considered a branch of the operations function of a larger chart (**Figure 17-8**).

EMS must be represented in the command post, and it has that right under the concept of unified command. This is easier to accomplish if the individuals involved have trained and exercised together previously.

Legal Requirements

An ICS or IMS is not just a good idea; there is often a legal requirement to implement it. Both the Superfund Amendment and Reauthorization Act (SARA) of 1986 and OSHA (29 CFR 1910.120(q)(3)(i–ix)) have regulations that require the use of ICS at all hazardous materials incidents. The Environmental Protection Agency Oil Control Pollution Act has adopted regulations that impose the same requirements in non–OSHA states. The regulation states, "The incident command system shall be established by those employers for the incidents that will be under their control and shall be interfaced with the other organizations or agencies who may respond to such an incident."[17]

The National Fire Protection Administration adopted standards 1500, 1521, and 1561 that relate to fire department occupational health and safety programs. They essentially state that all fire departments will have written procedures for using ICS, and that all department members will be trained in and familiar with the system. The standards place strong emphasis on scene safety and require a method of tracking and accounting for personnel.

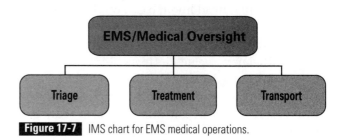

Figure 17-7 IMS chart for EMS medical operations.

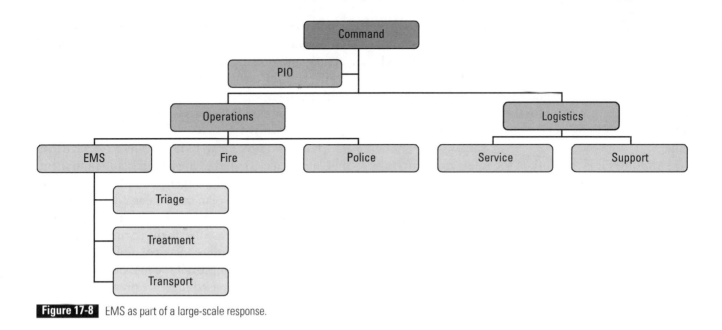

Figure 17-8 EMS as part of a large-scale response.

Comprehensive Emergency Management

All of the items discussed so far in this chapter are pieces of a comprehensive emergency management (CEM) plan. A CEM plan brings all the parts of disaster management into focus in one plan. There are four parts in a CEM plan — mitigation, planning, response, and recovery. The basic idea of CEM is to take the HVA and ask the following questions: How do I reduce the medical consequences of disaster related to a high-risk event? If I cannot reduce the medical consequences to almost nonexistent, how do I plan for my response? What is my response? How do I recover to an augmented "normal" state?

Mitigation

The concept of mitigation is to reduce the medical consequences of a disaster. Much of mitigation occurs in building codes, laws, and regulations. EMS can participate in this process by having an active role in regional planning. In addition, based on the HVA, EMS can preposition specific antidotes and supplies. For example, one large city has chosen to predeploy multiple MARK-I nerve agent kits to its EMS crews. These can be used immediately on scene to save lives. EMS can assist in early evacuation of people in a floodplain or hurricane area. These actions will help reduce or mitigate the medical consequences of a disaster.

Planning

As discussed earlier, training and exercising are part of planning. One of the most important parts of the planning phase is to develop the relationships with other responding agencies that are called on during a disaster. The other point that bears repeating is that a plan must be dynamic and be reevaluated frequently.

Response

The response phase consists of three parts. These parts, as previously discussed, include activation, implementation, and definitive scene management.

Safety must be worked into each part of the disaster plan. EMS units must never enter a situation that is not secure or is possibly unsafe. EMS personnel must have proper personal protective equipment available to them for responses based on the community HVA.

Another aspect of the response phase is medical triage. Triage is the process of sorting patients based on the immediacy of their medical needs. There are many patient triage and tracking systems.[18,19] One of the most prevalent is the **START (simple triage and rapid treatment) system**, which rapidly assesses breathing, pulse, and neurologic function and sorts victims into emergent (red), urgent (yellow), and nonurgent (green) categories.[19] The START protocol is shown in **Figure 17-9**.

The START protocol does not work in young children, so various other triage schemes have been pro-

START Triage

Walking wounded are directed to go to treatment area. (All are triaged as Green.)

Those unable to walk are assessed by the "RPM" method:

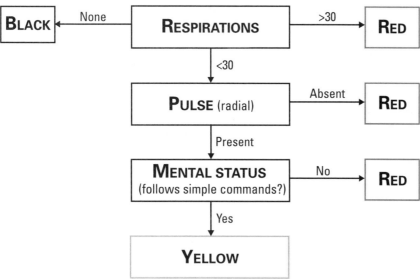

Important:

Once any RED criteria are met, tag patient and MOVE ON!
Triage is sorting, not treatment. Only 2 interventions may be made during triage:
1) Open/clear airway.
2) Apply direct pressure to major bleeding sites.
Patients will be reassessed at treatment area(s).

Figure 17-9 Summary/adaptation of the START triage system, originally developed by Hoag Hospital and the Newport Beach Fire Department.[19]

posed. One such system is **JumpSTART** (**Figure 17-10**), which modifies the START protocol for nonverbal children.[20]

One difficulty with START and JumpSTART is that the triage is not tied to outcomes. Current triage systems are being modified to tie them closer to patient outcome.

A key concept that separates disaster triage from normal triage is that, in a disaster, the idea is to provide minimal medical care to the maximal number of people. Conversely, normal, everyday triage assumes maximal care for a minimal number of people. This distinction can be difficult for medical personnel who are accustomed to providing maximal care to each patient.

Recovery

The recovery phase, as discussed earlier, includes the following:

- Return to normal operations with incorporation of lessons learned
- Support for response personnel
- Victim tracking and notification of relatives

- Equipment resupply and repair
- Reimbursement

Communications

One of the commonly recognized problems in all disaster responses and full-scale exercises is communications.[21] There are several types of communications failures, including technologic failures (equipment) and human failures (not conveying messages as they were intended).

Technologic Failures

Factors that contribute to technologic failure are:

- Insufficient number of radio channels for all the functions needed during a response, leading to crowding. In a large response, radio channels are needed for command, scene operations, support agencies, dispatching, talking to hospitals, and normal operations such as routine dispatch, medical direction, and so on.

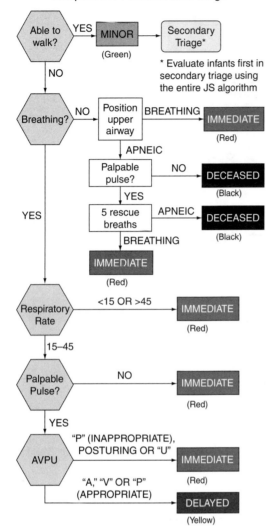

JumpSTART Pediatric MCI Triage©

Able to walk? — YES → MINOR (Green) → Secondary Triage*

* Evaluate infants first in secondary triage using the entire JS algorithm

NO ↓

Breathing? — NO → Position upper airway — BREATHING → IMMEDIATE (Red)

APNEIC ↓

Palpable pulse? — NO → DECEASED (Black)

YES ↓

5 rescue breaths — APNEIC → DECEASED (Black)

BREATHING ↓

IMMEDIATE (Red)

YES ↓

Respiratory Rate — <15 OR >45 → IMMEDIATE (Red)

15–45 ↓

Palpable Pulse? — NO → IMMEDIATE (Red)

YES ↓

AVPU — "P" (INAPPROPRIATE), POSTURING OR "U" → IMMEDIATE (Red)

"A," "V" OR "P" (APPROPRIATE) → DELAYED (Yellow)

Figure 17-10 JumpSTART pediatric MCI triage. © Lou Romig, MD, 2002. Reprinted with permission.

- Lack of radio interoperability among responding agencies. Many jurisdictions lack regional common frequencies that can be used in a large-scale event. Responding agencies have their own radio frequencies and cannot talk to other responding agencies. There are several devices available now that patch together different radio frequencies to create a seamless network. These devices can help alleviate this problem.
- Failure of the communications network due to the disaster. The radio infrastructure itself can be damaged by the disaster-producing event. For example, many radio antennae were on top of the World Trade Center build-

ings, and when those buildings collapsed several radio networks were adversely affected.

Human Factors

Communications failures can also result from the following human factors:

- Intended message is misunderstood. One of the principles of IMS is to speak in plain language and avoid 10-codes or signals. Responding agencies might not use the same codes and can interpret codes incorrectly.
- Lack of proper radio etiquette. People who are not trained in radio usage tie up radio channels by relaying unnecessary or confusing information. In addition, people who are not trained properly might not use the equipment correctly, resulting in mumbled or garbled words.
- Huge radio traffic volume due to channel crowding. If too few channels or frequencies are available, then people will begin interfering with each other as they try to use the overcrowded frequencies.

Proper Planning

There are several keys to improving communication in a disaster, as follows:

- Create a radio preplan that lists available frequencies and assigns functions to those frequencies. Remember to include both disaster functions and routine functions.
- Create a regional mutual aid common frequency that many or all responding agencies can use in a disaster.
- Develop a field communications resource with a patch box and/or a local repeater and handheld radios to bring together responding agencies.
- Plan for radio infrastructure failure. Develop alternative communication methods up to and including a messenger system in case no radio system is available.
- Train responders in proper radio etiquette and usage to reduce errors.
- Routinely test the radio network. For example, in New Jersey, there are three radio systems that can be used in a disaster — the EMS dispatch center network tying together all dispatch centers, the trauma/burn center network, and the Hospital Emergency Radio Network. Each system is routinely tested

once or twice a day so that staff members are comfortable using the radio equipment and speaking on the radio.

Summary

EMS plays a critical part in disaster response. The actions taken in the initial phases of a disaster response will dictate how the disaster response proceeds. Knowing community hazards and threats by performing a hazard vulnerability analysis and then applying comprehensive emergency management principles will allow an EMS system to take the correct initial and subsequent steps to provide timely and efficient patient care to the maximal number of patients.

References

1. International Federation of Red Cross and Red Crescent Societies. Volunteers combat climate change [IFRCRCS Web site]. Available at: http://www.ifrc.org/docs/news/03/03120502. Accessed January 5, 2005.

2. United Nations Office for the Coordination of Humanitarian Affairs. ReliefWeb Web site. Available at: http://www.reliefweb.int. Accessed January 5, 2005.

3. World Health Organization Collaborating Center for Research on the Epidemiology of Disasters (CRED). Emergency events data base (EM-DAT) [CRED Web site]. Available at: http://www.cred.be. Accessed January 5, 2005.

4. Murphy MF. Emergency medical services in disaster. In: Hogan DE, ed. *Disaster Medicine*. Philadelphia, Pa: Lippincott Williams & Wilkins; 2002:90–103.

5. American College of Emergency Physicians. Disaster medical services [policy statement]. June 2000. Available at: http://www.acep.org/1,435,0.html. Accessed January 5, 2005.

6. Koenig KL, Dinerman N, Kuehl AE. PICE nomenclature: a new system to describe disaster. *Prehospital Disaster Med*. 1994;9:S65.

7. Koenig KL, Dinerman N, Kuehl AE. Disaster nomenclature — a functional impact approach: the PICE system. *Acad Emerg Med*. 1996;3:723–727.

8. Nocera A. Australian major incident nomenclature: it may be a 'disaster' but in an 'emergency' it is just a mess. *ANZ J Surg*. 2001;71(3):162–166.

9. Reuters News Service. US germ detection system active in 31 cities. November 14, 2003.

10. Hogan DE, Dale CA, Osburn AE. The May 3, 1999 tornado in Oklahoma City. *Ann Emerg Med*. 1999;34(2):225–226.

11. Hogan DE, Waeckerle JF, Dire DJ, et al. Emergency department impact of the Oklahoma City terrorist bombing. *Ann Emerg Med*. 1999;34(2):160–167.

12. Simon R, Teperman S. The World Trade Center attack: lessons for disaster management. *Crit Care*. 2001; 5(6):318–320.

13. San Mateo County Department of Health Services Emergency Medical Services Agency. *The Hospital Emergency Incident Command System*. 3rd ed. [California EMS Authority Web site]. 1998. Available at: http://www.emsa.cahwnet.gov/Dms2/HEICS98a.pdf. Accessed January 6, 2005.

14. Firefighting Resources of California Organized for Potential Emergencies. FIRESCOPE Web site. Available at: http://www.firescope.org. Accessed January 5, 2005.

15. The FEMA Web site links to the USDA Forest Service Web site, which has downloadable PDFs of ICS forms 201–225, among others. Available at: http://www.fs.fed.us/fire/planning/nist/ics_forms.htm. Accessed January 5, 2005.

16. Mountain-Valley Emergency Medical Services Agency. *Operational Area EOC Medical/Health Branch Manual* [California EMS Authority Web site]. Available at: http://www.emsa.ca.gov/dms2/oadmhc.pdf. Accessed January 6, 2005.

17. Oil Pollution Act of 1990. Pub L No. 101-380. 57 *Federal Register* 15201 (1992).

18. Bozeman WP. Mass casualty incident triage [letter]. *Ann Emerg Med*. 2003;41(4):582-583.

19. Super G, ed. *START: A Triage Training Module*. Newport Beach, Calif: Hoag Memorial Hospital; 1984.

20. Romig LE. JumpSTART Web site. Available at: http://www.jumpstarttriage.com. Accessed January 5, 2005.

21. Garchnek V, Burkle FM. Telecommunications systems in support of disaster medicine: applications of basic information pathways. *Ann Emerg Med*. 1999;34(2):213–218.

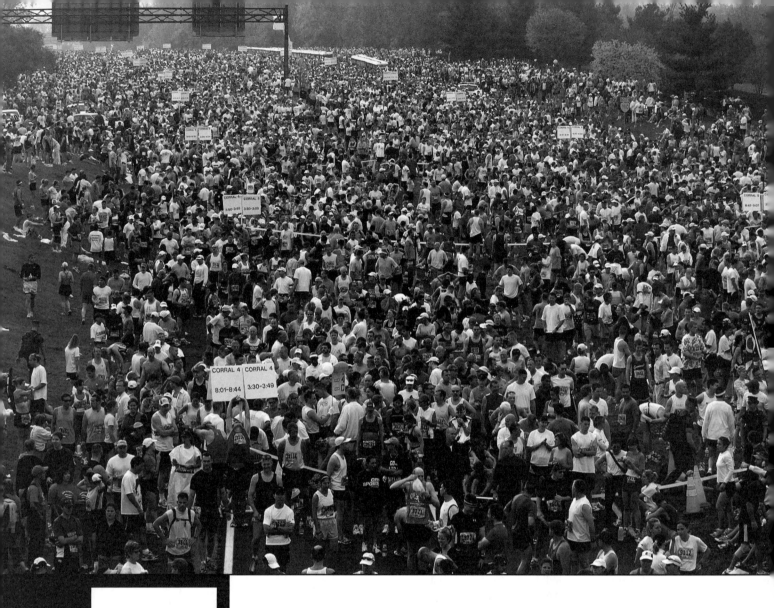

18

Emergency Medical Care at Mass Gatherings

Arthur H. Yancey II, MD, MPH, FACEP

Principles of This Chapter

After reading this chapter, you should be able to:

- Recall the medical director's responsibilities at mass gatherings.
- Describe the level of care and the medical staffing considerations at mass gatherings.
- List the equipment, medications, treatment facilities, and patient transportation resources that are used.
- Discuss environmental elements.
- Discuss access to care and the elements of communications.
- Describe prospective quality management.

EVENTS AS DIVERSE AS FAIRS, POLITICAL RALLIES, AIR SHOWS, parades, festivals, concerts, and sports competitions attract voluntary and temporary attendees. They also generate the same emergency medical care needs that exist in the general population, in addition to needs that are specific to the event. The development of organized emergency medical care for such events is recent; documentation can be traced to football games at the University of Nebraska, where two spectators died without benefit of CPR during the 1965 season.[1] Following the institution of timely CPR, defibrillation, and airway management, eight of nine subsequent arrest victims at that venue over the next 8 years survived to hospital discharge. As early as 1976, mass-casualty guidelines were developed.[2] The 1984 Los Angeles Olympics[3] and the 1996 Atlanta Olympics[4] were examples of well-developed mass-casualty preparation and guidelines. The sentinel information paper of the American College of Emergency Physicians (ACEP) was published in 1990,[5] followed by the position paper[6] and medical director's checklist[7] of the National Association of EMS Physicians (NAEMSP) in 1999.

A **mass gathering** has been informally defined as an event attended by 1,000 or more people. Unique variables in event and crowd characteristics contribute to significant variations in the number of patient incidents at a mass-gathering event. These factors produce demands for emergency medical care that have little relationship to crowd size. They include exposure to adverse weather conditions, alcohol and/or illicit drug use, inadequate intake of potable water combined with environmental temperature extremes, consumption of contaminated food, and violent behavior. Statistics from major rock concerts demonstrate a higher incidence (0.96 to 17 per 1,000) of demand for medical care among spectators than at sporting event mass gatherings (0.3 to 1.6 per 1,000).[8] In the largest known "concert medicine" study (405 concerts, five venues, over 5 years), risk factors predictive of patient load were examined.[9] Music type was identified as the best predictor, with 2.5 times more medical care required at rock concerts than at non–rock concert events. Younger spectators, alcohol abuse, and illicit drug use were implicated as factors largely responsible for this difference, either directly or as a result of associated injuries.

As our society has encouraged a healthier lifestyle and more adults have begun participating in athletic activities such as walking, running, and biking marathons, related mass-gathering events in which participants outnumber spectators have become more common. In these events, the incidence of demand for medical care (24 per 1,000) can far exceed that associated with events at which spectators are the majority present.[10]

Several unique features distinguish medical care at mass gatherings from medical care in other settings. Mass-gathering incidents can overwhelm onsite resources. There are densely clustered crowds, physical barriers that prevent access to and care of ill and injured patients, special communications technology requirements, and the need to coordinate care with jurisdictional public resource managers. As is true of EMS in general, the successful care of patients at mass gatherings depends on understanding public health, public safety, clinical emergency medicine, public relations, telecommunications, logistics, business negotiations, and disaster preparedness.

Medical Direction

Planning for medical care at a mass gathering should begin with the appointment of a medical director for the event. The goal of medical direction should be to

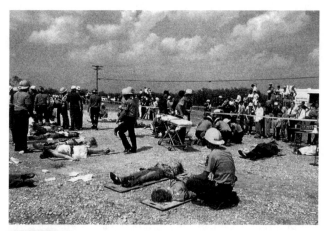

Figure 18-1 Distance communications technology is most vulnerable to breakdown when it is needed most — in disaster circumstances most likely involving multiple casualties.

provide medical care according to a standard that is at least commensurate with that provided in the surrounding community. Accomplishing this goal requires integrating the position of the medical director into the overall administrative structure of the event, with clear lines of responsibility for event management and authority over health care providers. Similar to the organization of an EMS system's medical oversight function, mass-gathering events have indirect versus direct and onsite versus offsite components. Onsite direct medical oversight is preferable for several reasons.[11] Although it is ubiquitous, distance communications technology is most vulnerable to breakdown when it is needed most — in disaster circumstances most likely involving multiple casualties (**Figure 18-1**). An onsite medical director can expeditiously resolve critical medical issues that would otherwise be made worse by communications technology problems. Also, decision-making regarding triage and transport is enhanced by having first-hand information. Most important, the medical director's presence symbolizes a commitment to the highest level of care possible. However, despite these benefits, at least one study has documented that, for small-to-moderate sized, "low acuity" events, whose medical direction is online but offsite, with arrival times of less than 30 minutes, physicians do not need to be present.[12] When onsite, the medical director must be easily identifiable by uniform or vest. Because of the potential conflict with oversight duties, the medical director should usually avoid direct patient care responsibilities.

Medical Director– Event Manager Negotiations

The medical director must meet with the event manager and/or venue owner to impart a clear understand-ing of all elements of mass-gathering medical care and to gain their full support in planning and executing this care. The first meeting should address the organizer's vision of the event issues relevant to medical coverage. Subsequent meetings should cover the medical team's reconnaissance of the event venue and research into medical demand and care at similar events.

The medical director and the event manager also must meet to address the agreement upon which planning will be based. This agreement must be documented in the form of a contract for risk management and medical-legal reasons. It should address the following crucial elements: personnel issues covering medical-legal liability, credentialing, scope of practice, compensation, labor laws, logistical support covering potable water, meals, sanitation facilities, parking, lodging, work cycle assignments, communications system design for physician supervision of all event medical personnel, and medical equipment. The details of each element should be described in the medical care organization plan for the event.

Venue Reconnaissance and Prospective Event Research

The medical team should conduct a thorough inspection of the event venue in search of risk factors for morbidity or mortality. Weather, attendance capacity, spectator density, terrain, fire code specifications, exit and aisle space capacities, and emergency vehicle ingress and egress route capacities must be investigated. At both the 1984 and 1996 Olympics, medical care was required most often in venues where spectators were ambulatory.[13,14]

The medical team also must investigate the jurisdictional EMS system's capabilities and operations to know how to plan for patient evacuation. Distances from the venue to hospitals serving the event and EMS transport times (time-sensitive traffic pattern considerations) must be measured. Issues regarding VIP-dedicated transport and division of spectator and performer-dedicated transport resources also must be investigated.

To be prepared to handle a **mass-casualty incident (MCI)**, the medical team must know the jurisdictional 911 EMS system's patient capacity, augmented capacity provided by mutual aid provisions, and patient demand levels that would trigger a jurisdictionally declared disaster response. The event medical director and coordinator should meet with the administrative and medical directors of the jurisdictional EMS service to obtain this information.

The medical director and event coordinator should attend events similar to the one being planned to observe and/or estimate the risk factors and potential for injury or illness. This assessment should lead to specific requests of event management regarding the level of care, personnel, equipment, treatment facilities, and transportation and public health resources.

Level of Care

The level of expertise available for medical care at any event will depend on two factors: the ideal, which is appropriately determined by reconnaissance, and the possible, which is limited by available financial support and community resources. The EMT-Basic should be the minimal acceptable level of care, with CPR and early defibrillation deliverable to anyone at the event within 4 minutes of notification. Planning for response to presumed cardiac arrest must be based on distances when the venue is at capacity. Cardiac arrest at mass gatherings is infrequent (0.01 to 0.04 events per 10,000 people), and resuscitation can be successful: three studies have shown an 85% success rate based on return of spontaneous circulation.[15] The chance of survival demands that ALS (paramedic) care be immediately available to follow up BLS care.

The medical director must require that all non-physicians deliver care according to protocols and standing orders that he or she developed or approved. These must be consistent with and provided at the level of EMS care in the surrounding community. Formal pre-event education on all medical policies and protocols must be conducted for all event medical providers.

Human Resources

The number of medical care providers at an event should be determined by reconnaissance and preplanning, statistical estimates, records of previous similar events, and the number of attendees that can be realistically cared for by the community. In terms of the relationship of crowd size to patient volume, no correlation has been found for football or basketball games. A small but statistically significant increase in patient volume with increasing crowd size was detected for rock concerts according to a 7-year study of major collegiate events.[16]

No known, universally acceptable, practical formula can predict accurate staffing requirements, either in terms of number or level of expertise. The medical director must collaborate with the event coordinator to distinguish the unique attributes of different types of providers and arrange them into appropriate level of care and duty assignments.

The assignments should be documented in an or-ganizational chart designed in collaboration with event management. The chart should show the numbers and describe the functions of each medical care staff position. Each position's reporting pathway to the medical director should be illustrated. The following sections describe the various strengths of different types of providers.

Physicians

Onsite physician care is desirable in the following circumstances: onsite diagnostics require physician interpretation (ECGs, x-rays); patient transportation to offsite definitive care is limited; a large number of spectators is expected, implying a broad array of medical problems; participants are at significant risk of life- or limb-threatening injury (motor vehicle racing, skiing, boxing, equestrian events); and transport times to definitive care facilities are long.

An event medical director must have, at a minimum, an active medical license in the state where the event is to be held and experience in the care of patients with life- or limb-threatening illnesses and injuries. A residency-trained, board-certified or board-prepared emergency physician would have the ideal training.

Physician Extenders

As physician extenders, experienced certified nurse practitioners and physician assistants can have a valuable role in caring for ambulatory patients in fixed treatment facilities, especially when large numbers of patients must be evaluated and treated expeditiously. They must be licensed in the state in which the event is to take place and should be certified in CPR and ACLS.

Nurses

At fixed facilities, nurses should be used to triage patients and follow up on patients under observation. A nurse who is credentialed as a flight or critical care nurse in the out-of-hospital arena might also be able to evaluate and treat patients outside fixed facilities. Nurses also can dispense, track, and restock medications when applicable at larger mass gatherings. As is true for all providers, they must be licensed in the state where the event is taking place and should be CPR and ACLS certified.

Emergency Medical Technicians

The expertise of EMT-Intermediates and EMT-Paramedics is most valuable when event participants and spectators are at significant risk of injury, large numbers of spectators preclude easy access or adequate onscene coverage by other providers, or long transport times to definitive care facilities demand extended care en route. Their role is primarily the evaluation and treatment of patients with life- or limb-threatening conditions on scene and, secondarily, within fixed facilities. They must be appropriately trained and credentialed. EMT-Basics should be used primarily to respond on scene to ill and injured victims. All EMTs must know the appropriate response to MCIs, including a working knowledge of the incident command system.

Other Event Personnel

Ushers and security personnel can be valuable as "spotters" of medical events. Because of their large numbers, they will most likely be the first to discover spectators in need of immediate medical attention. They should undergo pre-event training in how to survey spectators and how to communicate discovery of a medical incident to the event medical system.

Personnel Identification

All medical personnel should wear photo identification badges and, if applicable, should have clearances permitting them to enter specific areas to which they are assigned. Field personnel should wear brightly colored vests or uniforms. In events that involve significant risk of injury to performers, medical personnel should be assigned to either spectators or performers so that care to one sector does not interrupt coverage of the other.

Personnel Deployment

A specified time for deployment of medical personnel must be determined in conjunction with event management. Determination of this time should depend on when the gates open and the time needed for medical personnel to arrive at their assigned positions, organize their equipment, and test their communications links to medical command. Similarly, their demobilization time should be determined based on how long it will take spectators to leave the venue.

Medical Equipment, Medications, and Supplies

The scope and level of medical care depends on the medical personnel available and on the equipment and pharmaceutical resources available. This availability should be based on the medical director's assessment of the level of care likely to be needed. Collaboration with event managers might be needed to organize fund-

Figure 18-2 Equipment and supplies that are essential for a BLS ambulance or temporary facility covering a mass-gathering event.*

Airway adjuncts
- Nasopharyngeal
- Oropharyngeal
- Ambu bags
- Bag-mask devices

Alcohol swabs
Backboards
Bandages, elastic
Bandages, triangular
Band-aids
Cervical collars, rigid
Cold packs, disposable
Defibrillators, automatic
Gauze pads, multiple sizes
Gloves, nonsterile, non–latex
Gloves, sterile, non–latex
Kling dressing
Obstetric pack
Oxygen delivery devices
- Nasal cannula
- Nonrebreather mask

Restraints, soft
Sheets
Scissors, trauma style
Sling and swath
Splints — finger, wrist, forearm, lower extremity traction
Stethoscope
Sphygmomanometer
Suction device, portable and rechargeable
Tape, adhesive
Tongue blades
Additional equipment, desirable in a stationary facility:
- Bedpan
- Facial tissues
- Feminine hygiene products
- Lip balm
- Sunscreen

*List is not all-inclusive. Equipment should be stocked in sizes appropriate for both children and adults.

ing support and/or donations for specific equipment. Equipment resources must correspond to and not exceed the available personnel's level of expertise. **Figures 18-2** and **18-3** are equipment lists distinguished by items typically stocked on BLS and ALS ambulances. Unlike the equipment listed for use in fixed facilities (**Figure 18-6**), where a nurse or physician presence is desirable, the lists in **Figures 18-2** and **18-3** apply mainly to mobile responders and, secondarily, to temporary stationary facilities managed on an EMT-Paramedic level (eg, an ambulance dedicated to event care).

Figure 18-3 Equipment and supplies that are mandatory for the provision of ALS-level care.*

Blood glucose test strips and meter
Cardiac monitor with manual defibrillator and external pacer
Cricothyrotomy kit or supplies
Endotracheal tubes
Intravenous bags, tubing, and access cannulas
Intubation confirmation devices (end-tidal CO_2 or esophageal detectors)
Laryngoscope with an array of blades
Magill forceps
Pulse oximeter
Thoracostomy kit or supplies
Additional equipment, desirable depending on the venue:
- 12-lead ECG
- Alternative advanced airway devices (eg, Combitube, lighted stylet)
- Automated blood pressure monitor
- Automated ventilators for out-of-hospital use
- Broselow tape
- Intravenous fluid infuser

*List is not all-inclusive. Equipment should be stocked in sizes appropriate for both children and adults.

Figure 18-4 is a list of common medications to consider stocking. This list corresponds to a standard ALS level of care for out-of-hospital intervention.

ALS providers must be prepared to use any of these and other medications approved through the medical director's event protocols. The medical director, in formulating event protocols, must respect all jurisdictional (municipal, county, state) regulations regarding medication administration by paramedical personnel.

Figure 18-5 is a list of nonmedical supplies that are essential when reconnaissance indicates and resource allocation allows the use of a stationary facility.

Fixed-Facility Equipment

The use of emergency department equipment and pharmaceuticals is rare at mass-gathering events. It usually is limited to extremely large (hundreds of thousands), well-funded (millions), regular (at least annual) events that have constant physician and support staff presence and a permanent fixed facility. Many motor racing and some horse racing facilities have such onsite facilities. Stocking most of the medical equipment listed in **Figure 18-6** should be considered only if physicians charged with direct patient care will staff the facility.

Figure 18-4 Medications to support ALS care.*

ACLS medications
- Adenosine
- Atropine
- Amiodarone
- Calcium chloride
- Diltiazem
- Dopamine (preferably premixed)
- Epinephrine (1:10,000 concentration)
- Lidocaine
- Sodium bicarbonate

Analgesics
- Aspirin (ischemic chest pain, use per event medical protocols)
- Morphine (parenteral only)

Anaphylaxis medications
- Diphenhydramine (parenteral and oral)
- Epinephrine (1:1,000 concentration)
- Glucocorticoid

Antiepileptics
- Lorazepam
- Midazolam

Asthma medications
- Albuterol
- Glucocorticoid

Cardiac medications
- Nitroglycerine, sublingual
- Furosemide

Diabetic medications
- Dextrose, 25% and 50%
- Glucagon

Intravenous solutions
- Lactated Ringer's solution or normal saline

*List is not all-inclusive.

Fixed-Facility Medications

In addition to the items on the ALS list **(Figure 18-4)**, stocking the medications listed in **Figure 18-7** should be considered if physicians charged with direct patient care will staff the event facility, or if other medical personnel will dispense them under a combination of standing orders and online medical direction.

All of the lists provided in this chapter are suggestions. They are not intended to be either all-inclusive or prohibitive of other medications and equipment. The event medical director has ultimate responsibility for all equipment and medications. If planning reveals this crucial aspect of care to be more intricate and time-consuming than can be managed by one person, consideration must be given to appointing a lo-

Figure 18-5 Other nonmedical supplies for a stationary facility.*

Stretchers, cots, or examination tables
Sheets
Blankets
Dedicated hazardous waste receptacles with clear signage
Non–hazardous waste receptacles
Spare batteries for devices (defibrillators, suction devices, flashlights)
Pens
Paper
Patient care report (PCR) forms
Additional desirable items:
- Bathroom with sink and toilet dedicated to the treatment facility use
- Chairs for medical staff
- Diapers
- Linen disposal or recycle bin
- Patient identification bracelets
- Pillows
- Refrigerator (essential for cold-chain storage pharmaceuticals)
- Safety pins
- Towels

*List is not all-inclusive.

Figure 18-6 Equipment and supplies for fixed facilities staffed by physicians.*

Benzoin
Betadine
Burn wound dressings
Cotton applicators and balls
Tissue adhesives
Eye patches
Chest tubes, tray, and Pleurevac suction
Intravenous poles
Intravenous pumps
Nasogastric tubes
Ophthalmoscope
Otoscope
Prescription pads
Ring cutters
Splinting supplies
Steri-strips
Sutures and kits
Thermometers
Vaseline gauze
Woods lamp

*List is not all-inclusive.

gistician or assigning these duties to the event coordinator. Responsibilities involved in this position include the following:

- Procuring planned quantities of equipment and medications
- Distributing supplies at the venue prior to the beginning of the event
- Ensuring the continuous availability of supplies through replenishment
- Preserving cold-chain storage where necessary
- Protecting them from theft or misuse
- Managing their collection and disposition following the event
- Ensuring access to medications by appropriately credentialed personnel only
- Distributing patient care report (PCR) forms
- Collecting the completed PCRs for risk-management and CQI purposes

Treatment Facilities

Onsite Fixed Facilities

Onsite treatment facilities must be constructed primarily for the most efficient care of expected patient volume and potential acuity based on reconnaissance.

With onsite treatment, most ill and injured spectators will be able to return to the event. Onsite treatment facilities are indicated in the following circumstances: large-attendance events that have the possibility of complicated medical presentations; physician expertise available to address these events and presentations; events of long duration; considerable risk of time-sensitive, life-threatening injury to competitors or performers; long transport times to definitive care facilities; and limited definitive care (hospital) facility capability.

If an onsite facility is established, the following should facilitate its accessibility: location prominently displayed (eg, balloons with medical symbol); location and access path announced by public affairs at regular intervals; prominent signage (eg, on the scoreboard) displayed at regular intervals; access path secured to prevent obstruction; clear markings in all appropriate languages to indicate that it is an emergency medical facility; and entrances and exits clearly marked according to jurisdictional fire codes.

Structures range from simple tents to complex freestanding emergency departments. The structure must be capable of withstanding predictable weather conditions, protecting its occupants, and reducing their exposure to extremes of temperature. It should provide privacy for at least one patient at a time. Its construction must allow clear communications with the medical director and have backup modes of communication

Analgesics
- Acetaminophen
- Ibuprofen
- Morphine

Anesthetics
- Lidocaine
- Tetracaine or procaine (for the lidocaine-allergic patient)

Antacids
- Ointment
- Oral

Antidiarrheals

Antiemetics

Antiepileptics
- Phenytoin

Airway management agents
- Etomidate
- Ketamine
- Midazolam
- Succinylcholine
- Rocuronium
- Vecuronium

Burn medications
- Gentamicin ointment
- Silver sulfadiazine cream
- Xeroform gauze

Cardiac medications

Diabetic medications
- Insulin, regular

Intravenous solutions
- Dextrose

Ophthalmic Agents
- Anesthetic
- Antibiotic ointment
- Fluorescein strips
- Irrigating solution
- Morgan lens
- Mydriatic agent

Poisoning
- Activated charcoal (ALS use as per event protocols)

*List is not all-inclusive.

such as radio and landline or cell telephone. Sufficient floor area must be available to accommodate a dedicated supply of medications. If mobile units are to be stocked or restocked from the fixed facility, these supplies should be kept separate.

The medical director must ensure that medical providers capable of delivering the highest predetermined level of care are available for the duration of the event. Staff assignments should be made according to expected patient volume and morbidity type. All facility medical staff should know where the closest se-

curity personnel are stationed and the communications pathway to access them.

Offsite Facilities

The medical director must know all the offsite definitive care facilities available for the more critically ill and injured at the event, their technical expertise, and their bed resource capacities. The medical director should meet with key administrative and medical personnel at selected hospitals to inform them of medical plans for the event, explore their participation in event medical care, and discuss their ability to care for patients if an MCI occurs.[4,17]

Hospitals for the specialized care of burn, eye, obstetric, pediatric, psychiatric, spinal cord, and other life- and limb-threatening conditions should be designated, as should a receiving facility for suspected victims of weapons of mass destruction (WMD). The specialty receiving hospital designations for the event should, with rare exceptions, be consistent with those of the state and local EMS system. Bed capacity information should be included in an MCI contingency plan.

The medical director and key event medical staff must also meet with the administrators and medical directors of all jurisdictional EMS services to brief them on patient destination facilities.

Transportation Resources

Intravenue

Venue reconnaissance and event research should identify transportation needs in terms of number and type of vehicles. The modes of intravenue patient transportation resources and the settings in which they are suitable are listed in **Table 18-1**.

These nontraditional transportation resources must be staffed to the BLS level, and preferably to the ALS level. The vehicle operators must have experience in their handling and maneuverability prior to the event. The vehicles or vessels must be clearly identifiable and highly visible. They should be dedicated for exclusive medical use throughout the duration of the event.

Extravenue

The mode of transportation for a given patient from the event to an offsite definitive care facility depends on the clinical indications for transport and the resources available. The medical director must approve

Table 18.1	Intravenue transportation resources.
Mode	**Setting**
Pedestrian-provider gurney	Close (less than 5 minutes) destination (eg, bleachers)
Stretcher-bearing golf cart	Large area, smooth terrain (eg, golf, motor racing)
Stretcher-bearing offroad vehicles	Large area, uneven terrain (eg, cross-country running, biking, motorcycling, equestrian events)
Boats	Aquatic events (eg, rowing, sailing, triathalon)

the means, time, and destination of all patient transports because he or she bears ultimate responsibility for the patient's condition until arrival at the destination facility.

The medical director should design protocols governing nonemergency vehicle usage. The protocols should address the following issues:

- A process initiating mandatory screening examinations by onsite medical personnel
- Clinical conditions for eligibility (eg, normal airway, breathing, circulation, mental status, and partial ambulatory status)
- Classes of eligibility (eg, spectator, performer, official, media)
- Criteria for personnel accompanying the patient
- Onboard radio or cell phone communications capability and patient comfort resources (eg, wheelchair lift)
- Periodic online reporting requirements from the driver to the medical director
- Arrangements for patient return from the hospital to the venue

Ambulances are the mainstay of transport from mass-gathering events to hospitals. The event medical coordinator and medical director must address the following planning issues: number of ambulances needed versus number allocated; augmentation of state-regulated medical equipment, medications, and staffing for specific event needs; and labeling to help spectators identify emergency vehicles. Protocols should address provisions for staging, refueling, and restocking; locations within the venue to reduce response times to high-morbidity areas (the playing field) and to venue exits; financial and logistical arrangements for a replacement vehicle when a transporting ambulance leaves the venue; and finally, agreements with the jurisdictional 911 EMS service to support event emergency medical transportation.

Air medical transportation, usually helicopters, is beneficial in the following limited circumstances: victim's injury or illness is life threatening and time sensitive; weather conditions are acceptable; safe landing zones exist at the venue and the destination institution; total out-of-hospital times are significantly diminished compared to ground transportation; and the appropriate level of care can be provided en route. These circumstances require careful consideration by the medical director, leading to the formulation of clear protocols that define the indications and procedures for recruiting an EMS helicopter service.

Environmental Elements

In planning for any mass-gathering event, the potential for environmental factors to affect the health of participants and spectators, including reckless or violent behavior and the use of potentially toxic substances, must be investigated. As part of the reconnaissance and planning process, the medical director should explore the elements described in the following sections with jurisdictional public health authorities to determine the degree that responsibilities and oversight will be shared with the event organization. Prevention measures directed toward the management of these elements and the treatment of illness and injury resulting from them must be governed through the event medical protocols.

Heat

Victims of hyperthermia syndromes frequently present for medical care at mass gatherings. Educating spectators in prevention measures through the public address system should reduce demand for treatment.

Insufficient potable water intake is a major contributor to hyperthermia syndromes. A strategy used in the 1996 Atlanta Olympics to prevent hyperthermia syndromes was based on stratifying levels of environmental heat for which an escalating response was planned (**Table 18-2**). Level 4 was defined as any heat index at which the emergency plan was instituted. The emergency plan could be instituted by the venue medical officer in conjunction with the venue manager. This decision was based on a demand for hyperthermia prevention resources exceeding the supply and/or a sentinel event occurring. The State of Georgia Division of Public Health and the Centers for Disease Control and Prevention identified a **sentinel event** as, "Three heat-related illnesses in one venue/day requiring emergency transport to the hospital." At the declaration of a sentinel event, additional prevention resources were to be added.[18]

Table 18.2	Stratified levels of environmental heat and corresponding cumulative interventions for the 1996 Atlanta Olympics.

Level	Heat Index	Responses (cumulative)
I	<90°	Water stations operational Mobile hydration teams operational Shade structures erected Signage and spectator wellness guides (brochures) refer to the foregoing
II	90° to 95°	Additional water stations operational Additional hydration teams operational Public address announcements encouraging hydration
III	>95°	Water distribution by recruited nonmedical staff Increased frequency of public address announcements encouraging hydration Identification of shaded and air-conditioned shelters at the venue Free distribution of bottled water by concessionaires
IV	Emergency plan in effect	Extravenue resource recruitment to include churches, schools, and buses in the vicinity

Water

Potable water must be considered both a preventive and therapeutic public health necessity. A mechanism for obtaining and administering free, safe, potable water in adequate amounts to persons in need is mandatory.

Medical personnel must attempt to identify those most at risk of dehydration or hyperthermia and administer water and electrolyte-containing sports beverages. The medical director must coordinate with public affairs regular announcements and signage for everyone to drink an appropriate amount of water. Provisions must be made for adequate amounts and distribution. Prior to the 1996 Atlanta Olympics, the State of Georgia enacted the Department of Human Resources–Public Health Water Regulation 290-5-55-03, which states, ". . . Special event sponsors must provide an adequate number of potable water supplies as set forth by the local plumbing code." The Department of Health interpreted this to mean that the special event sponsor had to provide one available water source for every 1,500 people.

Food

Enteric pathogens can be transmitted efficiently and widely at mass-gathering events. This was well documented at the Rainbow Family Gathering of 1987, attended by approximately 12,700 people.[19] *Shigella sonnei* accounted for an outbreak of enteritis among those who

attended. All medical personnel should be informed of the relevant aspects of appropriate food handling, the reporting mechanism for violations, food-borne disease presentation patterns, and their treatment.

Waste and Ecology

Given the implications for disease transmission through vectors such as hymenoptera or rodents that are attracted to waste material, all medical personnel must be educated about both the injury and illness patterns possible as a result of flawed waste management and their treatment.

Prevention strategies for avoiding a range of harmful offenders, from poison ivy to snakes, hymenoptera, deer ticks, raccoons, and mosquitoes, must be developed. The medical director must collaborate with public affairs to plan for dissemination of appropriate information specific to the event through brochures and announcements. Medical protocols must include treatment plans for addressing the sequelae of transmitted injurious toxins and disease vectors as varied as poison ivy dermatitis, rabies, tetanus, West Nile fever, Lyme disease, and hymenoptera and snake or spider envenomation.

Abused Substances

From the earliest published literature on planning medical care at mass gatherings, authors have indicated that potentially abused substances have a role in producing morbidity.[2,20] Rock concerts present a significantly higher demand for onsite medical care than sporting events.[16] The relatively high correlation of alcohol and illicit drug use with demand for medical care (48% of patients presenting for care) due to clinical intoxication (32% of patients) as well as injuries (30% of patients) in one series of five major rock concerts[8] illustrates the importance of the issue.

Several initiatives have been instituted to address this issue. At University of Arizona football games, no alcohol was ever sold inside the stadium, and it was banned from being brought inside beginning in 1985.[21] The National Highway Traffic Safety Administration, in association with private industry, developed the program, "Techniques for Effective Alcohol Management" (TEAM) in 1985.[22] With the realization that the effects of alcohol can affect injury rates before, after, or away from the event to subsequent traffic incidents, this program deserves consideration for all types of events. This program's alcohol-management policies serve as a risk-management tool to address the safety of all spectators threatened by the violent behavior of an intoxicated few as well as the legal liability borne by event management and venue ownership.

Traffic

Initial event planning must include coordination between the medical director and the event security director charged with securing ingress and egress routes for emergency medical, water, food, and supply vehicles. The mapped details of these routes must be transmitted to event-dedicated personnel responsible for these event needs and for evacuating patients to extravenue facilities. Delineating ingress and egress routes is crucial to placement of both intravenue fixed care facilities and ambulance staging areas. Equally important are the safety measures for pedestrians who will be in close proximity to motorized traffic entering and exiting the venue.

Access to Care

Informed negotiations should result in a plan ensuring that all event spectators and participants have timely access to emergency care regardless of their ability to actively seek such care. Accomplishing this task requires public education: informing all spectators of what they should do if they witness anyone becoming a victim in need of medical care, including themselves. The public address system (audio and video) is critical to ensuring appropriate access to medical services. Announcements (optionally augmented with large screen displays or illustrations) regarding how to find medical care facilities and personnel must be scripted and regularly repeated, descriptive or illustrative, and instructive.

Children younger than 8 years should be provided wrist bracelets with their names and telephone numbers when they enter the event. Event personnel who find lost children can broadcast their identity on the public address system or call their homes to reunite them with their adult chaperones or parents.

Protocols for a notification system must be designed to facilitate communication between nonmedical personnel without radios (such as vendors and ushers) who will likely discover victims and radio-equipped medical or security staff. This is a crucial interface in the emergency care process. Messenger, whistle, voice, flare, and flag systems have been used. In well-financed venues, scanning surveillance cameras feeding images into event command centers can be used to help staff discover victims.

Finally, the plan to ensure access to care must be in compliance with the Americans with Disabilities Act and pertinent local, regional, and state guidelines.

Communications, Medical Control, and Event Command

The medical control center must be linked by cellular telephones, landline telephones, or radio resources to the directors of the following jurisdictional services: public safety answering point (PSAP, 911 service), MCI plan (local emergency management agency), public health, fire, EMS, all area emergency departments, and event-dedicated public transportation.

The medical control center should be wherever the medical director is located. It represents the medical communication system's hub, linking victims of injury and illness to both the event and surrounding jurisdictional systems of emergency medical care. Whether mobile or fixed, the center must also link the medical director with event service directors whose personnel and expertise might be needed for medical care support. The communications network used for medical care should be dedicated to that purpose.

From the medical control center, the medical director must be linked by radio, cellular telephone, or landline telephone to all event field medical providers, any intravenue fixed facility providers, and all ambulance staff dedicated to event service. The center should contain a roster of all medical staff, their respective functions, and maps of their coverage areas and/or positions. Communications protocols must specify the following information: reporting pathways for information feedback from medical incident scenes; rules of etiquette maximizing efficiency and minimizing interference; the care to be executed under standing orders versus online communication; and each patient's destination outside of the venue. All medical personnel should participate in its testing prior to the event to ensure its effectiveness and reliability.

All of the communications links must be reviewed and tested in conjunction with the jurisdictional officials of these services and approved by them for technical and protocol compatibility with event resources and operations. Additionally, the medical director or event medical coordinator must ensure that the jurisdictional 911 center has entered the official event venue address into its computer-aided dispatch system and has the correct telephone number to the event's medical control center. Staff at the 911 center should maintain and update information on the diversion status of acute care facilities in the area.

The medical control center should be part of an event command center so that the medical director can instantaneously access directors of event services integral to managing a health or medical crisis, including the following: event management, facility maintenance (to include logistics and parking), public relations (to include the public address system), security, and ushers. These service directors should be stationed in close physical proximity within the command center. A slightly less reliable alternative involves intravenue radio links between directors not in close proximity. Whether the medical control center and event command center are geographically integrated or separate, they must be clearly and readily identifiable to all medical personnel. They must be staffed continuously from a predesignated time prior to the event to one following the event based on spectator ingress and egress periods. If the scope of the event precludes oversight of communications logistics by the medical director, a communications manager or the event medical coordinator should be designated to accomplish the required duties.

Special Emergency Medical Operational Features

The following details also should be included in the operational plans.

Mobile Events

"Moving venues" such as parades, running and cycling events, and wheelchair marathons present unique organizational challenges (**Figure 18-8**). Medical resources for these events cannot remain stationary for the du-

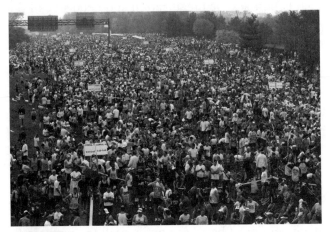

Figure 18-8 Parades, running and cycling events, wheelchair marathons, and other "moving venues" present unique organizational challenges.

ration. The event route, in relationship to the surrounding geography, should determine the type of vehicles chosen to access and evacuate participant and spectator victims. These must be close enough for personnel to extricate victims in a timely manner, yet removed enough for timely scene evacuation without spectator interference. Ambulances should be strategically prepositioned along the route at regular intervals in streets that intersect the event route. Vehicles should face away from the route and be parked in reserved spaces protected by event security. Ambulances must not cross the event route during the event. They should be positioned on both sides of the route, although not necessarily at the same level. They must be prohibited from being dispatched "upstream," against the direction of the event.

Radio communication is vital. If enough event-dedicated ambulances can temporarily staff the entire route, they can return to previous duty assignments as the event passes their positions. Or, since the number of victims will likely increase as the event proceeds, they can be "stacked" toward the finish line.

Physician Intervener

Physicians often attend events as spectators or participants. Those who witness medical events as bystanders are likely to intervene as first responders. The event medical staff should understand that this is entirely appropriate. If a physician bystander wants to continue care after the arrival of an official event medical staff member, the responding staff should immediately contact the medical director for guidance on how to include the physician in the patient's care. But if the bystander physician's participation is detrimental to the patient, the medical director must explain his or her ultimate responsibility for the patient and recruit security personnel to ensure uninterrupted care by official event medical staff. An exception to this would occur if the person is accompanied by a personal physician. Ideally, in the case of a dignitary or VIP, event management would have known this before the event.

Dignitary and VIP Care

During negotiations with event management, the medical director should ascertain the likelihood that VIPs or dignitaries will be in attendance. For medical care purposes, the qualification for VIP status should be anyone for whom management wants medical care delivered separately from other participants or spectators.

The medical director's most important liaison with regard to dignitaries is the assigned tactical emergency medical support (TEMS) provider.[23] Planning for such contingencies also requires coordination with the security and law enforcement details assigned to VIPs and dignitaries to ensure their safe passage to indicated medical care. A separate treatment area might be required. Extra medical provisions and personnel will prevent the VIP's care from interfering with that of other patients, and vice versa.

Mass-Casualty Incident Preparedness

Along with event security and event management, jurisdictional fire, law enforcement, emergency operations center, and PSAP managers, the medical director must contribute to a cohesive plan of action in response to an MCI. The jurisdictional disaster plan must be studied and reviewed with the responsible personnel prior to the event.

In general, there are two types of MCIs: those requiring only resources within the venue or dedicated to the event but in reserve outside the venue, and those requiring resources in the public domain. One designated intravenue official should be the link between the event and public resources to ensure an expeditious, coherent transfer of MCI management from event personnel to city, county, state, and/or federal personnel. This person should be responsible for making the call for outside resources. This arrangement supports accountability as well as communications security. Before the event, the medical director and the selected event personnel must agree on who will inform the link and what information will be provided, such as approximate number and injury type of casualties, scene accessibility, known hazards to responders, and any specific resource requests. Consistent with their responsibilities, event managers and the link will ultimately decide when public resources must be recruited. Event security will then be expected to expedite the scene arrival of public emergency resources and the orderly evacuation of spectators, if indicated.

Event personnel must have clear roles within the MCI response. These roles must be consistent with jurisdictional incident command system positions. **Table 18-3** lists examples.

Triage tags for these categories must be uniformly designed, consistent with those used by the surrounding jurisdiction, and distributed to all event field providers before the event. All event medical personnel should remain responsible to the event medical director until the onscene arrival of an incident commander.

Table 18.3	MCI response roles.	
Position title or function	**Role can be assigned to**
Triage officer	Emergency physician, emergency nurse, paramedic supervisor
Treatment officer	Event medical director
Immediate victim category officer	Spectator care physician
Delayed category officer	Athlete or performer care physician
Minor category officer	Nurse or EMT-B
Deceased category officer	Security, law enforcement
Ambulance staging, loading	EMTs
Transportation recorders	Red Cross, administrative personnel

Assignments will vary according to the nature and extent of the incident and the available event medical personnel.

To prepare for an MCI scene that is unsafe for triage, the security manager and medical director should designate contingent casualty collection areas within the venue. The safety of responders is paramount. Arrangements should be made for intravenue or public domain firefighting expertise to inspect any MCI scene for residual hazards that prevent safe triage.

Security must ensure the safety of both victims and medical personnel. These areas should optimally be no more than 4 minutes' walking distance from triage sites (time from cardiac arrest to anoxic brain death)

Quality Management

Medical Care Organizational Plan

The medical care organizational plan is the document that comprises the organization and details of all the components described so far. All of the plans within the document should meet or exceed local, regional, and state guidelines and statutes.[24] The medical director and event manager must agree on its final contents, and the plan should be finalized at least 30 days before the event. Copies (minus the proprietary business information) must be forwarded to local, regional, state, and federal officials who have responsibility for any aspect of the event or emergency care in the surrounding jurisdiction. Copies should also be distributed to all event medical staff to inform them of the available medical resources. Any modifications to the document must be agreed on by both the medical director and the event manager and then redistributed to the same personnel.

Prospective Phase

All of the planning for medical care at an event is part of the prospective phase, as are the medical staff hiring, orientation, and training processes. Implementation of the medical organizational plan occurs in this phase. Optimally, all event medical personnel will simultaneously participate in orientation and training sessions on site. All medical personnel must know their assigned geographic postings and coverage areas, as well as the locations of the medical control center, any fixed facilities, ambulances, and security personnel relative to their coverage areas. They must receive instruction in radio use and practice efficient, effective transmissions. Practical scenarios for rehearsal include a mock MCI requiring discovery, intravenue management, and then jurisdictional intervention; hyperthermia and hypothermia casualty prevention and treatment; cardiac arrest in the venue's most difficult extrication site; event participant injury; and dignitary/VIP emergency care. Within each of these scenarios, radio communications and intravenue routes to optimal care should be rehearsed. Event briefings and training sessions should translate into high-quality medical care. The only way to confirm this and improve it for subsequent events is through detailed documentation.

Given the crucial need for uniform documentation, the medical director must be responsible for designing or adopting a **patient care report (PCR)** form suitable for the event. It is a legal as well as a medical record form, and its contents have important implications for both purposes. Medically, uniformly completed PCRs allow the retrospective analysis of organized data on the event population's medical needs and its treatment. This generally serves the quality of the practice of medicine, specifically emergency medicine, and especially mass-gathering medical care.

The simplest method of addressing this issue is to adopt the standardized state (if one exists) or local system's EMS PCR form. Such a form can be tailored for documentation of time-sensitive, out-of-hospital, brief patient encounters. At a minimum, the PCR form must include the information listed in **Figure 18-9**.

A **patient encounter** must be defined so that all patient encounters will be recorded on event PCR forms. Orientation must include training on refusal of medical assistance and leaving against medical advice documentation, as well as a uniform categorization of chief complaints. Instruction on the system of PCR collection and storage is crucial to the quality management process. This process must include strict protection of patient confidentiality. For onsite, fixed medical facilities, delegating scribe duties to well-oriented ancillary personnel might improve efficiency.

Figure 18-9 Required elements of a PCR form for a mass-gathering event.

Time of first alert to the medical sector
Time of arrival at patient's location
Encounter date, time, location within the venue
Patient name, sex, age
Chief complaint or mechanism of injury, pertinent medical and allergy history
Pertinent physical examination findings
Diagnostic impression
Treatment rendered, supplies used
Time from scene to disposition
Followup instructions or disposition with time of event staff departure from patient

Retrospective Phase

For the future well-being of all who attend or participate in mass-gathering events, the medical director should conduct a systematic review of the care rendered. This review should take place as soon as possible following the end of the event. All PCRs should be reviewed, either by the medical director or a multidisciplinary audit committee.

Occasionally, because medical care should always take precedence over its documentation, means other than the PCR reviews must be used to critique medical care. This is especially true in regard to MCIs. Review of these incidents will likely rely on interviews with involved event medical, security, and usher staff as well as EMS responders in the public sector. Any incidents involving jurisdictional EMS should be jointly reviewed with those authorities and event management. All event debriefings should be structured and conducted in a way that emphasizes education and improvement rather than blame and punishment.

Data should be summarized not only in terms of absolute case numbers but also in terms of population incidence. Wherever possible, meaningful comparisons should be made to the incidence of similar cases in the general public. Only at this point can event risk be assigned so that corrective measures can be instituted for the next event. The medical director should formally report his or her conclusions and recommendations regarding the cases encountered and treated. A written document should be distributed to all involved parties, medical and nonmedical, with a message of appreciation for their dedication and care.

Summary

Mass gatherings of people occur every day in the United States. They require a commitment to develop medical care planning tailored to attendees. EMS systems have the expertise and the responsibility to care for these populations. This chapter can serve as a blueprint for planning expeditious, efficient, high-quality emergency care for all who attend and participate.

References

1. Carveth SW. Eight-year experience with a stadium-based mobile coronary care unit. *Heart Lung.* 1974;3:770.

2. Whipkey RR, Paris PM, Stewart RD. Emergency care for mass gatherings: proper planning to improve outcome. *Postgrad Med.* 1976;76(2):45–52.

3. Weiss BP, Mascola L, Fannin SL. Public health at the 1984 Summer Olympics: the Los Angeles County experience. *Am J Public Health.* 1986;78:686–688.

4. Meehan P, Toomey KE, Drinnon J, et al. Public health response for the 1996 Olympic Games. *JAMA.* 1998; 279(18):1469–1473.

5. Disaster Medical Services Subcommittee, American College of Emergency Physicians. *Provision of Emergency Medical Care for Crowds.* Dallas, Tex: American College of Emergency Physicians; 1990.

6. Jaslow D, Yancey AH, Milsten A. Mass gathering medical care. *Prehospital Emerg Care.* 2000;4(4):359–360.

7. Jaslow D, Yancey AH, Milsten A, for the NAEMSP Standards and Clinical Practice Committee. *Mass Gathering Medical Care: The Medical Director's Checklist.* Lenexa, Kan: National Association of EMS Physicians; 2000.

8. Erickson TB, Aks SE, Koenigsberg M, et al. Drug use patterns at major rock concert events. *Ann Emerg Med.* 1996;28(1):22–26.

9. Grange JT, Green SM, Downs W. Concert medicine: spectrum of medical problems encountered at 405 major concerts. *Acad Emerg Med.* 1999;6(3):202–207.

10. Friedman LJ, Rodi SW, Krueger MA, et al. Medical care at the California AIDS Ride 3: experiences in event medicine. *Ann Emerg Med.* 1998;31(2):219–223.

11. Parrillo SJ. Medical care at mass gatherings: considerations for physician involvement. *Prehospital Disaster Med.* 1995;10(4):273–275.

12. McDonald CC, Koenigsberg MD, Ward S. Medical control of mass gatherings: can paramedics perform without physician on-site? *Prehospital Disaster Med.* 1993;8(4):327–331.

13. Baker WM, Simone BM, Niemann JT, et al. Special event medical care: the Los Angeles Summer Olympics experience. *Ann Emerg Med.* 1986;15(2):185–190.

14. Wetterhall SF, Coulombier DM, Herndon JM, et al. Medical care delivery at the 1996 Olympic Games. *JAMA.* 1998;279(18):1463–1468.

15. Spaite DW, Criss EA, Valenzuela TD. A new model for providing prehospital medical care in large stadiums. *Ann Emerg Med.* 1988;17(8):825–828.

16. DeLorenzo RA, Gray BC, Bennett PC, et al. Effect of crowd size on patient volume at a large, multipurpose, indoor stadium. *J Emerg Med.* 1989;7:379–384.

17. Klaucke DN, Buehler JW, Thacker SB, et al. Guidelines for evaluating surveillance systems. *MMWR Morb Mortal Wkly Rep.* 1988;37(suppl 5):1-18.

18. Epidemiology Section of the Epidemiology and Preventive Branch, Division of Public Health, Department of Human Resources. 1996 Centennial Summer Olympic Games: heat-related illness. *Georgia Epidemiology Report.* 1996;12(6):1–3.

19. Wharton M, Spiegel RA, Horan JM, et al. A large outbreak of antibiotic-resistant shigellosis at a mass gathering. *J Infect Dis.* 1990;162:1324–1328.

20. James SH, Calendrillo B, Schnoll SH. Medical and toxicological aspects of the Watkins Glen rock concert. *J Forensic Sci.* 1974;1:71–82.

21. Spaite DW, Meislin HW, Valenzuela TD, et al. Banning alcohol in a major college stadium: impact on the incidence and patterns of injury and illness. *J Am Coll Health.* 1990;39:125–128.

22. Apsler R. *Responsible Alcohol Service Programs Evaluation: Final Report.* Washington, DC: National Highway Traffic Safety Administration; 1991.

23. Heck JJ, Kepp JK. Protective services: medical equipment selection for protective operations. *The Tactical Edge.* Spring 2000:68–69.

24. Jaslow D, Drake M, Lewis J. Characteristics of state legislation governing medical care at mass gatherings. *Prehospital Emerg Care.* 1999;3(4):316–320.

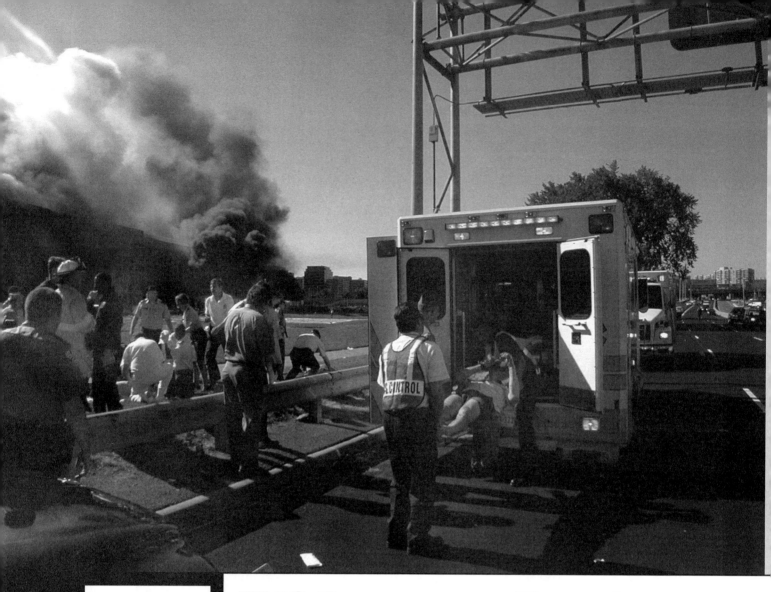

19 EMS Response to Terrorist Incidents and Weapons of Mass Destruction

Jerry L. Mothershead, MD, FACEP
Thomas H. Blackwell, MD, FACEP

Principles of This Chapter

After reading this chapter, you should be able to:

- Discuss the use of weapons of mass destruction throughout history.
- Define nuclear, biological, and chemical agents.
- Recall the current federal preparedness initiatives.
- Describe the differences between a WMD incident and other mass-casualty incidents and how EMS personnel respond to a WMD incident.
- Discuss EMS considerations for radiologic incidents.

NONCONVENTIONAL WEAPONS DESIGNED TO PRODUCE MASS casualties, frequently referred to as weapons of mass destruction, or WMD, have been used in warfare throughout history. In 600 BC, Assyrians poisoned enemy wells with ergot alkaloids. During the Peloponnesian War, allies of Sparta used a combination of sulfur, coal, and pitch smoke against Athenian forts. At the Siege of Kaffa in 1346 AD, bodies of Tartarian soldiers infected with plague were catapulted into the walled city, subsequently infecting those who had not yet escaped. In an attempt to inflict disease on Native Americans loyal to the French, Sir Jeffrey Amherst delivered variola-infested blankets to Indians defending Fort Carillon during the French and Indian Wars.[1] More recently, Germany used chlorine gas during World War I, and Britain, France, and the United States began offensive chemical weapons programs as a result.[2] Agent Orange was used as a defoliant during the Vietnam War,[3] and chemical agents were deployed during the Iran-Iraq War against Kurdish insurgents.[4] During Operation Desert Storm and Operation Desert Shield, it was feared that Iraq might use chemical or biological agents against coalition or Israeli forces.

The first civilian use of WMD by a terrorist group occurred in 1994 when members of a Japanese cult, Aum Shinrikyo, disseminated sarin gas outside a courthouse to poison several judges hearing a land fraud suit brought against the group. Four people were killed, and 150 became ill. In a more publicized attack, other members of this same group released diluted sarin gas in a central Tokyo subway about a year later. Although only 12 persons died from this incident, more than 5,000 were inflicted and sought medical care.[5]

Several incidents involving terrorist use of WMD have recently occurred in the United States. In 1984, followers of the Bhagwan Shree Rajneesh religious cult deliberately contaminated restaurant salad bars in The Dalles, Oregon, with *Salmonella* in an effort to influence a local legislative initiative.[6] In New York City, an incendiary device was detonated in the subbasement level of the World Trade Center, resulting in six fatalities and more than 1,000 injuries.[7] A 4,800-lb fuel-oil fertilizer bomb was detonated in front of the Alfred P. Murrah Federal Building in Oklahoma City in 1995, killing 169 and injuring more than 500.[8] Certainly the most catastrophic intentional disaster in US history occurred on September 11, 2001, when two hijacked planes were crashed into the World Trade Center twin towers in New York City, followed by a third intentional crash into the Pentagon, followed by yet another plane crash outside of Pittsburgh. The mailing of envelopes containing anthrax spores subsequent to those attacks qualifies as bioterrorism; although the legislative definition would also refer to these as WMD events, the paucity of actual casualties does not permit these incidents to be categorized as true catastrophic disasters.

Definitions and Overview of Nuclear, Biological, and Chemical Agents

Terrorism

Terrorism is defined by federal statute as "premeditated, politically motivated violence perpetrated against noncombatant targets by subnational groups or clandestine agents."[9] A terrorist incident, therefore, must have political motivations.

Weapons of Mass Destruction

Weapons of mass destruction are defined in public law as nuclear, biological, or chemical materials, weapons, or devices deliberately used by terrorists that produce a nuclear yield or disseminate a significant quantity of biological or chemical agent over a wide area for purposes of maiming or killing populations.[10] Elements of WMD include immense lethality, portability, and ready accessibility. The results of WMD events can include massive casualties, a contaminated environment, widespread panic (mostly out of proportion to the actual effects), a myriad of responses by government officials, and social and economic damage. WMD agents can be ingested, injected, or absorbed dermally or through the pulmonary system, with the latter posing the greatest threat. Early detection and identification of the offending agent are required for optimal therapy and might require symptom-based diagnosis and treatment. Most chemical and many biological agents cause death through respiratory failure and shock.

Nuclear Weapons

A nuclear weapon would release vast amounts of energy through nuclear fission (splitting of element nuclei) or a combination of fission and fusion (combining nuclei from higher elements with lower elements, with release of energy). Of the two, fusion is more destructive (due to the greater amount of energy that is released) but is technologically more difficult and more expensive to achieve.

These devices cause damage through three primary mechanisms: blast, thermal energy, and radiation. Blast accounts for 50% of the bomb's energy output,[11] and thermal energy is approximately 35%. First-, second-, or third-degree burns are typical and frequently present in combination with the blast injuries.[12] Exposure to radiation occurs at the time of the blast and later from exposure to contaminated dust, of fallout. Initial survivors of nuclear explosions might subsequently succumb to acute radiation sickness, which produces symptoms proportional to the dose of radiation absorbed and ranges from mild, nonspecific symptoms to rapid demise.[13]

Radiologic Weapons

Radiologic weapons release radioactive material without yielding a nuclear explosion. These weapons cannot produce a nuclear reaction. Hazards of exposure include short-term radiation exposure and longer-term increase in cancer risk.[14] Release of radiologic agents would require extensive environmental decontamination and, if strategically released at critical locations (such as a Federal Reserve Bank or major stock exchange), could significantly affect the national economy through the disruption of services.

Biological Weapons

Biological weapons disseminate pathogenic microorganisms or biologically produced toxins to cause illness or death in human, animal, or plant populations. The most effective biological agents are generally released in aerosol form and can be lethal in minute quantities. Infectious agents include bacteria, viruses, and fungi. Common threats include those organisms that produce anthrax, plague, brucellosis, cholera, tularemia, viral hemorrhagic fevers, and smallpox. Because rapid diagnostic capabilities do not exist or are not widespread, identification of the offending biological agent might rely on specific clinical or epidemiologic clues.[15] **Toxins** are poisonous substances produced by living organisms and include such substances as botulinum toxin, ricin (derived from castor beans), and *Staphylococcus* enterotoxin B. Such substances are ideal terrorist tools in that they are odorless, colorless, and tasteless. Most toxins are less deadly than living pathogens, can be chemically synthesized, and cannot be transmitted person to person.

Chemical Weapons

Chemical weapons, including toxic industrial chemicals, are manmade poisons that can be disseminated as gases, liquids, or aerosols. Chemical agents can be highly toxic, usually must be delivered in large doses to achieve the desired effects, can persist in the environment (rendering a site contaminated and uninhabitable), and typically require extensive decontamination and cleanup procedures. **Nerve agents** represent the greatest chemical threat from terrorism. Their effects, similar to organophosphate toxicity, result from acetylcholinesterase inhibition. Other chemicals posing significant risk include **pulmonary agents** (phosgene, chlorine), **vesicants** (mustard, lewisite), and **cyanide**. Successful treatment for chemical agent exposure is exquisitely time dependent and includes gross and technical decontamination. Further, rapid agent detection and identification dictate treatment algorithms. Antidotes exist for nerve agents but are unavailable for pulmonary agents or vesicants, which might require extensive supportive measures. Antidotes exist for cyanide but are expensive, have limited shelf lives, and require rapid postexposure delivery and close patient monitoring.

Federal Programs, Initiatives, and Response to WMD and Terrorism

Most Americans probably now know that the federal government has implemented several major initiatives to protect America from terrorist attacks, especially those caused by the use of WMD. What they might not know is that the federal government had already gradually increased funding, resources, and initiatives against terrorism in the decade before the events of the fall of 2001.

Until the 1990s, terrorism primarily occurred in third-world countries and affected individuals, not whole societies. Principal tools of terrorism included car bombings and assassinations. Hijackings, although not rare, were not generally used for terrorism.

A number of geopolitical events occurred in the last decade of the 20th century, beginning with the dissolution of the USSR into what is referred to as Former Soviet Union states. With a more open society, the extent of the Soviet biowarfare program became more apparent. Although this threat of direct state use of WMD had declined, security — of the weapons, technology, and intellectual capital — was in jeopardy, and many experts considered the possibility of wholesale sell-off of these commodities to nations not so friendly to US interests.

The number of terrorist organizations increased worldwide, and these organizations began using larger and more devastating conventional weapons. The frequency and severity of terrorist attacks against direct US interests were increasing as well. Additionally, overt protectionism of terrorists by "rogue nations" represented an unholy alliance of resources, technology, and motivation to cause great harm to the United States.

The use of sarin nerve agent by the Aum Shinrikyo religious sect showed that terrorist organizations could have both the will and the technology to obtain and deploy WMD against a civilian population. The safety and security of US residents also became more tenuous. The 1993 World Trade Center bombing was the first time US soil had been threatened by attacks since World War II, and the first time since the War of 1812 that the continental United States had been threatened. The destruction of the Alfred P. Murrah Federal Building, albeit by a domestic terrorist, further highlighted this threat.

In response to these events, the federal government took a number of steps to protect the homeland. Beginning in 1995, President Clinton promulgated a number of executive orders, referred to as **presidential decision directives (PDDs)**, specifically targeting terrorism and WMD incidents. Three of these documents collectively provided direction to federal agencies in developing and implementing actions to prevent or respond to terrorist acts against US interests or citizens.[16-18]

Congress also passed a number of laws that paralleled White House efforts. The most significant of these was the **Defense Against Weapons of Mass Destruction Act**,[10] commonly referred to as the Nunn-Lugar-Domenici legislation, enacted in 1997. One of its many purposes was to provide resources needed to train and equip local response personnel for mitigating a WMD incident. One component, the **Domestic Preparedness Program**, was offered to 120 cities across the United States and was the first of many training and equipment programs offered to civilian emergency response agencies and personnel. The US Department of Health and Human Services (HHS) also received funding to support 27 cities in the development of Metropolitan Medical Strike Teams (MMSTs). These local or regional assets consisted of law enforcement, fire, and emergency medical personnel. Eventually reconfigured as the **Metropolitan Medical Response System (MMRS)**, this initiative incorporated a broader scope of health care, medical planning, and program development and was expanded with a target goal of 200 communities.

Other legislative efforts sought to tighten security of biological or chemical weapon precursors, strengthened sanctions against terrorists or those who might support terrorism, and provided targeted funding to federal agencies for a variety of demonstration programs or specific initiatives, such as vaccination development or education programs.

Thus, by the turn of the millennium, the federal government had already taken significant actions to defend America and Americans against terrorism. Unfortunately, these were retrospectively not enough.

In the aftermath of the terrorist attacks of 2001, President Bush issued a number of executive orders, referred to as **Homeland Security Presidential Directives**.[19] These orders, in conjunction with Public Laws — the most notable of which are the Uniting and Strengthening America by Providing Appropriate Tools Required to Intercept and Obstruct Terrorism (USA PATRIOT ACT) Act of 2001,[20] the Homeland Security Act of 2002,[21] and the Public Health Security and Bioterrorism Preparedness and Response Act of 2002[22] — strengthened all aspects of defense against and response to terrorism and the use of WMD.

The newly established **US Department of Homeland Security (DHS)** consolidated 22 agencies and 180,000 employees, unifying many federal functions into a single agency dedicated to protecting America. Included in these numbers were the US Coast Guard, the Federal Emergency Management Agency (FEMA), and the newly created Transportation Security Administration. FEMA's traditional role as the lead coordinating agency for all disaster response in the United States continues, but under the oversight of DHS.

Federal response to terrorism (or other national disasters) or WMD events will henceforth follow the concepts of operations outlined in the **National Response Plan (NRP)**,[23] a major revision of the Federal Response Plan (FRP) first issued in 1994. The NRP follows the same framework of the FRP but adds three emergency support functions and attempts to eliminate duplicity or variation between the old FRP and other national response plans, such as the Federal Radiological Emergency Response Plan (FRERP). The second major document outlining response operations is the **National Incident Management System (NIMS)**.[24] Again, this document is a major revision of an existing concept, that being the original incident management system first developed as the result of lessons learned during a series of wild land fires in the western United States in the 1970s.

From a public health and medical perspective, there are four major federal agencies that drive programs and initiatives related to prevention or response to terrorism. These are DHS and HHS, the Department of Veterans Affairs (DVA), and the Department of Defense (DOD).

DHS assumed cognizance over several important health and medical programs. Principal among these are the MMRS program, discussed earlier, the **National Disaster Medical System (NDMS)**, and the **Strategic National Stockpile (SNS)** program.

The NDMS, established in partnership with DOD, DVA, FEMA, and the Public Health Service Commissioned Corps Readiness Force, has three components that assist in providing needed services to disaster victims. More than 7,000 volunteer health and support professionals can be deployed as members of 44 **Disaster Medical Assistance Teams (DMATs)** to provide onsite medical triage, patient care, and transportation to medical facilities. Four **National Medical Response Teams (NMRTs)** have capabilities to detect illness-causing agents, decontaminate victims, provide medical care, and remove victims from scenes. Out-of-area transportation (the second component) is coordinated through the DOD **Global Patient Medical Requirements Center (GPMRC)**, and US Transportation Command can provide airlift services, primarily fixed wing. Definitive care, the third component, is provided through more

than 1,500 volunteer civilian hospitals that have collectively agreed to make available close to 100,000 hospital beds. The participation of these facilities is coordinated through 67 **Federal Coordinating Offices (FCOs)** operated by DVA and DOD medical facilities.

The SNS program was designed as a cost-effective method of providing large amounts of medical equipment and supplies, including prophylactic antibiotics or vaccinations, in the event of a large, overwhelming disaster. Through this program, states may request immediate (within 12 hours) delivery of SNS "push packages" that are air transportable, palletized caches. In addition to these prepackaged supplies, ventilators and vaccines are available. Should only a specific antibiotic be needed or additional supplies be required, these may be handled separately from the push packages, through contracted Vendor Managed Inventories (VMI) that can be delivered within 24 to 36 hours from approval. The Centers for Disease Control and Prevention, which provides day-to-day management of the SNS, also has training packages and mans a Technical Assistance Response Unit that would be deployed with any cache. Regionally placed CHEMPAKS, containing chemical agent antidotes, is a current SNS program initiative.

HHS operates 11 centers, institutes, and offices (CIOs), ranging from the National Institute of Health (NIH) to the Food and Drug Administration (FDA). Virtually all CIOs have a role in terrorism preparedness, ranging from reach-back or onsite expertise to medical research and development. Several research grant programs have been offered by the Agency for Healthcare Research and Quality (AHRQ) or the Health Resources and Services Administration (HRSA). US Public Health Services personnel, who have been deployed to disasters in the past, also fall under HHS. From a response perspective, the most important CIO is probably the **Centers for Disease Control and Prevention (CDC)**. The CDC has developed programs and plans addressing the threat posed by biological agents or emerging infections that include a public health communication infrastructure; a multilevel network of private, state, and federal diagnostic laboratories; an integrated disease surveillance system, and a deployable **Epidemiological Investigation Service (EIS)**.[25] The Agency for Toxic Substances and Disease Registry (ATSDR) operates many similar programs related to chemical threats.

Although the primary mission of the DOD is homeland defense (ie, the protection from threats through actions taken *outside* the US), it has an important backup role in virtually all potential federal response functions. A new organizational structure has evolved in response to terrorism and WMD threats against the homeland. DOD policy related to terrorism is directed at the headquarters level, but operationally, all DOD functions are coordinated through the US Northern Command (USNORTHCOM). A subordinate unit, Joint Task Force for Civil Support (JTF-CS), has also been established as the tactical command at the scene of the incident. Neither USNORTHCOM nor JTF-CS has significant resources; rather, personnel, equipment, and supplies to accomplish missions are requested from the component military services. JTF-CS controls and directs all military forces responding to the scene once they are assigned operational control under USNORTHCOM.

DOD has numerous public health and medical resources that can be mobilized in response to terrorism. These range from medical treatment facilities, either fixed or mobile, to smaller response teams similar but not identical to DMATs. Fixed capabilities include more than 75 military hospitals within the United States. Mobile treatment facilities can be large, exemplified by 1,000-bed hospital ships, or smaller, modular, and more agile, such as the US Air Force air transportable EMEDS platforms. All services have modularized response teams, such as the US Navy Special Psychiatric Intervention (SPRINT) Teams, the US Army Chemical and Biological Special Medical Augmentation Response (CB/SMART) Teams, the US Air Force Radiation Assessment Teams (AFRATs), or the US Marine Corps Chemical and Biological Immediate Response Force (CBIRF).

Finally, DOD has a number of highly specialized research and operational facilities and commands that can be called on during preparedness or response initiatives. These include the Armed Forces Radiobiological Research Institute (AFRRI), Armed Forces Institute of Pathology (AFIP), and the US Army Medical Research Institutes on Infectious and Chemical Defense (USAMRIID and USAMRICD). These and other service-specific organizations can be called in to assist other federal agencies, as well as JTF-CS. The Guardian Brigade has been developed to manage and coordinate DOD's chemical and biological defense support to civil authorities during an event. Teams are capable of dismantling, transporting, and providing disposition or disposal and neutralization of agents or devices; environmental monitoring, hazard prediction, detection, analysis, mitigation, and containment of the incident; and providing advice and support for patient decontamination, triage, transport, and treatment.

Military installations can also have an integral role in assisting local communities in the event of a terrorist incident, and directives allow for this local assistance without prior higher authority approval. A military commander might provide any and all assistance to a local community to prevent loss of life or severe property damage as the result of a disaster, including a WMD event. Capabilities and concurrent military requirements will dictate what resources are available from local military installations and medical facilities.[26]

Prior to 2001, Congress also funded approximately 40 **WMD Civil Support Teams (WMD-CSTs)**. These 22-member teams, consisting of full-time National Guard personnel, are trained and equipped by the federal government but are considered state resources unless federalized. They have the capability for initial detection and identification of a variety of WMD agents and have an extensive communication network to assist in establishing early state and federal linkages.[27] Recently this number has been expanded so that every state and territory will have at least one WMD-CST.

A third key federal partner in community preparedness is the **Veterans Health Administration (VHA)**, one of the three principal branches of DVA. The VHA, with more than 150 hospitals, 800 clinics, and 200,000 physicians, nurses, and ancillary staff, is the largest provider of health care in the country. In addition to NDMS participation, the VHA serves as a repository for the SNS "push packages" and maintains the **Disaster Emergency Medical Personnel System (DEMPS)**, a database of VHA medical personnel who have volunteered and are approved by their medical center directors to be deployed in the event of a disaster.[28] VHA operates the Medical Emergency Radiological Response Team (MERRT), and several of the regional Veteran Integrated Service Networks (VISNs) have more nonspecific Medical Emergency Response Teams (MERTs). Many local VHA hospital personnel also assist community health care resources in preparedness, exercises, and drills.

Offices and organizations and their roles at the federal level continue to evolve. From a local perspective, particularly as it relates to first responders (including EMS personnel), the following conclusions can be drawn:

- The federal government is an important source of expertise, funding, and response capabilities to communities affected by terrorism or WMD.
- Federal capabilities, while immense, will require a finite amount of time to activate and mobilize and become fully operational at the scene of an event.
- In all cases, federal personnel and resources are there to assist and augment state and local

authorities, who remain in charge of mitigating the effects of the disaster.

- Most communities have access to federal funds for equipment, supplies, planning, and education and training. The key to success is identifying the sources of this assistance.

Responding to a WMD or Terrorist Incident

A terrorist incident involving use of a WMD agent or device will present in one of two ways: either as a sudden-impact, defined-scene incident producing mass casualties, or, in the case of a covert release of a biological pathogen or radiologic or chemical agent with delayed effects, as a progressive community health catastrophe with ill-defined endpoints. Although any incident resulting in massive casualties generates an emergency response, inherent differences exist between a WMD incident and other mass-casualty incidents. These differences could adversely affect the ability of communities and emergency personnel to respond. Most natural hazards are known geographically due to prior incidents, and hazard and risk assessments can be performed on community and regional toxic industrial materials. Many natural disasters allow some degree of warning, and certain epidemics can be anticipated temporally. A WMD attack typically occurs without warning and can occur anywhere. Most disasters are not prone to false alarms, whereas most potential WMD reports are hoaxes. Following the September 11, 2001, incidents, there were more anthrax threats and hoaxes than actual releases. These posed potential threats to life and consumed valuable community resources for response and evaluation.

Another issue unique to a WMD incident is its criminal nature. In most disasters, the cause is known and the final or projected extent of damage is either established or can be predicted with a high degree of accuracy. Although there are obvious concerns about the safety of responders, the risks encountered are normally well understood, and danger to rescue personnel is reduced by additional safeguards. The criminal nature of a terrorist WMD event, however, adds several concerns, such as secondary devices, crime-scene control, and evidence collection.

EMS Integration

A WMD incident involving chemical or explosive (including nuclear) agents would produce an immediate **mass-casualty incident (MCI) (Figure 19-1)**. An MCI typ-

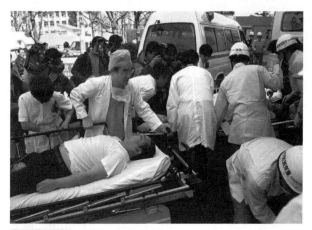

Figure 19-1 Mass-casualty incidents such as the Aum Shinrikyo attack in Tokyo typically involve multiple response agencies.

ically involves multiple response agencies from the local jurisdiction with mutual aid resources responding as needed from surrounding regions. A WMD incident would involve local, regional, state, and federal agencies. However, only local resources would be available during the first several hours because of the inherent delay in mobilization of outside resources. Decisions for securing appropriate federal and state resources might also be delayed because of political hesitancy or bureaucratic barriers.

The MMRS program provides a model, even for those communities that do not qualify for federal resources due to size. Various MMRS programs have established alternative methods to prepare emergency response agencies for a WMD incident. The **integrated approach** requires training all law enforcement, fire, and emergency medical personnel in the characteristics of a WMD response. A **mixed or augmented approach** includes a separate team composed of response personnel that can be called while on or off duty to supplement the existing emergency agencies. Some systems incorporate a separate team whose sole purpose is to respond to these events. System design clearly must be individualized to the municipality and will depend on local planners, existing resources, and inherent risks. Regardless of design, EMS must be an integral component of the system, and all EMS personnel should be trained in MCI response procedures and the risks inherent to and unique procedures required for a WMD incident.

Scene Arrival

As might be expected, an incendiary or other dispersal device releasing a chemical agent would likely be quickly detected. Numerous patients with multiple but similar complaints would be immediately identified. Conversely, a covertly released biological or radiologic agent (such as food or water contamination or aerial spray) would not produce such a defined scenario. Patients would become infected or exposed, but symptoms would not appear until some time later, depending on the incubation (biological) or degree of exposure (radiologic). Thus, the response to each type of agent is dependent on the type of agent released. In these latter instances, there might not be a scene identified until significant time has passed.

When multiple symptomatic patients are encountered in a single location, it should be intuitive that some form of exposure has occurred. Containment of the hazard and responder and bystander safety are the most important initial actions. For the initial responder, it is imperative that safety concerns be addressed prior to entering the scene. Factors such as wind direction and terrain must be considered in order to limit exposure and contamination of rescue personnel.

When a WMD incident has occurred with the possibility of contamination, the risk of contamination to rescuers and bystanders in general decreases as the distance from the scene increases. Stratification of the areas of risk and subsequent necessary protective measures are accomplished through the establishment of **contamination zones**, referred to as the "hot/red" zone, "warm/yellow" zone, and "cold/green" zone. **Table 19-1** defines these zones and the level of protection required for entering each. In a typical hazardous materials incident response, it might take up to an hour to identify and establish these zones. Although such containment measures might delay treatment of victims in the hot zone, it could also provide time for bomb disposal specialists to clear the area. A common tactic of the modern terrorist is to plant a secondary device, hidden from view but in direct proximity to the involved area and designed to detonate after rescue personnel have arrived. Terrorists might also perform a secondary attack where fire suppression, rescue, or other patient care activities are taking place. Such strategies are demoralizing and limit further response activities. An example of a secondary device would be the second airplane that crashed into the World Trade Center on September 11, 2001. Establishing safety zones and using canines specially trained to identify bombs might be worthwhile procedures for initial scene entry.

Once a scene is contained and rendered safe, multiple activities can occur. Perhaps the most important duty is to establish a unified command structure. Generally, this brings leadership staff from all participating agencies together for information-gathering, consultation, decision-making, resource management, and informa-

Table 19.1	Contamination zones and level of protection required.	
Designation	**Definition**	**Highest Level of Protection**
Hot (Exclusion) RED	Area where contamination or exposure might occur	Fully encapsulated chemically protective suit; closed-system, positive-pressure breathing apparatus
Warm YELLOW	Decontamination area; exposure or contamination from victims or equipment egressing the hot zone might occur	Chemically resistant garments; liquid resistance "splash suit"; closed-system, positive-pressure breathing apparatus
Cold GREEN	Uncontaminated (clean) area	Chemically resistant garments, including gloves

tion and task dissemination. Such structure opens lines of communication to achieve consistent scene management and resource allocation. Ensuring safety and preventing further loss of life should be the primary responsibility for all responders and commanders.

While patient evacuation, decontamination, triage, and treatment activities are ongoing, agent detection and initial identification must occur simultaneously. Identification of the offending substance, which might dictate treatment algorithms, is usually performed by hazardous materials personnel familiar and experienced in entering a contaminated environment and using detection devices or instruments.

Triage

The principles of triage, or classifying and assigning priority according to type and critical nature of injury, apply to most MCIs even under contaminated conditions. Various types of triage systems are used and should be individualized by each system. In a WMD incident where contamination might be present, triage and initial patient movement should be performed expeditiously to remove ambulatory patients from the source while assisting those who are nonambulatory. Thus, an initial identification and designation of ambulatory and nonambulatory might serve as a useful starting point.

Quickly mobilizing patients is paramount; however, these patients must be corralled into an area usually designated as a casualty collection point. Once there, decisions regarding decontamination must be made. For noncontaminated incidents, formal triage might take place immediately. If contamination were present, it would be reasonable, given sufficient personnel, to triage prior to decontamination procedures. Limited treatments might be considered during triage. Airway support and hemorrhage control are important initial considerations. If nerve agents are involved, initial doses of atropine, 2-pralidoxime, and a benzodiazepine might be considered prior to further movement. Triage may always be performed prior to decontamination in the event of a radiologic incident.

Decontamination

Once patients are assembled at a casualty collection area and an initial triage has separated contaminated from noncontaminated casualties, victims who are not contaminated may be further triaged according to conventional protocols. Decontamination procedures for victims requiring them should commence. EMS agencies should work with the fire services to develop protocols for establishing and staffing gross and technical **decontamination corridors** for both ambulatory and nonambulatory victims. These procedures should be performed in a warm zone where personal protective equipment, including filtered or supplied air, is required.

Gross decontamination usually includes disrobing of the victims and an initial high-volume water rinse. This can be accomplished by placing fire engines alongside or across from each other and providing high-volume water spray from a side port or deck gun (**Figure 19-2**). Protocols should specify whether victims should be undressed, either fully or down to their underwear, or just enter the wash fully clothed. The purpose is to quickly remove any gross liquid product that might be adherent to the body or clothes. It is estimated that removing clothes and undergoing a general rinse with large volumes of water could potentially remove 85% to 90% contamination. Gross decontamination in this manner might be provided to ambulatory patients who simply walk through the water flow, and for nonambulatory patients who might be carried through on litters.

Technical decontamination includes meticulous removal of contaminant by physical measures. Complete clothing removal and cycles of rinsing, soap application, and light scrubbing are part of this procedure. Ambulatory patients should be able to perform these measures by themselves, but nonambulatory patients will most likely need to be decontaminated by onscene personnel trained in these procedures. One method to accomplish nonambulatory victim decontamination includes a system of rollers within a tent structure with water booms overhead. As patients are moved on the rollers, a series of rinsing, soap application, and repeat rinsing are performed. Technical decontamination

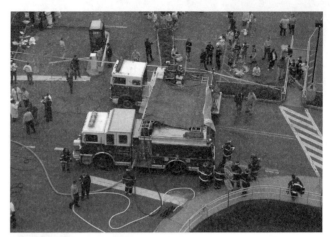

Figure 19-2 Decontamination corridor.

should occur on scene as soon as possible, prior to transport to receiving facilities. This limits the risk of contamination of ambulances, which renders them useless for future conventional transport.

Once victims have been decontaminated, a secondary triage should be performed to determine if their conditions have changed and to ensure that the appropriate triage category has been assigned. As stated earlier, several triage methods are available and should be tailored to individual systems. As part of the Domestic Preparedness Program, the **Simple Triage and Rapid Treatment (START)** algorithm was modified specifically for chemically contaminated patients and serves as an example of such tailored triage models.[29]

Treatment

As patients are triaged into a priority category, treatment can be initiated. Treatment teams should be assembled for all categories of patients. As patients arrive in the treatment area from triage, a repeat primary and secondary assessment should be performed. Treatment measures should include airway management, hemorrhage control, burn care, and fracture immobilization. If chemical nerve agents have been involved, antidote therapy should be considered, if not already performed, prior to decontamination or repeated if symptoms are still present. Most other agents require supportive care only.

Transportation

Critical patients should be transported initially, followed by those less severely injured or ill. An individual knowledgeable about receiving hospital capability should coordinate transportation. Depending on local protocol, the transportation officer should receive a status update from each hospital capable of receiving casualties so as to appropriately allocate patients and resources. Depending on the local health care environment, specialty hospitals might be available (such as a trauma center and/or a burn center). Such designations and capabilities should be factored into decisions regarding patient destination. For multiple ambulatory, nonpriority patients, alternative transportation assets such as public transit or school buses could be considered.

Ambulance contamination is a consideration. It would be prudent to consider complete decontamination of all patients prior to transport; however, when an MCI involves hundreds or thousands of patients, this might not be plausible. Contamination barriers could be placed in the patient compartment to isolate the interior and equipment. Alternatively, commercially available patient protective wraps can be used to isolate the patient from the ambulance environment. If patients are transported while still significantly contaminated, however, there might be a risk to providers accompanying them in patient compartment areas.

Incident Termination

The decision to terminate or stand down should be made by incident command. Further duties of EMS should be directed toward rehabilitation of other rescue workers, ensuring both rest and hydration. Decontamination procedures for all workers should also be completed. Depending on the magnitude of the catastrophe and the numbers and severity of the casualties, critical stress incident debriefing might be necessary for large numbers of responders.

EMS Considerations for Biological or Covert Radiologic Incidents

The previous discussion focused on EMS issues in responding to a chemical or explosive incident. Such incidents would be obvious and at a defined location. Whenever an explosion has occurred, responders should be concerned about the possibility of a terrorist incident. If that is the case, the possibility of terrorist use of a "dirty bomb," one in which the explosion is used to disperse radioactive material, must not be overlooked. While the immediate risk of a **radiologic dispersion device (RDD)** would be minimal due to spread of the material over a relatively large area, long-term complications such as the increased risk of cancer must not be overlooked. Unlike chemical agents, however,

there is virtually no risk of harm to responders from contamination from victims from an RDD. There are no documented cases of death of any responder to a radiologic incident in which the death was caused by or related to radiation exposure.[30] If possible, radioactively contaminated individuals should be decontaminated prior to transportation to receiving facilities, but it must be stressed that all lifesaving interventions in the field should take precedence over decontamination. At least one community hospital in the area should be equipped and designated to receive and decontaminate such patients while resuscitative efforts continue in the emergency department. The greatest risk to such patients, beyond the trauma encountered, is from internal, unrecognized radiation due to shrapnel or from accidental ingestion.

Health care providers and public health agencies will likely be concerned with communities affected by a biological agent. Unless the release is overt, infected and possibly contagious victims will likely be treated and transported prior to the recognition that such an event has occurred. Fortunately, most biological warfare pathogens are not contagious, and standard precautions will exclude the risk of blood or body fluid transmission. Two notable exceptions are plague and smallpox, both of which could be transmitted by a patient with respiratory distress and paroxysms of coughing. Well-fitting **high-efficiency particulate air (HEPA) filters** will reduce this risk substantially but will not totally eliminate it because these pathogens do survive outside the host, creating fomites for potential disease spread.

Another issue that would affect EMS agencies is the ever-increasing demand for services at a time when personnel and vehicles are reduced. Personnel resources could be limited due to personal illnesses, disease in their families, or fear. Vehicles suspected of being contaminated will have to be vigorously decontaminated after each transport to ensure that uninfected patients do not acquire the illness nosocomially. Finally, it is possible that, during a time of austere resources, EMS personnel might be tasked to provide services within the receiving facilities. Any plans addressing bioterrorism must include provisions for rapid expansion of services through mutual-aid agreements, expedient certification or credentialing of volunteers, and augmentation of vehicle fleets with alternative forms of transportation.

Summary

An incident involving a nuclear, biological, chemical, or incendiary weapon of mass destruction brings a new set of parameters not typical of a mass-casualty event.

Issues of agent detection, contamination, personal protection, and treatment modalities take on a new focus and have a more important role. Successful response and mitigation will depend on detailed planning and preparedness, program organization, interagency consensus, and personnel and government commitment. Financial and logistical resources are available at the state and federal levels. Depending on future appropriations, sustained allocations might need to be developed locally.

References

1. Smart JK. *History of Chemical and Biological Warfare Fact Sheets*. Aberdeen Proving Ground, Md: US Army Chemical and Biological Defense Command; 1996. Special Study 50. Not cleared for public release.

2. Brophy LP, Fisher GJB. *The Chemical Warfare Service: Organizing for War*. Washington, DC: Office of the Chief of Military History; 1959.

3. Smart JK. History of chemical and biological warfare: an American perspective. In: Zajtchuk R, Bellamy R, eds. *Medical Aspects of Chemical and Biological Warfare*. Washington, DC: Borden Institute; 1997.

4. Dingeman J, Jupa R. Chemical warfare in the Iran-Iraq conflict. *Strategy & Tactics*. 1987;113:51–52.

5. Okumura T, Takasu N, Ishimatsu S, et al. Report on 640 victims of the Tokyo subway sarin attack. *Ann Emerg Med*. 1996;28:129–135.

6. Torok TJ, Tauxe RV, Wise RP, et al. A large community outbreak of salmonellosis caused by intentional contamination of restaurant salad bars. *JAMA*. 1997;278: 389–395.

7. Maniscalco PM. Terrorism hits home. *Emerg Med Serv*. 1993; 22(5):31–32, 34–37, 40–41.

8. Nordberg M. Oklahoma City remembers. *Emerg Med Serv*. 2000;29(4):39–44.

9. Requirement of annual country report on terrorism, 22 USC 2656f(d)(2).

10. Defense Against Weapons of Mass Destruction Act of 1997, Pub L No. 104-201.

11. Zajtchuk R, ed. *Medical Consequences of Nuclear Warfare*. Washington, DC: Department of the Army; 1990.

12. Grace C. *Nuclear Weapons: Principles, Effects and Survivability*. London, England: Brassy's Ltd; 1995.

13. Army Field Manual FM 8-283 Treatment of Nuclear Warfare Casualties and Low level Radiation Injuries. *AMEDD*. San Antonio, Tex; April 2000.

14. Jarrett DG. *Medical Management of Radiological Casualties*. Bethesda, Md: Armed Forces Radiobiology Research Institute; 1999.

15. Wiener SL, Barrett J. Biological warfare defense. *Trauma Management for Civilian and Military Physicians*. Philadelphia, Pa: WB Saunders; 1986:508–509.

16. *US Policy on Counterterrorism*. Washington, DC: The White House. June 21, 1995. Presidential Decision Directive 39.

17. *Protection Against Unconventional Threats to the Homeland and Americans Overseas*. Washington, DC: The White House. May 22, 1998. Presidential Decision Directive 62.

18. *Critical Infrastructure Protection*. Washington, DC: The White House. May 22, 1998. Presidential Decision Directive 63.

19. National security presidential directives [NSPD]. George W. Bush Administration. Federation of American Scientists Web site. Available at: http://www.fas.org/irp/offdocs/nspd/. Accessed January 26, 2005.

20. Uniting and Strengthening America by Providing Appropriate Tools Required to Intercept and Obstruct Terrorism (USA PATRIOT ACT) Act of 2001, Pub L No. 107–56, 115 Stat 272.

21. Homeland Security Act of 2002, HR 5005-8.

22. Public Health Security and Bioterrorism Preparedness and Response Act of 2002, Pub L No. 107–188, 116 Stat 594.

23. US Department of Homeland Security. National response plan [DHS Web site]. Available at: http://www.dhs.gov/dhspublic/interapp/editorial/editorial_0566.xml. Accessed January 26, 2005.

24. US Department of Homeland Security, Federal Emergency Management Agency. National incident management system [FEMA Web site]. Available at: http://www.fema.gov/nims. Accessed January 26, 2005.

25. Centers for Disease Control and Prevention. MMWR Recommendations and Reports. *Biological and Chemical Terrorism: Strategic Plan for Preparedness and Response*. April 21, 2000;49(No. RR–4).

26. *Military Assistance to Civilian Authorities*. Washington, DC: Department of Defense. Department of Defense Directive 3025.12.

27. Larsen EV, Peters JE. *Preparing the US Army for Homeland Security: Concepts, Issues, and Options*. Arlington, Va: Rand Corporation; 2001:85–87.

28. Emergency Management Strategic Healthcare Group. Fact sheet. Veterans Health Administration. Washington, DC. Available at: http://www.va.gov/emshg. Accessed October 28, 2001.

29. US Army Soldier and Biological Chemical Command. *Guidelines for Mass Casualty Decontamination During a Terrorist Chemical Agent Incident*. Aberdeen Proving Ground, Md: SBCCOM; 2000.

30. Chief, Bureau of Medicine and Surgery. *Initial Management of Irradiated or Radioactively Contaminated Personnel*. Washington, DC: Department of the Navy. December 7, 1998. Instruction 6470.10A.

Additional Reading

EmergencyNet News. Bomb Explodes at Atlanta Nightclub. ENN Intelligence Report. February 22, 1997; 3(53). Available at: http://www.emergency.com/atlnabm2.htm. Accessed January 18, 2005.

Macintyre AG, Christopher GW, Eitzen E Jr, et al. Weapons of mass destruction events with contaminated casualties: effective planning for health care facilities. *JAMA*. 2000; 283:(2)242–249.

Waeckerle JF. Domestic preparedness for events involving weapons of mass destruction. *JAMA*. 2000;283(2): 252–254.

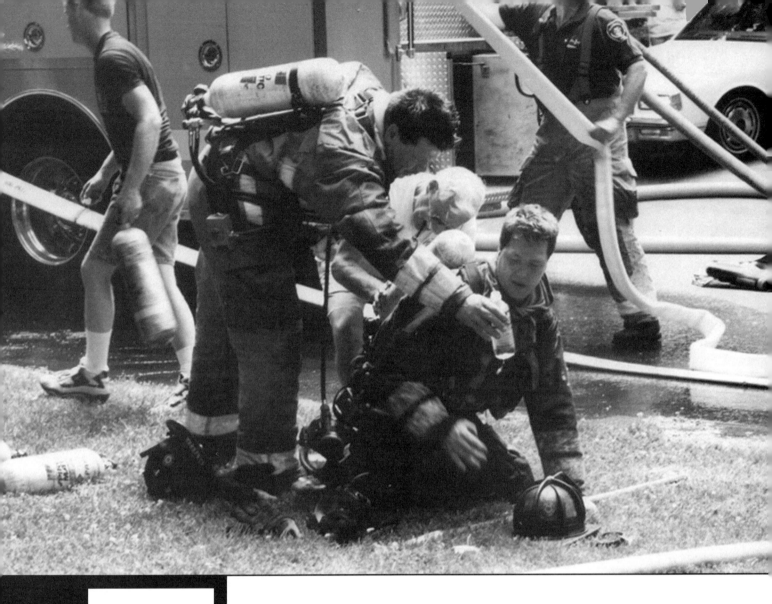

20 Operational EMS

Mary S. Bogucki, MD, PhD, FACEP
Joseph J. Heck, DO, FACOEP, FACEP

Principles of This Chapter

After reading this chapter, you should be able to:

- Recall the components of a tactical EMS program, including health maintenance, forensic evidence collection, care under fire, weapons safety, and personal protective equipment. .
- Explain the components of a fire ground EMS program, such as prevention, onscene care, rehabilitation, monitoring, apparatus, and personal protective equipment.
- Describe the military EMS program, which involves casualty management, conservation of fighting strength, and assistance during humanitarian, disaster relief, and peacekeeping operations.
- Discuss HazMat EMS, including phases of response, entry and rescue, treatment, transport, recovery, and equipment.

OPERATIONAL EMS COMPRISES A BODY OF KNOWLEDGE, SPE-cially trained providers, dedicated protocols, and applied technology organized into a medical support system for personnel working in hazardous, austere, and/or tactical environments. Its emphasis is on prevention of occupational morbidity and maintenance of optimal operational capability.[1,2]

In operational EMS, out-of-hospital medical care or monitoring can be directed to either civilian casualties or to emergency response personnel. It generally represents only one component of a larger mission. Operational EMS is frequently performed under hazardous conditions, and prevention of injury or incapacitation among team members is a primary goal. Examples that will be discussed in this chapter include:

- Tactical EMS
- Fire ground EMS
- Military EMS
- HazMat EMS

The fact that operational EMS implies a mission context means that EMS providers are likely to require additional skills, sometimes unrelated to typical EMS activities, in order to optimize the chances of successful completion of the mission. For example, battlefield medics are also war fighters because both self-defense and offensive support could be essential in any given action. The operational environment could be hostile, austere, or both, meaning providers will frequently be encumbered by **personal protective equipment (PPE)** or by limited resources. This impedes delivery of medical care by interfering with the dexterity of providers, hindering access to victims, and complicating medical monitoring of working responders.

Medical monitoring of personnel engaged in emergency operations raises interesting questions. EMS providers monitoring the condition of those working in the operational environment must consider that these are generally healthy young adults engaged in physical exertion, and not patients at rest. Further, they might be operating in hazardous or extreme environments, with attendant thermal stress and catecholamine excess. Assessment of ongoing operational fitness and work capacity based on the normal vital signs associated with patient care might not be appropriate. Alternative parameters that correlate with functionally significant fatigue or impairment of physiologic compensatory mechanisms are under investigation.

The spectrum of illness and injury encountered in operational EMS will reflect the practice milieu. For example, HazMat team EMS providers require chemical protective garments and special toxicologic expertise, while **tactical emergency medical support (TEMS)** providers for **special weapons and tactics (SWAT)** teams require ballistic protection and expertise in evaluation of penetrating trauma. Both have specialized training curricula available for EMS personnel.[3,4]

The primary prevention objective of operational EMS arises from both its mission context and its environmental challenges. Typically, each member of a small and highly specialized team is mission critical, or he or she would not be included on the team. Thus, sudden incapacitation of one team member threatens not only that individual's health but also the success of the mission and the safety of other team members. These threats might be amplified by hazards imposed by the environment in which the team is operating. Structural firefighters, for example, operate in small teams surrounded by intense heat and smoke. An incapacitated firefighter destroys the functional integrity of the team and diverts its attention from rescuing civilian victims or saving property. Each of these situations will be discussed in this chapter.

Tactical Emergency Medical Services

Over the past decade, law enforcement agencies have increasingly sought the aid of EMS in high-risk situations. Unfortunately, in many communities, EMS providers and physicians are ill prepared to deal with the requirements of medical care in the environment of law enforcement special operations.

Unprepared to respond to the civil unrest and disorder of the 1960s, police departments developed SWAT teams.[5] These teams are composed of highly trained officers capable of assuming varied roles and prepared to handle high-risk situations that are beyond the scope of traditional police officers. Inherent to these high-risk situations is an increased risk of injury; SWAT teams sustain casualty rates of 33 injuries per 1,000 officer-missions.[6] Recognizing the need for specialized medical support, representatives from law enforcement, emergency medicine, and EMS conducted national conferences in 1989 and 1990 to develop the concepts necessary for providing medical support to tactical, or special operations, teams.[7,8] In 1993, the National Tactical Officers' Association published a position statement in support of TEMS, stating: "The provision of TEMS has emerged as an important element of tactical law enforcement operations."[9] Further support for specialized medical support followed the results of a 1995 survey of SWAT commanders that documented their most common form of medical support was a civilian ambulance on standby at a predesignated location, and that 94% of the out-of-hospital care providers taking part in these activities had no specific training in this area. These results suggested a need for TEMS protocols, medical oversight, and specialized training.[10]

Operational Roles and Responsibilities

Although the responsibility for the success or failure of a mission rests with the incident commander, that individual will most likely have neither a background in nor be cognizant of the important issues relating to maintaining the health of the team. Yet these issues are vital to mission success. In addition to having expertise in providing acute medical care in hostile and functionally austere environments, the law enforcement special operations medic must be a technical expert in medical matters that can potentially have an impact on the team's performance. In this capacity, the medic functions as the commander's "medical conscience."

Health Maintenance

Keeping the team healthy begins with the baseline medical preparations that are continually taking place, regardless of mission activity. This includes collecting and maintaining emergency medical information on team members. Having this information on file can permit the medic to screen for underlying medical problems or medication use that might predispose an operator to injury. Having the information readily available will also expedite an injured officer's medical treatment if he or she is otherwise unable to provide the information. Health surveillance, to include immunization status and occupational exposure to diseases such as tuberculosis, is another area that requires the attention of the team medical provider. Ensuring team members are adequately immunized against tetanus, hepatitis B, measles-mumps-rubella, and influenza will reduce potential illness and keep the team operational.

Preventive Medicine and Performance Integrity

Although most SWAT activities are of short duration, some operations last several hours or days. Planning for personal hygiene needs, provision of food and water, and mitigating the effects of temperature extremes are some of the preventive medicine activities that the tactical medic should undertake. In addition, the performance decrement of team members engaging in sustained or continuous operations will affect the rate of injury. Recommending work-rest cycles to the incident commander could prevent unnecessary injuries.

Primary Care

Many injuries sustained in the course of tactical operations are sprains, strains, abrasions, and contusions.[6] A law enforcement medic who can expeditiously evaluate and treat these injuries will help prevent further injury and eliminate time lost to the officer and to the agency. The ability to offer symptomatic treatment for simple illnesses such as upper respiratory infection or environmental allergies can provide the same benefits to the team. This can be significant in remote tactical team operations, where access to other medical care is limited.

Forensic Evidence Collection

Evidence collection and preservation is primarily a job for the evidence recovery technicians or crime scene analysts. It is not uncommon, however, for medical providers to uncover perishable evidence during the course of patient treatment, such as soot from a firearm on clothing or skin. One study concluded that emergency care providers often overlooked, lost, or discarded forensic evidence that required appropriate securing, handling, and documentation.[11] The tactical medical provider must have knowledge of principles and procedures used to maintain evidence integrity.

Hazardous Materials

With the increased focus on terrorist use of weapons of mass destruction and on clandestine drug laboratory interdiction, an array of hazardous materials can be encountered during the execution of law enforcement special operations. Law enforcement personnel can also be exposed to hazardous substances through their use of riot control agents, accidental exposure from routine industrial and residential storage, and response to transportation accidents. Many of these materials are flammable or explosive, and the use of equipment or procedures common in law enforcement such as weapons fire, distraction devices, flashlights, or photography equipment can ignite a volatile atmosphere. The supporting medic should be capable of providing consultative services to the incident commander on the medical risks of operating in these environments.

Care Under Fire

The primary mission of EMS is to provide acute medical care and transportation to the suddenly ill or injured. Providing these services during a law enforcement operation will be the responsibility of the tactical medic. The inherent danger of assessing and treating patients in potentially hostile situations precludes the use of standard EMS providers who are not trained to function under these conditions. Decisions concerning immediate patient extraction versus treatment and the method of treatment must be made after assessing the ongoing risk to the provider versus the potential benefit to the patient.

Apparatus, Equipment, and Personal Protective Equipment

Equipment for the tactical medic can be divided into two categories: personal and medical. Personal protection is essential and includes a Kevlar helmet, ballistic eye protection, ballistic vest, protective mask, gloves, and supportive footwear; the medic should have the same level of protection as the team. The medic should carry water to maintain personal hydration and should be provided with a radio to monitor the tactical channel and communicate with the tactical team and local EMS assets.

Just as standard medical treatment procedures will be adapted for the tactical environment, so will the

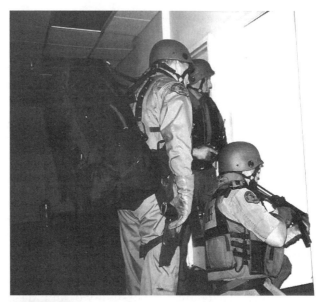

Figure 20-1 TEMS medic, with trauma bag on his back, waits at guarded perimeter during SWAT operations in an apartment building. In this service, TEMS personnel are armed and stationed in proximity to the hot zone. Many teams opt to keep EMS functions further away so that providers do not require firearms or ballistic protection.

medical equipment. Important considerations in selecting equipment are functionality and compactness. Carrying a standard ambulance trauma kit in a hostile environment will burden the medic with excess weight and impede maneuverability. The usual EMS containers are brightly colored, large, bulky, and not useful for covert movements. The ideal tactical device will allow the hands to remain free and will provide easy access. The pack should be soft-sided and waterproof. Coloring should be subdued; tactical black is preferred. Backpacks or fanny packs fulfill this requirement, and several variations are commercially available (**Figure 20-1**). Load-bearing vests are another good alternative; vests with modular pockets can be designed to accommodate mission-specific equipment.

Much of the equipment in a standard EMS kit will not be useful in a tactical situation, in which the time for intervention is short. The amount and type of medical supplies will depend on the provider level and should be tailored to the mission. An inner-city raid might not require the same resources as a barricaded subject with hostages in a remote location. Therefore, a method of carrying the essential elements to provide initial treatment should be augmented by a rapid resupply mechanism.

Emphasis should be placed on equipment that is used in the treatment of immediate life threats. The selected airway device will vary based on provider level but should include a basic and a more advanced device. Ventilation will require a pocket mask or bag-mask device. Carrying an oxygen cylinder in this environment is impractical due to the added weight and danger of damage. Methods to control hemorrhage such as direct pressure dressings and tourniquets, as well as intravenous access supplies, are mandatory.

Other items that warrant consideration, based on provider level, local protocol, and medical director approval, include over-the-counter comfort medications, dental repair kits, and cricothyrotomy and needle thoracostomy equipment.

Scope of Practice Compared With Routine EMS

Basic EMTs provide most of the medical support to law enforcement. Therefore, the possibility of an EMT-B performing certain advanced procedures such as needle thoracentesis and advanced airway management requires consideration. Paramedic skills might require changes in technique specifically adapted for the tactical situation; lifesaving interventions commonly performed in the routine setting might not be feasible in a tactical environment due to the provider's inability to assess and treat a patient while maintaining a critical perspective of the progress of the action.[12]

Regardless of level of certification, all providers should have an enhanced scope of practice that includes an expanded pharmacy and preventive medicine skills, as well as the additional skills described in the previous sections, that are necessary to accomplish the medical tactical mission.

Medical Threat Assessment
The medical threat assessment is a tool that can be used to determine and plan for potential health hazards inherent to an operation. This assessment, provided to the tactical commander in advisory format, includes evaluation of local medical resources and preparation for evacuation of casualties. Information regarding terrain, site hazards, known disease threats, and forecasted weather must be gathered. The medical threat assessment is designed to increase mission effectiveness, command credibility, and team morale while decreasing personnel attrition, costs due to injuries, and legal liability.[13]

Rapid and Remote Assessment Methodology
Wounded individuals are sometimes located beyond the zone of safe medical care. In this situation, the ability to accurately assess the patient from a distance could provide the tactical commander with needed information to direct the operation.

Remote physical assessment is a method in which the care provider can attempt to ascertain patient injuries and condition by visualizing and talking to the victim from a remote, safe location. The injured person could also be verbally directed in basic lifesaving intervention such as hemorrhage control, or might be instructed to proceed to an area that provides greater cover. The medic might also be able to determine lethal injuries and obviate a rescue attempt in a hostile location.

Medicine Across the Barricade
During a hostage-taking or barricade incident, the tactical medic might encounter situations in which individuals who are not accessible require medical care. Providing medical advice to those inside the unsecured area, via telephone or radio, might open the door to further negotiations, provide intelligence information to the incident commander, and facilitate care that could mean the difference between life and death.

Medicine across the barricade must follow an organized approach to evaluation and treatment according to a protocol designed to deliver immediate lifesaving care, possibly through a layperson, if extraction of the victim is not possible. EMS dispatch prearrival instructions provide an excellent template. These instructions can easily be used to provide instructions for patient care to those in the unsecured area.

Hasty Decontamination
Rapid physical removal of a contaminant from an individual is the single most important action in decreasing the potential of medical consequences from toxic exposures. Due to the types of activities law enforcement special operations teams conduct, they are at increased risk for hazardous exposure. A tactical medic who quickly and effectively begins the decontamination process prior to the arrival of HazMat teams or transport to a medical facility greatly decreases the toxicity of absorbed toxins.

Weapons Safety
The tactical medic will likely encounter a variety of weapons. Improper handling of a firearm mishap can have devastating consequences. One strategy to prevent a firearms mishap is to prohibit medics from handling weapons. This, however, leaves the medic untrained to manage an injured yet armed individual. Medical providers operating with a tactical team should at least be familiar with the weapons used by the team and know how to render them safe. A weapon in the hands of a wounded, distressed, possibly obtunded patient increases the likelihood of injury to the medic and team members.

Specialized Training

Before EMS personnel undertake the challenges of providing emergency medical care in the tactical environment, additional training is required. A basic understanding of tactical operations will help providers understand the overall mission plan and roles of each team member. Familiarity with individual team member responsibilities and law enforcement technologies will help prepare for likely injuries. Planning for medical contingencies such as patient evacuation is simplified if the medical provider can adequately assess the direction and objective of the mission. Much of this tactically oriented training can be obtained by attending a basic SWAT school or through on-the-job training with the supported team. The additional medical training is best obtained through a recognized TEMS training program.

One area that will require additional training is the physical assessment of injured patients in a tactical situation. The protective equipment worn by SWAT team members impedes palpation and visual assessment. Poor lighting and the inability to safely illuminate the patient are additional restrictions. In an active, hostile mission, extraneous stimuli from weapons fire, distraction devices, and radio communications could interfere with concentration. All of these factors will force the provider to use additional techniques to accurately survey the patient.

Training techniques pioneered by the Uniformed Services University of Health Sciences and the US Park Police to address this issue include the **sensory-deprived physical assessment (SDPA)** and the **sensory-overload physical assessment (SOPA)**. These techniques are designed to reinforce physical examination skills with emphasis on senses other than vision. The examiner is blindfolded during the SDPA and is forced to rely on tactile and aural clues to complete the physical assessment. In the SOPA, flashing lights, loud noises, and crackling radios force increased concentration on the part of the provider and emphasize tactile examination.[14]

Considerations for Medical Directors

Medical oversight is a standard and essential component of any EMS activity, and a TEMS program is no exception. A physician functioning as the medical director of a TEMS program should have all the characteristics and knowledge of a traditional EMS medical director, but he or she must also possess a rudimentary knowledge of law enforcement operations, procedures, and techniques. The previously discussed unique attributes of TEMS demand the attention of medical oversight for development of appropriate protocols and teaching of additional skills.

The desired scope of practice for the tactical medic will depend on the mission and operations of the supported team. Teams that execute a large number of missions in rural locations might require more advanced skills than a team that operates primarily in an urban location. Whatever the desired range of skills, the training to properly perform them in a safe and effective manner must be provided, and they must be clearly delineated in written protocols. A review of the applicable statutes and governing regulations is essential in the development of tactical EMS protocols, with preventive medicine, primary care, and advanced intervention skills requiring particular attention.

Supporting tactical law enforcement operations is a unique practice environment that requires skills beyond the scope of traditional physician education. National education programs exist to address this body of knowledge, and completion of this training is highly recommended. A variety of courses is available, and a national standard for training is emerging. The medical director should review the curricula of the programs and select one that provides the best training suited to the mission requirements. The completion of a core curriculum course cannot guarantee concept and skill retention, so a continuing education curriculum should also be developed.

Because of the exigent circumstances under which medical care is provided, the medical director of the tactical support team must have an understanding of the enhanced scope of practice, care of patients under fire, and other influences of the operational environment on patient management. These issues must be addressed in the quality review and improvement process. Tactical medical support programs are much smaller than traditional EMS programs and therefore provide a unique opportunity for a close relationship between the medical director and providers.

Hostile conditions are commonly encountered in the law enforcement special operations arena. Barricaded subjects, hostage-taking, military-type weapons, and organized opposing forces are some of the dangers that SWAT teams face in the performance of their missions. These teams are composed of highly trained and highly motivated individuals operating on the edge of the safety envelope. Manpower maintenance and appropriate medical support are essential to mission accomplishment.

Relying on standard EMS resources in these situations places the officers and the out-of-hospital care providers at risk. Medical care providers who are unprepared and unequipped could become patients rather than caregivers.

So to summarize, TEMS is nonmilitary EMS modified for the law enforcement special operations environment, providing the full spectrum of medical services necessary to establish and maintain the health, welfare, and safety of special operations law enforcement officers. It is recognized as an emerging new subspecialty with nationwide application in out-of-hospital care.[15]

Fire Ground Emergency Medical Services

Rescue squads and companies have a long tradition in the fire service because of the extreme danger involved in structural firefighting. Their roles included searching for and removing civilian victims from burning structures, but they were primarily organized to rescue their own department members when they were overcome by toxic products of combustion or trapped in structure collapses. This fire service rescue tradition represents one of the evolutionary pathways that eventually joined with initiatives in out-of-hospital cardiac support and trauma care to form modern EMS.

Despite recent decreases in the incidence of structure fires and improvements in firefighter protective equipment, fire suppression remains the most hazardous duty performed by fire service personnel. In most years, more than 100 firefighters die in the line of duty in the United States, and tens of thousands are injured.[16] Although structure fires account for less than 10% of fire department call volume nationally, 50% of the deaths and more than 70% of the injuries occur on the fire ground.[17] Not surprisingly, many of the injuries are orthopedic, with extremity or back sprains and strains being the most common. The fire ground fatalities, however, are predominantly cardiac or otherwise related to the physiologic stresses of the job and represent an important target for medical support by EMS.

Operational Roles and Responsibilities

Prevention
Like TEMS, fire ground medical support starts long before emergency operations occur. Because of the epidemiology of line-of-duty fire service fatalities, it is essential that comprehensive occupational medical programs with particular emphasis on identification of cardiac risk factors be implemented by fire departments. Additionally, participation in fitness and well-

ness programs aimed at long-term modification of risk factors in fire service personnel should be mandatory. Examples of comprehensive medical, fitness, and wellness programs for fire departments include NFPA 1582[18] and 1583,[19] as well as the IAFF/IAFC Labor-Management Initiative.[20] It is not expected that EMS providers will personally perform these preventive functions. They typically are the responsibility of the department and its occupational health provider. As consultants to or part of fire department leadership, however, EMS personnel should make every effort to ensure that these functions are consistently performed by properly qualified medical providers.

Onscene EMS
A transport-capable EMS unit should be automatically dispatched to any working structure fire, particularly if fire personnel are engaged in an interior attack. An EMS unit dispatched for a report of civilian victims trapped or injured does not satisfy the requirement for a dedicated unit supporting fire service operations. This requirement is based on federal regulations governing emergency responses to hazardous materials incidents (29 CFR 1910.120). The interior of a burning structure is considered an "immediately dangerous to life or health" (IDLH) environment that mandates the use of **personal protective equipment (PPE)**. For this reason, the provisions of 29 CFR 1910.120 apply to emergency operations on the fire ground. Other implications of this interpretation by the federal Occupational Safety and Health Administration (OSHA) include minimal staffing in full PPE required for entry into the burning structure and medical monitoring of firefighters. Transport-capable EMS support on the fire ground is also specified in NFPA Standard 1500.[21] The NFPA standard indicates that a minimum of BLS-level support is required, but the technical committee indicates in appendix language that ALS is preferable where it is available.

EMS assets on the fire ground can be assigned certain functions without compromising their ability to rapidly treat and transport an injured firefighter. They should not, however, be part of the interior fire attack unless other EMS providers are on scene to serve the medical support and rapid transport function.

Rehab Science
Fire ground rehabilitation (rehab) provides periodic rest, rehydration, shelter from environmental extremes, and repletion of calories for personnel during protracted incidents. The rehab area should be situated close enough to the incident to provide easy access for

working firefighters but far enough from smoke or hazardous materials so that PPE can be safely doffed.

EMTs can and should be deployed to the fire ground rehab area for medical assessment of firefighters who are resting between work rotations. NFPA 1500 and 1582 further specify that the fire department physician, who oversees the occupational medical program, and the EMS medical director should assist the fire department's administration in the development of protocols for medical evaluation and treatment of personnel in onscene rehab areas. To do this effectively, some understanding of the physiology of structural firefighting is necessary.[22]

Interior structural firefighting involves extreme physical exertion. Examples of the activities involved in the initial attack on a burning structure include climbing ladders or stairs while carrying heavy tools or equipment; advancing charged hose lines of up to 2.5 inches in diameter; using chain saws or axes to ventilate roofs; using pike poles to pull down ceilings and drywall; and carrying or dragging victims from the structure to safety.

These tasks are accomplished while personnel are fully encapsulated in fire- and thermal-protective turnout gear and **self-contained breathing apparatus (SCBA)** weighing as much as 50 pounds. The SCBA is a positive-pressure, demand-type respirator. This, plus the fact that the SCBA is worn using a backpack-style harness, adds significantly to the firefighter's work of breathing. The work is performed in a hot environment; temperatures during interior operations can transiently exceed 750°F[23] (**Figure 20-2**).

Finally, many firefighters are in poor aerobic condition; many are smokers, overweight, or simply not conditioned to safely engage in this level of activity. In sum, then, fire ground morbidity and mortality statistics can be understood in the following context: a large, predominantly male population of inadequately conditioned firefighters rushing to perform tasks involving instantaneous, maximal exertion in extremely hot environments while wearing heavy, insulating PPE that completely prevents evaporative heat loss and complicates breathing. It is probably also significant that all of this occurs in an atmosphere of excitement and fear that is known to invoke a state of protracted adrenergic hyperactivity.

The earliest reports of cardiac monitoring in firefighters[24,25] documented increased heart rates beginning at the time of alarm, followed by achieving and sustaining maximal or near-maximal heart rates in all personnel engaged in structural firefighting. Subsequent experimentation using various simulation models has

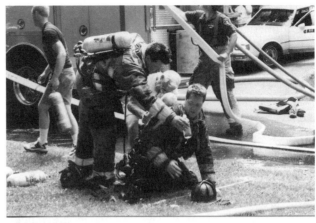

Figure 20-2 Fire ground EMS responders must be prepared to care for firefighters who are fully encapsulated in protective gear, carrying heavy equipment, and working in environments where temperatures can exceed 750°F.

confirmed the sustained maximal heart rates.[26-40] In addition, oxygen demand and consumption were shown to be at or near maximal,[26-29,33-40] while core temperatures rise as high as 40°C,[28,29,35,37,38,40] at which point most studies are stopped for ethical reasons but clearly indicate profound, uncompensable heat stress.

Classical understanding of the physiology of exercise in the heat suggests that firefighters probably experience the following sequence of changes during an initial fire attack. First, the combination of excitement and donning the protective ensemble causes the heart rate to increase. With the onset of exertion, the heart rate virtually immediately reaches maximal levels. Muscular activity produces heat at the same time the firefighter enters the heated environment. The peripheral capacitance vasculature dilates and sweating begins, but there is no effective heat loss due to the nature of the firefighter's PPE. Additional central blood volume is redistributed to the working muscles. These events result in a very early decrement in stroke volume, and hence in cardiac output, because the heart rate is already maximal and cannot increase to compensate for the decreasing stroke volume. Sweating remains profuse despite its futility, and the core temperature rises while the fluid loss further exacerbates the decreasing cardiac output. These events are the hallmarks of uncompensable heat stress and lead to rapid physical exhaustion.

Uncompensable heat stress due to exercise in protective clothing has been studied using young military volunteers on treadmills in environmental chambers.[41] Under these conditions, heart rates, core temperatures, and oxygen demand rose more gradually than in firefighters, although they eventually reached the point where exercise was stopped due to core temperature elevation or due to clinical signs of heat-related illness. The so-called anaerobic threshold was reached much later in the military/treadmill tests than was observed in tests on firefighters, where venous lactate levels began to rise nearly concomitantly with onset of exercise.[34] This is likely due to the high static load intrinsic to fire ground tasks compared with the largely aerobic components of field combat that are simulated in the treadmill exercises. In the studies involving soldiers, cardiac output also increased, along with heart rate, throughout the trials. It was suggested earlier that, in firefighting, the heart rate reaches maximal so quickly that the predicted blood redistribution and rapid loss of volume through sweating can only compromise cardiac output. This hypothesis was supported by preliminary results reported by Smith et al.[42]

Medical Monitoring

It is easy to appreciate the complexity of the physiologic stressors inherent to structural firefighting. The excess cardiovascular morbidity associated with performance of fire ground activities by older or inadequately conditioned personnel might also be understood in this context. The need for frequent periods of rest and repletion of fluids between work cycles to maintain work capacity and prevent heat-related illness or cardiovascular complications is obvious.[43] The roles and components of medical monitoring associated with fire ground rehab are not as clear.

Many departments routinely obtain and record heart rates and blood pressures of firefighters during rehab. Some also track body temperature.[44] OSHA mandates medical monitoring of responders before and after hazardous entries requiring the use of PPE. In most instances, the time-critical functions of rescue and initial fire attack make getting vital signs for firefighters before suiting up impractical. Furthermore, these practices are based entirely on intuition and the known relationship between hemodynamic parameters and hydration status. There are no data that support the routine use of vital signs to monitor firefighters, and no data guiding rational medical or tactical decision-making based on heart rate or blood pressure values measured under these circumstances. The sole advantage might result from the fact that breathing apparatus and turnout coats must be removed by firefighters to have their blood pressures checked. This helps to cool the individual by allowing some evaporation via the skin.

Although there are no prospective studies proving effectiveness of routine body temperature monitoring of firefighters in rehab, this practice might be appropriate for departments located in climates where personnel are at increased risk for heat-related illness.[44] Certainly, discovery of a body temperature higher than 101°F in the rehab area indicates that heat production and storage have exceeded an individual's physiologic compensatory mechanisms. By protocol, this finding requires rest, oral rehydration, and continued observation and should preclude further exertion or use of PPE on the fire ground. Intravenous hydration and transport for further medical evaluation, treatment, and observation might be advisable in some cases.

The lack of data supporting routine vital sign monitoring during fire ground rehab should not deter deployment of EMS staff to this area. EMS personnel should be present and equipped to rapidly assess, treat, and transport firefighters who exhibit signs and symptoms of heat-related illness, cardiorespiratory decompensation, or other evidence of medical emergency. EMTs assigned to rehab must be familiar with clinical manifestations of these processes and their management. They should also be vigilant in ensuring that firefighters are appropriately rehydrating while under their supervision, as failure or inability to do so might suggest that clinically significant dehydration has already occurred, which can result in incapacitation during subsequent work cycles.

Rest

Optimal **work-rest cycles** during structural firefighting depend on many factors. The weight and thermal properties of the firefighter's protective ensemble increase the physiologic workload for any given task. Firefighting tasks require heavy exertion characterized by large static and dynamic, or aerobic, components. Work periods must be shortened with increasing environmental temperature and humidity.[45,46] This is especially true for a nonacclimated work force. Physiologic acclimation to heat occurs over 5 to 7 days of exposure, so firefighters in most parts of the United States have the greatest risk of heat stress during early summer. Work-rest cycles, or time spent in fire ground rehab, should be adjusted to climate and season accordingly.

The best predictor of exercise tolerance in the heat is aerobic capacity.[47,48] Body mass negatively affects exercise tolerance in the heat, especially when climate conditions or PPE restricts evaporative cooling.[48] Work-rest cycles must therefore also consider fitness of the workers along with ambient temperature and humidity. Finally, it is essential that firefighters remove their PPE and that the environment in the rehab area promote evaporative loss of the heat stored during the previous work cycle. Intermittent exertion without opportunity to release stored metabolic heat imposes a greater physiologic strain than does continuous, low-intensity exercise.[49]

Rehydration

The subject of fluid volume replacement in firefighters has been recently reviewed along with published recommendations for fire and EMS personnel.[22] Consequently, only a few rudiments of fire ground rehydration will be discussed here.

Firefighters and others experiencing body fluid loss through exercise-induced sweating must maintain a positive fluid balance, especially during acclimation to warmer work conditions.[50,51] Although it is possible to fluid load prospectively under experimental conditions or prior to athletic competitions, fire responses are typically unplanned events, requiring firefighters to make a major lifestyle commitment to maintain optimal prehydration. This practice should be facilitated wherever possible by providing water and/or sports drinks in fire stations and on fire apparatus. On-duty and volunteer fire personnel should be encouraged to limit consumption of alcohol and caffeine-containing and other beverages that have diuretic effects to prevent negative fluid balance prior to initiation of fire operations. Habitual intake of fluids before and during exercise conditions the gastrointestinal tract and reduces stomach cramps and other discomfort sometimes associated with prehydration and rehydration.[52]

Similarly, water and/or sports drinks must be available in rehab areas to replace fluid volumes lost during firefighting. Much has been written about the choice of oral rehydration fluids in both trade journals and the scientific literature. To avoid dehydration during structural firefighting, average-sized firefighters must replace fluids at rates of approximately 1.6 kg/hr.[53] For this to occur, oral rehydration fluids must be cool, palatable, and noncarbonated. Although the benefits of electrolytes (sodium) in oral fluids used by adults are controversial, low concentrations of carefully chosen carbohydrates improve taste and help replace calories. Higher concentrations of carbohydrates delay gastric emptying and might trigger osmotic diarrhea and are therefore contraindicated.[52]

Treatment and Transport

Roughly 50% of line-of-duty firefighter fatalities have cardiovascular origins. Accordingly, aggressively treating early evidence of coronary syndromes and defibrillating nonperfusing arrhythmias on scene are high priorities. Where available, 12-lead ECG capability on the fire ground can decrease time to definitive intervention. Most injuries are orthopedic sprains and strains, but some require immobilization and pain control en route to the hospital.

EMS personnel must be prepared to handle burns and toxic inhalations. Where distance to the nearest hospital dictates long transport times, EMS providers should have standing orders to draw a tube of blood when they obtain intravenous access in firefighters who might have been exposed to carbon monoxide. This will ensure that a "time zero" carboxyhemoglobin level is obtained before the accelerated washout associated with administration of high-flow oxygen. In addition, fire ground EMS providers should be aware of the potential for cyanide poisoning, methemoglobinemia, and other toxidromes that can result from smoke inhalation at some structure fires. Although nitrates, cyanides, and a variety of other toxic chemicals have been identified among products of combustion in fires involving synthetic materials and agricultural products, there have been few reports of clinically significant acute exposures of firefighters.

Finally, consideration of predetermined destination hospitals is sometimes appropriate when access to specialized burn units, invasive cardiac care, trauma care, or hyperbaric oxygen therapy would not substantially compromise time to hospital arrival.

Apparatus and Personal Protective Equipment

Those who provide medical support should work with department leadership to implement fire ground safety measures that will decrease the risk of serious exposure or injury to personnel. All apparatus, equipment, and PPE used for fire suppression or other hazardous duty should be in compliance with relevant NFPA standards, as well as state and federal regulations. Their use should be governed by department standard operating procedures that are implemented through documented training and enforced through progressive discipline.

The level and type of PPE required for EMS responders to fire incidents depends on several factors. In general, if responders are tasked solely with staffing the rehab area or treating and transporting injured personnel, their PPE need only protect them from the weather, blood, and body fluids. Alternatively, dual-role firefighter/EMTs who are called on to carry out fire suppression, extrication, or other rescue activities require full fire protective ensembles, including respiratory protection in some cases.

Medical equipment available to treat ill or injured firefighters on scene should conform to state regulations and local protocols for ALS providers established by EMS medical directors.

Specialized Training

EMS responders and physicians who provide fire ground medical support require minimal training in addition to their baseline EMS competencies. To operate safely and effectively at an incident scene, providers should be trained and experienced in the incident command system (ICS) used by the local fire department. For example, one essential aspect of a fire ground ICS is an accountability system that keeps track of the identities and locations of all personnel present. This system must be maintained in all sectors and divisions, including rehab areas, to be effective.

If EMS responders serve in expanded roles involving fire suppression or rescue, they must be trained and certified as required by OSHA, state statute or regulation, and by department policy.

The medical director should periodically review the common causes of injury and incapacitation to firefighters with EMS personnel who might be called on to provide medical support on the fire ground. This should include strategies for primary prevention; recognition of clinical syndromes such as heat stress, coronary insufficiency, and carbon monoxide toxicity through clinical signs and symptoms; and optimal medical care in the field.

Considerations for Medical Directors

Most of the fire ground EMS considerations for medical directors have already been discussed. It is extremely important that the physicians providing EMS medical oversight and those responsible for fire department occupational health programs work together with fire department administrators to develop fire ground medical support and rehab protocols. EMS providers must be familiar with and trained in these procedures.

Medical directors who become part of the medical response configuration supporting fire ground operations must also be trained in ICS, fire ground safety, and proper use (including limitations) of PPE. Physician roles and limitations on scene must be prospectively established by department administration and must reflect the specific skills, training, and experience of individual response physicians. Dispatch criteria and procedures and arrangements for safe conveyance to incident scenes must be established in advance, as should communications mechanisms and designations. Without these preparations and precautions, physicians and other EMS providers can become liabilities rather than assets in the emergency operational environment.

Military Emergency Medical Services

Military EMS has its roots in the Napoleonic Wars with the development of a systematic process for clearing the battlefield of casualties.[54] In the Unites States, military EMS can be traced back to the Civil War and the efforts of William Hammond, Surgeon General of the Union Army, and Jonathan Letterman, the medical director of the Army of the Potomac. These men were the leaders in the effort to restructure chaotic wartime emergency services into an organized system.[55]

Through the 20th century, the military was a leader in out-of-hospital care, developing EMS systems long before the National Academy of Sciences 1966 landmark white paper, *Accidental Death and Disability: The Neglected Disease of Modern Society,* and before the Emergency Medical Services Systems Act of 1973. Advances in military EMS led to innovations in extraction, stabilization, resuscitation, and transport modalities. In the latter half of the century, however, the military lost its leading edge as civilian agencies more quickly embraced newer technologies and practices.[56]

Military EMS during peacetime is characterized by a single-tiered, low-volume, BLS response system staffed by corpsmen or medics trained to a level equivalent to the EMT-Basic. Few military EMS systems respond to calls outside their installations, and most of the runs are for medical complaints. During wartime, however, an echeloned approach to casualty management exists, where the patient volume can increase greatly, and the medics are more likely to use skills not usually associated with the civilian EMT-Basic (intravenous cannulation and administration of opioid analgesia). The emphasis shifts to managing penetrating trauma and assisting in the care of victims suffering from disease and nonbattle injury.[57]

Corpsmen and medics who support special operations receive advanced training to provide a higher level of medical care. Currently, this training is based on the principles taught in the Advanced Trauma Life Support (ATLS) course, but the appropriateness of extrapolating ATLS guidelines to the battlefield has been called into question.[58]

Operational Roles and Responsibilities

The primary mission of military medicine is to conserve the fighting strength. To that end, the primary role of military EMS providers has historically been to extract, stabilize, and transport the wounded during tactical operations. It is here, on the battlefield, that the initial care provided to the wounded will have the greatest impact on survival. As stated by LTC Douglas Lindsey, US Army, in remarks to the Army Medical Service Graduate School in 1951:

> It is difficult to emphasize sufficiently the importance of initial treatment on the battlefield. What the wounded soldier does on his own behalf, or what his infantry colleagues do for him; and what the company aidman does for a traumatic amputation or gaping wound of the chest. In the thick of battle, in dust and heat or in blowing snow — on these simple procedures depend life and death . . . A slight improvement in the skill and judgment of the company aidman will save . . . more human lives than will the attainment of 100% perfection in the surgical hospital.[59]

Combat casualty care encompasses a great deal more than the care of high velocity bullet wounds. The combat medic encounters mass-casualty incidents in austere and remote locations, with large numbers of casualties from shrapnel, blast, burns, and traumatic stress. There will be a mismatch between demand and available resources, along with delayed transportation to definitive care.[2] Therefore, the military medic must be experienced in caring for multiple trauma patients who have complex wounding mechanisms.

However, just as world politics have evolved over the past decade, so, too, has the mission of the military medical community: providing assistance during humanitarian, disaster relief, and peacekeeping operations has replaced taking care of battlefield casualties. Several reports from recent military operations demonstrate the need for medics and corpsmen to be adept at evaluating and treating diverse populations, including children, the elderly, and handicapped patients.[60-62] This further emphasizes the importance of recognizing and treating disease and nonbattle injury, along with experience in infectious disease and a working knowledge of tropical medicine, parasitology, epidemiology, preventive medicine, and environmental health.[2,63]

The military medic must maintain his or her general military skills and medical skills. The ability to treat patients under combat conditions will not increase the medic's personal survivability. Marksmanship, land navigation, and donning and operating in a chemical and biological protective suit are just a few of the skills all soldiers, sailors, airmen, and marines must maintain, regardless of military occupational specialty.

HazMat Emergency Medical Services

Spectacular incidents involving hazardous materials (HazMat) have occurred throughout history. In the United States, many of the recorded incidents involved transportation mishaps. In 1988, two improperly secured railroad cars rolled backward down a mountain for 13 miles until they crashed into a passenger train in the Fountain, Colorado, train station. The first car, a tanker filled with liquid naphtha, split open on impact and burst into flames, and the fire flowed through the depot with the leaking chemical. The second car was loaded with dynamite and exploded when it hit the burning tanker, killing three people and injuring 28.

In 1947, ammonium nitrate in the hold of a ship docked in Texas City, Texas, caught fire. Shipboard firefighters did not use enough water to control the fire for fear of damaging the cargo, and the hold exploded. The concussion blew an adjacent ship off the dock and into a third ship, which was fully loaded with ammonium nitrate; that ship also exploded. The combined explosions of the two ships produced a 25-mile radius damage and sent a tidal wave 15 feet high into the port city. There were 468 fatalities, more than 2,000 injuries, and property damage estimated in excess of $40 million.

A 1978 train derailment in Waverly, Tennessee, was initially handled with proper precautions. The local volunteer fire department ordered appropriate evacuation zones around a derailed and damaged tank car containing 27,871 gallons of liquid propane. Over the ensuing days, local fire department procedures were apparently countermanded by others working at the scene. The evacuation perimeter shrank, water cooling was discontinued because the underlying mud was creating problems for salvage workers, and vehicular traffic was allowed into the incident area. Two days after the derailment, pressure from the warming liquid caused a dented area of the tank to rupture. The resulting high-pressure gas leak found an ignition source and exploded, killing 16 people and injuring about 100 more.[64]

The main impetus for improved response capabilities for chemical emergencies and increased federal regulation of HazMat incidents in both fixed facilities and transportation appears to have been the incident that occurred in Bhopal, India, in December 1984. There, the release of methyl isocyanate from a Union Carbide plant killed more than 2,500 people and injured approximately 150,000.

Two years after this catastrophe, Congress passed the **Superfund Amendments and Reauthorization Act (SARA)**.[65] SARA Title III, Emergency Planning and Community Right to Know, directed establishment of **state emergency planning commissions (SERCs)** and **local emergency planning committees (LEPCs)** to draw up jurisdiction-specific emergency response plans.

At about the same time, OSHA was instructed to develop new guidance for personnel responsible for responding to HazMat emergencies, as well as those remediating Superfund sites. It expanded its regulations within Subpart H of the Occupational Safety and Health Standards dealing with hazardous materials (29 CFR 1910.101-126). The **HAZWOPER Standard**[66] and its subsequent interpretations define hazardous materials and responders; characterize types of responses; prescribe levels of training, staffing, and PPE; mandate medical monitoring of responders; and direct incident management methods.

Federal regulations promulgated by the US Department of Transportation (DOT) give the Secretary of Transportation authority to

> designate material (including an explosive, radioactive material, etiologic agent, flammable or combustible liquid or solid, poison, oxidizing or corrosive material, and compressed gas) or a group or class of material as hazardous when the Secretary decides that transporting the material in commerce in a particular amount and form may pose an unreasonable risk to health and safety or property.[67]

Other federal entities, including the Environmental Protection Agency (EPA) and the Federal Emergency Management Agency (FEMA), have other terms and definitions designed to delineate jurisdiction and categorize materials according to planning and regulatory requirements.[68]

HazMat incidents are frequently divided into categories according to the nature of the hazard or potential mechanisms of injury. For example, the DOT and the United Nations have nine classifications based largely on their physicochemical properties: explosive, flammable gases, flammable liquids, flammable solids, organic peroxides, poisonous materials, radioactive materials, corrosives, and miscellaneous. The FEMA categories reflect pathophysiologic mechanisms, and materials are considered to represent thermal, etiologic, asphyxiant, mechanical, chemical, psychological, or radioactive hazards.[68] Hazardous materials thought to be threat agents or those that might be released intentionally as a weapon of mass destruction are categorized by the Department of Defense and the Department of Justice as biologic, nuclear, incendiary, chemical, or explosive.

Operational Roles and Responsibilities

To create a context for the various EMS functions associated with HazMat emergencies, a prototypical incident can be arbitrarily divided into four roughly chronological phases of EMS response: early, entry/rescue, treatment/transport, and recovery/termination. Not all incidents include all of these phases or require completion of all the tasks commonly associated with them.

Early Phase

During the early phase of a HazMat incident, several tasks must be executed. These include recognition, establishment of incident command system and demarcation of zones, research, notification, and initiation of onsite medical monitoring.

Recognition

Recognition can sometimes be the most challenging aspect of a HazMat incident. If it is not dispatched as such, it is often easy to overlook evidence that hazardous chemicals are present at an incident scene. The clues to HazMat presence are discussed in detail during standard first responder awareness training and are only briefly reviewed here.

As part of scene safety, responders should consider the possibility that hazardous materials might be present as they approach any incident. Both location and occupancy of the site can offer clues. The size and shape of any containers at the scene should be noted, and, where appropriate, responders should look for placards or labels indicating chemical cargoes. Shipping papers on trucks and other transportation modalities and **Material Safety Data Sheets (MSDS)** in fixed facilities are also useful clues. The most dangerous method of detecting hazardous chemicals is through the senses. Once chemicals have been smelled, exposure to extremely hazardous substances might have already occurred, and toxicity might be unavoidable. An audible hiss of escaping gas could provide evidence of proximate hazard, as might seeing persons or animals down without evidence of trauma. Adequate use of PPE and adherence to protocols should prevent acquisition of sensory cues through touch or taste.

Monitoring devices such as home carbon monoxide alarms or radionuclide dosimeters might detect the incident and alert responders to the presence of hazards. Fire departments and specialized HazMat teams increasingly rely on portable instrumentation that quantifies explosive, oxygen-deficient, and other **IDLH (immediately dangerous to life or health)** atmospheres. Portable and mobile devices for detection and identification of chemical and biological threat agents are used by military personnel. Some of these technologies have been transitioned into civilian emergency response arenas to augment domestic preparedness for events involving chemical or biological weapons. More importantly, this is an area of active research and rapid technology development, with significantly increased detection capabilities at the near-market stage.

Establishment of Incident Command System and Demarcation Zones

EMS responders will seldom be responsible for establishing a scene ICS or serving as the incident commander. It is essential, however, that EMS personnel be aware of the federal requirement for management of all emergencies involving hazardous materials using an ICS.[66] This enhances the effectiveness of the multiagency responses typically required for HazMat incidents.

Likewise, demarcation of zones will not likely be the responsibility of EMS responders on scene. Such responders, however, must understand the significance of the zones, the location of the decontamination corridor, and where they will be deployed. Positioning of EMS operations depends on the characteristics of the hazard agent, the magnitude of the incident, the acuity and severity of injuries sustained at the scene, and the PPE available to EMS personnel. EMS personnel should not don chemical protective clothing or respiratory protection unless they have been trained, medically cleared, and fit-tested for it.[66,69]

Research

The next critical function during the early phase of a HazMat incident is research. Research can begin en route to the alarm if a hazardous product was identified at the time of dispatch. Responders en route to any incident should always check department preplans prepared for the origin of the alarm. If review of the preplan discloses potential hazards at the site, then the incident must be handled as a HazMat incident until proved otherwise.

Once the incident commander knows what products are involved, he or she might request assistance from EMS personnel in determining physicochemical properties and specific medical risks posed by the chemical. This research is essential prior to making decisions regarding levels of PPE, staging distances and strategies, resources that will be necessary to effect mitigation, and implications for victims of the incident.

The reference that is consulted first by responders in most emergency situations is *Emergency Response Guidebook* published by the DOT.[70] This small, paperback book is found in the glove compartment of almost every fire department apparatus in the country. Using just the chemical name or a placard number, a provider can obtain basic information regarding the product, including evacuation perimeters and initial medical treatment protocols.

Historically, the next most common source of information is the toll-free number for the **Chemical Transportation Emergency Center (CHEMTREC)** operated by the Chemical Manufacturer's Association. In recent years, CHEMTREC has been most helpful in situations where the product cannot be identified on scene. Under these circumstances, the CHEMTREC operator will contact the shipper, the manufacturer, and any other source of information responders need to manage the incident. Other resources accessible by telephone from the field include the **Agency for Toxic Substances and Disease Registry (ATSDR)** maintained by the CDC, state or local poison centers, and local online medical oversight.

Computers have profoundly altered the way most services perform HazMat field research. The first program used extensively by fire services at chemical emergencies is referred to as **CAMEO (Computer Aided Management of Emergency Operations)**. This software product represents collaboration by the EPA's Chemical Emergency Preparedness and Prevention Office and the Office of Response and Restoration at the National Oceanographic and Atmospheric Administration (NOAA). In addition to providing common chemical databases, CAMEO allows responders to input local weather conditions and geographic features in order to generate dispersion models and to more precisely map evacuation and/or hot zone perimeters. With the advent of more powerful, less expensive laptop computers and wireless modems, the same medical and chemical databases used by hospitals and poison centers are now frequently available to responders on scene.

Notification

Field research and notification can be concurrent events. If medical oversight or the receiving medical facility's emergency department is used during the research phase, notification has essentially already occurred. Regardless, it is crucial that the receiving hospital be notified at the earliest possible point that there are or might be chemically contaminated patients at the scene. The hospital, like a HazMat team, requires considerable lead time to prepare its staff and decontamination facilities. Not all hospitals are prepared to manage chemical emergencies, so community preplans should designate hospitals that have this capability as chemical casualty destinations. Since the fall of 2001, federal funding available for development and maintenance of decontamination capabilities has increased, which should result in expansion of the number of designated HazMat receiving facilities. The following information should be provided to the hospital at the time of notification and updated throughout the incident as necessary:

- The correct name of the chemical(s) involved. Protocols should require that chemical names be spelled over the radio or telephone because mispronunciation can implicate chemicals with very different properties, toxidromes, and treatments.
- The size of the incident, both the volume of product released and the number, nature, and severity of casualties that will eventually be transported.
- Whether field decontamination has occurred or will occur before transport.
- The estimated time of hospital arrival for the casualties.[68]

If online medical oversight is provided by an entity other than the destination hospital, this entity should also be notified of the incident as early as possible. Base stations should have access to toxicology texts and computerized databases to ensure optimal prescription of medications and antidotes when contacted by field providers.

Initiation of Onsite Medical Monitoring

Initiation of onsite medical monitoring completes the early phase. Medical monitoring refers to an organized, protocol-driven process of evaluating personnel wearing PPE and operating in the hot zone. Federal regulations mandate this function anytime PPE is worn by personnel in IDLH environments (29 CFR 1910.120). Onsite medical monitoring should be just one component of a comprehensive occupational medical surveillance program for HazMat responders. The exact constituents of such programs have not been defined.[71] **NFPA 1582, Medical Requirements for Firefighters,** has been used as a template for this surveillance function,[72] although the essential job tasks of fire suppression and HazMat response are not the same.[73]

Most onsite medical monitoring is performed by EMS providers and comprises a brief history to rule out current medical problems that would predispose the HazMat responder to injury, mission failure, heat-related illness, and other adverse medical outcomes. Examples of items that might be addressed in the presuit history include alcohol consumption in the pre-

vious 24 hours; current medications (both prescribed and over-the-counter); upper respiratory, cardiac, gastrointestinal, or neurologic symptoms experienced in the previous 24 hours; and subjective assessment of present condition.

Responders' vital signs should be recorded before they don PPE, then again in the rehab area during protracted incidents, and after decontamination and suit removal. Personnel are not released by EMS staff to suit up again or to leave the site until postsuit parameters approximate the presuit readings. Actual values of temperature, heart rate, and blood pressure that are considered permissible in the hot zone vary by department and protocol. Vital sign limits requiring local rehab (including rest and rehydration) and those requiring transportation for further medical evaluation also vary by region and department but should be specified in EMS protocols.

Federal regulations require the monitoring outlined here, although its value is intuitive and unproven. Many HazMat teams and affiliated fire or EMS departments have added parameters including 3-lead or 12-lead ECG, pulse oximetry, orthostatic hemodynamics, and chest auscultation to their medical monitoring protocols. These are not required and are of unproven value, and some could be considered medically counterintuitive.

It is also important to remember that the documents generated during medical monitoring of HazMat responders are medical records and must be handled as such. Provisions must be made to maintain confidentiality of these records and for appropriate and confidential medical followup of any conditions encountered. Without such safeguards, personnel cannot reasonably be expected to comply with the spirit of the program.

Entry/Rescue Phase

By definition, the entry/rescue phase occurs in the hot zone. EMS personnel might also be HazMat responders, and as such wearing PPE, entering the hot zone, and rescuing victims. However, little if any medical treatment will occur during this phase. Wearing PPE severely restricts a responder's ability to communicate with, medically evaluate, or treat a victim. Repositioning of an airway, basic CPR, delivery of supplemental oxygen, pressure hemostasis, and spinal or limb immobilization are the only emergency medical interventions that are practical in the hot zone or before gross field decontamination. Even these maneuvers are compromised by limited dexterity, which makes it difficult to determine whether a victim has a pulse. Intubation should never be attempted, even by qualified person-

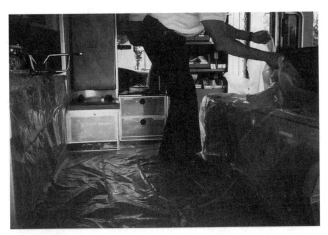

Figure 20-3 Before transporting victims of a HazMat incident, it might be necessary to cover the inside of the ambulance with plastic sheeting to prevent secondary contamination.

nel, in the hot zone: the likelihood of success is decreased when the responder is wearing PPE, and chemical contamination of the airway must be avoided.

During this phase, other EMS functions such as research, medical monitoring, and updating medical destination facilities should be ongoing. EMS should also be preparing to receive victims. If the danger of secondary contamination persists despite gross field decontamination, the transporting ambulance should be emptied of all unnecessary equipment and supplies and then draped with nonabsorbent plastic sheeting before victims are put on board (**Figure 20-3**). Transporting EMS personnel must don appropriate level PPE; level C is usually adequate following decontamination in the field.

Treatment/Transport Phase

During the treatment/transport phase, decontaminated victims are evaluated by EMS personnel and treated and/or transported as needed. This phase is conducted outside the hot zone. It might involve trauma care if the incident involved a transportation accident, fall, explosion, or burns. Emergency treatment of toxidromes associated with exposure might also be required. ALS protocols and pharmaceutical lists should provide for field use of time-sensitive antidotes to immediately life-threatening poisons that are known hazards.

Recovery/Termination Phase

The recovery/termination phase of a HazMat incident corresponds to completion of the emergency interventions required to mitigate the chemical hazard. It involves getting ready for the next incident and returning the incident site to civilian authorities or its original occupants. This phase occurs after emergency response personnel no longer require PPE.

From a medical standpoint, much of this phase involves final assessment of clinical conditions of entry personnel and completion of documentation. Final disposition of records maintained by EMS personnel must be orderly and specified by department standard operating procedure. Records of patient encounters should be managed in the same way as any other EMS call. Some civilians will be assessed and/or decontaminated but not medically treated or transported. The department should institute a system for archiving a record of these cases as part of the incident report. The medical monitoring records of department personnel, including any known or suspected toxic exposure, must be maintained in confidential files until they are forwarded by a secure modality to the department's occupational medical provider for inclusion in their personnel medical records. OSHA requires that such records be maintained for a minimum of 30 years beyond an employee's termination date with a particular department.[66]

In general, EMS staff responsible for treatment and transportation of victims will have left the scene by the time the recovery/termination phase begins. If they transported contaminated victims or were required to wear PPE to complete their assignments, both the transporting personnel and the apparatus must be decontaminated. Depending on protocol and facilities this might occur at the hospital. Alternatively, protocol might call for personnel to return with the apparatus to a location previously designated by the service for this purpose. Sometimes decontamination capability for apparatus, equipment, and personnel is already established at the incident scene. Regardless of where apparatus and personnel decontamination occurs, it is essential that rehabilitation and medical monitoring of personnel occur when they complete their suit time.

Like the early stages of the incident, this final stage requires a high level of vigilance for development of conditions likely to result in additional toxic exposures. Typically, by this stage, emergency personnel, bystanders, and media representatives have been on scene for a protracted period. Familiarity with circumstances of the incident can lead to relaxed enforcement of hazard zones and doffing or loosening of PPE even if there is a persistent hot zone.

Apparatus, Equipment, and Personal Protective Equipment

Many different types of apparatus and equipment and various levels of PPE have been developed for management of HazMat incidents. The EMS medical di-

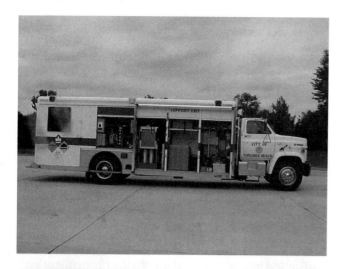

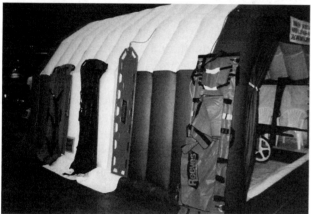

Figure 20-4 A HazMat team's response vehicle, with easily accessible exterior storage compartments (top) and a commercially available, inflatable, portable decontamination facility (bottom).

The other major type of dedicated HazMat response apparatus comprises a variety of mobile or portable decontamination facilities (**Figure 20-4**). Once again, few small or mid-sized jurisdictions have such resources available, although regional assets are currently being assessed and upgraded by most states through federal antiterrorism initiatives. In most locations, the definitive HazMat response apparatus is still the fire engine. Decontamination is typically set up using small-caliber hose lines with low-pressure tips and kiddie pools to contain hazardous runoff. To provide privacy and a modicum of environmental control, tarps draped over ladders extended from aerial trucks can form an adequate decontamination corridor (**Figure 20-5**).

Equipment can generally be divided into detection/identification, mitigation, communication, and medical categories. A detailed discussion of HazMat equipment is beyond the scope of this chapter, but readers should be aware that a significant armamentarium of relevant equipment exists. It is an area of intense and aggressive technology development, particularly as it applies to chemical and biological agent detection and countermeasures. Through the **Metropolitan Medical**

rector or other person responsible for selecting types and levels for an incident should be guided by two concepts: use of the minimum apparatus, equipment, and personnel that are consistent with safe mitigation of the hazards, and use of the lowest level of PPE that affords definitive protection from the hazards involved. These critical decisions must be made by officials who are knowledgeable in the capabilities and limitations of apparatus (ie, specially designed and equipped vehicles) equipment, and PPE and familiar with operational procedures and specific threats associated with the full spectrum of HazMat incidents.

Regional HazMat teams or teams that operate as part of large, metropolitan fire departments usually have dedicated apparatus (ie, specially designed and equipped vehicles) for HazMat response. Such apparatus typically provides storage space for PPE and equipment required for mitigation of common chemical releases (**Figure 20-4**). Many also provide interior workspace that can serve as a command and communications center and facilitates online field research.

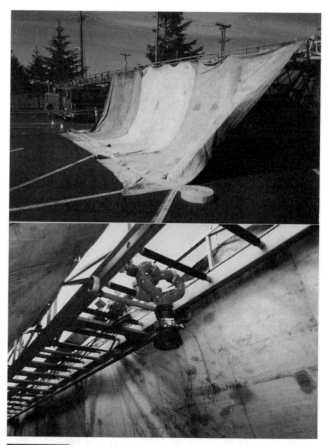

Figure 20-5 Salvage tarps draped from the ladder of a fire department truck using S-hooks can form an acceptable decontamination corridor, providing some privacy and a little protection from the weather.

Response System, a federal program within the Department of Homeland Security, fire and HazMat services in many large jurisdictions have acquired and trained with substantial arrays of chemical and biological agent detection instrumentation.[74] Medical directors must be aware of the precise applications and limitations of these devices. Many have very short track records in the civilian out-of-hospital arena, and their reliability should be considered unproven pending further study and experience. Decisions regarding responder or civilian health and safety should not be based exclusively on results from detection/identification technologies or methods that have not been evaluated and validated by either regulatory agencies or well-designed scientific studies.

Communications are mentioned briefly as they are required by OSHA for personnel operating in IDLH or confined-space environments.[66] Although direct voice contact is not required by regulation, many teams have adopted commercially available solutions that incorporate radio communication into PPE. As HazMat teams become better equipped through federal funding, there will continue to be an infusion of advanced communications technologies. Both mitigation procedures and medical protocols must keep pace with equipment improvements, optimizing both the safety and effectiveness of responders.

Medical equipment, like apparatus and personnel, should be deployed to HazMat incident scenes with their inherent risk of contamination only if absolutely indicated. Expensive electronics such as cardiac monitors are difficult to decontaminate and should be used only for specific indications, not as part of routine ALS protocols on contaminated patients. Provisions for common requirements such as supplemental oxygen following inhalation injuries, care of chemical and thermal burns, management of other wounds, and toxidromes in contaminated, multiple casualty environments must be tailored to local hazard assessments, response capabilities, and provider levels.

The EPA classifies the PPE used in HazMat operations into four levels: A, B, C, and D. In general, the higher the level of protection, the higher the heat strain index associated with wearing it. **Level A** PPE is a fully encapsulating liquid- and vapor-resistant suit that is worn over SCBA. It represents the highest level of protection and must be worn in any chemical IDLH environment or where potentially toxic unknown chemical threats are present. The materials comprising the suits vary and differ in the qualitative and quantitative protection offered against specific products. The composition of the level A suit to be worn at a given incident must be selected by knowledgeable personnel follow-

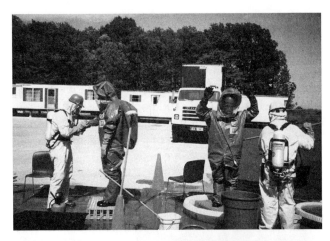

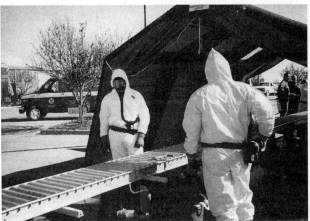

Figure 20-6 HazMat technicians in fully encapsulating, level A, chemical protective PPE are decontaminated with soap and water by responders wearing level B protection, where the SCBA is worn outside the suit (top). Responders in level C protection with powered, air-purifying respirators staff a decontamination corridor equipped with conveyor apparatus for multiple, stretcher-confined victims (bottom).

ing appropriate research. **Level B** PPE also includes use of SCBA (or supplied air respirators) but it is worn outside of the vapor- and liquid-resistant suit. The level B suit includes integrated hood and foot coverings and is worn with chemical-resistant disposable boots and gloves. These are frequently duct-taped to the suit to make the ensemble more impervious to liquids and vapors, though by definition, level B protection is worn when respiratory protection is a higher priority than skin protection. Level B suits are used when investigating spills or other circumstances suspected to represent biological threats.[75] They are also used by personnel responsible for decontamination of other responders who have made level A entries into a hot zone (**Figure 20-6**). As discussed previously, personnel tasked with medical responsibilities during a HazMat emergency should rarely be in level A or B protection. The suits severely inhibit the ability to perform medical evaluation or treatment.

Level C PPE (**Figure 20-6**) typically includes hooded chemical-resistant suits similar to those used for level B protection but with a lower level of respiratory protection. Portable air-purifying respirators or cartridge respirators are most commonly used with level C ensembles. Hoods, gloves, and boots are used in level C as they are in level B protection. Level C PPE is appropriate for decontamination of responders who made a level B hot zone entry, and in most instances for staff in hospital decontamination facilities. EMS personnel might use level C PPE for treatment and transport of contaminated victims following gross field decontamination.

Level D PPE refers to work outfits that offer little or no respiratory or skin protection from hazardous chemicals. It is important to point out that structural firefighting ensembles do not fit into the EPA PPE classification scheme. SCBA does offer a high degree of respiratory protection, and the coats, pants, and gloves used for fire suppression provide some vapor and water protection, but the materials are not chemical resistant. Chemicals capable of producing toxicity to or through the skin can generally penetrate turnout gear, although it might provide brief protection in order to effect a rescue if no immediate alternative exists. Exposure to chemicals can also compromise the thermal and vapor protective properties of the gear, rendering it unfit for subsequent firefighting. Turnout gear is not appropriate for entry into biohazard zones, although it does offer some initial protection. Gear that has been inadvertently exposed to biological agents should be destroyed; it is highly unlikely that it could be successfully decontaminated except through the use of chemicals that can affect its protective properties.

Specialized Training

Training for HazMat EMS responders must conform to the requirements of 29 CFR 1910.120. This document prescribes the level of certification (First Responder–Awareness or First Responder–Operations, depending on responsibilities of providers in the local system) and the hours required but not the content of the training. **NFPA 473, Standard on Hazardous Materials Competencies for EMS Responders**, provides curriculum guidance.[76] ALS providers can take advantage of additional training opportunities. Proprietary field toxicology courses are offered at some venues, and the National Fire Academy offers a 2-week residential course that is equivalent to a one-semester college course in ALS for HazMat responders.[77] Such training could expand the capabilities of paramedics during HazMat incidents at the discretion of physician medical directors who remain responsible for protocols, training, and quality maintenance. A 2-day advanced HazMat life support course is also available for EMS personnel.

Considerations for Medical Directors

Much of what currently takes place during HazMat incident responses has developed with very little input or oversight by EMS medical directors. Consequently, medical directors should take the time to become familiar with all aspects of HazMat response, with particular emphasis on where there is or is not science to support the traditions. This level of expertise is essential before safe and rational protocols for patient care and medical monitoring of responders can be put into effect.

Summary

Operational EMS involves providing out-of-hospital medical care of victims and medical support for those engaged in hazardous missions, frequently in austere or hostile environments. Military, or battlefield, EMS is one example of medical care performed in a mission context under uncontrolled conditions. In the civilian setting, fire ground, tactical, and HazMat EMS present largely analogous circumstances. Each of these has been discussed from the standpoint of the operational roles and responsibilities, specialized training, apparatus, PPE, and other considerations that must be understood for effective EMS medical oversight. The foregoing discussion should be considered introductory rather than comprehensive. Medical support for many forms of technical rescue, including swift water, confined space, high angle, and urban search and rescue are all examples of operational EMS with inherent hazards, distinct protocols and training, and dedicated apparatus, equipment, and PPE. Although space does not permit inclusion of these disciplines in this chapter, the same issues must be addressed before committing EMS personnel to such operations. Medical directors should conduct hazard assessments in their jurisdictions to determine which of these specialized response capabilities should be included in their scopes of practice.

References

1. Bogucki MS. More expanded scope: operational EMS. *Prehospital Emerg Care.* 1998;2:330–333.
2. Zimble J. Military medicine: an operational definition. *Milit Med.* 1996;161:183–188.

3. *Counter Narcotics Operational Medical Support Emergency Medical Technician–Tactical.* Bethesda, Md: Uniformed Services University of Health Sciences; 2001.

4. *Advanced Life Support Response to Hazardous Materials Incidents.* Emmitsburg, Md; National Fire Academy, 1995.

5. Kolman JA. *A Guide to the Development of Special Weapons and Tactics Teams.* Springfield, Ill: Charles C. Thomas; 1982.

6. CONTOMS incident summary report [database online]. Bethesda, Md: Casualty Care Research Center, Department of Military and Emergency Medicine, Uniformed Services University of Health Sciences; July 8, 1990–June 7, 1997. Available at: http://www.casualtycareresearchcenter.org/data_injury_page.htm. Accessed January 26, 2005.

7. Rasumoff D. EMS at tactical law enforcement operations seminar a success. *The Tactical Edge.* 1989;7:25–29.

8. Carmona R, Brennan K. Tactical emergency medical support conference (TEMS): a successful joint effort. *The Tactical Edge.* 1990;8:7.

9. NTOA position statement of support for counter narcotics tactical operations medical support. *The Tactical Edge.* 1993;11:71.

10. Jones JS, Reese K, Kenepp G, et al. Into the fray: integration of emergency medical services and special weapons and tactics (SWAT) teams. *Prehospital Disaster Med.* 1996;11(3):202–206.

11. Carmona R, Prince K. Trauma and forensic medicine. *J Trauma.* 1989;29(9):1222–1225.

12. Rasumoff D, Carmona R. Echeloned field medical care: definition and justification. *The Tactical Edge.* 1993; 11(4):72–76.

13. Heck J, Kepp J, Walos G, et al. Medical threat assessment. In: Gibbons M, Tan L, Krebs D, et al, eds. *Counter Narcotics Operational Medical Support Emergency Medical Technician—Tactical.* Bethesda, Md: Uniformed Services University of Health Sciences; 2001.

14. Vayer J, Hagmann J, Llewellyn C. Refining prehospital physical assessment skills: a new teaching technique. *Ann Emerg Med.* 1994;23:786–790.

15. Heiskell LE, Carmona RH. Tactical emergency medical services: an emerging subspecialty of emergency medicine. *Ann Emerg Med.* 1994;23:778–785.

16. *Fire in the United States, 1987-1996.* Emmitsburg, Md: National Fire Data Center, US Fire Administration, FEMA; 1999. FA–173.

17. International Association of Fire Fighters. *1994 IAFF Death and Injury Survey.* Washington, DC: IAFF; 1995.

18. National Fire Protection Association. *NFPA 1582: Standard on Comprehensive Occupational Medical Program for Fire Fighters, 2003 Edition.* Quincy, Mass: NFPA; 2003.

19. National Fire Protection Association. *NFPA 1583: Standard on Health-related Fitness Programs for Firefighters.* Quincy, Mass: NFPA; 2000.

20. International Association of Fire Fighters, International Association of Fire Chiefs. *The Fire Service Joint Labor-Management Wellness-Fitness Initiative.* 2nd ed. Washington, DC: IAFF; 2000.

21. National Fire Protection Association. *NFPA 1500: Standard on Fire Department Occupational Safety and Health Program, 2002 Edition.* Quincy, Mass: NFPA; 2002.

22. Dickinson ET, Wieder MA. In: *Emergency Incident Rehabilitation.* Upper Saddle River, NJ: Brady/Prentice Hall Inc; 2000: 129.

23. Lawson JR. *Fire Fighter's Protective Clothing and Thermal Environments of Structural Fire Fighting.* Washington, DC: US Department of Commerce. NISTIR 5804, 1996.

24. Abeles FJ, Del Vecchio RJ, Himel VH. *A Firefighter's Integrated Life Protection System.* New York, NY: Fire Department of the City of New York; 1974. Report of Contract 219454.

25. Barnard RJ, Duncan HW. Heart rate and ECG responses of fire fighters. *J Occup Med.* 1975;17:247–250.

26. Gledhill N, Jamnik VK. Characterization of the physical demands of firefighting. *Can J Spt Sci.* 1992;17:207–213.

27. Louhevaara V, Smolander J, Tuomi T, et al. Effects of an SCBA on breathing pattern, gas exchange, and heart rate during exercise. *J Occup Med.* 1985;27:213–216.

28. White MK, Vercruyssen M, Hodous TK. Work tolerance and subjective responses to wearing protective clothing and respirators during physical work. *Ergonomics.* 1989;32:1111–1123.

29. Faff J, Tutak T. Physiological responses to working with fire fighting equipment in the heat in relation to subjective fatigue. *Ergonomics.* 1989;32:629–638.

30. Kuorinka I, Korhonen O. Firefighters' reaction to alarm, and ECG and heart rate study. *J Occup Med.* 1981;23: 762–766.

31. Motohashi Y, Takano T. Influence of age on cardiorespiratory responses of firefighters during exercise in the heat. *Industrial Health.* 1985;23:289–293.

32. Lim CS, Ong CN, Phoon WO. Work stress of firemen as measured by heart rate and catecholamine. *J Hum Ergol.* 1987;16:209–218.

33. Pipes TV. Physiological responses of fire fighting recruits to high intensity training. *J Occup Med.* 1977;19:129–132.

34. Smith DL, Petruzzello SJ, Kramer JM, et al. Phsiological, psychophysical, and psychological responses of firefighters to firefighting training drills. *Aviat Space Environ Med.* 1996;67:1063–1068.

35. Bennett BL, Hagan D, Banta G, et al. Physiological responses during shipboard firefighting. *Aviat Space Environ Med.* 2004;65:225–231.

36. Manning JE, Griggs TR. Heart rates in fire fighters using light and heavy breathing equipment: similar near-maximal exertion in response to multiple work load conditions. *J Occup Med.* 1983;25:215–218.

37. Romet TT, Frim J. Physiological responses to fire fighting activities. *Eur J Appl Physiol.* 1987;56:633–638.

38. Duncan HW, Gardner GW, Barnard RJ. Physiological responses of men working in fire fighting equipment in the heat. *Ergonomics.* 1979;22:521–527.

39. Sothmann MS, Saupe K, Jasenof D, et al. Heart rate response of firefighters to actual emergencies. *J Occup Med.* 1992;34:797–800.

40. Skoldstrom B. Physiological responses of fire fighters to workload and thermal stress. *Ergonomics.* 1987;30:1589–1597.

41. Montain SJ, Sawka MN, Cadarette BS, et al. Physiological tolerance to uncompensable heat stress: effects of exercise intensity, protective clothing, and climate. *J Appl Physiol.* 1994;77:216–222.

42. Smith D, Petruzzello SJ, Kramer JM, et al. Physiological, psychophysical, and psychological responses of firefighters to firefighting training drills. *Aviat Space Environ Med.* 1996;67:1063–1068.

43. Miles DS, Gotshall RW. Impedance cardiography: noninvasive assessment of human central hemodynamics at rest and during exercise. *Exerc Sport Sci Rev.* 1989;17:231–263.

44. Stanley T. *Heat Stress Management Guidelines.* Phoenix, Ariz: City of Phoenix Fire Department; June 2000.

45. US Department of Health and Human Services, National Institute for Occupational Safety and Health. Working in hot environments [NIOSH Web site]. Available at: http://www.cdc.gov/niosh/hotenvt.html. Accessed January 26, 2005.

46. Smith MJ, Duffy RM, Beer AR, et al. *Thermal Stress and the Fire Fighter.* Washington, DC: IAFF Department of Research, Health and Safety Division; 1982.

47. Kenny WL, Johnson JM. Control of skin blood flow during exercise. *Med Sci Sports Exerc.* 1992;24(3):303–312.

48. Havenith G, Coenen JML, Kristemaker L, et al. Relevance of individual characteristics for human heat stress response is dependent on exercise intensity and climate type. *Eur J Appl Physiol.* 1998;77:231–241.

49. Kraning KK, Gonzalez RR. Physiological consequences of intermittent exercise during compensable and uncompensable heat stress. *J Appl Physiol.* 1991;71(6):2138–2145.

50. Convertino VA, Armstrong LE, Coyle EF, et al. Exercise and fluid replacement. *Med Sci Sports Exerc.* 1996;28(1):i–vii(F9-F37).

51. Kristal-Bonch E, Glusman JG, Shitrit R, et al. Physical performance and heat tolerance after chronic water loading and heat acclimation. *Aviat Space Environ Med.* 1995;66(8):733–738.

52. Horswill CA. Effective fluid replacement. *International J Sports Nutrition.* 1998;8:175–195.

53. Faff J, Tutak T. Physiological responses to working with fire fighting equipment in the heat in relation to subjective fatigue. *Ergonomics* 1989;32(6):629–638.

54. Richardson GR. *Larrey: Surgeon to Napoleon's Imperial Guard.* London, England: John Murray; 1974.

55. Rice MM, Brown JF. Military systems. In: Kuehl AE, ed. *Prehospital Systems and Medical Oversight.* 2nd ed. St Louis, Mo: Mosby Lifeline; 1994;59–65.

56. Jagoda A, Pietrzak M, Hazen S, et al. Prehospital care and the military. *Milit Med.* 1992;157:11–15.

57. DeLorenzo RA. Improving combat casualty care and field medicine: focus on the military medic. *Milit Med.* 1997;162:268–272.

58. Butler FK, Hagmann J, Butler G. Tactical combat casualty care in special operations. *Milit Med.* 1996;161:S1–S16.

59. Lindsey D. Professional considerations of patient evacuation. Paper presented at: The Course on Recent Advances in Medicine and Surgery, Army Medical Service Graduate School, Walter Reed Army Medical Center. April 19, 1951, Washington, DC.

60. Pretto EA, Begovic M. Emergency medical services during the siege of Sarajevo, Bosnia and Herzegovina: a preliminary report. *Prehospital Disaster Med.* 1994;9:S39–S45.

61. Vujovic B, Mazlagic D. Epidemiology and surgical management of abdominal war injuries in Sarajevo: State Hospital of Sarajevo experience. *Prehospital Disaster Med.* 1994;9:S29–S34.

62. VanRooyen MJ, VanRooyen JB, Sloan EP, et al. Mobile medical relief and military assistance in Somalia. *Prehospital Disaster Med.* 1995;10:118–120.

63. Shemer J, Heller O, Adler J. Lessons from the Israeli Defense Force Medical Corps' experience in the organization of international medical disaster relief forces. *Prehospital Disaster Med.* 1992;7:282–284.

64. Cashman JR. *Hazardous Materials Emergencies. Response and Control.* Rev, 2nd ed. Lancaster, Pa: Technomic Publishing Company Inc; 1988.

65. Superfund Amendments and Reauthorization Act (SARA), Pub L No. 99-499, October 17, 1986.

66. Occupational Safety and Health Administration, US Dept of Labor. Hazardous waste operations and emergency response, 29 CFR 1910.120.

67. Transportation of Hazardous Material. General Regulatory Authority. 49 USC 5103(a).

68. Bogucki S, Costello D. *Advanced Life Support Response to Hazardous Materials Incidents: Student Manual.* Washington, DC: FEMA/USFA/NFA-ALSRHMI-SM; 1995.

69. Occupational Safety and Health Administration, US Dept of Labor. Personal protective equipment; respiratory protection, 29 CFR 1910.134, Subpart I.

70. US Department of Transportation, Transport Canada, Secretariat of Communications and Transportation of Mexico. *2004 Emergency Response Guidebook* [DOT Web site]. Available at: http://hazmat.dot.gov/pubs/erg2004/gydebook.htm. Accessed January 26, 2005.

71. Kales SN, Polyhronopoulos GN, Aldrich JM, et al. Prospective study of hepatic, renal and haematological surveillance in hazardous materials firefighters. *J Occup Environ Med.* 2001;58:87–94.

72. Kales SN, Aldrich JM, Polyhronopoulos GM, et al. Fitness for duty evaluations in hazardous materials firefighters. *J Occup Environ Med.* 1998;40:925–931.

73. Samo DG, Bogucki MS. Fitness for duty evaluations of firefighters [letter]. *J Occup Environ Med.* 1999;41:213–214.

74. US Fire Administration, Federal Emergency Management Agency. Hazardous materials response technology assessment [FEMA Web site]. Available at: http://www.usfa.fema.gov/downloads/pdf/publications/fa-199.pdf. Accessed January 26, 2005.

75. US Department of Health and Human Services, Centers for Disease Control and Prevention. Interim recommendations for the selection and use of protective clothing and respirators against biological agents [CDC Web site]. Available at: http://www.bt.cdc.gov/DocumentsApp/Anthrax/Protective/10242001Protect.asp. Accessed January 26, 2005.

76. National Fire Protection Association. *NFPA 473: Competencies for EMS Personnel Responding to Hazardous Materials Incidents.* Quincy, Mass: NFPA; 2002. (Available as a free download from the NFPA Web site, www.nfpa.org.)

77. National Fire Academy, US Fire Administration, FEMA. *Advanced Life Support for Hazardous Materials Incidents.* Washington, DC: NFA/USFA/FEMA; 1995.

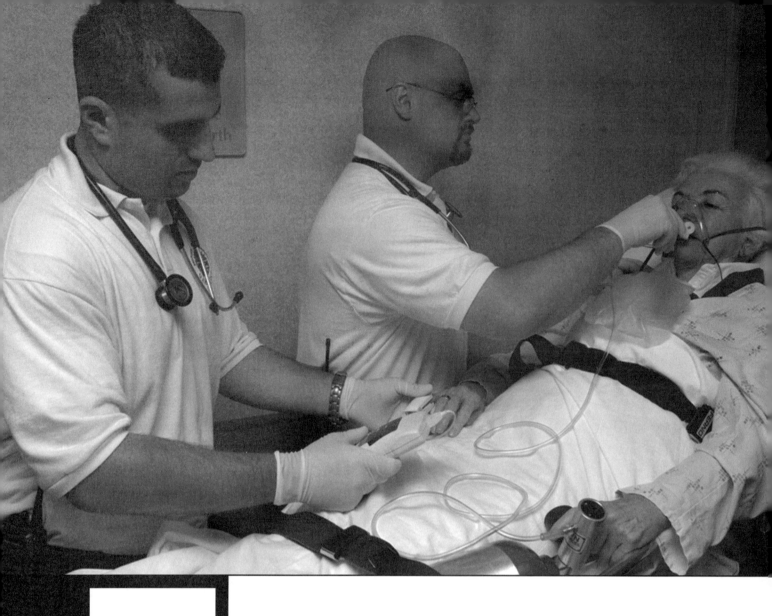

21 EMS and Public Health

James V. Dunford, Jr., MD, FACEP
Theodore C. Chan, MD, FACEP

Principles of This Chapter

After reading this chapter, you should be able to:

- Discuss the reform of both public health and EMS.
- Explain prior EMS–public health relationships.
- List the potential benefits to public health from a partnership with EMS, and the potential benefits to EMS from a partnership with public health.
- Describe the barriers to an EMS–public health partnership, including traditional roles and stereotypes, education and cross-training, new performance standards and measures, limited civic and business support, and lack of common forums.

PRIOR TO SEPTEMBER 11, 2001, MANY IN THE MEDICAL COMmunity would likely have been surprised to learn that EMS and public health were forging a partnership. EMS usually connotes images of ambulances and fire engines responding with lights and sirens, while public health suggests carefully coordinated plans to stem communicable diseases. Despite differences of reputation, in the wake of the terrorist attacks, the overlapping missions of EMS and public health in providing essential fabric for the public safety net is much more evident. In the 21st century, EMS and public health share fundamental health care concerns rooted in poverty, violence, substance abuse, family disintegration, environmental degradation, and poor education. As the tragic events of September 11 have demonstrated, their common charges clearly include planning for and managing the effects of terrorist acts as well. Both disciplines must work closely and cooperatively in effectively planning domestic preparedness response activities.

The American Public Health Association (APHA) and the National Association of EMS Physicians (NAEMSP) have initiated a series of steps to bring these disciplines into more formal alignment.[1] The purpose of this chapter is to review the common ground between EMS and public health and explore the advantages of enhanced EMS–public health collaboration. A closer alliance between EMS and public health can provide powerful new strategies for addressing some of today's most challenging health issues.

Background

American public health has its roots in epidemiology, prevention, health policy, and regulation and has achieved recognition and respect over the past 200 years. Conversely, it has taken just three decades for EMS to also find itself an acknowledged, essential community health care service. The philosophical and operational approaches of EMS and public health are very different: public health addresses its mission in a proactive manner, and EMS is, to a large degree, reactive.

The traditional approach of public health, or PH, follows the three basic steps of assessment, policy, and assurance. **Assessment** involves careful and systematic analysis of indicators of community health. This process typically begins with the identification of an important health issue. Epidemiologic investigation of individual events surrounding that issue then occurs, followed by analysis of the contributing factors and determinants of the issue. Ultimately, there must be advocacy to effect corrective actions. **Policy** refers to the step in which PH enacts rules to codify the desired care in order to sustain its effect. **Assurance** is the final step in PH practice; it uses tools such as surveillance to track compliance to policy. Effective immunization and water and air quality programs are examples of ongoing PH programs that protect and serve the health of the community.

By contrast, EMS is based on the care of individual patients and is designed to be a reactive delivery model. Although EMS uses data-driven status plans to anticipate demand, its primary role is to rapidly deploy staff and equipment to mitigate specific and unique events. EMS relies on advanced public access communication systems to identify emergencies and target responses. A common organizational structure, the incident command system, is typically used to ensure that necessary resources are rapidly assigned to meet dynamic and often unpredictable conditions.[2]

Public Health Reform

During the course of the 20th century, the infrastructure of the US public health system underwent a series of striking evolutions to provide the elements required for successful PH intervention.[3] At the beginning of the century, PH initiatives (typically begun and supported by nongovernment organizations) were related to infectious diseases associated with poor hygiene and sanitation, diseases of poor nutrition, and injuries due to unsafe working conditions. As successful interventions (eg, vaccinations) affected these issues, chronic diseases and traffic-related injuries received more intense focus. The demonstrated benefits of community action to address PH concerns progressively recruited support for the growth and involvement of government, community, professional, voluntary, and academic organizations. PH acquired quantitative analytic techniques, standardized health surveys, morbidity and mortality surveillance, and training. External analyses have caused PH to refocus its efforts recently,[4,5] and a new process using measurable, 10-year objectives has been adopted. EMS leaders will recognize many of their own goals in the current PH objectives.

In 1990, the national initiative **Healthy People 2000** was introduced. This project contained 319 specific national health promotion and disease prevention objectives targeted for achievement by 2000. By 1993, 70% of local health departments were using Healthy People 2000 objectives. In 1998–1999, 15% of the objectives had been reached or exceeded, and progress had occurred in 44% of the remainder.[6] In January 2000, **Healthy People 2010** was released.[7] The current second edition lists 10 leading health indicators based on their ability to motivate action, availability of data to measure progress, and on their importance as PH issues, as follows:

- Physical activity
- Overweight and obesity
- Tobacco use
- Substance abuse
- Responsible sexual behavior
- Mental health
- Injury and violence
- Environmental quality
- Immunization
- Access to health care

Each of the targets is to be attained by 2010. It is significant that EMS objectives are identified as essential components of the nation's health care (**Figure 21-1**).

Figure 21-1 Healthy People 2010 objectives related to EMS.

Reduce the proportion of persons who delay/have difficulty getting emergency care.
Increase the proportion of persons who have access to rapid out-of-hospital EMS.
Establish a single toll-free number for poison centers, 24-hours/day.
Increase the number of states with trauma care systems that maximize survival and functional outcomes of trauma patients and help prevent injuries from occurring.
Increase the proportion of local health service areas that have established community health promotion and disease prevention programs.
Ensure that states establish training, plans, and protocols and conduct annual multi-institutional exercises to prepare for response to natural/technological disasters.
Increase the proportion of adults aware of the early warning symptoms and signs of heart attack and the importance of accessing rapid emergency care by calling 911.
Increase the proportion of eligible patients with heart attacks who receive artery-opening therapy within an hour of symptom onset.
Increase the proportion of adults who call 911 and administer cardiopulmonary resuscitation when they witness an out-of-hospital cardiac arrest.
Increase the proportion of eligible persons with witnessed out-of-hospital cardiac arrest who receive first electrical shock within 6 minutes after collapse recognition.
Increase the proportion of adults aware of the early warning signs of stroke.
Reduce nonfatal head injury/spinal cord injury hospitalizations, firearm-related deaths and injuries, nonfatal and fatal poisonings, and suffocation deaths.
Increase the number of statewide emergency department surveillance systems that collect data on external causes of injury through hospital discharge data systems.
Reduce fatal and nonfatal unintentional injuries, motor vehicle crash injuries, pedestrian injuries, injuries from falls, deaths from residential fires, and drowning incidents.
Increase use of safety belts, child restraints, motorcycle and bicycle helmets, and protective equipment in school sports.
Increase the proportion of major health data systems that promote geographic information systems; increase proportion of HP 2010 objectives for which national data for all population groups are available and tracked regularly nationally.
Increase the proportion of state/local health agencies that provide continuing education to develop specific competencies in the essential public health services.
Increase the proportion of agencies that meet national performance standards for essential public health services; ensure comprehensive epidemiology/laboratory services to support essential public health services.
Reduce deaths, hospitalizations, and emergency department visits for asthma.
Reduce injuries/deaths related to substance abuse and motor vehicle crashes.
Reduce drug-induced and alcohol-induced emergency department visits and deaths and intentional injuries from alcohol and illicit drug-related violence.
Increase the proportion referred for followup for alcohol/drug problems or suicide attempts after treatment in a hospital emergency department.
Increase the number of communities using partnerships or coalition models to conduct comprehensive substance abuse prevention efforts.

PH leaders now believe they are most effective when functioning as a complex partnership with federal agencies, state and local governments, nongovernment organizations, academia, and community members. In 1994, the APHA and the American Medical Association created a working alliance called the **Medicine and Public Health Initiative**.[8] This partnership nurtures a more fully integrated health system. The initiative established seven goals, as follows:

- Engaging the community in an effort to change existing thinking within academic health centers, health-oriented community organizations, health care delivery systems and providers, and among health care purchasers to focus them on improving the health of the community.
- Changing the education process by expanding public health's understanding of medicine and medicine's understanding of public health.
- Creating joint research efforts by educating clinical and public health researchers, focusing on significant health issues, and promoting public and private funding of research supporting conceptual and institutional linkages between public health and medicine.
- Devising a shared view of health and illness that provides a conceptual framework for collaboration between the professions.
- Working together in health care provision by developing a framework, including standards and strategies, for integrating health promotion and prevention services and activities into both clinical and community settings.
- Jointly developing health care assessment measures to improve the quality, effectiveness, and outcome measures of health care.
- Creating networks to translate ideas into actions by outlining processes for translating and implementing proposals from the Medicine/Public Health Initiative.

EMS Reform

In 1996, the National Highway Traffic Safety Administration (NHTSA) and the Health Resources and Services Administration (HRSA) Maternal and Child Health Bureau convened a steering committee to set a course for EMS in the 21st century. The leadership group believed there was a need for EMS agencies and organizations to digest the accomplishments of the past three decades and to chart a new course that would improve the science, strengthen the infrastructure, and

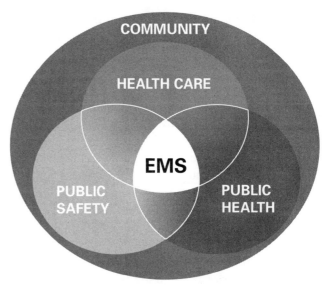

Figure 21-2 EMS as the "intersection" of public health, public safety, and health care. From NHTSA, "EMS Agenda for the Future."

broaden the involvement of EMS in the health of communities. In the landmark publication "EMS Agenda for the Future,"[9] EMS was identified as the intersection of public safety, PH, and health care systems (**Figure 21-2**). While providing a primary mission of serving as the public's emergency medical safety net, the agenda concluded that EMS should develop new and effective relationships with those responsible for the overall health care of the community. These new relationships would require discussions with managed care organizations, providers, other public service providers, and local PH agencies. New strategic partnerships could better integrate community expertise and produce measurable goals, long-term satisfaction, and even new financial sources. The agenda left little room for debate regarding the direction that EMS should travel to sustain itself and grow. A companion document, "EMS Agenda for the Future: Implementation Guide,"[10] provides examples of the tools, infrastructure, and strategic partnerships necessary to accomplish short-, intermediate-, and long-term agenda objectives.

A Health Care System in Flux

Over the past 10 years, many forces have affected the fundamental balance of emergency medical needs. Hospital closures, fewer oncall specialists, fewer inpatient beds, lack of access to primary care, and critical nursing shortages are fueling emergency department crowding and rising ambulance diversion. In 2001, there were more than 107 million visits to emergency departments in the United States.[11] Patients are increasingly becoming displaced from their physicians and hospitals, and EMS resources are being consumed for protracted periods of time as hospital emergency departments are increasingly saturated and going on diversion. The integrity of the PH safety net itself has been questioned.[12,13]

In addition, the quality of the nation's health care is under intense scrutiny.[14] Two Institute of Medicine reports criticized the basic oversight and management of health care and forced all health care providers to implement continuous quality improvement solutions.[15,16] The quality of care must now be formally managed using valid, measurable end points. While PH has long analyzed the "six Ds" (death, disease, disability, discomfort, dissatisfaction, and destitution) as indicators of performance, EMS is only now defining its own relevant performance measures.[17] The horrific events of September 11, 2001, and the subsequent anthrax attacks have brought into stark focus the need for all components of the health care system to collaborate more closely. Opportunities for emergency medicine and PH partnerships are emerging.[18] These dramatic times challenge EMS leaders to consider new ways of addressing their core missions. They must hone their administrative skills to more effectively manage the quality of care and consider redefining their roles and the roles of their personnel. Previous discussions often centered on expanded out-of-hospital care;[19-21] open-mindedness to any good idea is now the most appropriate attitude.

Prior EMS–Public Health Partnerships

The reason for the lack of a close association between PH and EMS is likely no different than the obstacles to communication between other health care entities. In many cases, individual disciplines have evolved in relative isolation from one another. In many smaller localities, EMS personnel have little outside contact beyond other public safety agencies and local hospitals. Similarly, PH departments have not focused on EMS to the degree that they attended to other efforts. Numerous individual reports of successful EMS–PH partnerships exist, but few have been replicated by other EMS systems.

Recently, the public health role of emergency medicine in surveillance of diseases, injuries, and health risks has been emphasized.[18] Emergency medicine (and EMS) offers new opportunities for monitoring health care access, delivering targeted preventive services, and developing PH policy improvements. The **Frontlines of Medicine Project**[22] is an exciting collaborative effort of emergency medicine, EMS, PH, clinical toxicology, emergency government, law enforcement, and informatics specialists. Its goal is to create an open systems approach for reporting emergency department data that could be used for such PH efforts as early warning syndromic surveillance (including acts of biological or chemical terrorism).

Primary Injury Prevention

EMS can have an important role in primary injury prevention.[23] In 1997, NHTSA, HRSA, and NAEMSP convened a consensus panel of 16 national organizations representing different components of EMS. The group concluded that primary injury prevention is an essential public safety service that should be provided by EMS personnel.[24] It was thought to be a natural duty for EMS because its primary role in the community combines elements of health care, public safety, and PH. Primary injury prevention was thought to be similar to other successful EMS and police programs targeting prevention of fire, burns, and impaired driving. Unique attributes of EMS that confer the ability to accomplish this goal were identified, including the following:

- EMS providers are widely distributed.
- EMS providers reflect the composition of the community.
- EMS providers enjoy high credibility.

EMS leadership was strongly encouraged to provide the needed education, support, and opportunity for health promotion and safety.

Successful primary injury prevention programs already exist. In Akron, Ohio, paramedics successfully identified and referred elderly persons at risk for social and medical problems.[25] This project involved the collaborative efforts of EMS, the fire department, local hospitals, and a local PH agency. Syracuse, New York, paramedics successfully identified and referred at-risk elderly persons to social services.[26] In addition, EMS crews were trained to identify child abuse, sexual abuse, sexual assault, isolation, and mental illness. EMS personnel in Philadelphia demonstrated that it is feasible to incorporate carbon monoxide monitors into routine medical equipment and detect occult exposure.[27]

Epidemiologic injury analysis can be accomplished using EMS run data. The **Crash Injury Research and Engineering Network (CIREN)**[28] is a multicenter research program involving a collaboration of clinicians and engineers in academia, industry, and government. The

CIREN database consists of multiple, discrete fields of data concerning severe motor vehicle crashes, including crash reconstruction and medical injury profiles. A North Carolina study demonstrated the utility of a computerized EMS database to assess rates of falls in the elderly.[29] The Maryland Institute for EMS Systems database has been beneficial in performing injury surveillance.[30] EMS personnel in Pinellas County, Florida, integrated surveillance, education, and a media outreach program on water safety and CPR that reduced pool drownings.[31] New York City EMS providers worked in conjunction with a Harlem Hospital injury prevention project called "Kids, Injuries, and Street Smarts" (KISS) to educate schoolchildren about injury and violence prevention.[32] The Tennessee Division of EMS used its statewide computerized database to both assess the demographics of home visits and analyze the value of surveillance programs.[33] Finally, it has been suggested that EMS data systems might one day provide regional community health monitoring and referral programs.[34]

Infection Control Surveillance

Links between EMS and infection control surveillance are now recognized as critical components of PH surveillance, particularly as a result of smallpox immunization and response planning activities. New York City's Office of Emergency Management (OEM) performs daily health surveillance to monitor for biological terrorism.[35] The critical daily OEM indicators include EMS call volumes for adult and pediatric asthma, difficulty breathing, respiratory, sick, sick minor, and sick pediatric cases. Other OEM monitors include total emergency department admissions through sentinel hospitals, a daily medical examiner census, rates of influenza-like illness in nursing homes, diarrheal illness (through sales of antidiarrheal medicines at sentinel pharmacies), and investigation of all unexplained deaths of persons younger than 49 years. EMS has also been successfully integrated into epidemic alert programs, allowing out-of-hospital personnel to use appropriate isolation procedures, prophylaxis of personnel, and predesignation of receiving facilities for patients suspected of having infection. EMS personnel used the model successfully during airport alerts for both suspected pneumonic plague and Ebola virus infection.[36]

Recent events have reminded EMS and PH leaders that terrorists can use both conventional and bioterrorist tactics, and that success in handling their effects is most likely when planning is both collaborative and inclusive. The fall 2002 planning activities regarding smallpox immunization and response plans are a classic example of the critical need (and opportunity) for EMS and PH organizations to work cooperatively at the local, regional, state, and national levels. Much progress has been made recently with increased interaction of EMS and PH agencies in domestic preparedness planning activities. The 2003 experience with severe acute respiratory syndrome (SARS) also provided the opportunity and reinforced the value of EMS and PH working together on surveillance activities.

Other EMS–Public Health Examples

There are numerous other examples of EMS activities that embody PH missions. For example, programs in some states now allow firehouses to be used as safe havens for unwanted newborns and infants. The **Alzheimer Foundation's Safe Returns Program** enables rapid identification and return of missing individuals by on-duty EMS and police. The **San Diego Serial Inebriate Program (SIP)** is a collaborative effort of police, EMS, and community leaders, using a coercive rehabilitation strategy to improve sobriety and reduce the frequency of EMS and emergency department visits.[37] Subsets of patients do overuse the EMS system and emergency departments for their primary care needs.[38,39] At San Francisco General Hospital, case management proved cost-effective in redirecting recidivist emergency department patients toward more appropriate resources and treatment.[40]

Many other EMS goals are clearly PH in nature, including the development of regional trauma centers and communitywide cardiovascular disease programs (such as the American Heart Association's Operation Heartbeat and Operation Stroke, as well as the implementation of public access defibrillation programs). In fact, many of today's important EMS agenda items incorporate PH themes.

EMS–Public Health Roundtable

In January 2000, Dr. Mohammed Akhter, former executive director of the APHA, enunciated a persuasive argument for beginning formal discussions between the APHA and EMS.[41] Dr. Akhter is the former director of emergency services and highway safety for the state of Illinois and is also a major trauma survivor. With joint sponsorship of the APHA, NAEMSP, NHTSA, and HRSA, a series of four meetings between EMS and PH leaders examined the potential benefits and challenges of such a proposed integration.[1]

Potential Benefits to Public Health From a Partnership With EMS

The EMS–PH roundtable[1] identified numerous benefits to PH from an affiliation with EMS, as follows:

- Use of EMS databases to enhance surveillance and assessment of specific populations, conditions, and diseases by neighborhood, community, or region
- Use of EMS infrastructure and workforce to more effectively implement community health initiatives and outreach efforts
- Improved visibility by aligning with the high-profile and credible voice of EMS

Following is a list of several of the PH opportunities from an EMS–PH partnership:

- EMS data for injury surveillance and infectious disease and epidemic surveillance
- EMS workforce involvement in immunization and education
- EMS data and workforce involvement in drowning surveillance, prevention, and education
- EMS data and workforce involvement in car seat use, surveillance, and education
- EMS data and workforce involvement in partner violence surveillance and prevention outreach
- EMS data and workforce involvement in elderly injury pattern surveillance and prevention
- EMS systems for surveillance of emerging epidemics or chemical/bioterrorism threats
- EMS data and workforce involvement to provide access to, surveillance of, and needs assessment of high-risk populations (eg, chronic alcoholics, the homeless, and the mentally ill)

Potential Benefits to EMS From a Partnership With Public Health

The participants[1] also identified benefits to EMS from an affiliation with PH, primarily through access to the expertise of PH personnel. Such an affiliation could bring the following to EMS:

- Enhanced epidemiologic analysis to assist in deploying and targeting EMS resources
- Resource alternatives for many of the health and social problems confronting EMS providers

- Increased job satisfaction through efforts focused on community health and injury and illness prevention
- Job satisfaction through accomplishment of long-term solutions
- Potentially new PH career options for EMS providers

Following is a list of several of the EMS opportunities from an EMS–PH partnership:

- Enhanced outcomes analysis of local EMS interventions
- More accurate analysis of regional EMS deployment and resource utilization
- Improved EMS triage through population-based, critical study
- More appropriate resources for special needs patients
- Expanded alternative care locations
- Reduced ambulance diversion and inappropriate use of services
- Improved scientific and epidemiologic EMS research

Barriers to an EMS–Public Health Partnership

The roundtable considered a number of barriers to EMS–PH collaboration.[1] The following obstacles were addressed:

- Traditional roles and stereotypes of EMS and PH could be difficult to overcome.
- Education and cross-training would require new funding and resources.
- New performance standards and measures might be perceived as a threat to job security.
- The current turmoil in health care and EMS delivery systems might retard efforts to collaborate.
- Civic and business support for such efforts could be limited, especially locally.
- Few common forums currently exist, making collaboration difficult.

Summary

Over the past 10 years, PH has identified the need to partner with many health care disciplines to solve the nation's health care needs. The Medicine and Public Health Initiative opened the door to collaboration with traditional medicine, and the EMS–PH roundtable began the same process for out-of-hospital care. Affiliations among PH, academic medicine, and the Centers for

Disease Control and Prevention will further strengthen the community safety net.[42,43] Following the September 11, 2001, attacks, Congress provided for $40 billion to be spent in recovery and preparedness efforts. Effective domestic preparedness activities require close interaction and cooperation between the EMS and PH systems. The opportunity now exists for a degree of unprecedented collaboration between PH and EMS. All EMS medical directors and administrators should now be undertaking an evaluation of their agencies' missions, values, customers, and needs. If it has not already occurred, conversations with their PH agencies should follow, exploring how EMS can assist their goals and objectives. A solid understanding of both Healthy People 2010 and the "EMS Agenda for the Future" will provide the common ground from which to begin this valuable partnership.

References

1. EMS & public health: building a partnership for community health care. National Highway Traffic Safety Administration Web site. Available at: http://www.nhtsa.dot.gov/people/injury/ems/emspublic/introduction.html. Accessed January 21, 2005.

2. Firescope. *Field Operations Guide. ICS 420-1 Incident Command System Publication.* Riverside, Calif: Firescope; 2004.

3. Centers for Disease Control and Prevention. Achievements in public health, 1900-1999. *MMWR Morb Mortal Wkly Rep.*1999;48(50):1141–1146. Also available at: http://www.cdc.gov/mmwr/PDF/wk/mm4850.pdf. Accessed January 21, 2005.

4. US Department of Health, Education, and Welfare, Public Health Service. *Healthy People: The Surgeon General's Report on Health Promotion and Disease Prevention.* Washington, DC: US Public Health Service; 1979. DHEW (PHS) Publication 79-55071.

5. Committee for the Study of the Future of Public Health, Division of Health Care Services, Institute of Medicine. *The Future of Public Health.* Washington, DC: National Academies Press; 1988. Also available at: http://www.nap.edu/books/0309038308/html/index.html. Accessed January 21, 2005.

6. US Department of Health and Human Services. *Healthy People 2000: National Health Promotion and Disease Prevention Objectives, 1991.* Washington, DC: US Department of Health and Human Services; 1991.

7. US Department of Health and Human Services. *Healthy People 2010.* 2nd ed. With Understanding and Improving Health and Objectives for Improving Health. 2 vols. Washington, DC: US Government Printing Office; 2000. Also available at: http://www.healthypeople.gov/document. Accessed January 21, 2005.

8. American Medical Association. Medicine and public health initiative [AMA Web site]. Available at: http://www.ama-assn.org/ama/pub/category/3621.html. Accessed January 21, 2005.

9. National Highway Traffic Safety Administration. EMS Agenda for the Future [NHTSA Web site]. Available at: http://www.nhtsa.dot.gov/people/injury/ems/agenda/emsman.html. Accessed January 21, 2005.

10. National Highway Traffic Safety Administration. EMS Agenda for the Future: Implementation Guide [NHTSA Web site]. Available at: http://www.nhtsa.dot.gov/people/injury/ems/agenda. Accessed January 21, 2005.

11. McCaig LF, Burt CW. National hospital ambulatory medical care survey: 2001 emergency department summary. *Advance Data from Vital and Health Statistics.* No. 335, June 4, 2003. Available at: http://www.cdc.gov/nchs/data/ad/ad335.pdf. Accessed January 21, 2005.

12. Lewin ME, Altman S, eds. *America's Healthcare Safety Net; Intact but Endangered.* Washington, DC: National Academies Press; 2000.

13. Hegner RE. The healthcare safety net in a time of fiscal pressures. Paper presented at: George Washington University, DC: National Health Forum; April 2001; Washington, DC. Available at: http://www.nhpf.org/pdfs/bkgr/1-110+(SafetyNet_4-01).pdf. Accessed September 12, 2001.

14. Chassin MR, Galvin RW, and the National Roundtable on Health Care Quality. The urgent need to improve health care quality. *JAMA.* 1998;280(11):1000–1005.

15. Committee on Quality of Health Care in America, Institute of Medicine. *Crossing the Quality Chasm: A New Health System for the 21st Century.* Washington, DC: Institute of Medicine, National Academies Press; 2001. Also available at: http://www.nap.edu/books/0309072808/html/. Accessed September 26, 2001.

16. Kohn LT, Corrigan JM, Donaldson MS, eds. *To Err Is Human. Building a Safer Health System.* Washington, DC: National Academies Press; 2000.

17. Dunford J, Domeier RM, Blackwell T, et al. Performance measurements in emergency medical services. *Prehospital Emerg Care.* 2002;6(1):92–98.

18. Pollock DA, Lowery DW, O'Brien PM. Emergency medicine and public health: new steps in old directions. *Ann Emerg Med.* 2001;38:675–683.

19. Spaite DW, Criss EA, Valenzuela TD, et al. Developing a foundation for the evaluation of expanded-scope EMS: a window of opportunity that cannot be ignored. *Ann Emerg Med.* 1997;30:791–796.

20. Bissell RA, Seaman KG, Bass RR, et al. Change in the scope of practice of paramedics? An EMS/public health policy perspective. *Prehospital Emerg Care.* 1999;3(2):140–149.

21. Bissell RA, Seaman KG, Bass RR, et al. A medically wise approach to expanding the role of paramedics as physician extenders. *Prehospital Emerg Care.* 1999;3(2):170–173.

22. Barthell EN, Cordell WH, Moorhead JC, et al. The frontlines of medicine project: a proposal for the standardized communication of emergency department data for public health uses including syndromic surveillance for biological and chemical terrorism. *Ann Emerg Med.* 2002;39:422–429.

23. Kinnane JM, Garrison HG, Coben JH, et al. Injury prevention: is there a role for out-of-hospital EMS? *Ann Emerg Med.* 1997;4:306–312.

24. Garrison HG, Foltin GL, Becker LR, et al. The role of EMS in primary injury prevention. *Ann Emerg Med.* 1997;30:84–91.

25. Gerson LW, Schelble DT, Wilson JE. Using paramedics to identify at-risk elderly. *Ann Emerg Med.* 1992;21(6):688–691.

26. Krumperman KM. Filling the gap: EMS social service referrals. *JEMS.* 1993;18(2):25–29.

27. Jaslow D, Ufberg J, Ukasik J, et al. Routine carbon monoxide screening by emergency medical technicians. *Acad Emerg Med.* 2001;8(3):288–291.

28. Crash Injury Research and Engineering Network. NHTSA Web site. Available at: http://www-nrd.nhtsa.dot.gov/departments/nrd-50/ciren/CIREN.html. Accessed September 27, 2001.

29. Wofford JL, Heuser MD, Moral WP, et al. Community surveillance of falls among the elderly using computerized EMS transport data. *Am J Emerg Med.* 1994;12:433–437.

30. Shankar BS, Dischinger PC, Cowley RA. The evolution of injury prevention and surveillance at MIEMSS. *Md Med J.* 1988;37:565–570.

31. Harrawood D, Gunderson MR, Fravel S, et al. Drowning prevention; a case study in EMS epidemiology. *JEMS.* 1994;19(6):34–41.

32. Minall GL. Wounded by violence: can a KISS make it better? *JEMS.* 1994;19:61–68.

33. Weiss SJ, Ernst AA, Phillips J, et al. Visits to home environments by emergency medical services: a statewide study. *Prehospital Emerg Care.* 2001;5(1):19–22.

34. Hsiao AK, Hedges JR. Role of the emergency medical services system in region wide health monitoring and referral. *Ann Emerg Med.* 1993;22:1696–1702.

35. Hauer JM. Preparing for biological terrorism: the New York City model. Paper presented at: the Western Regional Conference on Bioterrorism: The Medical and Public Health Response; February 3–5, 2000; San Diego, Calif.

36. McIntosh BA, Hinds P, Giordano LM. The role of EMS systems in public health emergencies. *Prehospital Disaster Med.* 1997;12(1):30–35.

37. Chan TC, Vilke GM, Bender S. Effect of a multidisciplinary community homeless outreach team on emergency department visits by homeless alcoholics [abstract]. *Acad Emerg Med.* 2001;8(5):486.

38. Purdle F, Honigman B, Rosen P. The chronic emergency department patient. *Ann Emerg Med.* 1981;10(6):298–301.

39. Chi CH, Lee HL, Wang SM, et al. Characteristics of repeated ambulance use in an urban emergency service system. *J Formos Med Assoc.* 2001;100(1):14–19.

40. Okin R. The effects of clinical case management on hospital use among ED frequent fliers. *Ann Emerg Med.* 2000;18(5);603–608.

41. Akhter M. 4th annual CJ Shanaberger memorial lecture and keynote address. Presented at: National Association of EMS Physicians Annual Meeting; January 6, 2000; Dana Point, Calif.

42. Baker EL. The AAMC/CDC partnership: linking academic medicine and public health. *Acad Med.* 2001;76(9):866–867.

43. Koplan JP. The AAMC and CDC as strategic partners: why? and why now? *Acad Med.* 2000;75:406–407.

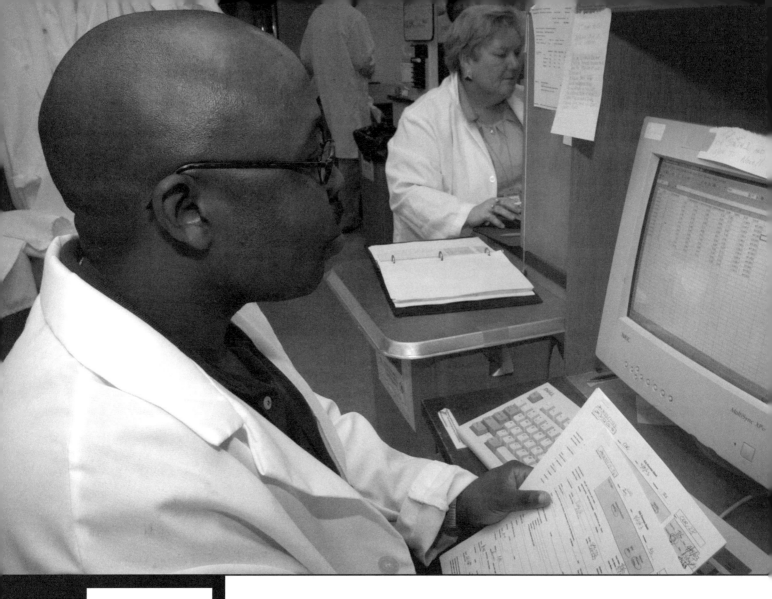

22 Research

Marianne Gausche-Hill, MD, FAAP, FACEP
Roger J. Lewis, MD, PhD, FACEP

Principles of This Chapter

After reading this chapter, you should be able to:

- Explain the basics of clinical research, including the research question, statistical concepts and methodology, informed consent, institutional review board evaluation, data collection and analysis, study monitoring, and results dissemination.
- List the six Ds of outcome measurement.
- Describe the challenges in conducting EMS research.
- Recall the categories and aspects of research design.

ORGANIZED EMS SYSTEMS HAVE BEEN IN EXISTENCE FOR more than 30 years.[1] Procedures, protocols, and medical interventions used in EMS systems have largely been adapted from emergency departments. These adaptations have not always worked as effectively as hoped in the out-of-hospital setting, where the environment is relatively uncontrolled and where patients must be transported, sometimes over long distances, for definitive care. The purpose of out-of-hospital research, therefore, is to find what works in the out-of-hospital setting.

Conducting research in the out-of-hospital setting is challenging for a number of reasons, including uncontrolled environmental factors, heterogeneous patient populations, variation in provider knowledge and skill, geographic issues, difficulty in obtaining informed consent, and difficulty in maintaining compliance with study protocols by a large number of study participants. Although there are many challenges, conducting well-designed clinical trials in the out-of-hospital setting is imperative if we are to improve the effective-ness of out-of-hospital emergency care. Because of their training and involvement in the administration and medical directorship of EMS systems, emergency physicians have a critical role in the design and implementation of clinical trials in the out-of-hospital setting.

This chapter will describe the basics of clinical research design, including discussions on choosing the research question, statistical concepts and methodology, obtaining informed consent, and institutional review board (IRB) evaluation, and will outline the logistical challenges in implementation of out-of-hospital research.

Components of a Research Project

The design and implementation of a research project can be divided into a number of components. These components will vary based on the complexity of the study. However, some basic parts make up most projects. These components include:

- **Developing the research question.** Selecting a good research question requires clinical experience, knowledge of the relevant literature, and the ability to define an important clinical question in terms of measurable variables.
- **Formulating the null and alternative hypotheses.** This is the process of translating the research question into statements that can be statistically evaluated using the data to be collected.
- **Designing the study.** Based on knowledge of possible research designs, consultation with other EMS and research experts, and accounting for logistical challenges, the investigator must select a research design for the study.
- **Seeking IRB approval for the study.** Approval and oversight help ensure protection of the human subjects involved in the study. It is a requirement if the results are to be published in a peer-reviewed journal.
- **Developing infrastructure for the study.** Required personnel might include an oversight committee, data collection personnel, data entry personnel, clerical support, EMS consultants (paramedics, EMTs, administrators, and others), and a data safety monitoring committee. Required equipment might include patient care supplies, computers, and database and statistical software.
- **Developing data collection instruments or case report forms.** Development of these

forms might sound easy, but it is not. It is important to involve experts in the development of the study forms. A definition for each data field must be created, along with data entry limits and value checks to reduce errors.

- **Implementing the study and collecting data.** Study participants must be educated with respect to the study protocol, patient entry criteria, patient exclusion criteria, and data field definitions. Study investigators must always be available to answer questions that come up during the course of the study. Rates of patient enrollment, the quality of collected data, and patient outcomes and safety should be continually monitored during the course of the study.
- **Analyzing the data.** This is a critical step in all research projects. Analyzing the data requires a close collaboration between study investigators and statisticians to ensure the data are being analyzed appropriately.
- **Assessing the results of the study.** Before any dissemination of study results, the study investigators, statisticians, and other consultants should meet to discuss the results obtained. This is important to ensure that all who report the data carry the same message about the study results and to avoid confusion.
- **Reporting the results.** Results can be disseminated by submitting abstracts for presentation at scientific meetings, giving reports of results to EMS agency committees, and, most importantly, by preparing a manuscript for publication in a peer-reviewed journal. However, widespread dissemination of study results before journal publication can make subsequent journal publication more difficult.

The Question

A good research question has the following characteristics:

- It is original, not previously studied. A conclusive answer to the question would result in a substantial change in the practice or administration of out-of-hospital care.
- It can be stated in terms of measurable outcomes.
- It can be answered using a study design that is practical in terms of logistics, financial resources, available personnel, available patient population, and projected duration.
- It is ethical and within the investigator's expertise.

- Its answer is likely to lead to other important research.

Ensuring that a research question is original requires thoroughly reviewing the literature to determine if it has been answered in the past and, if so, evaluating the previous study design and results to determine if further research in this area is warranted. Helpful Internet resources for literature and information review are listed in **Table 22-1.**

The next step in evaluating a question is to determine its importance in the practice of out-of-hospital care. Sometimes a simple question such as "Do soft collars provide better stabilization than no collar for transporting patients with potential cervical spine injury?" is potentially very important because, in this case, adequate methods for spinal immobilization are important to the everyday practice of out-of-hospital care.[2]

A good research question must also be stated in terms of outcomes that can be defined and measured. It also must be answerable using a study design that is within the capabilities of the investigators and, if possible, lead to other good research questions.

Hypothesis Testing

The research question must be stated in the form of a hypothesis that can be statistically evaluated.[3-5] The **null hypothesis** states that the treatment and control groups are not different with respect to the outcome being measured. In our example of a study of soft collar immobilization of the cervical spine, the null hypothesis would be that there is no difference in the frequency of complications of cervical spine injury in patients immobilized with a soft collar and a spinal board compared to those immobilized on a spinal board alone. (We are not claiming that either method is the current out-of-hospital standard of care. In general, however, the control treatment should be the current standard of care.) The **alternative hypothesis** is that the treatment has an effect on measured outcome; in this case, the effect is on the frequency of cervical spine injury complications occurring during out-of-hospital care. A statistical test is then used to determine whether the observed data from the study are consistent with the null hypothesis (**Figure 22-1**). The process of testing the null hypothesis involves determining the probability of obtaining the results observed in the study, *or* results more inconsistent with the null hypothesis, if the null hypothesis were true. This statistical probability is called the *P* value. If the *P* value is below some predetermined value (*A*), usually 0.05, then the null hypothesis is rejected as false.[3,4] If $P > 0.05$, then the null hypothesis is accepted as true.

Table 22.1   Resources for literature and information review.

Resource	Web site
Academic Emergency Medicine	http://www.aemj.org/
American Academy of Pediatrics (AAP)	http://www.aap.org/
American College of Emergency Physicians (ACEP)	http://www.acep.org/
Annals of Emergency Medicine	http://www.elsevier.com Follow "Journals" link to alpha list of journal titles.
Center for Pediatric Emergency Medicine	http://www.cpem.org/
Circulation	http://circ.ahajournals.org/
Emergency Medical Services for Children	http://www.ems-c.org/
Journal of the American Medical Association (JAMA)	http://jama.ama-assn.org/
JEMS [Journal of Emergency Medical Services] *Magazine*	http://www.jems.com/jems/
The Journal of Emergency Medicine	http://www.elsevier.com Follow "Journals" link to alpha list of journal titles.
Journal of Trauma	http://www.jtrauma.com/
Library of the National Medical Society	http://www.medical-library.org/library.htm
National Association of EMS Physicians (NAEMSP)	http://www.naemsp.org/
National Library of Medicine	http://www.nlm.nih.gov/
New England Journal of Medicine	http://www.nejm.org/
Pediatric Education for Prehospital Professionals	http://www.peppsite.com/
Pediatric Emergency Care	http://pec-online.com/
Journal of Prehospital and Disaster Medicine	http://pdm.medicine.wisc.edu/
Prehospital Emergency Care	http://www.elsevier.com Follow "Journals" link to alpha list of journal titles.
Society for Academic Emergency Medicine (SAEM)	http://www.saem.org/

The magnitude of the difference defined by the alternative hypotheses should be determined before beginning the study. This difference is usually the minimum difference that the investigators believe would be clinically significant, meaning that such a difference would warrant a change in clinical practice. The size of the difference defined by the alternative hypothesis is a principal determinant of the sample size required for the study. Because reliably detecting a small difference between groups requires a large sample size, investigators may choose an alternative hypothesis that defines a larger difference between the groups so that the trial can be completed with the available resources. In our example, the sample size calculations would take into account the rate of cervical spine injury, the difference in the rate of complications defined by the alternative hypothesis, the *P* value defined as statistically significant, and the desired power of the study.[4] **Power** is defined as the probability of detecting a treat-

ment effect equal to that defined by the alternative hypothesis. The power of a study should be 0.80 at a minimum; 0.95 is preferred. The required sample size can often be determined from published tables or by using commercially available software.[6]

Statistical hypothesis testing can lead to erroneous conclusions. There are two types of errors commonly considered: a **type I error** and a **type II error**. A type I error occurs when the investigator finds a difference between groups (ie, obtains $P < 0.05$) when no difference actually exists. The risk of a type I error, if there really is no difference between the groups, is equal to the maximum *P* value considered to be statistically significant (α). A type II error occurs when there is a difference between the groups as big or bigger than that defined by the alternative hypothesis but the study does not find such a difference (ie, $P > 0.05$). Type I errors can be considered **false-positive results** and type II errors **false-negative results**. The chance of a type II

Define the null and alternative hypotheses:

The null hypothesis is that there is no difference between the study groups with respect to the measured variable of interest.

The alternative hypothesis is that there is a difference between the groups, and it is of a defined size and is in the measured variable of interest.

↓

Calculate a *P* value or determine the difference between the groups (eg, raw difference, relative risk, odds ratio) and the associated confidence interval:

A *P* value is the probability of obtaining the data observed in the study or results more inconsistent with the null hypothesis if the null hypothesis were true.

The best statistical measure of the difference between the groups will depend on the type of study and the type of data being collected.

A 95% confidence interval is the range of possible values of the true treatment difference that is statistically consistent with the actual study results.

↓

Accept or reject the null hypothesis:

The null hypothesis is accepted if the *P* value is greater than the specified cutoff, or *P* > α, or when the 95% confidence interval includes no difference.

The null hypothesis is rejected if the *P* value is < α, usually 0.05, when the 95% confidence interval includes a difference.

Figure 22-1 Hypothesis testing and confidence intervals.

Table 22.2	Definitions of statistical terms.
Term	**Definition**
α	The maximum *P* value to be considered statistically significant; the risk of committing a type I error if the null hypothesis is true.
β	The risk of committing a type II error if the alternative hypothesis is true.
Type I error	Obtaining a statistically significant *P* value when, in fact, there is no effect of the studied treatment on the measured variable of interest; a false-positive result.
Type II error	Not obtaining a statistically significant *P* value when, in fact, there is an effect of the treatment on the measured variable of interest that is as large or larger than the effect the trial was designed to detect; a false-negative result.
P value	The probability of obtaining results similar to those actually obtained, or results more inconsistent with the null hypothesis, if the null hypothesis were true.
Power	The probability of detecting a treatment effect (ie, obtaining $P < \alpha$) if a true treatment effect exists equal to that defined by the alternative hypothesis. Power = 1- β.

Adapted from Lewis RJ. An introduction to the use of interim data analyses in clinical trials. *Ann Emerg Med.* 1993;22:1463–1469.

Table 22.3	Types of data.
Type of Data	**Definition**
Nominal or categorical	Values fall into unordered categories (eg, sex, race, or ethnicity).
Ordinal	Values fall into categories that have an inherent order. Differences between adjacent values are not quantifiable (eg, Likert scales).
Discrete	Values fall into specific categories with defined magnitudes. Differences have precise values (eg, the number of times a woman has given birth — two times is greater than one time and the difference between one and two births is the same as between three and four births).
Continuous	Data that represent actual numerical values. Values can be expressed as fractions (eg, weight, blood pressure, and time intervals).

error, when the difference defined by the alternative hypothesis truly exists, is equal to (1-power) denoted as β (**Table 22-2**).[3-5,7]

The type of statistical test used to calculate a *P* value depends on the characteristics of the data being analyzed (**Table 22-3**) and the number of groups being compared.[4] **Table 22-4** is a list of common statistical tests.[7]

Confidence Intervals

Although a *P* value gives information on whether the null hypothesis should be rejected, it does not provide an estimate of the magnitude of the difference between groups. A confidence interval, in contrast, provides the range of values that is statistically consistent with the study results.[8-10] The observed difference is statistically significant if the 95% confidence interval does not contain the value indicating no difference between the groups. For example, in studies in which proportions are being compared, an **odds ratio** might be used to measure the difference between the groups. The probabil-

Table 22.4	Statistical tests.
Statistical Test	**Description**
Student t test	Used to test whether the means of measurements from two groups are equal, assuming that the data are normally distributed and that the data from both groups have equal variance.
Wilcoxon rank sum test (Mann-Whitney or U test)	Used to test whether two sets of observations have the same median. These tests are similar in use to the t test, but they do not assume the data are normally distributed.
χ^2 test (chi-square test)	Used with categorical variables (two or more nominal treatments with two or more nominal outcomes) to test the null hypothesis that there is no effect of treatment on outcome. The χ^2 test assumes at least five expected observations in each combination of treatment and outcome under the null hypothesis.
Fisher exact test	Used in an analogous manner to the χ^2 test, the Fisher exact test can be used even when fewer than five observations are expected in one or more combinations of treatment and outcome.
One-way ANOVA (analysis of variance)	Used to test the null hypothesis that three or more sets of continuous data have equal means, assuming the data are normally distributed and that the data from all groups have equal variances. The one-way ANOVA can be thought of as a t test for three or more groups.
Kruskal-Wallis test	A nonparametric test analogous to the one-way ANOVA. No assumption is made regarding normality of the data. The Kruskal-Wallis test can be thought of as a Wilcoxon rank sum test for three or more groups.

Adapted from Young KD, Lewis RJ. Medical literature and evidence-based medicine. In: Marx JA, Hockberger RS, Walls RM, et al, eds. *Rosen's Emergency Medicine: Concepts and Clinical Practice.* 5th ed. St Louis, Mo: Mosby; 2002:2665. Copyright 2002, with permission from Elsevier.

ity of an event happening divided by the probability of the event not happening is known as the **odds** of an event. The odds ratio is equal to the odds of an event occurring in one group divided by the odds of the event occurring in the other group.[9] An odds ratio of 1 implies that the event is equally likely to occur in one group as the other, equivalent to the null hypothesis of no difference. For example, in a clinical trial comparing endotracheal intubation to bag-mask ventilation in children, survival rates were 26% in the endotracheal intubation group and 30% in the bag-mask ventilation group, yielding an odds ratio of 0.82.[11] The value of the odds ratio less than 1 indicates the lower survival rates in the experimental (endotracheal intubation) group, but the associated 95% confidence interval was 0.62 to 1.22. This implies that any odds ratio between 0.61 and 1.22 is consistent with the study results. Because the 95% confidence interval includes 1, the null hypothesis, one must conclude that there is no statistically significant difference in the survival rates of pediatric patients treated with bag-mask ventilation and those treated with endotracheal intubation.[11]

The Six Ds of Outcome Measurement

It is very important to identify and select meaningful and measurable outcomes. The most meaningful outcomes are those that measure whether an intervention resulted in a sustained change in life status for the patient, such as death, disability, or change in the quality of life. Such outcomes are ultimately what the patient and the patient's family care about. The six Ds of outcome measurement, as commonly defined in health services research, are death, disability, disease, discomfort, dissatisfaction, and destitution.[12] Although these have been described as the most important outcomes, very few published out-of-hospital studies have used one of these major outcomes.[12,13]

Researchers often collect data on the *process* of care under the assumption that the process of care has had an impact on patient outcome. Out-of-hospital researchers might be motivated to find outcome measures more proximate to the out-of-hospital care episode, and therefore easier to measure than long-term outcomes, or there might be a desire to use outcomes that are not influenced by differences in inpatient care between hospitals. These **process-of-care outcomes** could include out-of-hospital care time intervals, pulse oximetry measurements, success and complications of a procedure, minutes to CPR, or blood pressure on arrival to the emergency department. Although these variables might be important in some settings, it is not clear that they are meaningful out-of-hospital outcomes. For example, it is possible to have a group of trauma patients in which systolic blood pressure values are improved (eg, with the use of an antishock garment) and yet observe that a greater fraction of the patients die. The challenge for the researcher is to choose an outcome that is likely to reflect the intervention being evaluated and that is also a marker for change in long-term health status.

Categories of Research Design

Research designs used in out-of-hospital research can be divided into three main categories: retrospective, prospective, and interventional.[7,14]

In **retrospective** studies, data from one or more pre-existing sources are used to address specific research questions. The possible sources of information vary in the type and quality of data collected and might include EMS report forms (out-of-hospital patient care records), inpatient medical records, outpatient clinic notes, coroner's reports, trauma registry information, or hospital discharge data. These studies range from simple chart reviews, used to answer simple research questions, to complex analysis of administrative or national databases with thousands of records. Retrospective studies might also be used to determine the incidence of various diseases and injuries in the out-of-hospital setting, for example, the frequency and type of EMS calls for children.[15] Some of the advantages of retrospective studies are:

- They often do not require prospective written informed consent (IRB approval should always be sought before initiating such a study, however).
- They are relatively quick because the primary data collection has already occurred.
- They are relatively inexpensive to implement and can be often accomplished by one person.[7,16]

There are disadvantages as well, including:

- There is wide variability in the quality of the available data because of the lack of predefined criteria for recorded variables.
- The researcher cannot control for confounding variables that affect outcome.
- There might be missing and/or biased information.[7,16]

Consider a study of the use of high-dose versus low-dose epinephrine in the care of adults and children in cardiopulmonary arrest. You identify the sample population from EMS report forms for all patients in cardiopulmonary arrest over a 2-year period. You then record information on whether patients received no epinephrine, whether they received high-dose or

low-dose epinephrine (based on agreed-on definitions), and whether they had return of circulation in the field or in the emergency department. Whatever results are obtained regarding the association between the epinephrine dose and the return of circulation, the investigator must understand the limitations of this methodology to adequately answer the research question. There might be unmeasured or unanticipated factors that influenced which patients were given epinephrine, and at what dose. Possible factors include patient age, proximity to an emergency department, and the EMS provider's estimate of the likelihood of survival. Younger patients might also be less likely to have an intravenous line established in the field, and therefore be less likely to receive epinephrine. Even if an association between epinephrine dose and outcomes is found, you should still wonder whether the results are a reflection of the effects of epinephrine on survival, or whether there are other explanations for the differences in outcome, such as differences in age or prognosis among patients receiving the different treatments.

Furthermore, many of the EMS records might be missing important variables that could have affected outcome, such as down time, whether citizen CPR was performed, and presenting rhythm. Even more important, the pattern of missing information might not be random. Out-of-hospital personnel are less likely to record interventions or attempts at interventions if they are unsuccessful. Such informative censoring of information can severely bias the results of a study, and statistical analyses cannot adjust for such bias. One group of investigators conducting a retrospective study of the use of succinylcholine in the field to facilitate pediatric intubation was forced to discard almost 50% of the cases because of inadequate documentation.[17]

Prospective studies can be **observational** or **interventional**.[7] In a prospective observational study, patients are identified by preselected criteria and then followed to a preselected point in their care. These studies are sometimes called **cohort studies** because a defined group, or cohort, of patients is being followed. A prospective observational study conducted by Loffredo et al identified trauma patients in the out-of-hospital setting based on their presenting blood pressures and then followed these patients to discharge from an acute care hospital. Outcomes such as death, disability, and need for therapeutic surgery were measured, and a conclusion was drawn regarding the association between out-of-hospital hypotension and patient outcome.[18]

Interventional studies must be prospective and can be further divided into **controlled or uncontrolled studies.** If controlled, the study will be **randomized** or **nonrandomized.**[7] In an **uncontrolled interventional study**, all of the study patients receive the experimental treatment or intervention, and then preselected outcomes are measured. An example would be a single-armed study of out-of-hospital endotracheal intubation for patients in cardiopulmonary arrest, using survival as the primary outcome. Although the study results might show a high rate of survival in patients receiving the intervention, there is no way to know how those particular patients would have done with bag-mask ventilation or some other alternative airway management. In other words, a control group is lacking. The use of historical controls is not an adequate solution; the use of such controls has been shown to be unreliable, generally overestimating the effect of the treatment.[7,19]

In a **controlled clinical trial**, some of the study patients receive the experimental treatment or intervention, and the others receive standard treatment (**Figure 22-2**). Patients are prospectively identified and then assigned to treatment groups. Examples of controlled clinical trials in the out-of-hospital setting are the immediate versus delayed fluid resuscitation for hypotensive patients with penetrating torso injuries[20] and the pediatric airway management study.[11,21] In the pediatric airway management study, pediatric patients (with predefined selection criteria) identified as requiring out-of-hospital airway management were assigned to either the endotracheal intubation group or the bag-mask ventilation group based on calendar day of patient entry. Patients were then followed to discharge from an acute care hospital. Patient survival status and neurologic outcome were the primary and secondary endpoints, respectively. The study group was the endotracheal intubation group and the control group was the bag-mask ventilation group. This study could be conducted only because previous studies of the two treatments did not identify a superior therapy, ie, endotracheal intubation and bag-mask ventilation were both considered acceptable therapies for support of ventilation in the pediatric age group. In an interventional controlled trial, it would be unethical for the treatment group to receive a known superior therapy in order to ensure a positive effect on the outcome to be measured.[22,23]

There are many examples of randomized trials in the out-of-hospital setting. Brazier et al[24] and Sayre and Gausche-Hill[25] have reviewed the major randomized trials conducted in the out-of-hospital setting since 1991 and described many different randomiza-

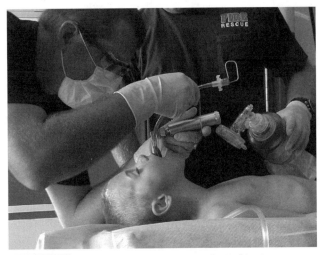

Figure 22-2 One example of a controlled clinical trial in the out-of-hospital setting is the pediatric airway management study,[11,21] which evaluated the effect of endotracheal intubation and bag-mask ventilation on patient outcome.

tion methodologies used. The best method for randomizing patients is to first identify the patient to be included and then to randomly assign that patient to one of the treatment groups. This method gives the out-of-hospital provider no opportunity to influence the treatment group assignment and reduces potential bias. Although this is the best method for randomization, it might not always be practical in trials in which the institution of lifesaving therapy should not be delayed. In these circumstances, a less rigorous randomization scheme or a pseudorandom allocation might be used, such as odd-even calendar day or even-odd medical record numbers.[25] The goal of randomization, regardless of the method used, is to equalize the number and types of patients in the treatment groups to ensure that the only systematic difference between the groups is the intervention itself.

Choosing a study design requires that the investigators consider logistic and cost constraints. Prospective interventional trials are the most difficult to implement because of the need to inform all out-of-hospital care providers of the study protocol before initiating the study, and they are more costly because of the need for dedicated staff to train providers and collect data.

Out-of-hospital research has been characterized by a lack of rigorous study design and limited consideration of different patient outcomes. Brice et al,[13] in a 10-year review of out-of-hospital research published in 2000, evaluated 285 studies. They found that case series represented 44% of the studies, and only 15% were randomized trials. Overall, 53% of the studies were retrospective. Death and the frequency of disease were the outcomes most often measured; other outcomes, such as disability and discomfort, were infrequently measured.

Callaham,[26] in a review of all randomized trials in out-of-hospital care published in 1997, found only 54 randomized trials in EMS since 1985, and that EMS controlled trials represented only 2% of the total number of randomized controlled trials on major emergency medicine topics, including myocardial infarction, cardiac arrest, trauma, and stroke.

Why are there so few controlled trials in EMS? The reason is difficult to ascertain, but the following are certainly factors[27-29]:

- Lack of qualified out-of-hospital investigators with training in research design
- Special logistic challenges, including large number of out-of-hospital providers enrolling patients, lack of supervision of out-of-hospital care, multiple potential receiving hospitals for patients, and difficulty with linkage of out-of-hospital and inpatient data
- Hesitance on the part of funding agencies to support out-of-hospital research
- Lack of time and personnel to obtain informed consent
- Poor understanding of the importance of conducting high-quality EMS research by out-of-hospital providers
- Problems in translating results of research into clinical practice

Relationship of the Topic to Logistic Issues

All emergency physicians must be able to read the medical literature critically; those pursuing clinical research as part of their practice must understand the basics of statistical methods and research design.[3,7] In 1992, a collaborative group that included the Resident Research Curriculum Subcommittee, the Research Fellowship Curriculum Subcommittee, and the Curriculum Subcommittee of the Research Committee for the Society for Academic Emergency Medicine assembled to develop research goals and objectives for residents and fellows in emergency medicine. The group believed that residents in emergency medicine should understand the following topics as part of their residency training:

- Study critique
- Hypothesis generation and testing
- Study design and methodology
- Consent
- Basic statistics

Figure 22-3 Topic areas for a model research curriculum.[30]

Overview
Reading the literature
Study design
Study planning and implementation
Animal research
Ethics of research
Statistical analysis
Manuscript writing
Presentation skills
Grants and funding issues

- Computer applications
- Ethics in research
- Manuscript preparation and presentation

A model research curriculum was also proposed (**Figure 22-3**). It is a nice outline of topic areas to be covered for residents, fellows, and practicing emergency physicians who want to pursue a career in research.

Once a foundation of knowledge of research design and statistical methodology is established, the emergency physician, nurse, or paramedic will find that answering important questions in EMS requires collaboration with other experts in the field of emergency medicine research. The question might be easy to ask, but the methodology to answer the question often requires consultation with statisticians, academic-based researchers, or research center staff, such as those at the **National EMSC Data Analysis Resource Center (NEDARC)**. These experts have years of experience in research design and implementation, logistics of a clinical trial, and access to resources such as IRBs.

Using Statistical Consultants

Most investigators who are experienced in clinical or out-of-hospital research use statistical consultants to help them design their studies and analyze the resulting data. Statistical consultants often have extensive and diverse research experience and, based on this experience, might be able to anticipate potential difficulties in study design, data collection, and analysis that can be addressed before valuable time and effort are wasted.

The first step in using a statistical consultant is to find one. Statistical consultants can be found in local universities or medical schools, most commonly within departments of statistics, biostatistics, epidemiology, or public health. In addition, many large research groups have in-house statistical consultants who help them with study design, data management, and statistical analyses. Because most out-of-hospital research is relatively simple from a statistical and methodological point of view, it is more important that the statistical consultant have practical, real-world experience with medical research rather than being up-to-date on the newest and most sophisticated statistical methods.

Before the first meeting with the statistical consultant, the investigator should try to define the most important question to be answered by the proposed study in terms of quantifiable outcomes (eg, rate of survival to hospital admission or response time). If the study is comparative, it is important to define the minimum difference in the primary outcome the study should be designed to detect (the minimum clinically significant treatment effect). Next, the investigator should consider the likely outcomes in the control group. Predicting the likely outcomes in the control group, especially the variability in the data (eg, the standard deviation of response times), is necessary for the consultant to perform a sample size and power calculation. The statistical consultant will also need to know the desired power for the study and the maximum number of patients that could realistically be enrolled given time and resource constraints. If the proposed treatment effect size and desired power would require too many patients, the investigator should be prepared to discuss whether a lower power is acceptable, or whether it would be better to design the study to reliably detect only a larger treatment effect.[3,4]

The investigator should also consider whether there are important subgroups within the study population. For example, patients in medical cardiopulmonary arrest can be divided into important subgroups according to the initial rhythm or whether the arrest was witnessed. If there are clinically important subgroups that should be considered separately, the investigator should be prepared to identify the variables that define those subgroups.[31,32]

It is also important to consider whether there are multiple comparisons that will be conducted, such as comparing the treatment group outcomes in two or more important subgroups, or comparing more than one primary outcome between the different treatment groups. As a general rule, it is better to design a study with a single primary outcome so that corrections for multiple comparisons will not be required. Other potentially important comparisons should be considered as secondary outcomes.[33-38]

The investigator should also consider whether it would be feasible to conduct planned interim analyses of accumulating data during the course of the study to determine whether the study can be stopped early and a reliable conclusion drawn from the available in-

formation. Interim analyses are extremely important in protecting human subjects from unanticipated harm during comparative therapeutic studies.[39]

Finally, it is extremely useful to find examples of published studies similar to the proposed study that illustrate the type of statistical analysis the investigator wants the statistician to perform once the study is complete. Such published studies often include useful graphics or tables the statistician can use as a guide when preparing tables and figures for the final manuscript.

Informed Consent in the Out-of-Hospital Setting

All out-of-hospital research must be reviewed and approved by an IRB before study implementation. This is the process that ensures protection of human subjects. There are several issues related to obtaining informed consent in the out-of-hospital setting.

As a beginning, it is important to understand the ethical underpinnings of the requirement for consent for participation in research in the usual inhospital, nonemergency setting.[40] Regulations govern the protection of human subjects in the United States, but the ethical considerations cross all geographic borders.

A pivotal point in the development of protection for human research subjects was the publication of the **Belmont report**,[41] which elucidated three principles on which the protections should be based. These principles are respect for persons, beneficence, and justice. **Respect for persons** implies that each individual should have autonomy to make decisions regarding his or her own participation in research studies; subjects with reduced autonomy (eg, patients with altered mental status or minors) deserve special protection. A competent adult or a competent emancipated minor may make decisions regarding his or her own participation. Family members or other parties, regardless of their apparent good intentions, cannot take on this decision-making role for someone else who has decision-making capacity.[41]

Beneficence implies that participation in the research should have the potential to benefit either the individual participant or the class of subjects from which the participant is drawn, and the risks of the research should be minimized to the extent possible. If the research entails significant risk, participation is appropriate only if the patient himself or herself might benefit from participating (eg, a trial of a new implantable device that is potentially lifesaving). When the research entails less risk, participation might be appropriate if the knowledge to be gained has the potential to benefit an entire class, such as children or patients suffering with a particular disease.[41]

Justice implies that the population that participates in the research should also be the population that will benefit from the results. For example, it is not appropriate to test a new intervention in one location in the country or in one socioeconomic group when the benefits of the research will be applied only in another area or in another group. Similarly, it is not appropriate to test a therapy that is likely to be expensive and available to a privileged few in a population of medically indigent patients that happens to be the predominant population at the local county medical center.[41]

The exercise of autonomy (respect for persons) and the communication of potential risks and benefits (beneficence) traditionally occur during the process of obtaining prospective written informed consent. It is important to understand that consent is a *process*, not a written document. Although specific items of information must generally be present in the written informed consent document, the potential research subject must be given an opportunity to review the document; the key points should be explained orally to the patient in terms he or she understands, and the patient should be given the opportunity to discuss any concerns and to have any questions answered. An informed consent document, even when signed and witnessed, has no ethical or legal merit if the patient did not have time to adequately read it, did not understand its contents, or did not have an opportunity to have his or her questions answered.

Informed Consent Document

The elements required in an informed consent document are defined in federal regulations.[42,43] These regulations state, in part, that the information provided to each patient will include:

(1) A statement that the study involves research, an explanation of the purposes of the research and the expected duration of the subject's participation, a description of the procedures to be followed, and identification of any procedures which are experimental; (2) A description of any reasonably foreseeable risks or discomforts to the subject; (3) A description of any benefits to the subject or to others which may reasonably be expected from the research; (4) A disclosure of appropriate alternative procedures or courses of treatment, if any, that might be advantageous to the subject; (5) A statement describing the extent, if

any, to which confidentiality of records identifying the subject will be maintained and that notes the possibility that the Food and Drug Administration may inspect the records; (6) For research involving more than minimal risk, an explanation as to whether any compensation and an explanation as to whether any medical treatments are available if injury occurs and, if so, what they consist of, or where further information may be obtained; (7) An explanation of whom to contact for answers to pertinent questions about the research and research subjects' rights, and whom to contact in the event of a research-related injury to the subject; and (8) A statement that participation is voluntary, that refusal to participate will involve no penalty or loss of benefits to which the subject is otherwise entitled, and that the subject may discontinue participation at any time without penalty or loss of benefits to which the subject is otherwise entitled.[42]

Depending on the circumstances, there are additional, optional elements that might be required,[42,43] including additional information on risks, information on events that might result in termination of the subject's participation, any costs associated with participation in the research, procedures to be followed if the subject chooses to withdraw from the study, an assurance that any new relevant medical information will be communicated to the subject, and the number of subjects to be included in the study.

Elements of informed consent can be communicated in written form or, in some circumstances,[42,44] might be provided orally. In light of federal regulations, the IRB approving the proposed research determines whether written informed consent is required, or whether oral consent is appropriate.

Waiver of Informed Consent Requirements

Current federal regulations allow a narrow exception to the general requirement for prospective informed consent for the case of subjects participating in studies of therapies for emergent, life-threatening, and unexpected conditions that incapacitate them, making it impossible for them to participate in the process of prospective informed consent.[45,46] Examples of such conditions would include severe closed-head injury, respiratory failure, cardiopulmonary arrest, cerebrovascular emergencies, and major trauma.[47] Because patients incapacitated by sudden and unexpected illnesses represent a vulnerable population, they are given special protections in accordance with the principles of the Belmont report (respect for persons).[41] These additional protections are defined in the federal regulations and include consultation with community representatives, public disclosure of the planned research, public disclosure of the results of the study when it is complete, and the establishment of an independent data monitoring committee.[45,48-54]

The **emergency exception** to the requirement for informed consent is applicable only if the human subject is in a life-threatening situation, available treatments are unproven or unsatisfactory, or the collection of valid scientific evidence through a randomized placebo-controlled investigation is required to determine safety and effectiveness. The exception also applies if obtaining prospective informed consent is not feasible because the patient is incapacitated by the condition, the intervention must be administered before a legally authorized representative can be found, and there is no reasonable way to prospectively identify an individual before he or she is affected by the condition in question. Other exceptions are as follows: participation in the research might directly benefit the subject; the study cannot be practicably carried out without the waiver; there is a defined therapeutic time window, and, during that time, the investigator makes attempts to contact a legally authorized representative to seek prospective informed consent; and the IRB has reviewed and approved an informed consent procedure and document for use in those cases in which it is feasible.[40,45,46,50]

In order to initiate a study using a waiver of informed consent, the investigators, in cooperation with their IRB, must participate in processes of community consultation and public disclosure of the planned research. **Community consultation** is a process by which the research is discussed with representatives of the community in which the research will be conducted and from which the subjects will be obtained in order to obtain their views on the appropriateness of the research and the appropriateness of conducting the research without obtaining prospective informed consent from the subjects. Community consultation is a two-way dialogue. The community representatives *do not* provide surrogate consent for the ultimate subjects in the trial but, instead, provide the IRB with information on community sensibilities regarding the appropriateness of the proposed study.[50-52]

Public disclosure is a broader, one-way dissemination of information regarding the proposed research. The purpose of public disclosure is to ensure that potential subjects in the study and other members of the community in which the study will be performed are informed of the investigators' intent to conduct the re-

search. Public disclosure can be conducted through newspaper articles, other advertisements or flyers, over the radio, and so on.[45,50,53,54]

When planning either community consultation or public disclosure, it is important to ensure that the particular population to be studied is targeted. For example, when planning a study that is likely to involve elderly patients suffering medical cardiopulmonary arrest, it would be important to ensure that elderly patients in nursing homes, in board and care facilities, and living alone are contacted during the process of community consultation. In addition, when performing public disclosure, it would be important to ensure that the methods are effective in reaching the target population.

Studies using a waiver of informed consent must also have an independent **data monitoring committee** oversee the research.[45] The purpose of a data monitoring committee is to monitor the study progress and the accumulating data. The committee should also ensure that the study is terminated as soon as possible if a reliable conclusion can be drawn from the available data; if the research is futile, meaning that it is unlikely to yield useful information; or if the risks of participating in the study appear larger than originally anticipated. The structure and function of data monitoring committees is beyond the scope of this chapter, although many useful references are available.[55-67]

Development of an Infrastructure

The development of an infrastructure to support the implementation of a clinical trial is quite important. This infrastructure includes an organizational structure to manage all personnel related to the project, such as investigators, consultants, data gatherers, and those necessary for implementation. A committee structure, which, at a minimum, consists of a steering committee with representatives vested in the project, should be established. The steering committee is composed of study investigators, out-of-hospital provider agency directors, out-of-hospital providers, local EMS agency representatives, a statistician, and local physician experts. The steering committee oversees the study implementation and assists in problem-solving when difficulties arise. For controlled clinical trials, a larger committee structure might be necessary. A more extensive committee structure was developed for the pediatric airway management project (**Figure 22-4**).[21]

Study investigators are also responsible for providing feedback on the study developments to all study participants. This feedback can be provided at local

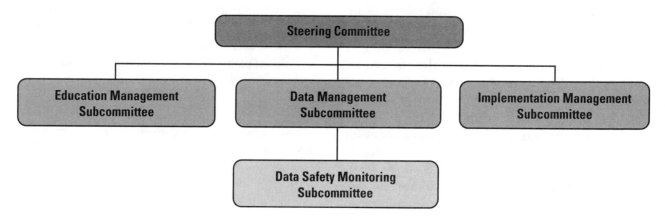

Figure 22-4 Committee structure for a controlled clinical trial in pediatric airway management. From Gausche-Hill M, Lewis RJ, Gunter CS, et al. Design and implementation of a controlled trial of pediatric endotracheal intubation in the out-of-hospital setting. *Ann Emerg Med.* 2000;36(4):356–365. Reprinted with permission.

committee meetings or through project or EMS agency newsletters, continuing education offerings, or Web sites or e-mail.

Monitoring Research

There are many ways an investigator can monitor the progress of the research project. The goals of monitoring vary depending on the research methodology but typically include overseeing rate of subject accrual, ensuring that all patients who qualify for the study are being entered into the study, ensuring that study procedures are being followed, monitoring patients for adverse events, and conducting planned interim data analyses. These goals can be achieved by going into the field and observing study procedures on a periodic basis, by being available to answer questions from out-of-hospital providers entering patients, and by gathering data on rates of patient accrual. They also can be achieved by working with quality improvement coordinators to evaluate the cases being entered into the study and ensuring that all cases that qualify are entered, by following all patients closely during and after their participation, and by working with a statistician to perform the planned interim analyses.

Funding Research

One of the most challenging aspects of research is getting it funded. The first step is to develop a solid project with sound research methodology, qualified investigators, and appropriate safety assurances. The next step is to identify possible funding agencies to submit the project for consideration of funding. There are many agencies, both private and public, that support research efforts. **Figure 22-5** is a list of some of these agencies. University-based researchers can also obtain information from their grants and contracts offices. Finally, it is important to begin the process of obtaining funding as early as possible to allow time for the application and review process, which can take more than a year.

Figure 22-5 Research funding agencies.

Local and national foundations
Corporate sponsors:
- Pharmaceutical companies
- Device manufacturers

State agencies (ie, federal block grant funds)
University-based medical centers and schools of medicine
Federal agencies:
- Agency for Healthcare Research and Quality
- Centers for Disease Control and Prevention
- Department of Defense
- Health Resources and Services Administration
- Maternal and Child Health Bureau
- National Fire Academy
- National Highway Traffic Safety Administration
- National Institutes of Health

Research Presentation and Publication

Once the research has been completed, it is important that the results be shared with the EMS community so that others can learn from the research project. Dissemination of results completes the research process.

Research results can be disseminated in several ways, most commonly in oral and written presentations. Most academic emergency medicine organizations, including SAEM, ACEP, NAEMSP, AAP, and state and local medical professional societies and organizations, hold periodic research forums to which the research project can be submitted for consideration for oral or poster presentation. Each of those organizations solicits requests for presentations and outlines the requirements that must be met in terms of content, structure, and organization. The abstracts for these presentations often will be included in the publication or proceedings from the specific meeting or will be published in the organization's journal. Some organizations accept presentations with the stipulation that the final manuscript will be submitted for publication in the organization's official journal (although a guarantee of acceptance is not made; the manuscript must be subjected to the same peer-review process as all other submissions).

There are several professional journals to which EMS-related research can be submitted for consideration for publication. In particular, *Annals of Emergency Medicine, Prehospital Emergency Care,* and *Academic Emergency Medicine* actively solicit EMS articles. Each of these peer-reviewed journals has specific submission requirements and processes for review and acceptance. The reviewers and members of the editorial boards of these journals are particularly knowledgeable and experienced in EMS research. In addition to peer-reviewed journals, there are several EMS trade journals that are not peer reviewed to which research can be submitted for publication.

Summary

Answering important questions in EMS will lead to future research. Increasing the number of qualified researchers who can implement controlled trials is a necessary step to improve the science of out-of-hospital emergency care. With the proliferation of researchers, additional studies will be performed, which can help evaluate the interventions, process of care, and educational methods used in out-of-hospital care.

Conducting well-designed clinical trials in the out-of-hospital setting requires training and preparation, collaboration and teamwork, and the willingness to dedicate significant time and energy over a prolonged period of time. Emergency physicians can have a vital role in EMS research by serving as research investigators, collaborators, EMS medical directors, and EMS administrators. Ultimately, the maturation of EMS depends on the integration of results of clinical trials into evidence-based, out-of-hospital practice.

References

1. Boyd DR, Edlich RF, Micik SH. *Systems Approach to Emergency Medical Care.* Norwalk, Conn: Appleton-Century-Crofts; 1983.

2. Podolsky S, Baraff LJ, Simon RR, et al. Efficacy of cervical spine immobilization methods. *J Trauma.* 1983;23: 461–465.

3. Lewis RJ, Bessen HA. Statistical concepts and methods for the reader of clinical studies in emergency medicine. *J Emerg Med.* 1991;9:221–232.

4. Pagano M, Gauvreau K, eds. *Principles of Biostatistics.* Belmont, Calif: Wadsworth Publishing Company; 1993.

5. Kelen GD, Brown CG, Ashton J. Statistical reasoning in clinical trials: hypothesis testing. *Am J Emerg Med.* 1988;6:52–61.

6. Fleiss JL, ed. *Statistical Methods for Rates and Proportions.* New York, NY: John Wiley & Sons; 1981.

7. Young KD, Lewis RJ. Medical literature and evidence-based medicine. In: Marx JA, Hockberger RS, Walls RM, et al, eds. *Rosen's Emergency Medicine: Concepts and Clinical Practice.* 5th ed. St Louis, Mo: Mosby; 2002: 2658–2672.

8. Young KD, Lewis RJ. What is confidence? Part 1: the use and interpretation of confidence intervals. *Ann Emerg Med.* 1997;30:307–310.

9. Young KD, Lewis RJ. What is confidence? Part 2: detailed definition and determination of confidence intervals. *Ann Emerg Med.* 1997;30:311–318.

10. Simon R. Confidence intervals for reporting results of clinical trials. *Ann Intern Med.* 1986;105:429–435.

11. Gausche M, Lewis RJ, Stratton SJ, et al. Effect of out-of-hospital pediatric endotracheal intubation on survival and neurological outcome: a controlled clinical trial. *JAMA.* 2000;283:6:783–790.

12. Maio RF, Garrison HG, Spaite DW, et al. Emergency medical services outcomes project I: prioritizing conditions for outcomes research. *Ann Emerg Med.* 1999;33:423–432.

13. Brice JH, Garrison HG, Evans AT. Study design and outcomes in out-of-hospital emergency medicine research: a ten-year analysis. *Prehospital Emerg Care.* 2000;4: 144–150.

14. Meinert CL. *Clinical Trials: Design, Conduct, and Analysis.* New York, NY: Oxford University Press; 1986.

15. Seidel JS, Henderson DP, Ward P, et al. Pediatric prehospital care in urban and rural areas. *Pediatrics.* 1991;88:691–690.

16. Stapczynski JS. Conducting prehospital research. In: Roush WR, ed. *Principles of EMS Systems.* 2nd ed. Dallas, Tex: American College of Emergency Physicians; 1994:433–449.

17. Brownstein DR, Shugerman R, Cummings P, et al. Prehospital endotracheal intubation of children by paramedics. *Ann Emerg Med.* 1996;28:34–39.

18. Loffredo AJ, Gausche M, Brueske PJ, et al. Field hypotension in trauma patients is an independent predictor of the need for emergent therapeutic surgery. *Acad Emerg Med.* 1997:4:348.

19. Sacks H, Chalmers TC, Smith H. Randomized versus historical controls for clinical trials. *Am J Med.* 1982;72:233–240.

20. Bickell WH, Wall MJ, Pepe PE, et al. Immediate versus delayed fluid resuscitation for hypotensive patients with penetrating torso injuries. *N Engl J Med.* 1994;331:1105–1109.

21. Gausche-Hill M, Lewis RJ, Gunter CS, et al. Design and implementation of a controlled trial of pediatric endotracheal intubation in the out-of-hospital setting. *Ann Emerg Med.* 2000;36(4):356–365.

22. Edwards SJ, Lilford RJ, Hewison J. The ethics of randomised controlled trials from the perspectives of patients, the public, and healthcare professionals. *BMJ.* 1998;317:1209–1212.

23. Passami E. Clinical trials — are they ethical? *N Engl J Med.* 1991;324:1589–1592.

24. Brazier H, Murphy AW, Lynch C, et al, on behalf of the Ambulance Response Time Sub-Group of the National Ambulance Advisory Committee. Searching for the evidence in pre-hospital care: a review of randomised controlled trials. *J Accident Emerg Med.* 1999;16(1):18–23.

25. Sayre MR, Gausche-Hill M. Conducting randomized trials in the prehospital setting. *Prehospital Emerg Care.* 2002;6(suppl 2):S38–S47.

26. Callaham M. Quantifying the scanty science of prehospital emergency care. *Ann Emerg Med.* 1997;30:785–790.

27. National Highway Traffic Safety Administration, Maternal and Child Health Bureau. National EMS research agenda [NHTSA Web site]. Available at: http://www.nhtsa.dot.gov/people/injury/ems/EMS03-ResearchAgenda/home.htm. Accessed January 22, 2005.

28. Heller MB, Melton JB, Kaplan RM, et al. Data collection by paramedics for prehospital research. *Ann Emerg Med.* 1988;17:414–415.

29. Warnke WJ, Bonnin MJ. Direction and motivation of prehospital personnel to do research: how to do it better. *Prehospital Disaster Med.* 1992;7:79–83.

30. Cline D, Henneman P, Van Ligten P, et al. A model research curriculum for emergency medicine. *Ann Emerg Med.* 1992;21:184–192.

31. Yusuf S, Wittes J, Probstfield J, et al. Analysis and interpretation of treatment effects in subgroups of patients in randomized clinical trials. *JAMA.* 1991;266:93–98.

32. Oxman AD, Guyutt GH. A consumer's guide to subgroup analysis. *Ann Intern Med.* 1992;116:78–84.

33. O'Brien PC, Shampo MA. Statistical considerations for performing multiple tests in a single experiment; 1: introduction. *Mayo Clin Proc.* 1988;63:813–815.

34. O'Brien PC, Shampo MA. Statistical considerations for performing multiple tests in a single experiment; 2: comparison among several therapies. *Mayo Clin Proc.* 1988;63:816–820.

35. O'Brien PC, Shampo MA. Statistical considerations for performing multiple tests in a single experiment; 3: repeated measures over time. *Mayo Clin Proc.* 1988;63:918–920.

36. O'Brien PC, Shampo MA. Statistical considerations for performing multiple tests in a single experiment; 4: performing multiple statistical tests on the same data. *Mayo Clin Proc.* 1988;63:1043–1045.

37. O'Brien PC, Shampo MA. Statistical considerations for performing multiple tests in a single experiment; 5: Comparing two therapies with respect to several endpoints. *Mayo Clin Proc.* 1988;63:1140–1143.

38. O'Brien PC, Shampo MA. Statistical considerations for performing multiple tests in a single experiment; 6: Testing accumulating data repeatedly over time. *Mayo Clin Proc.* 1988;63:1245–1250.

39. Lewis RJ. An introduction to the use of interim data analyses in clinical trials. *Ann Emerg Med.* 1993;22:1463–1469.

40. Fish SS. Research ethics in emergency medicine. *Emerg Med Clin North Am.* 1999;17:461–474.

41. US Department of Health, Education, and Welfare, The National Commission for the Protection of Human Subjects of Biomedical and Behavioral Research. The Belmont report: ethical principles and guidelines for the protection of human subjects of research [National Institutes of Health Web site]. Available at: http://ohsr.od.nih.gov/guidelines/belmont.html. Accessed January 22, 2005.

42. 21 CFR §50.25.

43. 45 CFR §46.116.

44. 45 CFR §46.117.

45. 21 CFR §50.24.

46. Department of Health and Human Services. Waiver of informed consent requirements in certain emergency research. 61 *Federal Register* 51531 (1996).

47. Sloan EP, Koenigsberg M, Houghton J, et al, for the DCLHb Traumatic Hemorrhagic Shock Study Group. The informed consent process and the use of the ex-

ception to informed consent in the clinical trial of di-aspirin cross-linked hemoglobin (DCLHb) in severe traumatic hemorrhagic shock. *Acad Emerg Med.* 1999; 6:1203–1209.

48. Biros MH, Runge JW, Lewis RJ, et al. Emergency medicine and the development of the Food and Drug Administration's final rule on informed consent and waiver of informed consent in emergency research circumstances. *Acad Emerg Med.* 1998;5:359–368.

49. Passamani ER, Weisfeldt ML. Task force 3; special aspects of research conduct in the emergency setting: waiver of informed consent. *J Am Coll Cardiol.* 2000;35:862–880.

50. Biros MH, Fish SS, Lewis RJ. Implementing the Food and Drug Administration's final rule for waiver of informed consent in certain emergency research circumstances. *Acad Emerg Med.* 1999;6:1272–1282.

51. Baren JM, Anicetti JP, Ledesma S, et al. An approach to community consultation prior to initiating an emergency research study incorporating a waiver of informed consent. *Acad Emerg Med.* 2000;6:1210–1215.

52. Kremers MS, Whisnant DR, Lowder LS, et al. Initial experience using the Food and Drug Administration guidelines for emergency research without consent. *Ann Emerg Med.* 1999;33:224–229.

53. Alpert S. Implementing the final rule. *Acad Emerg Med.* 2000;6:1188–1189.

54. Santora TA, Cowell V, Trooskin SZ. Working through the public disclosure process mandated by use of 21 CFR 50.24 (exception to informed consent): guidelines for success. *J Trauma.* 1998;5:907–913.

55. Armstrong PW, Furberg CD. Clinical trial data and safety monitoring boards: the search for a constitution. *Circulation.* 1995;91:901–904.

56. Dixon DO, Lagakos SW. Should data and safety monitoring boards share confidential interim data? *Control Clin Trials.* 2000;21:1–6.

57. Freidlin B, Korn EL, George SL. Data monitoring committees and interim monitoring guidelines. *Control Clin Trials.* 1999;20:395–407.

58. Friedman LM, Furberg CD, DeMets DL. Monitoring response variables. In: *Fundamentals of Clinical Trials.* 3rd ed. New York, NY: Springer-Verlag; 1998.

59. Korn EL, Simon R. Data monitoring committees and problems of lower-than-expected accrual or events rates. *Control Clin Trials.* 1996;17:526–535.

60. Meinert CL. Masked monitoring in clinical trials — blind stupidity? *N Engl J Med.* 1998;338:1381–1382.

61. Fleming TR, Harrington DP, O'Brien PC. Designs for group-sequential tests. *Control Clin Trials.* 1984;5: 348–361.

62. Geller NL, Pocock SJ. Interim analyses for randomized clinical trials: ramifications and guidelines for practitioners. *Biometrics.* 1987;43:213–223.

63. Lan KKG, Simon R, Halperin M. Stochastically curtailed tests in long-term clinical trials. *Communications in Statistics; Sequential Analysis.* 1982;1:207–219.

64. O'Brien PC, Fleming TR. A multiple testing procedure for clinical trials. *Biometrics.* 1979;35:549–556.

65. Pocock SJ. Interim analyses for randomized clinical trials: the group sequential approach. *Biometrics.* 1982;38: 153–162.

66. Pocock SJ. When to stop a clinical trial. *BMJ.* 1992;305: 235–240.

67. Lewis RJ, Berry DA, Cryer H III, et al. Monitoring a clinical trial conducted under the Food and Drug Administration regulations allowing a waiver of prospective informed consent: the diaspirin cross-linked hemoglobin traumatic hemorrhagic shock efficacy trial. *Ann Emerg Med.* 2001;38:397–404.

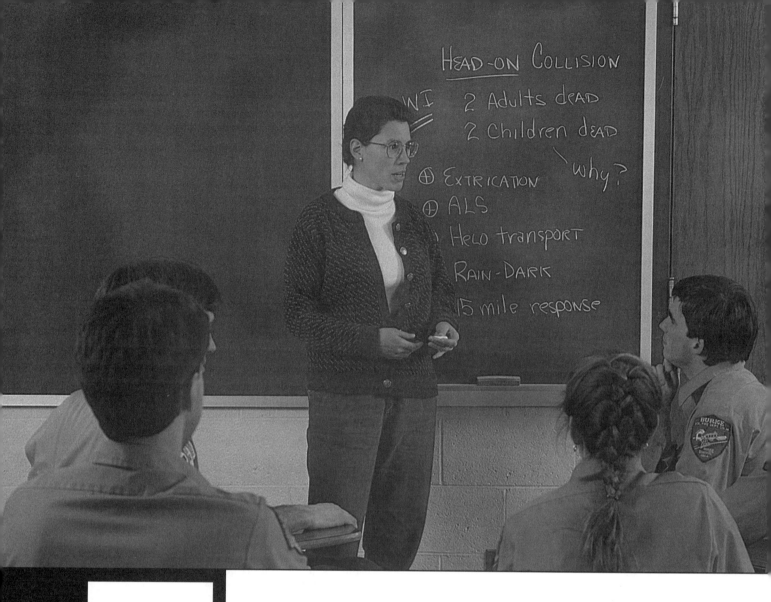

23

EMS Education Programs

Daniel L. Storer, MD, FACEP

Principles of This Chapter

After reading this chapter, you should be able to:

- Describe the components of the national "EMS Education Agenda for the Future," such as core content, scope of practice, standards, program accreditation, and certification.
- Explain the characteristics of an EMS education program, including sponsorship, medical oversight, administrative policies and procedures, evaluation, and curriculum.

IN ANY FIELD OF ENDEAVOR, EDUCATION IS ESSENTIAL TO the success of the final product. The provision of EMS is no exception. Emergency medical services are provided under the auspices and involvement of physician medical directors. Therefore it is essential that physicians be actively involved in the education process for all levels of EMS personnel.

Before standard EMS curricula were established in the 1970s, most EMS education courses were conducted by pioneering EMS physicians seeking to extend themselves through their students. Then, with the proliferation of education programs following the development of national standard curricula, physician involvement diminished to the point of being nonexistent at some levels. The lack of physician involvement was most notable with the first responder and EMT-Basic levels. However, more recently, the need for medical oversight in the development and implementation of education programs at all levels has been acknowledged.[1]

EMS Agenda for the Future

In August 1996, the "EMS Agenda for the Future" was published by the National Highway Traffic Safety Administration (NHTSA).[2] This project was supported by NHTSA and the Health Resources and Services Administration, Maternal and Child Health Bureau. It provides a vision for out-of-hospital EMS, including education issues. Recommendations within this document related to education include a standard that all EMS education be conducted with the benefit of qualified medical directors. The physician medical director should be involved in all aspects of education program planning, presentation, and evaluation, including evaluation of faculty and students.[2] The agenda has formed the basis of many of the planning activities that have occurred in EMS since then, including those related to education issues.

EMS Education Agenda for the Future: A Systems Approach

In September 1999, NHTSA released the "EMS Education Agenda for the Future: A Systems Approach."[3] This document provides a vision for the future of EMS education with an improved system structured to educate the next generation of EMS professionals. It was developed by a task force representing the full range of professionals involved in EMS education, including EMS administrators, physicians, regulators, educators, and providers. The proposed education system has five integrated primary components, as follows:

- A national EMS core content
- A national EMS scope-of-practice model
- National EMS education standards
- National EMS education program accreditation
- National EMS certification

A critical aspect of the EMS education agenda is that all of these components are interrelated and depend on each other to varying extents. One component cannot be considered without the other components. All components come together to complete the entire EMS education spectrum (**Figure 23-1**).

The **national EMS core content**, released in early 2004, describes the entire domain of out-of-hospital emergency medical care. It is important to understand that not all components of the core content will be appropriate for all EMS personnel or in all EMS systems. The purpose of the core content is to define what is potentially appropriate and not appropriate for the out-of-hospital environment by dependently licensed

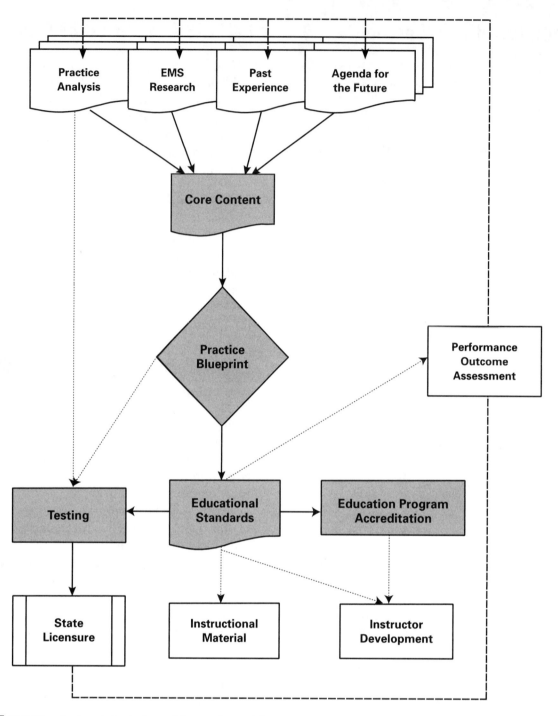

Figure 23-1 EMS Education Agenda for the Future: A Systems Approach.[3]

care providers. The national EMS core content includes a schedule and the methods for updating core content components. This will obviate the need to revisit the medical appropriateness of each procedure or cognitive domain when individual standards are revised. As a result of this framework, the architects of the other system components can focus on their specific areas of responsibility rather than on defining and redefin-

ing the overall domain of practice each time there is a revision of the curriculum.

The **national EMS scope-of-practice model** will drive the national education standards. Scope of practice defines the parameters of various duties and services that may be provided by an individual with specific credentials. Whether by rule, statute, or court decision, it tends to represent the limits of services an individual may perform. EMS education programs most commonly face this differentiation with the following levels of EMS practice: first responder, EMT-Basic, EMT-Intermediate, and EMT-Paramedic. This practice model will define, by name and by function, the levels of out-of-hospital EMS providers based on the national EMS core content. The national EMS scope-of-practice model, rather than the curricula, will drive the scope of practice and national provider level nomenclature and establishment of the entry-level competencies for each level of provider. With this model, there will be considerable flexibility in designing EMS education programs. It is expected that the scope of practice will be completed and released to the EMS community in 2005.

The **national EMS education standards** will define terminal learning objectives for each EMS provider level. **Terminal learning objectives** include desired educational endpoints of understanding, psychomotor skill capability, and behavior appropriate for the level of EMS professional that students must achieve by the end of the education program. These education standards will be updated regularly and will serve as a basis for the development of detailed declarative instructional materials and lesson plans. Publishers, education institutions, instructors, and others will develop these materials. The national EMS education standards will be published in the national EMS education document, but the detailed declarative education materials will not; publishers and educators will develop these. With the instructional system developed in this manner, a greater variety of lesson plans will be available. The national EMS education standards will encourage enhanced flexibility for instructors, allowing multiple instructional methods while maintaining consistency of learning objectives.

National EMS education program accreditation will provide the greater assurance of quality and national consistency in both the process and outcomes of EMS education. **Accreditation** is defined as a nongovernmental, independent, collegial process of self-assessment and peer assessment. The purpose of accreditation is to provide a system of public accountability and continual improvement of academic quality. EMS education program accreditation represents a method to assure students and the community that the education program meets uniform, nationally accepted standards. Accreditation review includes assessment of structure, process, and most important, outcomes of the education program. Accreditation stimulates self-assessment and encourages self-improvement. It promotes sound educational change and provides institutions with validation to obtain the resources they need to improve. The essential values of accreditation are continual self-improvement, professional excellence, peer review and collaboration, and civic responsibility.

National EMS education program accreditation is the major mechanism for verifying education program quality for the protection of students and the public by ensuring the entry-level competence of EMS providers as they complete their education and enter the field. The EMS education agenda suggests that all students must graduate from an accredited program.

National EMS certification, along with national EMS education program accreditation, will provide greater assurance of quality and national consistency of EMS education and EMS providers. **Certification** is the process of verifying personnel competency at a predetermined level of proficiency.

National EMS certification should be conducted by one independent national agency composed of a board of directors with multidisciplinary representation. Having one certification agency will provide a consistent evaluation of recognized EMS provider entry-level competencies. Certification examinations should be based on nationally recognized standards and a practice analysis. A nationally recognized, validated, and reliable examination should be used by all state EMS agencies as a basis for state licensure. This national EMS certification will not replace a state's right to license but would be used as a component of eligibility for licensure to practice within that state. It also should allow for greater flexibility and reciprocity when EMS personnel move to other states.

The proposed EMS education agenda system will align the primary responsibilities for developing and maintaining current standards for each component with the appropriate content experts (eg, physicians, regulators, and educators) while recognizing that the entire system is a fully cooperative effort among many EMS personnel with diverse backgrounds. The EMS education agenda describes an interdependent relationship among the five system components and recommends specific lead groups for development and revision responsibilities. The national EMS core content is based primarily on medical knowledge and will be led by the medical community, with input from system regulators, educators, and providers. The national EMS scope-of-practice model is fundamentally a system issue, with system regulators leading its development with input from other stakeholders. National EMS education standards represent an educational focus, with development coming primarily from EMS educators with input from other stakeholders.

With this systems approach, curriculum revision will be simpler. Changes can be made to one component without revising all components. This increases efficiency, consistency of instruction quality, and student competence by prescribing a high degree of structure, coordination, and interdependence among the five components.[3]

Role of the EMS Education Program Medical Director

The physician medical director of an EMS education program is responsible for all of the medical aspects of the program and must commit an adequate amount of time to ensure the success of the program. The medical director should review and approve the education content of the program curriculum to certify its ongoing appropriateness and medical accuracy. To do this, the medical director should review and approve the quality of medical instruction, supervision of instruction, and evaluation of the students in all areas of the program. The medical director should review and approve the progress of each student throughout the program and help develop appropriate corrective measures when a student does not show adequate progress. The medical director should attest to the competence of each graduate of the program in the cognitive, psychomotor, and affective domains.

The physician medical director should establish a cooperative interaction with the program director. The medical director can delegate responsibilities to associate medical directors as appropriate. However, the medical director must have adequate controls to ensure the outcome quality resulting from the delegated responsibilities. For example, the medical director might delegate lab station audit to an assistant medical director. The medical director would remain responsible for the process, even though another physician is performing the task. The final authority would rest with the medical director.

Qualifications of the EMS Education Program Medical Director

To optimize medical oversight of EMS education programs, the physician medical director should be qualified as follows:

- A physician licensed to practice medicine who has current knowledge of emergency care of acutely ill and injured patients
- Adequately trained or experienced in the delivery of out-of-hospital emergency care, including the proper care and transport of patients, medical direction, and quality improvement

- An active member of the local medical community who participates in professional activities related to out-of-hospital care
- Knowledgeable about the education of EMS professionals, including related legislative and regulatory issues

Authority

A written agreement or contract defining the job description and authority of the physician medical director should be established. Unless otherwise defined or limited by state or local requirements, the physician medical director for EMS education programs should have full authority over all clinical and patient care aspects of the program, including the authority to:

- Determine the appropriate medical care content of courses provided and ensure that the content meets or exceeds the national standard curricula
- Set or approve minimum education and ethical standards for potential students
- Ensure the competency of personnel who provide instruction in patient care
- Ensure the adequacy of cognitive knowledge evaluation
- Ensure the adequacy of clinical and field internship experiences and evaluations
- Access all relevant records necessary to validate student competency and fitness for patient care activities
- Remove a student from a course for reasons related to inadequate knowledge, clinical ability, or suitability using an appropriate review and appeals mechanism
- Recommend certification and recertification of students to the appropriate certifying agencies

Program Obligations

The EMS education program is obligated to provide the physician medical director with the resources and authority commensurate with his or her responsibilities, including the following:

- Appropriate compensation for the time required (as determined by local standards)
- Necessary material resources and personnel support
- Appropriate academic appointment, if applicable
- Liability insurance for duties or actions performed as physician medical director

- Written agreement or contract delineating the medical director's authority and responsibilities to the program and the program's obligations to the physician medical director

EMS Education Program Characteristics

Medical directors of EMS education programs should have a basic understanding of the characteristics typical of EMS education programs, as described in the following sections.

Sponsorship

EMS education has historically been provided in a variety of settings. The early programs were conducted primarily in a hospital setting that could provide both cognitive and psychomotor education. As the education for EMS providers has become more professional rather than technical, education institutions have become more important in the overall scheme of EMS education. Hospitals, however, are still critical components in the provision of clinical training. The ideal EMS education arrangement results from a close working relationship among an education institution, a hospital or hospitals, and a high-volume EMS agency.

The sponsoring institution (and affiliates, as appropriate) should be accredited by recognized agencies or meet equivalent standards for postsecondary education institution accreditation. The sponsoring institution and affiliates should be authorized under applicable law or other acceptable authority to provide a program of postsecondary education. EMS education programs should be designed to provide maximal opportunity for students to obtain formal academic credit and continue their formal education with minimal loss of time and duplication of learning experiences. Programs not offering associate's or bachelor's degrees are encouraged to establish articulation agreements with institutions that do to provide for maximal transfer capability of clinical and clinically related course work. Course work in general education, social sciences, and health sciences should parallel courses offered in colleges and universities.

Admission Policies and Procedures

Admission policies for students, including advanced placement, should be consistent with clearly defined and published practices of the institution. Any specific academic and technical standards required for admission to the program should be clearly defined and published. These should be readily accessible to prospective students and the public.

Evaluation of Students

Evaluation of students should be conducted on a recurring basis, often enough to provide both the student and the program faculty with valid and timely indicators of the student's progress toward achievement of the entry-level competencies. **Entry-level competencies** are the cognitive, psychomotor, and affective competencies that a newly graduated EMS provider would be expected to possess and are required for entry into the practice environment.

The methods used to evaluate students should be valid and reliable and should verify the achievement of the cognitive, psychomotor, and affective objectives stated in the curriculum. Evaluation methods should include direct assessment of student competency in all areas of clinical experience, including field and inpatient care environments.

Validity refers to how well the evaluation instrument focuses on the intended subject. **Reliability** is present when the results of one evaluation tool compare well with the results of another evaluation tool used for the same student. For example, written examination results should compare well with the evaluation instruments used in a skill station addressing the same medical problem.

The **cognitive domain** refers to the factual information learned from lectures, reading, and other sources. The **psychomotor domain** includes the skills portion of the education program. The **affective domain** encompasses the behavioral aspects of the student's education program.

Testing instruments and other evaluation methods should be reviewed frequently to ensure effectiveness. Quality improvement reviews should result in updates, revisions, and formulation of more effective test instruments or evaluation methods.

Program Evaluation

The program should have a system for ongoing review to make sure that the education program is achieving its stated goals and objectives and to illustrate that measured outcomes are consistent with national guidelines. Program evaluation methods should emphasize the gathering and analyzing of data on the program's success with regard to developing competencies that are consistent with stated program goals and objectives.

Program evaluation methods should include preparing timely self-study reports to help the staff, sponsoring institution, and accrediting agency assess program qualities and needs. The program should use a minimum of two valid and reliable measurements for each domain of learning to demonstrate that program goals and objectives are being met.

Outcomes

Programs should routinely secure sufficient qualitative and quantitative information regarding program graduates to demonstrate ongoing evaluation of outcomes. Sources of data should include, where appropriate, course completion, state licensing examination results, national registration, and job placement rates.

The community of interest consists of individuals or agencies that interface with the program's graduates, such as employers, EMS system administrators and medical directors, program directors, didactic instructors, skill laboratory instructors, hospital clinical instructors, and field internship instructors, and possibly even EMS consumers. This list is neither all-inclusive nor mandatory. Program officials might want to establish an advisory committee to assist in program development and review. The membership of the advisory committee should reflect the groups listed and the type of service provided by the EMS community, as well as the needs of the general community.

Curriculum

The goal of the program should be to produce competent, entry-level EMS professionals. Objectives should be measurable indicators of attainment of graduate success in competencies of the cognitive, psychomotor, and affective domains. Although no sequence of instruction is prescribed, the order of subject presentation and learning experiences should be based on a logical relationship between the basic and applied aspects of the didactic and clinical curriculum. Clinical instruction should begin early enough in the curriculum to allow maximal application of other subjects and to provide sufficient hands-on practice.

Accredited paramedic programs typically range from 1,000 to 1,300 clock hours, including the four integrated phases of education (didactic, laboratory, clinical, and field) to cover the stated curriculum (**Figure 23-2**). Further prerequisites and/or corequisites might be required to address competencies in basic health sciences such as anatomy and physiology and in the basic academic skills such as English and mathematics. Together with the core content of the EMT-Basic

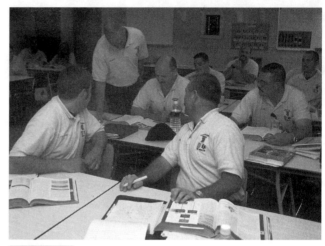

Figure 23-2 Accredited paramedic programs include the four integrated phases of education. The didactic phase includes lectures, reading, and other forms of cognitive learning.

training, the EMS-Paramedic professional's education might lead to an academic degree, typically an associate's or bachelor's.

Curriculum Content

The curriculum should be designed to ensure that the students acquire the knowledge and skills necessary to fulfill the entry-level competencies appropriate for the level of graduation. It should follow planned outlines and the appropriate sequence with lecture, laboratory, hospital, field clinical, and field internship experiences. The curriculum should include content that provides the basis for knowledge and skill development pertaining to the out-of-hospital emergency care of geriatric, adult, adolescent, and pediatric patients. Increasing focus is being placed on disaster management and issues of terrorism response. The curriculum content should be consistent with the current national education document.

Skills Laboratory

The skills laboratory content should include those portions of the curriculum that require psychomotor activity and learning. The labs provide an excellent opportunity for the medical director to interact directly with students.

Clinical Instruction

Clinical instruction should be aimed at developing entry-level competence in psychomotor skills and knowledge applicable to actual patient situations. It should provide adequate opportunity for patient contact to give students a foundation in clinical decision-making and role-modeling of professional attitudes. Clinical instruction should occur in both the hospital and field settings. The program should track the number of times each student successfully achieves each of the objectives. A suggested process involves tracking age, sex, complaints, pathologies, and interventions.

Field Internship

The field internship should verify that the student has achieved entry-level competence and is able to serve as team leader in a variety of out-of-hospital life-support emergency medical situations. The field internship should occur after the student has achieved the desired didactic and clinical competencies. Some less critical didactic material might be taught concurrently with the field internship.

The field internship is primarily limited to paramedic level training. It can exist at other levels of EMS training but is absent or abbreviated in most lower levels.

Challenges

Several challenges face EMS education. With the advent of satellite transmission of courses, Internet-based courses of instruction, and telemedicine over high-speed, high-quality phone lines, the demand for distance learning opportunities has increased. These education methods generally are appropriate for cognitive learning but problematic for skill labs, clinical training, and field internships. Some EMS education programs routinely send their clinical coordinators to the distant clinical and field internship sites to meet with clinical and field preceptors to ensure that the goals and objectives of the program are being met.

Another education challenge is the development of accreditation for all levels of EMS education programs. Much work will be focused on this area as the EMS education agenda is further implemented and education activities evolve.

Summary

The EMS education program medical director must be intimately involved in the education program to be able to attest to the entry-level competency of each graduate. This involvement is more than having the medical director's name on a program application or pharmacy license. The required involvement includes getting to know the students; verifying that the education is appropriate by reviewing the quality of instruction in the curriculum; and reviewing the laboratory, clinical, and field internship experiences. The medical director should be aware of any tracking system the program uses to ensure that each student meets the terminal objectives of the program. The medical director should attest to the entry-level competence of each graduating student by initialing or signing documentation that certifies that the student has met all of the terminal objectives of the education program.[4]

References

1. American College of Emergency Physicians, National Association of EMS Physicians. Physician medical direction of emergency medical services education programs [joint policy statement]. ACEP Web site. Available at: http://www.acep.org/1,639,0.html. Accessed January 23, 2005.

2. National Highway Traffic Safety Administration. EMS agenda for the future [NHTSA Web site]. Available at: http://www.nhtsa.dot.gov/people/injury/ems/agenda/emsman.html. Accessed January 23, 2005.

3. National Highway Traffic Safety Administration. EMS education agenda for the future: a systems approach [NHTSA Web site]. Available at: http://www.nhtsa.dot.gov/people/injury/ems/EdAgenda/final/. Accessed January 23, 2005.

4. Commission on Accreditation of Educational Programs for the EMS Professions. Standards and guidelines [CoAEMSP Web site]. Available at: http://www.coaemsp.org/standardspolicies.htm. Accessed January 23, 2005.

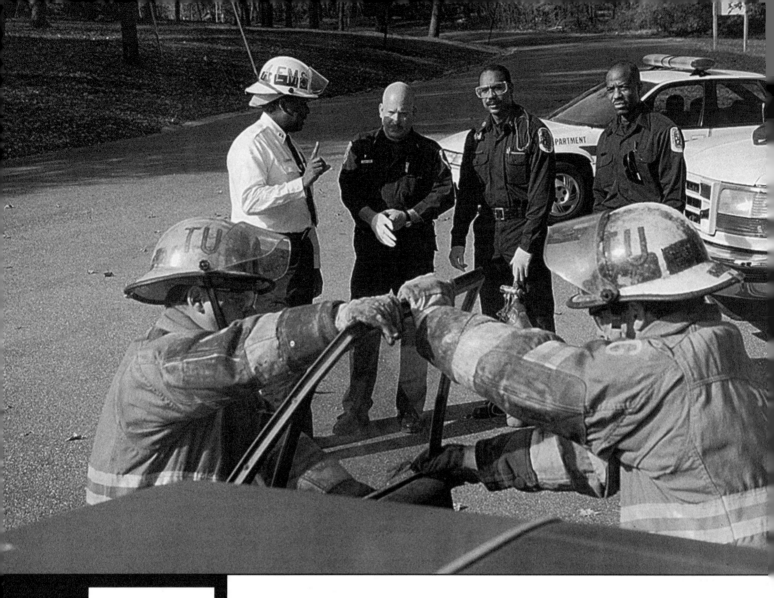

24

EMS Providers and System Roles

Michel A. Sucher, MD
Jennifer L. Waxler, DO, FACOEP, FACEP

Principles of This Chapter

After reading this chapter, you should be able to:

- Define the different types of EMS providers and describe their roles within the EMS system.
- Define the role of EMS medical directors.
- Define the role of higher education as it relates to increasing EMS professionalism.
- Describe career opportunities and work settings for EMS providers.
- Explain future challenges surrounding EMS manpower issues.
- Describe the role of EMS personnel and the EMS system in prevention, public health, community intervention, and disaster preparedness.
- Explain why the data generated from EMS research should drive the operation of the EMS system.

WHAT KIND OF PERSON CHOOSES EMS AS A CAREER? Is there a personality type that is drawn to EMS? Is that positive, negative, or both?

Most people who choose EMS as a career will say that the main reason for their choice is to help people and to make a difference. The personality of a person who chooses EMS is someone who is dedicated and committed and wants to help people. Other common traits include those who like excitement and are idealistic and self-motivated.

The work of EMS is often mundane and routine, but the excitement of the unknown and the potential for being in a heroic situation make EMS a calling, not just a job. As in most industries, those who will be most successful are well trained, have a sense of purpose, and truly like what they do. It is also helpful to have confidence, high self-esteem, and a strong ability to deal with stress.

In surveys, EMS providers consistently rank at the top of the most trusted and admired of all occupations.

But what will future EMS systems and providers look like? The development of the "EMS Agenda for the Future" began in 1992 by the National Association of EMS Physicians (NAEMSP) and the National Association of State EMS Directors (NASEMSD). The EMA agenda provided an overall vision for EMS as a "community-based health management system that is fully integrated with the overall health care system." The agenda encouraged the continued evaluation of the current EMS system and the development of steps for its improvement. This chapter embraces the work that has been done through this valuable process.

Types of EMS Providers

First Responders

The most basic field provider in EMS is the first responder. First responders undergo training that includes first aid and CPR. This training can be provided in a multiday course that exceeds 40 hours. In many states, the first responder is a certified position. First responders are used primarily as the initial responder, both in two-tiered urban EMS systems and in rural systems. They are critical in rural settings when higher-level providers are unavailable or have delayed response. They are trained in the operation of emergency vehicles and are used in some states as designated ambulance drivers.

EMT-Basic

The EMT-Basic (EMT-B) is the most common EMS field provider throughout the United States. They are the primary providers in BLS (basic life support) EMS systems. EMT-Bs undergo more than 120 hours of training. This includes first aid, CPR, basic trauma care, and extrication procedures. EMT-B training courses are commonly provided through EMS agencies or community colleges, with the local EMS system providing clinical and operational training. In most states, EMTs are certified.

In addition to the primary role of basic field provider, EMTs might also be employed in industry, emergency departments, and other settings requiring this level of training. This generally occurs outside of the state's EMS legislation and oversight system. The EMT-B level is a prerequisite to becoming an EMT-Intermediate or EMT-Paramedic.

There is a national EMT-B curriculum published by the National Highway Traffic Safety Administration (NHTSA) and adopted by most states. It outlines the various areas of training required for the EMT-B position.

EMT-Intermediate

The EMT-Intermediate (EMT-I) is the next level of EMS provider. The EMT-I position was originally envisioned to provide a response to the need for advanced providers in rural settings when paramedics were not available.

The training includes all training required of an EMT-B plus additional skills and knowledge established by the specific state. This might include advanced cardiac life support, including significant training in cardiac arrhythmias and in the administration of pharmacologic agents. The drug list authorized for the EMT-I varies by local protocol and might include 50% dextrose, epinephrine, and numerous cardiac medications. This list is not nearly as extensive as that allowed for paramedics.

The EMT-I is also trained in endotracheal intubation and intravenous line placement. The training ranges from 300 to 500 hours, above that of an EMT-B. Most states account for this level of provider with state certification.

Use of the EMT-I extends well beyond the originally intended rural setting. In some areas with shortages of paramedics, there are significant employment opportunities for the EMT-I.

EMT-Paramedic

Paramedics are the highest level of EMS provider and have truly provided the backbone of modern EMS care at the advanced life support (ALS) level. The EMT-Paramedic (EMT-P) (or EMT-Advanced) undergoes 750 to 1,500 hours of training beyond the EMT-B level. Becoming a paramedic generally requires a year or more of EMT-B field experience. Training as a paramedic lasts 1 to 2 years. States generally certify paramedics, although licensure is becoming more prevalent.

Paramedics are trained extensively in pharmacology and the administration of emergency medications. This includes training to establish intravenous access, both peripheral and central. Paramedics receive training in advanced airway management, including oral and nasal intubation and cricothyrotomy. Paramedics also receive more advanced training in trauma, pediatrics, and geriatrics.

Paramedics are used as the initial responders in some EMS systems, and in others are second-tier responders. This varies among systems. Paramedics work under close medical oversight with standing orders or online medical direction, or both. Historically, paramedics were the only EMS personnel who worked under medical oversight. Based on the national "EMS Agenda for the Future," all levels of providers are now expected to work under medical oversight. (See Chapter 6, "Medical Oversight and Accountability.")

Critical Care Paramedics

There is a relatively new level of provider known as critical care paramedic. Critical care paramedics are the traditional EMT-Ps with additional training in the monitoring, treatment, and transport of critically ill patients. Additional training involves an understanding and use of medications beyond the scope of standard paramedic practice, as well as the ability to monitor infusion pumps. These individuals might also receive training in monitoring the use of respirators, intra-aortic balloon pumps, and other advanced medical devices.

Critical care paramedics have not been widely used in EMS systems. They are primarily used in interfacility critical care transports and on fixed-wing and rotor-wing air transports (Figure 24-1). Training varies and is provided by universities and hospitals. The University of Maryland, Baltimore County (UMBC), founded one of the first critical care paramedic training programs at the university level. This course has spread to other areas of the country, on a limited basis, and has helped to establish some degree of standardization, although there are critical care training programs. Also, there are specialized paramedics trained in the transport of critically ill infants and children.

As the number of interfacility critical care transports increases, the need for this level of provider is likely to increase. As sophistication of EMS care continues to evolve, there might be a use for critical care paramedics in the EMS/911 arena as well.

Emergency Medical Dispatchers

Emergency medical dispatchers provide a critical communication link in the EMS system. These personnel were traditionally EMS providers who were trained informally. Fortunately, there has been increased recognition of the importance of the dispatcher, and training has now become more formalized.

The National Academies of Emergency Dispatch (NAED) has endorsed a high level of emergency medical dispatch training and the use of its priority medical dispatch protocols. It also has established training and certification standards for both emergency medical dispatchers and dispatch centers. (See Chapter 10, "Emergency Medical Dispatch.")

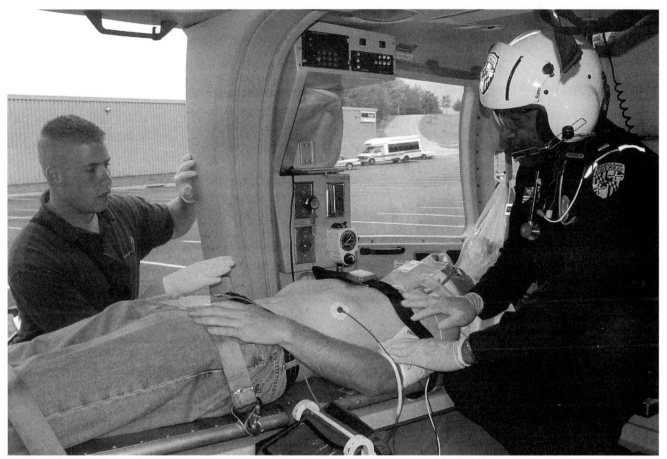

Figure 24-1 Critical care paramedics are used most commonly by air medical transport services.

Roles of EMS Providers

EMS providers can assume many roles within their profession. These include field provider, supervisor, administrator, dispatcher, and educator.

Field Provider Roles

Field providers are the cornerstone for any EMS system. The largest number of providers nationally are EMT-Bs; the others are first responders, EMT-Is, and paramedics. They are allowed to function within their scope of practice in the systems they staff. The specific configuration of providers varies greatly around the country, with some ambulances staffed with EMT-Bs and first responders. Some systems incorporate basics, intermediates, and paramedics; some use only paramedics.

Supervisory Roles

There are various levels of supervisory positions depending on the size and complexity of the EMS sys-
tem. Most systems rank supervisors from field supervisor through general manager, with one to three levels of supervision in between.

Supervisory roles provide a career ladder for field personnel as they grow more experienced and pursue advanced education degrees. This career ladder might include field supervisors, operational managers, quality improvement managers, education coordinators, and agency administrators. Some EMS personnel also pursue other health care-related professions, including nursing and medicine.

Dispatch Roles

Dispatch is a very important role in every EMS system, but it often is the most undervalued. Dispatch is often the first point of contact for patients and is the point in the system that prioritizes calls and provides instruction to callers.

The advent of advanced call triage systems has been a major development for emergency medical dispatch. Systems and organizations such as Priority Medical

Dispatch and the Association of Public-Safety Communication Officials (APCO) have revolutionized the standards and consistency of dispatch systems.

Management and Administrative Roles

Effective management and oversight of EMS operations are critical. Most of the individuals in these positions worked their way up from a field position to supervisor and then to a manager role without any formal training in management. This is particularly problematic for individuals who have not undergone training in human resources, finance, and leadership skills. Fortunately, there are now some graduate programs in EMS management, as well as specialized courses offered by the American Ambulance Association and others.

Teaching Roles

EMS providers gain a wealth of experience while on the job. "Street skills" coupled with higher/continuing education contribute to a more well-rounded provider. Some providers have a strong desire, along with an inherent ability, to teach others. EMS providers who want to teach can become authorized to do so through established state and national avenues. EMS providers can have the opportunity to teach extensive initial training programs such as EMT-B, EMT-I, EMT-P, or shorter specialty courses, or continuing education programs such as ACLS, BTLS, PALS, APLS, and PEPP.

The Role of the Medical Director

Medical directors provide the medical and professional direction for EMS providers. They also develop and authorize protocols for clinical practice, set quality improvement standards, and lead education and training programs for out-of-hospital providers. It is under the supervision of the medical director that out-of-hospital providers are allowed to function in their roles. The medical director also is responsible for controlled drugs and other pharmaceutical products, as well as the use of medical devices and equipment requiring medical oversight.

Medical directors are typically emergency physicians who have experience and interest in EMS. Most are board certified in emergency medicine and are licensed MDs or DOs in the states in which they provide medical direction. NAEMSP is examining the possibility of offering a subspecialty certification process for qualified EMS physicians.

The role of the medical director is an essential one, and it will expand as EMS continues to evolve. More part-time EMS medical directors will become full-time with the evolution of high-performance EMS systems that require significant and consistent medical direction.

Finally, the role of the medical director of an EMS system has changed dramatically. In the past, many services simply looked for a physician to sign off on certification and protocols. This is no longer the trend. As EMS systems become more sophisticated with new equipment, drugs, and devices, the role of the experienced medical director is vitally important in achieving a quality EMS system. In this capacity, the EMS medical director certifies the status of field providers, ensures that they receive continuing education, and manages the quality improvement process, which includes the necessary timely revision of medical protocols.

The Role of Higher Education

Advanced degree programs for out-of-hospital care providers are becoming available on a more widespread basis. These include baccalaureate and advanced degree programs with clinical, educational, and administrative tracks.

The most significant benefit of these advanced degree programs is the increased skills, knowledge, resources, and job opportunities a degree can provide for EMS personnel. It also offers more advanced roles, possibly leading to tenure in universities, and it allows for advancement in the business and corporate world. With the consolidation of ambulance and emergency service companies, individuals who have both clinical experience and administrative advanced degrees have a unique opportunity for advancement into management and other leadership positions.

In larger, more advanced systems, there are dedicated roles for out-of-hospital providers in the areas of education, training, quality improvement, and clinical research. This is a particularly viable option for those trained at universities. There are undergraduate and graduate degree programs in EMS with a focus on quality improvement and education. There are also many opportunities for research in EMS. With the increased interest in outcome data and evidence-based medicine, EMS research will have an important role in the development of EMS systems and definition of out-of-hospital clinical care in the future.

Career Opportunities and Work Settings

Public and Municipal Fire Departments

Municipal fire departments are among the largest employers of EMS personnel. This includes all the roles mentioned. Although most fire departments did not initially envision EMS as part of their role, it has now become the primary activity for most of them. In fact, approximately 80% of fire department calls are now EMS related. Most fire departments have embraced EMS as a significant part of their mission.

Third Services

Some municipalities have an EMS service that is independent, distinct from the fire department, other municipal agencies, and private companies. In this arrangement, the EMS service, known as a third service, assumes the primary responsibility for patient care in the EMS setting. These systems have a similar structure to municipal fire departments. Where these third services exist, they provide excellent employment and career growth opportunities for all levels of providers.

Private EMS and Ambulance Services

Private services are present in almost every municipal area. They might provide 911 transport services (often in conjunction with the local fire department) independently, via contract with the government jurisdiction, or through an arrangement known as the **public utility model**, in which there is a partnership through an authority or agency that provides both emergency and nonemergency transport in a given area. Public utility models exist in many major metropolitan areas. The EMS system model in Fort Worth, Texas, is an example of a public utility model.

In many areas, private ambulance services (either for-profit or not-for-profit) almost exclusively provide nonemergency and interfacility transport in the geographic areas they serve. Usually this is by contract with hospitals, nursing homes, and insurance companies and is on a private fee-for-service basis. These services usually provide both BLS and ALS care. Often critical care, neonatal, and other specialty services are among the offerings of private ambulance services. Private ambulance services can be small and locally owned or part of large corporations that operate in multiple states.

There are some private ambulances, however, that are primarily responsible for emergency service response in their communities.

Career growth opportunities might be limited at smaller and family-owned ambulance services, but these companies can provide a family-like atmosphere. The larger, multistate companies provide significant career opportunities as personnel are able to assume leadership roles at local, regional, and corporate levels. In addition, many of these companies provide specialty services such as critical care and neonatal transport, which allows employees to receive additional training and responsibilities.

Volunteer Services

Volunteer ambulance services still outnumber private and municipal services, particularly in suburban and rural areas of the United States. Most are small and rural services and might be the only EMS opportunity for individuals who live in small towns or rural areas. There is a trend to combine both volunteer and paid services in an effort to provide better EMS coverage for communities. Paid EMS/fire paramedics are integrated into traditional volunteer systems in an effort to provide ALS care 24/7 for communities that have experienced large growth. This integration of paid personnel into the volunteer ranks might at first pose administrative or morale problems, but it can also lead to an increase in professionalism that will continue over time. Also, municipal services from nearby larger cities and private ambulance services are partnering with volunteer services in many areas to provide resources that might not be available in all volunteer sectors.

Air Ambulance Services

Much like the specialty areas, air ambulance services offer unique opportunities. Most provide scene response as well as interfacility transfers as part of their service offerings. These are usually critical care or other specialized types of services that offer true career professional growth opportunities through specialization. A common configuration for many air ambulance programs is a nurse and paramedic crew.

Air ambulance companies are either private companies, which usually have multiple operations, or are part of hospital systems. For those EMS personnel who want to move into other careers such as nurse, physician assistant, or nurse practitioner, these system-type positions provide the entrée into this type of professional growth.

Medical Groups

Out-of-hospital providers have limited opportunities to work in medical groups. This type of work setting might increase in the future due to the shortage of nurses and other health care providers. Also, it is becoming more common for out-of-hospital providers to work with emergency physician groups in hospitals and primary care providers in urgent care centers. This area has significant growth potential and offers the opportunity to work directly with physicians.

Education Settings

As mentioned earlier, there is a growing need for out-of-hospital providers to educate future providers. There will be more opportunities for teaching positions within universities and community colleges for those with the proper combination of experience and education. Higher learning institutions often partner with local fire or EMS services to assist in training new providers.

Many public and private services also provide education benefits to their employees and will hire educators to meet the need for ongoing training and continuing education.

■ The Future of EMS Manpower

Advanced Providers

As medical transportation needs grow and the level of care provided increases, there will be an increased need for advanced providers. There also will be an increased regionalization of specialty care that will require transfer of patients with more complicated conditions.

There will be a need for multiple advanced providers. The most common will be a paramedic with advanced critical care training, as described earlier. This will include training to manage an expanded list of drugs, ventilators, multiple intravenous infusions, balloon pumps, and other advanced medical devices (**Figure 24-2**). States will have to adopt legislation to allow this advanced scope of practice for paramedics and to define the required training.

There also could be out-of-hospital positions for **nurse practitioners** and **physician assistants**. As new models of care continue to evolve, including mobile primary care (ie, treating and transporting patients to alternative destinations), these providers will see a growth in the need for their services in the out-of-hospital environment.

With the increase in the number of patients being transported on ventilators, there might be an increase in the use of **respiratory therapists** in the out-of-hospital arena. There will be opportunities for cross-training to include paramedic and other critical care services.

In Europe and South America, physicians have long been used as providers on ambulances. This has not occurred in large numbers in the United States, but there has been limited use of neonatologists and pediatricians on pediatric and neonatal transport units. Intensivists and emergency physicians have been used in long-distance air ambulance transfers for quite some time. This trend might increase with the growth of patient repatriation, particularly in the critical care transport sector.

Expanded Service Models

In Argentina, ambulance services have been providing mobile primary and urgent care in the field for the past 18 years. They have models with multiple-tiered responses based on the severity of the patient's condition. Basically, the EMS priority dispatch-type protocols have been expanded to determine the time of response as well as the level of response. Physicians and nurses have been the primary providers in this

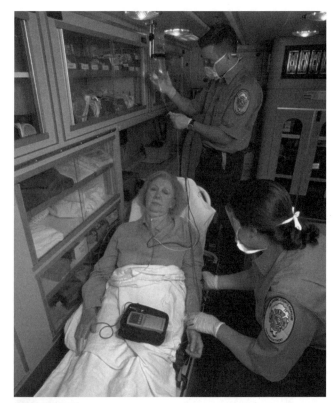

Figure 24-2 The increasing number of patients being transferred with complicated conditions will require more advanced care providers.

system. For example, if a patient has crushing chest pain, the system will produce a staffed, equipped ALS ambulance in 10 minutes or less. In the case of a sprain or bruise, a physician will respond in a car for home-based treatment within 90 minutes. There are also 15-, 30-, and 60-minute response times based on patient condition. Only the highest acuity situations will result in an ambulance response. In minor situations, a car is dispatched, with home treatment provided. This system has high patient satisfaction.

Such a system in the United States would be difficult to implement because of the liability climate and the use of mostly nonphysician providers in the out-of-hospital environment. However, in a climate of overcrowded emergency departments and scarce EMS resources, such a system bears consideration in some form. This would include true telephone/911 triage, tiered responses, scene treatment, and alternative destinations. A great deal of coordination and study would be required.

Also, with the advances in communication and telephone triage, there is an increasing role for **communications/911 call centers**. These advanced call centers could be the fulcrum for true integration of the EMS system with the emergency department. The expanded call center could become the health care information repository, providing past history and treatment records to the field, emergency department, physician office, and hospital. Such a model could align incentives among the various provider groups and the payers.

A truly integrated communications center in the future could also provide record-keeping and information exchange throughout the provider spectrum, including the hospital, physician practices, emergency department, EMS system, home health, and other parts of the health care system.

Any expansion similar to that described earlier would create significant new opportunities for EMS personnel for employment. Also, opportunities for additional training and career growth would abound. The future holds significant opportunity for out-of-hospital providers.

Certification, Licensure, and Registration

Currently, most states certify EMTs, paramedics, and other out-of-hospital providers. **Certification** is the process of verifying competency at a predetermined level, and **licensure** refers to a process in which a state agency declares that person is competent to "practice." Certification is not regarded as highly by some as li-

censure, which traditionally has been perceived as more professional. There has been some movement toward licensure in some areas that would pave the way for true professional growth for out-of-hospital providers. Licensure would open opportunities for hospital staff privileges, reciprocity with other states, and true specialization. Functionally, there is no significant difference between certification and licensure of out-of-hospital personnel.

Most state EMS regulatory agencies use the **National Registry of Emergency Medical Technicians (NREMT)** written and practical examinations to determine competency. Individuals who successfully complete the NREMT examinations are then **"registered"** with NREMT. It is the goal of the "EMS Education Agenda for the Future" that, by 2010, one national EMS certification will be administered by one independent national agency. This will provide a consistent evaluation tool that will provide certification accepted by all states for entry-level competency, and which will potentially lead to state licensure and the further enhancement of EMS as a profession. It will also greatly facilitate reciprocity between states, allowing more flexibility for EMS personnel.

Human Resource Shortages

Probably the biggest challenge in the out-of-hospital industry is the shortage of trained EMT-Ps. This is primarily a professional and pay issue. There is a disincentive for a paramedic to work in the field when he or she can earn more in another occupation.

Certainly with the popularity of EMS television shows and movies, not to mention the attention appropriately drawn to our fire and EMS services in the wake of September 11, 2001, there is a very high level of public trust and confidence in our EMS professionals. It is a highly challenging and satisfying career. This trend will likely continue.

When EMS is recognized and compensated appropriately, there will be less of a manpower shortage. However, until that time comes, shortages will be common and challenging to all types of out-of-hospital organizations.

There is significant attrition in the EMS field because of the lack of recognition as a profession and the current levels of pay. It is also a very high-stress occupation that can quickly produce burnout. The shift work schedules of 12 and 24 hours plus working nights, weekends, and holidays put additional pressure on both families and circadian rhythms. Our EMS employers must take into account the stresses of the job and the effects of the job on health and families.

Prevention and Public Health–Community Intervention and Integration

EMS must be an integrated health service component that does not exist on its own, but rather is fully integrated in the continuum of care for patients and their communities. In an excerpt from the "EMS Agenda for the Future," Alasdair K.T. Conn, MD, stated that,

> Out-of-facility care is an integral component of the health care system. EMS focuses on out-of-facility care and also supports efforts to implement cost-effective community health care. By integrating with other health system components, EMS improves health care for the entire community, including children, the elderly, and others with special needs.[1]

Back in 1996, those who developed the EMS agenda had the wherewithal to foresee the changing role of the EMS provider and its community outreach agenda.

To get to this model, many things will need to happen. First of all, EMS must expand its public health and prevention role in establishing strong ties with local public health agencies, active state and local surveillance programs, and social service and case management resources. Health care must be cost-effective by incorporating all of the local resources, including hospitals, clinics, and local and state EMS agencies, as well as state department of health agencies. By doing this, they will coordinate rather than duplicate their efforts in the continuum of care.

Second, EMS must get involved in community health fairs and in monitoring diseases prevalent to seasonal changes and also obtain data for health promotion and awareness. Educating the community is extraordinarily important, as is educating patients with myocardial infarctions to come in quickly for appropriate definitive therapy. The same is true for early stroke care and making sure the community is aware of potential stroke symptoms so that early intervention will be possible. From this early education, the next logical steps are clinical pathways and guidelines based on benchmarking and patient outcomes. Medical oversight and the relationship emergency physicians have with their physician colleagues is important in developing guidelines.

Just as the medical realms and hospitals are specializing in geriatrics, pediatrics, cardiothoracic care, and trauma, EMS must also incorporate these special-needs patients and incorporate protocols to ensure patients have the access they need to receive the most definitive and efficacious care. Because of the politi-

cal nature of these decisions, diplomacy and communication will be a key to make sure all of the involved parties have their interests included.

Theodore R. Delbridge, MD, MPH, in writing about prevention, summed this up best in the "EMS Agenda for the Future" by stating:

> In the future the success of EMS systems will be measured not only by the outcomes of their treatments, but also by the results of their prevention efforts. Its expertise, resources, and positions in communities and the health care system make EMS an ideal candidate to serve linchpin roles during multi-disciplinary, community-wide prevention initiatives. EMS must seize such responsibility and profoundly enhance its positive effects on community health.[1]

Disaster Preparedness

Since September 11, 2001, the **Department of Homeland Security** has been established, and millions of dollars have been and are being spent on disaster preparedness on federal, state, and local levels (see Chapter 19, "EMS Response to Terrorist Incidents and Weapons of Mass Destruction").

New communication and information Web sites, training, and education for all levels of health care providers have been extraordinarily helpful and are necessary to provide community stability and sound quality of care. Paramedics in the past have been trained in dealing with hazardous materials, have obtained more disaster training, and are providing community education. Many hospitals and states have invested in decontamination equipment and communications centers and have invested both financial and human resources into disaster preparedness training (**Figure 24-3**).

EMS Research

Although conducting EMS research is very challenging, it is necessary to improve the quality of patient care in an economically challenged health care market. In the past, out-of-hospital practice has been based on principles of care used in hospitals and on common practice. There has been little scientific justification for that common practice. In the future, EMS practice changes should be predicated on solid research in order to improve integrated EMS systems.

Lack of funding is one factor that has plagued out-of-hospital research. In addition, most academic institutions that provide research have found the overly

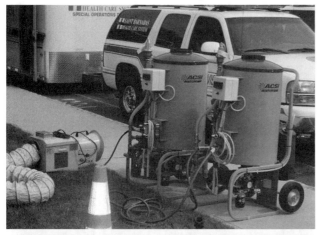

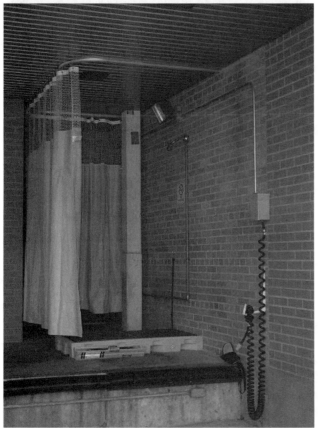

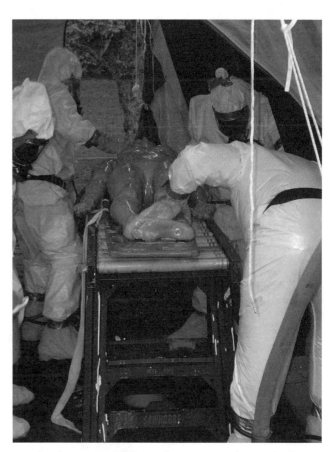

restrictive nature of the informed consent laws to be cumbersome enough to stay away from this important realm. Because the out-of-hospital realm is often not integrated with hospital systems and necessary informatics, data collection can be difficult.

Many EMS personnel are not trained in research, nor do they consider the importance of research. Education in research design and activities must be included in EMS education, starting with initial training to facilitate completing necessary and effective EMS re-

search that could improve the quality of health care provided to patients. (See Chapter 22, "Research.")

Summary

The EMS field has significant growth opportunities and professional and personal satisfaction. The increased specialization and growth of the industry will provide significant career opportunities for those who choose EMS as a career. There are advanced degrees such as critical care, public health, disaster medicine, and other specialties that paramedics are obtaining to further their education and skills. These degrees will give out-of-hospital providers the ability to teach, research, and pursue various other health care-related jobs. These are relatively new arenas that are wide open to EMS personnel, especially paramedics, and that make use of their medical skills.

Reference

1. National Highway Traffic Safety Administration. EMS agenda for the future: a systems approach [NHTSA Web site]. Available at: http://www.nhtsa.dot.gov/people/injury/ems/agenda/emsman.html. Accessed February 8, 2005.

Additional Reading

ASTM Committee F-30 on Emergency Medical Services. *ASTM Standards on Emergency Medical Services.* Philadelphia, Pa: ASTM; 1994.

Garrison HG, Benson NH, Whitley TW, et al. Paramedic skills and medications: practice options utilized by local advanced life support medical directors. *Prehospital Disaster Med.* 1991;6:29–33.

Gerson LW, Hoover R, McCoy S, et al. Linking the elderly to community services. *JEMS.* 1991;16(6):45–48.

Krumperman KM. Filling the gap: EMS social service referrals. *JEMS.* 1993;18(2):25–29.

Rosenberg M. *Program Briefing to Dr. David Satcher, Director, Centers for Disease Control and Prevention.* Atlanta, Ga: CDC, March 13, 1996.

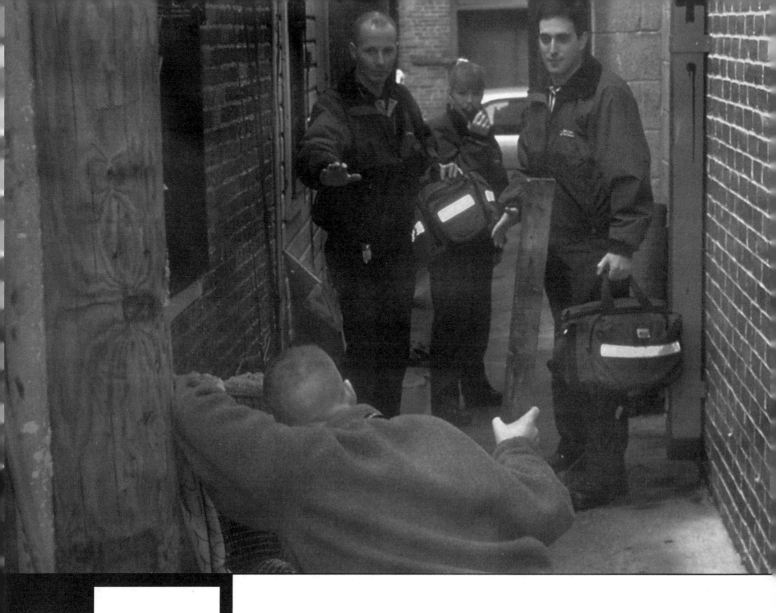

25 Occupational Health Issues

Deb Hogue, RN, ADN, EMT-P
Lynn Zimmerman, RN, BSN, Med

Principles of This Chapter

After reading this chapter, you should be able to:

- Describe the components of an EMS organization's health and safety program, such as fitness and musculoskeletal agility evaluations, drug testing, vision and hearing testing, immunizations, tuberculosis surveillance, and respiratory medical evaluation and clearance.
- Describe the occupational medical program for occupational injuries and illnesses, as well as wellness and employee assistance programs.
- Discuss health and safety programs and plans for bloodborne pathogen exposure, tuberculosis exposure, respiratory protection, workplace violence prevention, fire safety, and ergonomics.
- Explain some of the occupational issues specific to women in EMS.

EMS PERSONNEL ARE MEMBERS OF THE SERVICE OCCUPATION categorized as health care professionals.[1] As health care professionals, EMS personnel face unique occupational health and safety risks, including exposure to a variety of infectious diseases and hazardous chemicals, driving under emergency conditions, caring for and interacting with persons during some of life's most stressful periods, performing both heavy manual labor and highly technical skills, and working in uncontrolled environments. In addition, many EMS professionals have firefighting, search and rescue, hazardous material emergency response, and law enforcement responsibilities.

People who choose to enter the EMS profession should be aware of and prepared to manage these occupational issues. In addition, EMS organizations are obligated to ensure that they provide as safe and healthy a work environment as possible for their employees. This obligation is defined by the Occupational Safety and Health Administration (OSHA),[1] the National Fire Protection Agency (NFPA), and state and local regulatory agencies.

The following suggestions might be included in an EMS organization's health and safety program:

- Preplacement and periodic fitness evaluation for duty assessments
- Musculoskeletal agility evaluation based on essential job functions
- Drug testing, including prehire and for-cause testing; organizations might choose or be required to conduct random drug testing of personnel who provide services under contract with various government entities
- Vision testing
- Hearing and audiometric testing in conjunction with a hearing conservation program
- Per OSHA and Centers for Disease Control and Prevention (CDC) guidelines for health care workers, immunizations against the following:
  - Hepatitis B
  - Measles, mumps, and rubella
  - Chickenpox
  - Tetanus, diphtheria
  - Influenza vaccine, annual
  - Hepatitis A, when applicable
  - Anthrax and smallpox (under review)
- Tuberculosis surveillance, including skin testing and periodic health evaluations for positive skin tests
- Respiratory medical evaluation and clearance for the use of respirators (periodic fit testing and checking)
- Occupational medical program to manage occupational injuries and illnesses with persons trained and experienced in:
  - Managing EMS personnel issues
  - HIV/AIDS counseling for bloodborne pathogen exposures
- Wellness programs, including:
  - Weight management
  - Smoking cessation
  - Stress management
  - Aerobic and anaerobic exercise and conditioning
- Employee assistance programs, including critical incident stress debriefing services
- Development of appropriate health and safety programs and plans, including training in:
  - Bloodborne pathogen exposure control
  - Tuberculosis exposure control
  - Respiratory protection plan

- Workplace violence prevention plan
- Emergency plan and fire safety
- Hazardous communication plan
- Ergonomics

Infectious Disease Exposure

Prior to the early 1980s and the introduction of AIDS into our society, infection control practices were designed to protect patients. Since that time, we have looked more closely at how these issues also affect employees. Hepatitis B has been a significant occupational hazard for health care workers and had a major role in the federal legislation developed by OSHA. Airborne diseases such as drug-resistant strains of tuberculosis and the recent introduction of severe acute respiratory syndrome (SARS) also concern EMS providers.

Hepatitis B Virus

Hepatitis B virus (HBV) infection is a recognized occupational risk to EMS providers. It is a serious disease caused by a virus that attacks the liver. In the United States, it is estimated that there are between 1 and 1.25 million chronically infected persons. There are 5,000 to 6,000 associated deaths each year from chronic liver disease, including primary liver cancer. HBV infection occurs in 12,000 health care workers annually, with 200 to 300 deaths each year from chronic HBV infection. Needlestick exposure to HBV is among the most efficient modes of HBV transmission and carries a 6% to 30% risk of transmission. EMS providers are at high risk; other high-risk groups include injecting drug users, homosexual men, heterosexuals with multiple partners, infants born to infected mothers, and hemodialysis patients. The hepatitis B vaccine has been available in the United States since 1982. The OSHA regulations increased compliance with offering the hepatitis B vaccine, and there has been a sharp decline in incidence of HBV infection among health care workers. The effectiveness of hepatitis B immune globulin (HBIG) and/or hepatitis B vaccine in various postexposure settings has been evaluated by prospective studies. Multiple doses of HBIG initiated within 1 week after percutaneous exposure to HBsAg-positive blood provide an estimated 75% protection from HBV infection. The postexposure efficacy of the combination of HBIG and the hepatitis B vaccine series has not been evaluated in the occupational setting. Exposure prevention is still the best strategy for reducing occupational exposure to hepatitis B. Guidelines for postexposure

management have been published by the US Public Health Service.[2] With the revised bloodborne pathogen standard and the **Needlestick Safety and Prevention Act**,[3] there should be a further reduction in the number of occupationally acquired exposures to hepatitis B.

Human Immunodeficiency Virus

AIDS, or acquired immune deficiency syndrome, is caused by the human immunodeficiency virus (HIV). Once a person has been infected with HIV, it might be years before the symptoms of AIDS develop. HIV attacks the body's immune system so that it cannot fight deadly diseases. An estimated 60 million individuals worldwide have become infected with HIV. It is also estimated that 40 million are currently living with HIV, and more than 20 million[4] have died from AIDS since the epidemic started in the early 1980s.[5] Most of the infected individuals live in developing countries. Despite prevention efforts, HIV continues to spread rapidly. In the United States, it is estimated that there are more than 750,000 AIDS cases, with more than 435,000 associated deaths. There are more than 50 documented cases of occupationally acquired HIV infection in health care workers in the United States. In addition, there are more than 150 reported occupational HIV infections under investigation.

The greatest risk of HIV exposure to EMS providers is through needlestick injuries. To estimate the rate of HIV transmission, data were combined from more than 20 worldwide prospective studies of health care workers exposed to HIV-infected blood through a percutaneous injury. In all, 21 infections followed 6,498 exposures, for an average transmission rate of 0.3% per injury.[6] A retrospective case-control study of health care workers who had percutaneous exposures to HIV found that the risk of transmission was increased when the health care worker was exposed to a larger amount of infected blood.[7] The risk after mucous membrane exposure is estimated to be around 0.1%, and the risk after nonintact skin exposure is less than 0.1%. An Orange County (California) health care agency conducted a survey evaluating the knowledge and prevention of occupational exposure to police officers, paramedics, and firefighters. The results of the survey showed that the responders had an accurate knowledge of AIDS but incorrect perceptions of HIV transmission. Some still believed that HIV can be contracted through casual contact. Training was not given frequently. Preventive practices were also infrequent in the work setting, with precautions used less than 50% of the time. The survey concluded that there is a need for improved HIV/AIDS education programs for out-of-hospital personnel.[8]

HIV vaccine trials are being conducted, but there is still no vaccine available to prevent HIV infection.

Data on the timing and clinical characteristics of seroconversion in HIV-exposed health care workers are limited by the infrequency of infection following an occupational exposure. The US Public Health Service has published guidelines for postexposure prophylaxis for occupational exposure to HIV.[2] Considerations that influence the rationale and recommendations for prophylaxis include the pathogenesis of HIV infection, the biological plausibility that infection can be prevented by using antiretroviral drugs, the evidence of the efficacy of the specific agents used, and the risk and benefit of the prophylaxis. Information about primary HIV infection indicates that systemic infections do not occur immediately, leaving a brief window of opportunity during which postexposure antiretroviral intervention might modify or prevent viral replication. OSHA requires all EMS agencies to have exposure control plans in place. These plans should include postexposure prophylaxis recommendations. OSHA published the final rule for occupational exposure to bloodborne pathogens, needlesticks, and other sharps injuries in *Federal Register* on January 18, 2001. This rule conforms with the requirements of the Needlestick Safety and Prevention Act.[3]

Needlestick injuries are an important and continuing cause of exposure to HIV among EMS providers. With the revised bloodborne pathogen standard and the Needlestick Safety and Prevention Act, the hope is to reduce the number of occupationally acquired HIV infections to EMS and other health care professionals.

Hepatitis C Virus

Hepatitis C virus (HCV) infection is the most common chronic bloodborne infection in the United States. As of 2001, it was estimated that there were 170 million people chronically infected worldwide, and 3 to 4 million are newly infected each year. Of that, 3.9 million are in the United States. Chronic liver disease is the 10th leading cause of death in the United States.

Hepatitis C is transmitted primarily through large or repeated direct percutaneous exposures to blood. The good news is that HCV is not transmitted efficiently through occupational exposures to blood. Most new infections worldwide are due to unscreened blood transfusions and using contaminated needles and syringes. The average incidence of anti-HCV serocon-

version after accidental percutaneous exposure (needlestick) from an HCV-positive patient is 1.8%.

In 1999, the CDC received inquiries from state and local health departments about the prevalence of hepatitis C among medical first responders (firefighters, EMTs, and paramedics). There were five studies of HCV infection among first responders.[9] There were several limitations, and the studies could not exclude the possibility that some first responders had acquired HCV infection from occupational exposures. Routine HCV testing is not recommended for populations with a low prevalence of HCV infection (including first responders) unless they have an increased risk for infection (eg, receiving a blood transfusion before July 1992 or injecting drug use). A study done at Wayne State University examined the prevalence of anti-HCV by using an enzyme-linked immunoassay test in 2,447 volunteers (including 1,560 police officers, 678 firefighters, and 209 EMTs). Prevalence rates were found to be 1.1% and 1.3% among blacks and whites, respectively. Although firefighters and EMTs had a higher prevalence (2.3% and 2.8%) than police officers (0.6%), the overall prevalence was lower than that of most urban populations.[10]

Testing first responders for HCV is recommended after exposure to HCV-positive blood and should be considered if the source is unknown. Transmission of hepatitis C rarely occurs from mucous membrane exposures to blood. There are no clinical trials to assess postexposure use of antiviral agents to prevent HCV infection. In addition, there are no studies that have evaluated the treatment of acute infections in persons without evidence of liver disease. Interferon is used in the treatment of patients with ongoing, chronic hepatitis C. Long-term effects on disease progression and effect on the natural history of HCV infection are not known.

Tuberculosis

EMS providers also are at risk for occupational exposure to tuberculosis. In the 1940s, tuberculosis slowly began to disappear after scientists discovered the first of several drugs now used to treat it. In the mid-1980s, there was an increased incidence of tuberculosis in the US population, and strains of drug-resistant tuberculosis were identified. Since the mid-1990s, there has been a decrease in the overall number of tuberculosis cases in the United States. This is likely due to increased awareness and implementation of tuberculosis control measures recommended by the CDC and OSHA.

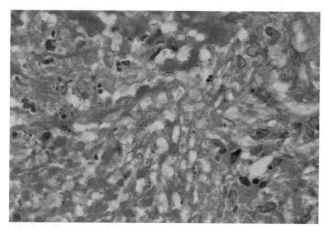

Figure 25-1 *Mycobacterium tuberculosis.*

Tuberculosis is caused by *Mycobacterium tuberculosis* (**Figure 25-1**). This bacterium usually attacks the lungs. It is spread through the air and can be infectious. Most people who breathe in the bacteria and become infected can fight the bacteria and keep them from growing. The bacteria become inactive, and the chance of the infection becoming active and infectious to others is approximately 10% in that person's lifetime.[11] People who have a weak or compromised immune system are at greater risk for developing disease.

In addition to other diseases, there are certain strains of tuberculosis that have become a serious concern. When tuberculosis patients do not take their medications, the bacteria can develop resistance to that antibiotic. Resistance is most common in people who have spent time with someone who has a drug-resistant tuberculosis disease; people who do not take their medicine; people who develop tuberculosis disease after having taken the medicine in the past; and people who come from areas where drug-resistant tuberculosis is common (southeast Asia, Latin America, Haiti, and the Philippines).[11]

Because the out-of-hospital environment is unpredictable, it is difficult to use engineering controls that are available to other health care workers (eg, isolation rooms and ventilation systems) to help prevent the spread of disease. The out-of-hospital provider must rely on identifying suspected tuberculosis patients through assessment and then apply a mask to prevent exposure. The National Institute for Occupational Safety and Health-approved mask for tuberculosis currently is the **N95 particulate respirator**. The OSHA standard for respiratory protection for *M. tuberculosis*[12] must be followed. OSHA is in the process of promulgating a separate standard for tuberculosis control and prevention. The standard will identify the scope (health care facilities, correctional institutions, long-term care facilities for the elderly, homeless shelters, and drug treatment centers); require education and training, engineering, and work practice controls (including respiratory protection); and require medical surveillance, tuberculosis skin testing, exposure evaluation, and followup and record-keeping.

Tuberculosis continues to be a major public health problem in some areas of the United States. Elimination of this disease will require coordinated efforts from public health and health care providers.

Hepatitis A and E

Hepatitis A and E are often confused by out-of-hospital care providers as bloodborne pathogens. Hepatitis A and E are transmitted via the oral or fecal route. These viruses are excreted in feces and transmitted in contaminated food and water. Hepatitis A can affect anyone. In the United States, hepatitis A can occur in situations ranging from isolated cases of disease to widespread epidemics. About one third of the US population has antibodies to hepatitis A.

Two inactivated whole virus hepatitis A vaccines are now available in pediatric and adult formulations. Neither vaccine is recommended for children younger than 2 years. Both vaccines recommend a booster dose 6 to 18 months after the administration of the first dose. In May 2001, the Food and Drug Administration approved a combination hepatitis A and B vaccine for people 18 years and older. The vaccine administration series is at 0, 1, and 6 to 12 months. The first and third doses must be at least 6 months apart. Postexposure management of people not vaccinated against hepatitis A is standard immune globulin (IG). IG should be given to exposed people not previously vaccinated as soon as possible but not more than 2 weeks after exposure.

Hepatitis A is a reportable disease in the United States. The CDC currently recommends the hepatitis A vaccine only for people traveling to or working in countries with high or intermediate prevalence of hepatitis A (ie, Central or South America, the Caribbean, Mexico, Asia [except Japan], Africa, and eastern Europe), children and adolescents who live in states or communities where routine vaccination has been recommended, men who have sex with men, people who use street drugs, people who have chronic liver disease, people who are treated with clotting factor concentrates, people who work with hepatitis A virus in research settings, and possibly children or adolescents in communities where outbreaks of hepatitis A are occurring.[13]

Hepatitis E is similar to hepatitis A and is transmitted by contact with contaminated food or water. It is estimated that 20% of people in the United States might be infected with hepatitis E. There is no vaccine available for hepatitis E.[14]

Hepatitis D

Hepatitis D, or Delta hepatitis, can replicate only by attaching to hepatitis B. It is not common in the United States except in intravenous drug abusers and people who require multiple blood transfusions. Those who have the antibody for hepatitis B are immune to further infection from both hepatitis B and D viruses.

Hepatitis G

Hepatitis G is transmitted via certain body fluids. Although only recently identified, hepatitis G is believed to have a mild chronic course, and the likelihood of liver damage is low. The risk factors for hepatitis G are probably similar to those of hepatitis C, although incidence among patients with multiple blood transfusions is much lower than it is with hepatitis C.

Multi–Drug-Resistant Organisms

Multi–drug-resistant organisms are pathogens that have developed the ability to resist antimicrobial drugs. Examples of these organisms include[15-19]:

- MRSA (methicillin/oxacillin-resistant *Staphylococcus aureus*)
- VRE (vancomycin-resistant enterococci)
- ESBLs (extended-spectrum β-lactamases, which are resistant to cephalosporins and monobactams)
- PRSP (penicillin-resistant *Streptococcus pneumoniae*)
- VISA/VRSA (vancomycin-intermediate/-resistant *Staphylococcus aureus*)
- DRSP (drug-resistant *Streptococcus pneumoniae*)

Most multi–drug-resistant infections are nosocomial in that they often develop in people who are hospitalized or are occupants or frequent users of other health care facilities, including nursing homes, hemodialysis centers, physician's offices, and clinics and child care centers.[16,19] They cause a variety of infections, including but not limited to pneumonia, bacteremia, otitis media, meningitis, peritonitis, and sinusitis.[16,17]

Transmission is person-to-person; direct contact is the most common means. Droplet spread can occur with some pneumonias, and indirect contact with objects contaminated with infected body fluids or substances rarely occurs. Risk factors include chronic disease states, presence of pressure ulcers, immunosuppression, malnutrition, presence of invasive devices, prolonged or frequent hospitalizations or institutionalizations, high prevalence areas such as burn units or CCUs, and indiscriminate use of antibiotics.[15-18]

Patients are the most important reservoir for multi–drug-resistant infections. Infected health care personnel can become carriers, but this is not a major source of infection. Health care personnel do become important transmitters of infection if they do not follow standard precautions (**Figure 25-2**) and good handwashing procedures.

If an institution's infection control committee or coordinator determines that a patient's condition is of special clinical or epidemiological significance, the patient can be placed under contact precautions. EMS personnel should follow the transferring institution's recommended precautions for the patient but, at a minimum, should observe standard precautions (or universal precautions) when treating and transferring patients with known or suspected multi–drug-resistant infection.

Multi–drug-resistant infections are becoming a very important public health issue. In response, the CDC and many state health departments are developing strategies to control the proliferation of drug-resistant organisms. Descriptions of several of the programs (including the Campaign to Prevent Antimicrobial Resistance and SEARCH) that are being developed can be found on the CDC Web site (http://www.cdc.gov/drugresistance/healthcare/default.htm).

Meningitis

Meningitis is an infection of the fluid surrounding the brain and spinal cord. Meningitis is usually caused by viral or bacterial agents. It is important to know whether meningitis is caused by a virus or bacterium because the severity of the illness and the treatment differ.

Viral meningitis is usually less severe and resolves without specific treatment. Bacterial meningitis can be severe and cause brain damage, hearing loss, learning disability, or death. When diagnosing bacterial meningitis, it is important to know which type of bacteria is causing it because antibiotics can prevent some types from spreading and potentially infecting other people. The signs and symptoms include headache, high fever, stiff neck, nausea, vomiting, and photophobia. These symptoms can develop over several hours or 1 to 2 days.

Figure 25-2 Standard precautions. Excerpted from "Guidelines for Isolation Precautions in Hospitals" [CDC Web site]. Available at: http://www.cdc.gov/ncidod/hip/ISOLAT/std_prec_excerpt.htm. Reviewed November 3, 2004. Accessed March 9, 2005.

Handwashing

Wash hands after touching blood, body fluids, secretions, excretions, and contaminated items, whether or not gloves are worn. Wash hands immediately after gloves are removed, between patient contacts, and when otherwise indicated to avoid transfer of microorganisms to other patients or environments. It may be necessary to wash hands between tasks and procedures on the same patient to prevent cross-contamination of different body sites. Use a plain (nonantimicrobial) soap for routine handwashing. Use an antimicrobial agent or a waterless antiseptic agent for specific circumstances (eg, control of outbreaks or hyperendemic infections), as defined by the infection control program.

Gloves

Wear gloves (clean, nonsterile gloves are adequate) when touching blood, body fluids, secretions, excretions, and contaminated items. Put on clean gloves just before touching mucous membranes and nonintact skin. Change gloves between tasks and procedures on the same patient after contact with material that may contain a high concentration of microorganisms. Remove gloves promptly after use, before touching noncontaminated items and environmental surfaces, and before going to another patient, and wash hands immediately to avoid transfer of microorganisms to other patients or environments.

Mask, Eye Protection, Face Shield

Wear a mask and eye protection or a face shield to protect mucous membranes of the eyes, nose, and mouth during procedures and patient-care activities that are likely to generate splashes or sprays of blood, body fluids, secretions, and excretions.

Gown

Wear a gown (a clean, nonsterile gown is adequate) to protect skin and to prevent soiling of clothing during procedures and patient-care activities that are likely to generate splashes or sprays of blood, body fluids, secretions, or excretions. Select a gown that is appropriate for the activity and amount of fluid likely to be encountered. Remove a soiled gown as promptly as possible, and wash hands to avoid transfer of microorganisms to other patients or environments.

Patient-Care Equipment

Handle used patient-care equipment soiled with blood, body fluids, secretions, and excretions in a manner that prevents skin and mucous membrane exposures, contamination of clothing, and transfer of microorganisms to other patients and environments. Ensure that reusable equipment is not used for the care of another patient until it has been cleaned and reprocessed appropriately. Ensure that single-use items are discarded properly.

Environmental Control

Ensure that the hospital has adequate procedures for the routine care, cleaning, and disinfection of environmental surfaces, beds, bedrails, bedside equipment, and other frequently touched surfaces, and ensure that these procedures are being followed.

Linen

Handle, transport, and process used linen soiled with blood, body fluids, secretions, and excretions in a manner that prevents skin and mucous membrane exposures and contamination of clothing, and that avoids transfer of microorganisms to other patients and environments.

Occupational Health and Bloodborne Pathogens

Take care to prevent injuries when using needles, scalpels, and other sharp instruments or devices; when handling sharp instruments after procedures; when cleaning used instruments; and when disposing of used needles. Never recap used needles, or otherwise manipulate them using both hands, or use any other technique that involves directing the point of a needle toward any part of the body; rather, use either a one-handed "scoop" technique or a mechanical device designed for holding the needle sheath. Do not remove used needles from disposable syringes by hand, and do not bend, break, or otherwise manipulate used needles by hand. Place used disposable syringes and needles, scalpel blades, and other sharp items in appropriate puncture-resistant containers, which are located as close as practical to the area in which the items were used, and place reusable syringes and needles in a puncture-resistant container for transport to the reprocessing area. Use mouthpieces, resuscitation bags, or other ventilation devices as an alternative to mouth-to-mouth resuscitation methods in areas where the need for resuscitation is predictable.

Patient Placement

Place a patient who contaminates the environment or who does not (or cannot be expected to) assist in maintaining appropriate hygiene or environmental control in a private room. If a private room is not available, consult with infection control professionals regarding patient placement or other alternatives.

Some forms of meningitis (eg, meningococcal) are contagious. The bacteria are spread through the exchange of respiratory and throat secretions. EMS personnel can become exposed while controlling an airway by suctioning or intubating. Mouth-to-mouth resuscitation is not recommended, but if it is performed, it should also be considered an exposure. Sometimes the bacteria are spread to others who have had close or prolonged contact; these people should be considered at increased risk of acquiring the infection and should receive antibiotic prophylaxis. There are vaccines against *Haemophilus influenzae* type B (Hib) and against some strains of *Neisseria meningitidis,* as well as many types of *S. pneumoniae.* The vaccines against Hib are very safe and highly effective. The vaccine that protects against *N. meningitidis* is not routinely used in the United States, although college freshmen are advised to consider the vaccine, which can decrease their risk.[20] Antibiotic prophylaxis can also be administered to people potentially exposed to these infectious agents.

Severe Acute Respiratory Syndrome

Severe acute respiratory syndrome (SARS) is a viral respiratory illness that was first identified in Asia in 2003. During 2003, there were approximately 8,000 cases identified worldwide, including the United States and Canada. There were 774 deaths; none occurred in the United States. The quarantine required as part of a surveillance program in Toronto resulted in many EMS personnel being quarantined for up to 10 days, significantly affecting the staffing in their EMS systems.

The virus that causes SARS, called **SARS-association coronavirus (SARS-CoV),** is most likely transmitted by close person-to-person contact via respiratory droplets or via contaminated surfaces. These patients have fever, headache, myalgias, and respiratory symptoms, including dry cough. Complications such as severe pneumonia and respiratory failure can be fatal.

There is no specific treatment for SARS other than appropriate supportive care. More important are an effective surveillance and screening program and use of appropriate PPE and respiratory protection for potentially exposed individuals. For more information, consult the CDC Web site.

■ Violence and Personal Injury

Violence

Violence and the injuries that can accompany it are all too common in today's society. EMS workers, by the nature of their jobs, are exposed to violence and the vic-

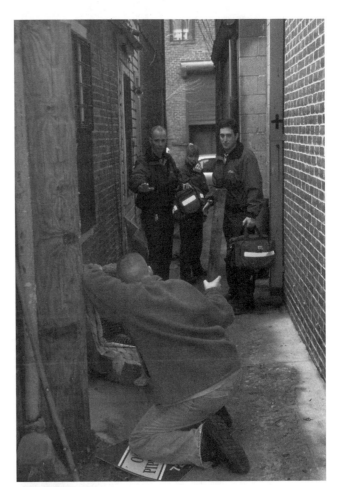

Figure 25-3 EMS workers are inevitably exposed to violence and the victims of violence every day.

tims of violence daily (**Figure 25-3**). OSHA and the Bureau of Labor Statistics reported that assaults and violent acts were the third leading cause of fatal occupational injury in the United States in 2003, and the second leading cause of fatal work injuries in women.[21]

Studies of violence in EMS indicate that personnel have been assaulted while on duty, including shot at while working and shot while on duty.[22] Workplace violence also includes beatings, psychological trauma, threats or obscene phone calls, intimidation, being followed, and harassment.

The frequency of nonlethal acts of violence is unknown. Gathering and analyzing data regarding these incidents are problematic because many events go unreported. But workplace violence research is becoming a priority for both government and private organizations as the toll becomes more apparent. The US Department of Justice National Crime Victimization Survey estimates that 1.7 million violent victimizations occur in the workplace every year.[23] However, the lack of good research on the causes and preventive measures hampers efforts to address the problem.

To better understand the problem, researchers have identified and divided workplace violence into four types or categories: criminal intent (Type I), customer or client (Type II), worker-on-worker (Type III), and personal relationship (Type IV). Service providers (eg, health care workers) are among the most common targets of Type II violence. For each of the violence categories, research topics have been created with the intention of better understanding and identifying prevention strategies.

Health care workers, including EMS providers, often face aggressive patients, visit clients in their homes in dangerous neighborhoods, encounter violent situations, and face other dangerous situations. Bureau of Labor Statistics data indicate that there were 69 homicides in the health services from 1996 to 2000, and that in 2000, 48% of all nonfatal injuries from occupational assaults and violent acts occurred in health care and social services.[24] The 2004 OSHA publication *Guidelines for Preventing Workplace Violence for Health Care and Social Service Workers* is designed to help employers establish effective workplace violence prevention programs. In this publication, OSHA has identified five elements that should be addressed in developing an effective workplace violence prevention program, as follows[24]:

- Management commitment and employee involvement
- Worksite analysis
- Hazard prevention and control
- Safety and health training
- Record-keeping and program evaluation

EMS organizations should be collecting and analyzing reports or data on the incidence and types of violence encountered by their employees and developing strategies to reduce their occurrence. More research is needed to determine the most appropriate and effective prevention strategies, but EMS organizations still should develop and implement violence prevention programs that include the OSHA guidelines, recommendations from local and/or state regulatory or training agencies, and other reputable organizations committed to preventing workplace violence.

Personal Injury Among EMS Personnel

EMS personnel often find themselves in unpredictable and uncontrollable environments. To do their jobs safely, they need to be in good physical and mental health. They are required to work both indoors and outdoors and in all types of weather conditions. Irregular hours and treating patients in life-or-death situations lead to job stress. They must perform rapid assessment of scene hazards while starting their patient assessment and delivery of care. Their daily jobs require them to kneel, bend, twist, and lift heavy equipment and patients. These tasks often are performed without the chance to stretch their cold, tight muscles. In an occupational injury study performed in New England, stress was identified as the most common occupational risk suffered, followed closely by back injuries.[25] According to an article published in the *American Journal of Emergency Medicine*, back strain is the leading cause of on-duty injuries among EMS personnel.[26] A study published in *Emergency Medical Services* indicated that 26 of 35 injured health care workers were injured as a result of bending forward or a combination of bending, twisting, and lifting.[27]

More EMS systems are creating positions for a health and safety officer. In addition to guiding the agency or department on the OSHA-required health and safety regulations, this person or department is charged with identifying and correcting safety hazards in the workplace and understanding factors related to physical and mental fitness and basic health, such as knowledge of exercise physiology, good nutrition, and stress management. The three major contributors to being out of shape are poor eating habits, lack of exercise, and emotional stress.[28] A safety officer would also conduct accident investigations and service record inspections and maintenance for equipment and vehicles, keep accurate, confidential personnel health records, and investigate job injuries and illnesses (including bloodborne pathogen exposures).

One of the basic duties of an EMS organization's manager is to ensure the well-being of his or her personnel. Being aware of the causes of personnel injuries is very important. It is important to reduce stress and back injuries in the workplace, and more research is needed.

Women and Careers in EMS

According to the National Registry of EMTs, in 1980, women accounted for 33.7% of nationally registered EMTs. By 1997, the total number of nationally registered EMTs had doubled, but the percentage of those who were women went down to 32%.[29]

EMS has been a male-dominated occupation from its beginning. In one study of occupationally related issues, a total of 49 EMTs (22 female, 27 male) completed a questionnaire. The identified gender-related issues were physical strength, assumption of authoritative roles, and organizational preparedness to implement gender-friendly working environments.[30]

Despite adversity, women continue to choose EMS

as a career. There is little literature that addresses issues related to women working in EMS. According to results of a survey conducted by the *Journal of Emergency Medical Services* (*JEMS*), women face major obstacles when trying to climb the EMS career ladder.[31]

One of the many obstacles women face in EMS is on-the-job sexual harassment. In the *JEMS* survey, almost half (44%) reported that they had experienced sexual harassment at work, including inappropriate comments and sexual advances. Only 38% reported that they had separate sleeping accommodations. Learning to live in a station house with men does not come easily for most women. EMS organizations should have in place a zero-tolerance policy regarding sexual harassment.

Another issue raised in the *JEMS* survey was how to balance the demands of a family with the responsibilities associated with a professional career. Working women are more likely than men to have the most responsibilities at home, including child-rearing.

The most common issue probably is the perception of physical strength. Concerns among EMS professionals about issues of physical strength are well documented. In the *JEMS* survey, 38% of respondents agreed that women have less physical strength than men do. However, researchers have noted that women might achieve a higher level of general fitness than men that enables them to overcome disparities of physical strength.[31]

Women have had a long road to travel in the traditionally male-dominated field of EMS. Women and men can better provide EMS services after reflecting seriously on what each sex can offer and addressing their careers as EMS team partners.

Summary

EMS professionals enjoy one of the most rewarding but challenging careers in today's rapidly changing world. Being properly prepared to perform their many duties in a safe and effective manner is the responsibility of every EMS professional and their employers. Since September 11, 2001, the risks associated with working in an EMS system have been more clear, and the job is viewed as more important. Today's EMS professionals and their respective organizations must work diligently to be prepared to respond and work as safely as possible in the hazardous conditions and environments they encounter.

References

1. US Department of Labor, Occupational Safety and Health Administration. Bloodborne pathogens. 29 CFR §1910.1030.

2. Centers for Disease Control and Prevention. Updated US Public Health Service guidelines for the management of occupational exposures to HBV, HCV, and HIV and recommendations for postexposure prophylaxis. *MMWR Morb Mortal Wkly Rep.* 2001; 50(RR11):1–42.

3. Occupational exposure to bloodborne pathogens; needlestick and other sharps injuries; final rule. 66 *Federal Register* 5317-5325 (2001).

4. Report on the global AIDS/HIV epidemic 2002. World Health Organization Web site. Available at: http://www.who.int/hiv/pub/epidemiology/pubepidemic2002/en/. Accessed January 23, 2005.

5. AIDS history project. University of California, San Francisco Web site. Available at: http://www.library.ucsf.edu/collres/archives.asp. Accessed January 23, 2005.

6. Gerberding JL. Incidence and prevention of human immunodeficiency virus, hepatitis B virus, hepatitis C virus, and cytomegalovirus among healthcare personnel at risk for blood exposure: final report from a longitudinal study. *J Infect Dis.* 1994;170:1410–1417.

7. Centers for Disease Control and Prevention. Case-control study of HIV seroconversion in healthcare workers after percutaneous exposure to HIV infected blood — France, United Kingdom and United States; January 1988-August 1994. *MMWR Morb Mortal Wkly Rep.* 1995;44:929–933.

8. Gellert GA, Maxwell RM, Higgins KV, et al. AIDS and prehospital personnel: knowledge and prevention of occupational exposure. *Prehospital Disaster Med.* 1996;11(2):112–116.

9. Centers for Disease Control and Prevention. Hepatitis C virus infection among firefighters, emergency medical technicians, and paramedics at selected locations, United States, 1991-2000. *MMWR Morb Mortal Wkly Rep.* 2000;49:660–665.

10. Upfal MJ, Naylor P, Mutchnick MM. Hepatitis C screening and prevalence among urban public safety workers. *J Occup Environ Med.* 2001;43:402–411.

11. Centers for Disease Control and Prevention. Core curriculum on tuberculosis (2000) [CDC Web site]. Available at: www.cdc.gov/nchstp/tb/pubs/corecurr/default.htm. Accessed January 23, 2005.

12. US Department of Labor, Occupational Safety and Health Administration. Respiratory protection. 29 CFR §1910.134.

13. Centers for Disease Control and Prevention, National Immunization Program. Hepatitis A vaccine: what you need to know [CDC Web site]. Available at: www.cdc.gov/nip/publications/vis/vis-hep-a.pdf. Accessed January 24, 2005.

14. Centers for Disease Control and Prevention, National Center for Infectious Diseases. Viral hepatitis E [CDC Web site]. Available at: http://www.cdc.gov/ncidod/diseases/hepatitis/e/index.htm. Accessed January 24, 2005.

15. Centers for Disease Control and Prevention, Division of Healthcare Quality Promotion. MRSA — Methicillin resistant *Staphylococcus aureus*: information for healthcare personnel [CDC Web site]. Available at: http://www.cdc.gov/ncidod/hip/aresist/mrsahcw.htm. Accessed January 24, 2005.

16. Centers for Disease Control and Prevention, Division of Bacterial and Mycotic Diseases. Drug-resistant *Streptococcus pneumoniae* disease [CDC Web site]. Available at: http://www.cdc.gov/ncidod/dbmd/diseaseinfo/drugresisstreppneum_t.htm. Accessed January 24, 2005.

17. Centers for Disease Control and Prevention, Division of Healthcare Quality Promotion. Multidrug-resistant organisms in non-hospital healthcare settings [CDC Web site]. Available at: http://www.cdc.gov/ncidod/hip/aresist/nonhosp.htm. Accessed January 24, 2005.

18. Centers for Disease Control and Prevention, Division of Healthcare Quality Promotion. Healthcare coalition successful in controlling vancomycin-resistant enterococcus (VRE) [CDC Web site]. Available at: http://www.cdc.gov/ncidod/hip/whats_new/nejm_vre.htm. Accessed January 24, 2005.

19. Centers for Disease Control and Prevention, Division of Healthcare Quality Promotion. VISA/VRSA–vancomycin-intermediate/resistant *Staphylococcus aureus* [CDC Web site]. Available at: http://www.cdc.gov/ncidod/hip/vanco/vanco.htm. Accessed January 24, 2005.

20. Centers for Disease Control and Prevention, Division of Bacterial and Mycotic Disease. Meningococcal disease [CDC Web site]. Available at: http://www.cdc.gov/ncidod/dbmd/diseaseinfo/meningococcal_g.htm. Accessed January 24, 2005.

21. US Department of Labor, Bureau of Labor Statistics. Census of fatal occupational injuries [BLS Web site]. Available at: http://www.bls.gov/news.release/cfoi.toc.htm. Accessed January 24, 2005.

22. Sayah AJ, Thomsen TW, Eckstein M, et al. EMS Providers and Violence in the Field. Presented at: ACEP Research Forum; October 11–12, 1999; Las Vegas, Nev.

23. US Department of Justice, Office of Justice Programs. Violence in the workplace, 1993-99 [OJP Web site]. Available at: http://www.ojp.usdoj.gov/bjs/pub/pdf/vw99.pdf. Accessed January 24, 2005.

24. US Deparment of Labor, Occupational Safety and Health Administration. Guidelines for preventing workplace violence for healthcare and social service workers [OSHA Web site]. Available at: http://www.osha.gov/Publications/osha3148.pdf. Accessed January 24, 2005.

25. Schwartz RJ, Benson L, Jacobs LM. The prevalence of occupational injuries in EMTs in New England. *Prehospital Disaster Med.* 1993;8:45–49.

26. Hogya PT, Ellis L. Evaluation of the injury profile of personnel in a busy urban EMS system. *Am J Emerg Med.* 1990;8:308–311.

27. Mitterer D. Back injuries in EMS. *Emerg Med Serv.* 1999;28:41–48.

28. Nordberg M. Looking good, feeling fit, staying strong: self-care in EMS. *Emerg Med Serv.* 1999;28:33–39.

29. Honeycutt L. Girl talk. *J Emerg Med Serv.* 1998;24:50–53.

30. Gonsoulin S, Palmer CE. Gender issues and partner preferences among a sample of EMT's. *Prehospital Disaster Med.* 1998;13(1):34–40.

31. Dernocoeur K, Eastman JN. Have we really come a long way? Women in EMS survey-results. *J Emerg Med Serv.* 1992;17:18–19.

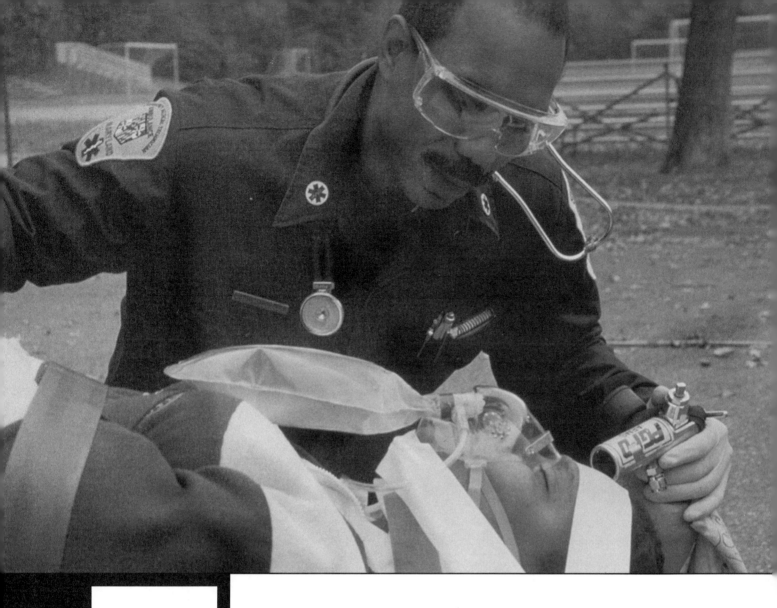

26 Medical-Legal Concerns in EMS

Leah J. Heimbach, JD, RN
Douglas M. Wolfberg, Esquire

Principles of This Chapter

After reading this chapter, you should be able to:

- Discuss the two basic types of law in the judicial system.
- Explain the overall liability risks of EMS providers and physician directors.
- Describe patient transport issues and how EMTALA affects EMS.
- Discuss system responsibility to act and refusal of care.
- List the antikickback issues.

OUT-OF-HOSPITAL CARE IN THE UNITED STATES WAS INITI-ated through efforts of individuals via self-designated rescue squads, fire department emergency responders, and volunteer emergency services to improve on the then-existing funeral home transport and poorly regulated private ambulance systems. Skillful out-of-hospital care gained popular support when the public became aware of the lifesaving possibilities through Seattle's "Medic One" and from television programs such as "Emergency!" Combat personnel returning from the Vietnam War brought to light the importance of field intervention by nonphysicians and medical evacuation systems, and medical command resulted in the realization of improved out-of-hospital care to trauma victims.

By 1970, Emergency Medical Technician-Ambulance (EMT-A) programs, funded by the US Department of Transportation (DOT), were implemented. The DOT also developed specifications regarding emergency transport vehicles that improved the quality of care. The use of station wagons (which also served as hearses) gave way to the use of the emergency transport vehicles of today. As advanced life support technology evolved, innovative and dedicated physicians from many areas and specialties committed to providing the medical expertise to direct such programs. These advocates of EMS worked within the medical community to obtain acceptance and permit the use of advanced and invasive skills in the out-of-hospital setting. Although dedicated and energetic, most physician leaders during the early years of EMS were not properly trained, nor were they prepared for the long-term administrative responsibilities that accompanied the developing EMS systems. However, in the late 1970s, with the development of emergency medicine as a specialty, medically appropriate care and medical accountability of the out-of-hospital provider became particularly significant for emergency physicians.

During the developmental years of EMS, there were minimal concerns about medical-legal liability. Although many agencies considered themselves to be covered by general Good Samaritan statutes or by specific immunity for government agencies, these legal immunities might not have actually existed. If they did, they were rapidly being eroded by case law in many jurisdictions. Some states found it necessary to pass immunity legislation to specifically cover the providers of EMS care, their sponsoring agencies, and in some cases the training and administrative agencies, physicians, and hospitals responsible for the systems. Medical malpractice actions against individual EMTs and paramedics are uncommon; however, incidents of litigation against out-of-hospital providers do occur and are increasing. Additional litigation directed toward EMS systems on the basis of training criteria, supervision, and medical direction make it clear that those involved in EMS must be aware of and concerned about legal and medical issues that confront them in the modern provision of EMS services.

The Judicial System

Before understanding the specific duties, obligations, and legal risks associated with EMS delivery, EMS providers must understand the basic concepts of the system of civil and criminal justice in the United States.

Criminal justice concerns are seldom involved in the administration of emergency medical care. Some states, however, indicate that actions beyond the scope of authorized practice for licensed individuals that result in harm or death might involve criminal violations. Also, some states mandate the reporting of child

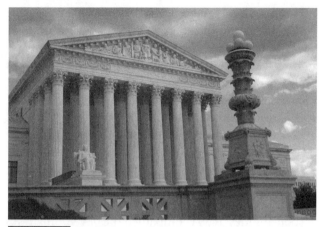

Figure 26-1 The US Supreme Court represents the highest level of the federal judicial system.

abuse and other forms of abuse and typically threaten criminal penalties for noncompliance.

The US legal system is unlike that in any other country in that it has two coexisting legal systems — **state and federal**. The differences between these two systems have to do with jurisdiction, authority, subject matter, limitations, and strategy, to name a few. In most states, the court system is divided into at least two different levels. Lower-level courts have more limited jurisdiction that is usually very specific. The upper-level courts have more general jurisdiction to hear matters that are more expansive. The federal system is divided into three levels: trial courts, courts of appeal, and, at the highest level, the US Supreme Court (**Figure 26-1**). Federal courts usually hear cases that involve federal rights and conflicts among citizens from different states.

Another factor that is unique to the United States is the **separation of powers**. The **legislative branch** of government makes law by passing statutes. The **executive branch** enforces and implements law through regulation. The **judicial branch** interprets and announces the meaning of law by hearing disputes. All of these branches take actions that can and do affect the function of emergency medical care and dictate how it can be delivered and directed.

There are two basic types of law — criminal (mentioned earlier) and civil (also known as tort law).

Negligence

The civil system, or the portion of the judicial system that deals with lawsuits, is familiar to physicians. Negligence is the basis of this system, which requires that every individual act as a reasonable person with the same or similar training would act under the same or similar circumstances. This includes both improper acts and the failure to act. Failure to meet this standard of care constitutes negligence.

In order to prove malpractice or negligence, a plaintiff must prove all four elements of the claim, as follows:

- That the defendant had a duty to the patient to provide care
- That the defendant breached that duty by failure to perform to the required standard of care
- That injury or damage to the patient resulted (which can include physical and/or psychological injury)
- That the damage or injury was caused by the failure to comply with the standard of care

If all four elements are not proved, there is no legal cause of action for negligence.

Willful and Wanton Conduct

There are concepts in the civil law system known as **gross negligence** or **willful and wanton conduct**. These terms are similar in concept but separated by the degree or extent of deviation from the standard of care. Willful and wanton conduct is based on showing a reckless disregard for safety; it is not a mere mistake or minor failure to meet the standard of care.

This differentiation is critical in some states. Statutes that provide legal protection under immunity might extend to negligence situations but afford no protection for willful and wanton actions or failures to act. Many insurance policies preclude protection for damages or judgments sustained in actions based on willful and wanton conduct.

Vicarious Liability

The civil law concept of vicarious liability is also known as **respondeat superior** ("let the master answer"). Under this concept, the "master" is responsible for the negligence or willful and wanton conduct of the "servant" within the scope and course of employment. This doctrine is sometimes applied in employment situations, or it could also apply to those who are in a position to give direction or exert control over EMS personnel. This has resulted in litigation directed toward medical directors of EMS systems for the alleged actions of EMS field personnel. Assertion of a claim based on vicarious liability is governed on a state-by-state basis.

Active negligence cases have been brought against EMS systems for failure to provide adequate training or supervision, failure to provide proper certification, and failure to remove an individual from duty when system administrators knew or should have known that the individual was not competent to provide emergency medical care.

Vicarious liability is a popular method by which a plaintiff's attorney will seek to draw the medical director of an EMS system into a negligence case to expand the financial resources from which to collect. Therefore, emergency physicians must ensure that their EMS medical direction activities are specifically and sufficiently covered by their medical malpractice insurance.

Although vicarious liability is the most common method of seeking to impose liability on a medical director for the alleged negligent acts of EMS personnel, plaintiffs' attorneys might also seek to impose direct liability on EMS system medical directors for breaches of specific duties, such as a failure to have proper policies, procedures, protocols, and training in place.

System Responsibility to Act

The creation of an EMS system and the delivery of care typically are regulated by state or local government. These rules and regulations, together with the written participation agreements with the providers in the system, constitute a legal set of conditions for the operation of the system. Failure to comply with those rules and regulations could result in administrative actions or civil lawsuits or both. Violation of statutes or regulations can constitute negligence per se in a tort lawsuit.

It is the EMS system's responsibility, and that of the medical director, to see that providers within the system are operating in a manner that is consistent with existing rules and regulations. The civil liability resulting from violations makes it extremely important for the medical director or other designated medical supervisory personnel to demand strict compliance with these regulations to avoid allegations of active negligence or vicarious liability.

When a system has announced its capability to provide advanced life support, it might be found that the public has the right to rely on that care and to expect the availability of such care 24 hours a day, 365 days a year. This might invoke the "duty to act" element of negligence. Volunteer staffing, service breakdowns, or difficult periods for staffing for that level of service might not constitute defenses to provide only BLS when an ALS response is indicated.

If a system provides for tiered response or allows waivers of certain standards, explicit policies and procedures must be in place and monitored to ensure that all units are in legal compliance and that the public is aware of the limited response capabilities.

Efforts to screen incoming calls to determine the existence of a true emergency have proved to be disastrous from a liability perspective. The general standard has evolved that an emergency exists if the caller deems it so, and that all callers receive an emergency response. As advocates for adopting the **prudent layperson definition of an emergency**, emergency physicians have achieved monumental success in getting the public to understand what constitutes an emergency. Through this advocacy, EMS might now be held to the same standard that has been so diligently asserted to, and in many cases adopted, by legislative bodies and insurance-related agencies. Given this new perception of what constitutes an emergency, great caution should be taken regarding screening calls.

Appropriate action should be guided by system policy and procedure, which includes EMS personnel's obligation to evaluate patients on scene and to provide appropriate care. The decision to release a patient without transport should be made only in consultation with the online physician or when the patient refuses treatment and/or transport against medical advice.

Refusal of Care

Frequently, patients at the scene of an emergency refuse care or transport by EMS personnel. Refusal of care or transport is a fundamental right of the competent adult, but it could also present potential legal problems. When this happens, protocols might direct the EMS provider to contact the online medical oversight physician. The EMS physician must provide guidance and direction in these situations.

An adult of sound mind has the right to refuse medical care or treatment, even when doing so puts the person at risk. This is often complicated when EMS personnel encounter patients with limited judgment or mental impairment that can result from alcohol or drug use, head injury, or other causes. Ultimately, it is the duty of the EMS personnel on the scene, and the online physician when consulted, to conclude whether the patient has the capacity to refuse care and to respond appropriately. This decision is made based on information communicated by the onscene EMS personnel to the physician.

If a patient refuses care, the online physician should ensure that the EMS personnel take the following actions:

- Calmly inform the patient of the possible consequences of refusing treatment. Refusal could stem from fear or emotional distress resulting from the current situation. Rational explanations and reassurance might dispel fear or denial and result in permission to treat.
- If this is not successful, carefully explain the possible diagnosis, the indicated treatment, and the possible consequences of not receiving treatment.
- If the patient persists in refusing care, urge the patient to seek medical attention from his or her personal physician.

At this point, documentation is of paramount importance. This includes specific observations that led the EMS personnel to conclude that the patient is an adult of sound mind, indicating that the person has mental capacity to make an appropriate decision. In making this assessment, the EMS personnel must be cognizant of the medical conditions and mechanisms of injury that can induce a patient to inappropriately refuse treatment. Typical among these are disorientation following a motor vehicle crash, diabetic conditions, head injuries, and stroke. Regretfully, poverty often is a cause of refusal of care, especially among the elderly. EMS systems owned and operated by hospitals must be particularly vigilant to ensure that concerns over financial responsibility do not prevent a person from receiving a medical screening examination; the medical-legal risk is a possible violation of the hospital's obligations under the Emergency Medical Treatment and Labor Act, or EMTALA.

Continuing with the list of actions onscene personnel should take:
- Document that the patient understands that care is being offered, that, in the EMS personnel's opinion, the care is necessary, and that the patient might sustain aggravated injury, disability, or even death as a result of refusing to permit treatment.
- Document that this was explained to family members or significant others, employers, supervisors, or anyone who might be present and in a position to exercise influence over the patient.
- Complete the against medical advice or release of liability form and have it witnessed and signed.

A caveat regarding the "AMA form": do not rely on it as anything more than evidence of the fact that the ramifications of refusing treatment were discussed with the patient. Consequently, it is critical to include references in the run report to support the fact that the nature and significance of the document were explained to the patient before he or she signed it. Merely handing it to the patient for signature is legally insufficient. It is also advisable to have at least two witnesses sign the document as well. Although it is legally acceptable to have a squad member sign as a witness, it is preferable to have as a signing witness a disinterested third party, whose testimony will carry greater weight in support of the EMS provider if a lawsuit results.

Other interesting dilemmas are presented when care is refused by parents or legal guardians or by minors. Parents or legal guardians can grant or refuse permission to treat their minor children, even against a child's wishes. In the event that a parent refuses treatment for a child, the same efforts used to obtain consent for an adult are appropriate. Some states have enacted laws that require EMS personnel to immediately report any case in which a parent refuses emergency care for a minor child. Special consideration must also be given to emancipated minors. A minor is emancipated if his or her parent or legal guardian relinquishes authority and control over the minor child. Usually, emancipation requires acknowledgment of both child and parent. When a child is then free from parental control, the child surrenders the right to maintenance and support from the parent. Emancipation frequently occurs when a minor child marries and might hold true for pregnant minor children. Some state laws allow an emancipated minor to consent to or refuse treatment.

Finally, refusal of care by a mature minor must be considered. Several states have enacted laws that allow mature minors to make health care decisions for themselves in certain circumstances. This often requires assessment by a physician (which can be accomplished with the online physician). Whether a minor is mature is a question of fact. Factors for the physician to determine whether the child has the capacity to consent depend on the age, ability, experience, education, training, and degree of maturity or judgment obtained by the child, as well as on the conduct and demeanor of the child at the time of the procedure or treatment. The determination also includes whether the child has the capacity to appreciate the nature, risks, and consequences of the treatment to be rendered or refused. A good-faith assessment of the minor's maturity level might absolve a physician from liability for looking to the minor for consent or refusal of care.

Belcher v Charleston Area Medical Center[1] is a case involving a 17-year-old boy (Larry Belcher) who died after hospital staff followed do-not-resuscitate orders. The patient suffered from muscular dystrophy and was confined to a wheelchair. On December 19, 1986, he stopped breathing. The father removed mucus from the patient's throat, began mouth-to-mouth resuscitation, and revived the patient. He was taken to Charleston (West Virginia) Area Medical Center by ambulance. He was admitted, intubated, and placed on a ventilator. The treating physician discussed the boy's prognosis with his parents. The parents had not yet decided what resuscitative efforts, if any, should be provided for their son. On December 23, 1986, he was extubated, and pain management was provided. The treating physician asked him if he wanted to be reintubated, and the patient motioned "no" with his head. The parents then told the physician not to reintubate their son unless he requested it. The physician wrote a do-not-resuscitate order in the record. The boy was not involved in this decision as the physician contends because he was emotionally immature due to his disease; he was on medication that diminished his capacity; involving him in the decision would have increased his anxiety, thus reducing his chances of survival; and the boy's parents told the physician that they did not want their son involved. On December 24, 1986, the patient went into respiratory arrest and died. The parents then filed a wrongful death action.

The West Virginia Supreme Court of Appeals held that:

> Except in very extreme cases, a physician has no legal right to perform a procedure upon, or administer or withhold treatment from a patient without the patient's consent, nor upon a child without the consent of the child's parents or guardian, unless the child is a mature minor, in which case the child's consent would be required. Whether a child is a mature minor is a question of fact. Whether the child has the capacity to consent depends upon the age, ability, experience, education, training, and degree of maturity or judgment obtained by the child, as well as upon the conduct and demeanor of the child at the time of the procedure or treatment. The factual determination would also involve whether the minor has the capacity to appreciate the nature, risks, and consequences of the medical procedure to be performed, or the treatment to be administered or withheld. Where there is a conflict between the intentions of one or both parents and the minor, the physician's good faith assessment of the minor's maturity level would immunize him or

her from liability for the failure to obtain parental consent.[1]

Impaired Patients

When a patient refuses treatment and that patient is, in the opinion of EMS personnel, mentally or physically unable to make such a decision, the emergency crew is placed in an awkward and potentially litigious position. In those situations, an against medical advice form should not be used, even if the patient is willing to sign one. Otherwise, it might appear that the EMT is "hedging" on the evaluation by stating that the patient is not capable of making the decision, yet allowing the decision to be made anyway.

It is frequently the duty of the EMS system to protect patients from themselves and from their medical or physical conditions. If a patient is mentally unstable, drug influenced, violent, hypoxic, or in any way impaired, it is the EMS provider's responsibility to provide appropriate treatment and transport. Depending on state law, this is often most appropriately accomplished in consultation with the online physician and local law enforcement. If treatment is to be rendered despite refusal, thorough documentation is indicated. In some circumstances, treatment is rendered under the concept of implied consent. Under this doctrine, consent for treatment is presumed on the basis that a conscious and competent patient would act in a reasonable manner and consent to medical care. If the patient physically resists, the EMS personnel must attempt to transport the patient against his or her will with the aid of law enforcement officers, taking care to avoid harming the patient without being harmed themselves.

EMS personnel are entitled to use reasonable force to defend themselves, but they must make every effort to appropriately restrain and contain the patient without inflicting harm. Use of force is justified only to the extent necessary to achieve control of the patient and protect the patient, EMS personnel, and others from harm.

If there is any indication of impending aggressive behavior on the part of the patient, every effort should be made to involve law enforcement personnel for the proper management of force. When this is not an option, as many personnel as possible should participate in the management of the patient so that the force used by any one individual is minimal. In addition to patient care skills, EMS personnel should be trained to recognize the signs of impending aggression, to deal with potentially violent patients with appropriate verbal means, and to use physical restraint methods suitable to achieve noninjurious patient control.

After an incident in which an aggressive patient has been managed or a refusing patient has been transported, particular care should be given to the thorough documentation of the incident in the run report. EMS personnel must document their nonphysical efforts to secure compliance by the patient, full details of all of the aggressive acts or actions of the patient, and all actions of a physical nature taken by EMS personnel. In writing this report, the tone must be one of concern for the patient's well-being. It should reflect that discomfort to the patient was reduced and that the only force used was what was necessary to contain the patient and provide needed medical care.

Patient Transport

Regardless of the nature of the EMS call, patients being transported require appropriate observation, evaluation, and treatment by out-of-hospital personnel from the time the provider arrives on the scene until the patient is delivered to the receiving facility. Out-of-hospital personnel should document the care given at the scene and during transport, as well as the patient's condition on transfer to the receiving facility. A complete and thorough narrative description of observations, sequences, events, and treatment should be completed for each patient encounter.

Destination Hospital

A competent, conscious adult who is not subject to immediate threat to life or limb has the general right to medical care of his or her choice. This includes selecting a destination hospital. If a patient expresses a preference, it is appropriate to make that choice known to the online physician. The choice of destination might also be subject to laws, regulations, or protocols within a state or a particular EMS system, creating tension between the choice of a competent, properly informed patient and those laws, regulations, or protocols.

In some states, the patient's right to select the destination hospital has been the subject of legislation. Also, many EMS departments have rules and policies directing emergency personnel to proceed only to the nearest available appropriate facility. When making a determination as to the nearest appropriate destination, EMS personnel should use predetermined system policies regarding facility capabilities or refer the decision to the online physician. Although compliance with local laws and regulations supersedes an EMT's personal judgment, compliance with the express wishes of a competent patient or a legally responsible decision-maker adds another dimension to the situation. It is critically important that the online physician participate in these decisions whenever there is a conflict.

All EMS personnel must recognize that a patient's preference must be disregarded if it would pose a risk to the life or safety of that patient. Again, however, the wishes of a competent patient or legally responsible decision-maker must be taken into account and should generally be followed unless these grave risks are present.

Interfacility Transfer

Interfacility transfer is now a substantial component of EMS operations. This service presents a unique set of challenges for which the EMS provider might not have been adequately trained or certified to handle.

Federal statutes now place interfacility transfers under the provisions of the **Emergency Medical Treatment and Labor Act (EMTALA)**. EMS personnel and physicians must be thoroughly familiar with this law and its regulations because they generally override any and all state or local rules or regulations involving patient transfer, including trauma center regulations (although EMTALA regulations do make some reference to local protocols in certain situations).

Under EMTALA, any person who comes to the "dedicated emergency department" of a Medicare-participating hospital and requests care must be provided a medical screening examination from that hospital, regardless of ability to pay. And, if the person is found to have an emergency medical condition, as defined in the law, the hospital must provide stabilizing treatment within its capabilities or effect an appropriate transfer (again, defined by law) to another hospital if it does not have the necessary capabilities.

EMTALA treats ambulances owned and operated by a hospital differently than those that are not hospital owned and operated. Although ambulances owned and operated by a hospital constitute hospital property for purposes of EMTALA, under regulations issued in 2003, a hospital-owned and -operated ambulance may transport a patient to a hospital other than that which owns and operates the ambulance if it does so under a communitywide EMS protocol that directs transport to a different facility. These regulations also permit transport to a hospital other than the one that owns and operates the ambulance if directed to do so by the online physician, so long as the physician is not affiliated with the hospital that owns and operates the ambulance.

According to the regulations, a hospital may by radio divert a non–hospital-owned and -operated ambulance to another facility when it is in diversion status — that is, it lacks the resources or staff to care for the patient. However, a decision of the US Court of Appeals, Ninth Circuit, suggests that a hospital can incur EMTALA liability when diverting even a non–hospital-owned and -operated ambulance to another facility when that diversion order is not based on an assessment of the facility's resources at the time, and further suggests that the *process* of getting to the hospital, as well as physical presentation at the hospital, might constitute coming to the hospital for EMTALA purposes.[2]

The EMTALA-mandated medical screening examination must be sufficient to determine whether the patient has an **emergency medical condition (EMC)**. An EMC is defined by law as:

> a medical condition manifesting itself by acute symptoms of sufficient severity (including severe pain) such that the absence of immediate medical attention could reasonably be expected to result in placing the health of the individual in serious jeopardy, serious impairment to bodily functions, or serious dysfunction of any bodily organ or part; . . .[3]

In the event that an EMC is identified by the medical screening examination, the hospital must provide stabilizing treatment within its capabilities. Under the law, the term **stabilized** has a special meaning and does not correspond to common medical terminology. Rather, under EMTALA, a patient's condition is stabilized when

> no material deterioration of the condition is likely, within reasonable medical probability, to result from or occur during the transfer of the individual from a facility, . . .[4]

Again, if the hospital does not have the capability to stabilize the patient's condition, it must arrange an appropriate transfer to a facility that does. **Transfer** means the "movement (including the discharge) of an individual outside the hospital at the direction of any person affiliated with the hospital."[5] In this situation, because the patient is unstable and the transfer is medically indicated, the transferring physician must certify that the risks of transfer are outweighed by the benefits to be obtained by transfer. If a transfer is to be made, the transferring facility must first verify that the receiving facility will accept the patient. Facilities providing a required higher level of care, including specialized facilities such as trauma centers, burn centers, or neonatal units, may not refuse an appropriate transfer if they have the capabilities and personnel to care for the patient.

The transfer must be effected using appropriate methods, equipment, and personnel. It is the responsibility of the transferring physician to determine and ensure that this occurs. Consideration must be given to the method of transport — whether a ground ambulance, a fixed-wing aircraft, or a helicopter is indicated. The benefits and risks of each must be weighed. EMTALA also requires the transferring facility to ensure that the transfer is effected using the appropriate life support equipment that is reasonably necessary to care for any *foreseeable deterioration* that might occur during transport. Case law throughout the United States has demonstrated that reliance on the basic equipment found in a standard ambulance might not be sufficient. The transferring physician must also ensure that the patient is accompanied by the appropriate personnel, including nurses or physicians, that would be required to care for *reasonably foreseeable complications* that could occur during transfer. Finally, the transferring physician is responsible for providing written orders for the care and treatment of the patient during the transfer. Copies of the patient's pertinent medical records, test results, x-rays, and other documents necessary for the receiving facility to adequately care for and treat the patient must be sent with the patient.

In many states, it is beyond the scope of EMS personnel to administer the drugs and procedures that might be required for a patient during transfer. An additional duty of the transferring physician is to be aware of the limitations of treatment that can be rendered by EMS personnel. If it is anticipated that a particular protocol, drug, procedure, or equipment might be reasonably required, the appropriate personnel to administer that treatment must accompany the patient.

Violations of EMTALA provisions can result in fines of up to $50,000 each against physicians (including on-call physicians) and hospitals responsible for an inappropriate transfer. In addition, a hospital or physician who has committed a gross and flagrant or repeated violation of EMTALA can also face termination from the Medicare, Medicaid, or state health programs. Although the actions of nurses or EMS personnel can contribute to what is determined to be a violation, they are not currently subject to fine under the provisions of the act.

However, violations can result in civil liability actions directed against a hospital in federal or state court. No direct EMTALA civil suits may be brought against physicians, EMS personnel, or nursing staff. If an EMTALA action is filed in federal court, state malpractice actions against physicians, EMS personnel, or nurses can be heard in federal court along with the EMTALA case against the hospital. Finally, liability for EMTALA violations is strict, meaning that proof of negligence or improper motive is not required once a violation has been proved.[6] (More information on EMTALA can be found in Chapter 27, "EMTALA and EMS.")

Advance Directives

There are situations in which EMS providers and online medical direction, in honoring the wishes of patients, withhold or limit resuscitation efforts. With increasing frequency, EMS providers responding to emergency scenes are presented with formal advance directive documents such as a do-not-resuscitate (DNR) order, living will, or medical power of attorney that grants authority to withhold, limit, or terminate treatment.

One reason for an increase in the use of advance directives is that federal law, through the **Patient Self-Determination Act**, requires all hospitals to inquire whether a patient has established an advance directive, and if not, to inform patients on arrival (possibly through the emergency department) of their right to do so. State laws vary as to the applicability of these provisions in the field.

Consequently, every EMS system must adopt policies and procedures that address the advance directive situation and outline procedures for EMS personnel to follow. While the details of such plans can vary from state to state, procedures must include communication with and direction from the online physician.

Most states have enacted statutes or established precedent through case law that permits resuscitative efforts to be withheld in cases such as decapitation, rigor mortis, extremity lividity, head injuries with exposed brain tissue, or other obvious signs of death. When death is obvious, CPR should not be initiated. EMS personnel must be trained to provide a clearly documented series of observations in the run report supporting such a decision. Ideally, EMS personnel should contact the online physician to obtain express authority for withholding resuscitative efforts. Documentation should include the lack of vital signs, including blood pressure, pulse, respirations, pupil response, and cardiac asystole. A history of the events surrounding the death is also required. Care must be taken to avoid confusing situations of acute drug overdose, hypoglycemia, hypothermia, and some poisonings, which might produce a death-like appearance.

Once CPR is initiated, it is extremely difficult to justify termination. Nevertheless, if a limit for resuscitation efforts is to be authorized, the policy should be consistent with do-not-resuscitate and advance directive guidelines. EMS personnel should not limit or terminate CPR under the direction of any physician on the scene unless that physician has been given on-scene responsibility by the online physician, or unless the physician making the determination is the patient's private physician. Even in the event of a private physician on scene, the decision to implement the DNR advance directives procedure should be made by an online physician. It is possible that further research and technological advances, such as correlating end-tidal CO_2 readings with ultimate survival probabilities, will enhance decision-making regarding the discontinuation of resuscitative efforts in the field. The authority of family members to terminate CPR in the out-of-hospital setting varies from state to state. EMS providers should be aware, however, that advance directives in the form of durable powers of attorney or medical powers of attorney might specifically grant designated individuals the right to make those decisions in some jurisdictions. Legal counsel should be actively involved in drafting EMS system policies and procedures to address this extremely complicated health care issue. Once such policies and procedures are in place, all EMS personnel should be thoroughly versed in their provisions and applicability.

Transporting Patients to Nonhospital Facilities

Transporting patients to freestanding or nonhospital facilities can create unique concerns and difficulties. When EMS personnel are managing a medical emergency, the patient should only be transported to a facility classified by the regional EMS system as a receiving facility. In most instances, only hospital-based emergency facilities should be used to receive emergency transports. Using a nonhospital facility as a destination would not be appropriate unless it is for prescheduled nonemergency care. Private ambulances routinely transport nonemergency patients to physician offices, ancillary care facilities, and hospital facilities. The freestanding urgent care facility should be viewed no differently in this situation than other nonhospital health care facilities.

There are rare situations in which a nonhospital facility may be used during an emergency transport. For example, it would be appropriate to use a nonhospital facility when the distance to a hospital emergency department is unusually long, the patient being transported is rapidly deteriorating, and the nonhospital facility is capable of providing emergency care that would benefit the patient. This should occur only under a preapproved regional EMS plan and under strict on-line medical direction. Once the patient has received necessary life-sustaining care at the freestanding facility, the EMS vehicle should proceed to the intended destination with appropriate medical staff and support from the freestanding facility. The nonhospital health care facility should not influence the ultimate destination of emergency patients. Online medical direction remains the authority over patient care and destination.

Physician on the Scene

Occasionally, EMS personnel will encounter a physician at the scene of an emergency who attempts to provide assistance to the EMS personnel. This physician could be an emergency physician or another physician who is adequately trained in emergency care, or a specialist in an area wholly unrelated to the treatment of trauma or medical emergencies.

When EMS personnel encounter the patient, they might have established a physician-patient relationship between the supervising online medical direction physician and the patient at the scene. EMS personnel must not deviate from their standard protocols for emergency care and treatment based on directions from an onscene physician. Such deviation could be construed as negligence in any subsequent court action based on that deviation.

The only exception to this provision is when the onscene physician has communicated with the online medical direction physician and has been authorized by the online physician to assume control of the scene. EMS personnel should verify this transfer of authority by confirming it over the radio or telephone and noting it in their report. Any instruction given by the onscene physician that deviates from the standard training and protocol of the EMS personnel could place them in legal jeopardy. If deviations from protocol result in an adverse outcome, the online physician is likely to be held legally responsible for inappropriately transferring authority to an individual who might not be trained and versed in the policies, procedures, and protocols of the EMS system.

If an onscene physician persists in attempting to interfere with EMS personnel's treatment of the patient, law enforcement assistance should be requested to remove that individual from the scene. In any incident where a physician is on scene and attempts to give direction, EMS personnel must thoroughly document all interactions and exchanges. Differences in medical opinion might be noted by bystanders and result in litigation regardless of the outcome of the case.

Under no circumstances should the onscene physician be allowed to assume control of the patient's medical care and then surrender this responsibility to the EMS personnel for transport. Once assuming medical responsibility, the physician must accompany the patient to the hospital. On the other hand, an onscene physician may assist with treatment that conforms to EMS protocols without assuming responsibility and being required to accompany the patient. For example, an anesthesiologist may help a paramedic who is having difficulty intubating a patient without being required to ride to the hospital in the ambulance. However, if this occurs, EMS personnel must document the name of the assisting physician and the extent of his or her participation in caring for the patient.

Religious Preference

EMS personnel and their medical direction physicians are occasionally confronted with patients whose religious beliefs challenge the appropriateness of emergency care or result in refusal of care. When this occurs, EMS personnel should be aware that competent and conscientious adults may refuse care for themselves but not necessarily for their minor children. EMS personnel are not expected to make legal or moral judgments on these issues.

If EMS personnel are required to provide appropriate emergency medical care to a minor child over the objection of parents, law enforcement personnel should be called to the scene to investigate possible child abuse or neglect. The decision of law enforcement personnel relieves the EMS personnel of making legal judgments for which they are not trained. If law enforcement personnel are not available, the online physician should be contacted. It is not likely that the child can be treated and transported without substantial objection of the parents. EMS personnel and the online physician should carefully consider the possibility of attempting to proceed with treatment and transporting the child to the hospital, where, once the child is stabilized, the matters of religion and legal rights can be resolved through appropriate legal channels. In so doing, however, EMS personnel must be prepared to be involved in litigation and must carefully document all conditions of the child that justify intervention.

When EMS personnel encounter this situation, they should make every effort to understand the nature of the parent's objection. Their concerns might involve only specific treatment and not transport, evaluation, and other possible treatment. Cooperation and consent can often be obtained once information and calm, rational explanations are provided.

Documentation

Documentation of out-of-hospital activities is of paramount importance. This is especially true in situations that might involve subsequent litigation such as motor vehicle crashes, assaults, personal injuries, alleged rape, child abuse, suspicion of foul play, patient refusal of treatment, patient refusal of transport, and a physician on the scene.

The necessary amount and type of documentation is increasing as the frequency of litigation increases throughout the EMS community. Clearly, documentation of the patient's condition on the scene, a brief history and physical examination, including vital signs, and changes in condition during transport are necessary. In certain cases, such as rape or child abuse, a brief, general description of the surroundings is indicated. If witnesses provide information, the information and the names of the witnesses should be documented. When two-way communication is established, the identity of the hospital and the online physician should be recorded. If therapy is provided, any complications and all changes in the patient's status should be noted.

When EMS personnel are on the scene for an extended time, they should document the patient's condition during the stay. They should also make subsequent documentation of the patient's condition when leaving the scene, as well as the condition on arrival at the receiving facility. Documentation requires narrative descriptions, not just check-off box entries.

The patient's destination as well as the method by which it was chosen should be noted. Changes in the patient's condition en route, or the absence thereof, must also be documented. The time the call was received, the time of arrival, the time on the scene, the time leaving the scene, and the time of arrival at the final destination should be recorded on every run. Recording all of this information might be time consuming, but it is necessary and might prove to be the best defense in a legal case. EMS personnel might find that it is not in their best legal interest to document only positive findings. Normal and negative findings must also be noted in the report. The legal assumption is that if a sign or symptom was not documented on the run sheet, then it was not observed. For example, if a patient is involved in any type of trauma and documentation of a cervical spine examination and stabilization does not appear in the chart, then, in the eyes of the courts, that examination did not occur.

Confidentiality

The EMS system, like the hospital, is bound to maintain confidentiality regarding any patient identifying information, medical condition, and treatment. Records maintained by the EMS system are deemed, in most states, to be medical records. As such, they must be preserved without disclosure unless there is patient consent, pursuant to an appropriate order from the court, when state law requires it, or when using the information for billing purposes. In addition, if the ambulance service is a covered entity under the **Health Insurance Portability and Accountability Act (HIPAA)** privacy rule, many additional restrictions on the disclosure of protected health information (PHI) apply.

State laws vary in requirements to access patient records, as well as to what constitutes patient records. However, if the entity is covered by HIPAA, EMS patient care reports clearly constitute PHI. The EMS system should adopt policies and procedures consistent with state law (and with HIPAA, if applicable) and protect confidential patient information. EMS personnel must be made aware of their responsibilities to maintain confidentiality (if the entity is covered by HIPAA, this training is mandatory). The patient is entitled to privacy as provided by law, and any inappropriate discussions of the identity, nature of conditions or illnesses, or treatment could result in personal liability for the EMS personnel involved and vicarious or direct liability for the EMS system, both under state law and HIPAA.

There are four areas that should be of particular concern. These are drug use, alcohol use, sexually transmitted diseases (including HIV), and psychiatric conditions. These conditions often carry additional legal protections because of the accompanying social stigma. In addition, some states have implemented more strict requirements to obtain information of this nature. In part, this is due to the overriding need to encourage citizens to seek medical care for these conditions. Patients often are reluctant to do so for fear of others finding out, the belief that they will be viewed in an unfavorable light, or the belief that they will be denied care. Divulging any confidential information, especially in these four areas, can result in substantial liability.

Bloodborne Pathogens

The federal Occupational Safety and Health Administration (OSHA) has issued regulations requiring that universal precautions be undertaken with regard to bloodborne pathogens.[7] Activities that might result in exposure must be identified so that employees know when the precaution must be observed. The burden of complying with OSHA regulations is on the employer of the EMS personnel.

This suggests that only ambulance services and fire departments employing EMS personnel are responsible for compliance. However, while under the medical direction of the EMS system, which overrides and supersedes the control by the employer, the EMS system could be considered the employer and EMS personnel or firefighters as borrowed servants. As such, OSHA liability rests on the EMS system, hospital, or medical director, rather than on the operator of the EMS service.

Therefore, the EMS system must develop universal precautions (protocols that specify those standards and procedures), including use of specific protective clothing and devices that are to be provided to and used by all EMS system employees during patient encounters (**Figure 26-2**). Continued participation in the EMS system would be contingent on ongoing compliance with those requirements. Compliance with appropriately drafted policies and procedures ensures compliance with OSHA regulations. The EMS system and the medical director should have the specific knowledge and expertise to provide information and counseling to EMS personnel that might not otherwise be available to them. The EMS system shares in the moral responsibility to protect all EMS personnel to the extent feasible and to prevent, if possible, any EMS personnel from being infected by deadly diseases. (More information about bloodborne pathogen issues can be found in Chapter 25, "Occupational Health Issues.")

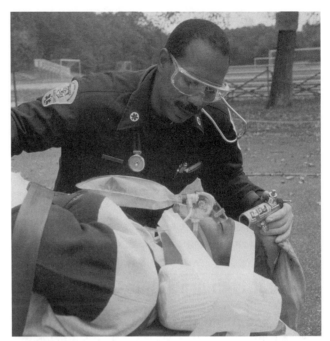

Figure 26-2 The EMS system must develop universal precautions that are to be provided to and used by all EMS system employees during patient encounters.

System Discipline

Along with the responsibility for medical direction of the EMS system comes the possibility that, at some point, it will be necessary to discipline or terminate individuals or services for noncompliance with system rules, policies, or procedures. Typically, that responsibility falls on the system medical director and/ or administrator and his or her subordinates.

The EMS system administrators and medical directors must be familiar with policies and procedures of the state agency that empowers them with the rights to discipline personnel. Additionally, they should be aware that an individual's ability to maintain licensure or certification to provide patient care services is increasingly critical to his or her continued employment. As a result, employees have acquired a property right under the US Constitution to that license or permit,

subject only to proper discipline effected through procedural due process. Inappropriate termination of employees without that due process could result in successful litigation against EMS medical directors. The EMS medical director, in conjunction with the employer, must provide a due process mechanism in applying discipline.

The policies and procedures of the EMS system should adequately detail those offenses for which EMS personnel can be suspended or terminated, the procedures for such suspension or termination, the rights of hearing and appeal, and the various steps included in state law or system policies for subsequent appeal. Discipline should be applied only on documented evidence of a specific violation, and only if applied uniformly in similar situations throughout the system. Personal animosities, defiant attitudes, insubordinate speech, and similar offenses that result in discipline to one party and not another are discriminatory and could present legal difficulties. Physicians acting to terminate EMS personnel based on personal animosity might find themselves and the system successfully sued for major losses.

At a minimum, EMS personnel charged with an offense that could result in suspension or termination should be entitled, within a reasonable time, to specific written charges, information on how to appeal any decision, and a hearing before a fair and impartial panel that is not subject to the control or retribution of the individual bringing charges. In addition, fundamental due process requires:

- The right to counsel at a hearing
- The right to present evidence in defense of the charges at a hearing
- A right to confront the witnesses and charges
- A procedural right to appeal

This process might seem complex and unnecessarily burdensome to most medical directors, but it represents the minimum standards of due process expected by most citizens in this country. In order to prepare policies and procedures that address these issues appropriately, legal counsel should be involved in both drafting and implementing these policies.

Quality Improvement

Regular and frequent review and audit of out-of-hospital run reports by EMS system personnel is imperative. Each report should be reviewed for appropriateness of medical care, adequacy of documentation, and compliance with rules and regulations. Evaluation protocols should be established, analyzed, and updated to remedy observed deficiencies discovered in the audit process. This process is often referred to as continuous quality improvement.

Frequent evaluation of run reports and a run review that includes the involved personnel is a necessary step in identifying problems of substandard performance and is an important step toward implementing corrective measures.

Due to legal confidentiality and protection requirements found in most state laws, it might be advisable to develop an EMS subcommittee under the direction of the hospital quality improvement committee. This might assist in providing peer review protection and thwart attempts by plaintiffs' attorneys to obtain this information through discovery. The quality improvement process must remain confidential and should not be discussed with other members of the EMS community, except as necessary to make effective correction of the problems ascertained. (More information on QI activities is found in Chapter 6, "Medical Oversight and Accountability.")

Antikickback Issues

EMS systems face several challenges with regard to compliance with applicable federal fraud and abuse laws, primarily the **antikickback statute (AKS)**.[8] The relationship between hospitals or health care institutions and out-of-hospital EMS agencies has especially come under close scrutiny by federal agencies and law enforcement authorities.

The AKS prohibits any knowing or willful solicitation or receipt of any remuneration (including any kickback, bribe, or rebate) directly or indirectly, in cash or in kind, in return for referrals of services reimbursable by any federal health care program. The statute provides for criminal penalties of up to 5 years imprisonment and a $25,000 fine for each violation. A separate statutory section also provides civil monetary penalties of up to $50,000 per violation for acts that violate the AKS.[9] A conviction under the AKS constitutes grounds for automatic exclusion from the Medicare and Medicaid programs.[10] A significant aspect of the AKS is that it is a two-way law — both parties to an unlawful arrangement can be found in violation and are thus equally at risk. In addition, violations have been found when only *one* purpose of the arrangement is to induce illegal referrals, even if the arrangement has other business-related purposes that are entirely legitimate.[11]

There are several common types of arrangements prevalent in many EMS systems that might implicate the AKS. The most common are ambulance restocking arrangements and contractual arrangements between hospitals or facilities and ambulance services.

With regard to ambulance restocking, the OIG has voiced its concern that the restocking of drugs and supplies by hospitals to ambulance services can be seen as illegal remuneration that might induce ambulance providers to bring patients to particular facilities.[12] This compliance concern is particularly prevalent in EMS systems where certain hospitals unilaterally engage in ambulance restocking and others in the area do not; in such instances the OIG believes that ambulance providers might be induced by restocking hospitals to bring patients to their facilities rather than to those that offer no restocking.

In recognition of the significant community benefits that derive from the prompt restocking of ambulances used in the provision of EMS, the OIG in recent years has signaled an increased willingness to permit ambulance restocking by hospitals as long as certain fraud and abuse safeguards are in place. For instance, the OIG approved restocking arrangements where all hospitals in a given EMS region participate equally in the restocking program and restock all incoming ambulances equally.[13] Further, the OIG has issued a set of safe harbor regulations that offer blanket protection to restocking arrangements that satisfy the regulatory criteria.[14] Hospitals and EMS systems that engage in ambulance restocking arrangements should consult with legal counsel knowledgeable in this area, but such arrangements can continue unabated where proper safeguards are in place.

Another area of AKS concern prevalent in EMS systems is in arrangements among ambulance services and hospitals, health care systems, and health care facilities. The primary concern is when ambulance services provide impermissible discounts for transports in which the facilities bear financial responsibility, while receiving referrals for Medicare or other federal health care programs and billing them substantially more. In such cases, the discounts given to the facilities can be seen as inducements by the ambulance service to the facility for the referral of more lucrative Medicare or other federal health care program business. Where one purpose of the discounting is to induce such referrals, the arrangement can be found to be in violation of the AKS. Individuals and organizations involved in such impermissible arrangements can suffer serious criminal, civil, and administrative penalties, so it is important that these arrangements be properly structured in conjunction with legal counsel knowledgeable in this area of the law.

Summary

Policies, procedures, and protocols must be drafted carefully and reevaluated frequently to ensure that an EMS system complies with the legal standards of medical care. A knowledgeable attorney can provide valuable assistance in formulating these standards, in conjunction with the EMS system directors, to ensure the legal adequacy of these documents. Exemplary policies, alone, are insufficient to ensure that appropriate care is rendered by appropriately trained EMS personnel. Monitoring and enforcement of the policies is paramount. Finally, the policies must be administered conscientiously to provide training to the EMS personnel as to their provisions, to physician and hospital staff on their application, and to ensure quality improvement in the identification and correction of deficiencies.

References

1. *Belcher v Charleston Area Medical Center,* 422 SE2d 827 (188 WVa 105 1992).
2. *Arrington v Wong,* 237 F3d 1066 (9th Cir 2001).
3. 42 USC §1395dd(e)(1)(A).
4. 42 USC §1395dd(e)(3)(B).
5. 42 USC §1395dd(e)(4).
6. *Roberts v Galen of Virginia, Inc,* 525 US 249, 119 SCt 685, 142 LEd 2d 648 (1999).
7. Occupational exposure to bloodborne pathogens; needlestick and other sharp injuries; final rule. 66 *Federal Register* 5317–5325 (2001) (codified at 29 CFR §1910.1030).
8. 42 USC §1320a–7b(b).
9. 42 USC §1320a–7a(a)(7).
10. 42 USC §1320a–7a(a)(1).
11. *US v Greber,* 760 F2d 68, 71 (3d Cir 1985).
12. Office of Inspector General, US Department of Health and Human Services. *Advisory Opinion No 97-6.* Washington, DC: US Dept of Health and Human Services; October 20, 1997.
13. Office of Inspector General, US Department of Health and Human Services. *Advisory Opinion No 98-7; 98-13, and 98-14.* Washington, DC: US Dept of Health and Human Services; June 11, 1998, September 30, 1998, and October 28, 1998.
14. 66 *Federal Register* 62979 (2001) (codified at 42 CFR §1001.952[v]).

Additional Reading

Flick GM. *Medical Malpractice: Handling Emergency Medicine Cases.* Colorado Springs, Colo: Shephard-McGraw-Hill; 1991.

Frew SA. *Street Law.* Reston, Va: Reston Publishing; 1983.

Goldstein AS. *EMS and the Law.* Bowie, Md: Brady Publishing; 1983.

Mancini MR, Gale AT. *Emergency Care and the Law.* Rockville, Md: Aspen Publishing; 1981.

Wilder S. *EMT Self Defense and the Aggressive Patient* [videotape]. Rockford, Ill: Stanstead Publishing; 1993.

Wilder S. *Compliance Guidelines for Fire Services and EMS Providers for Protection from Bloodborne Pathogens.* Bradley, Ill: S Wilder and Associates; 1992.

Wolfberg D, Wirth S. *The Ambulance Service Guide to HIPAA Compliance.* Mechanicsburg, Pa: Page, Wolfberg & Wirth, LLC; 2003.

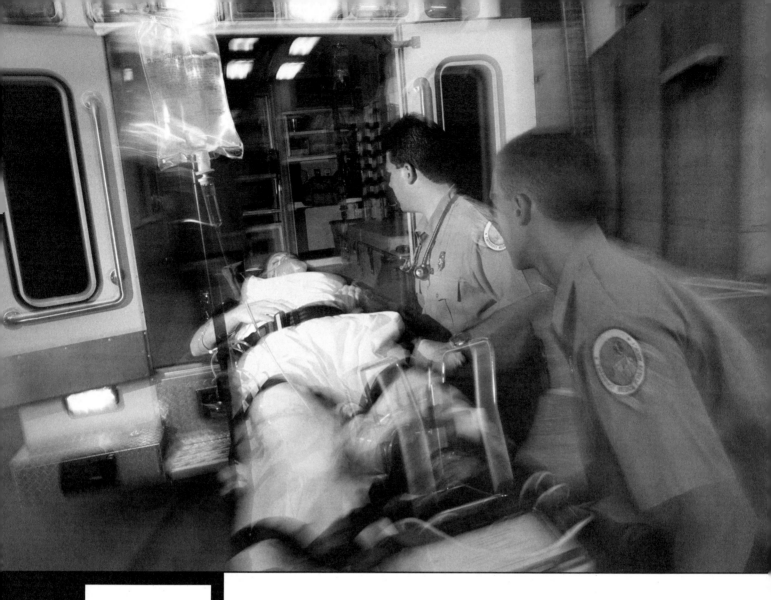

27 EMTALA and EMS

James C. Mitchiner, MD, MPH, FACEP

Principles of This Chapter

After reading this chapter, you should be able to:

- Explain the basic components of EMTALA, including the medical screening examination, stabilization, and transfer requirements.
- Describe how the revised regulations affect transport decisions for hospital-owned and non–hospital-owned ambulances.
- Discuss the EMS obligations for medically indicated transfers.
- List and explain the requirements of an appropriate transfer.

THE EMERGENCY MEDICAL TREATMENT AND LABOR ACT, commonly known by its acronym EMTALA, was enacted by the US Congress in 1986. Its purpose was to outlaw the common practice of patient "dumping," whereby indigent patients were denied access to initial or ongoing medical care in hospital emergency departments because they could not pay for it. EMTALA imposes several obligations on Medicare-participating hospitals. One of these is the requirement to offer a medical screening examination to any individual who presents to the hospital's "dedicated emergency department" (as defined in the regulations) for evaluation or treatment of a medical condition. As such, EMTALA guarantees universal access to all persons regardless of their insurance status or membership in a health maintenance organization (HMO) and irrespective of whether they are US citizens.

Because EMTALA governs out-of-hospital as well as interhospital medical care, it is incumbent on the EMS community to understand the law and its implications. In many ways, EMS agencies have generally maintained EMTALA compliance because of their longstanding tradition of providing emergency care without regard for a patient's financial status. Nevertheless, there are some important aspects of the EMTALA statute and the recently revised regulations that all EMS providers should understand. These aspects can be conveniently divided into two distinct topics: out-of-hospital transport of patients to hospitals, and interfacility transfer of patients from one hospital to another. These topics will be explored following a brief discussion of the EMTALA statute.

The Basic Components of EMTALA

Although the actual EMTALA statute is 4 pages long and has generated hundreds of pages of guidance and commentary, its three essential elements can be summarized as follows[1]:

- **Medical screening examination.** EMTALA mandates an appropriate and nondiscriminatory medical screening examination for any individual who presents to a Medicare-participating hospital's **dedicated emergency department*** for care in order to determine if an emergency medical condition is present.
- **Stabilization.** If an emergency medical condition is found, the patient must be stabilized within the capability of the hospital.
- **Transfer requirements if unstable.** If further stabilization is required and is beyond the capability of the hospital, the patient must be appropriately transferred to another hospital that is capable of stabilizing the emergency medical condition, and this receiving hospital must accept the transfer if it has the capacity and capability to treat the condition.

The purpose and scope of the medical screening examination can be summarized by the actual language of the EMTALA statute:

---

*The EMTALA final rule that went into effect November 10, 2003, defines the hospital's EMTALA duties depending on where an individual presents and the nature of the request for services. In brief, the four different presenting scenarios are the hospital's dedicated emergency department, hospital property other than the dedicated emergency department, hospital-owned and operated ambulances, and provider-based entities of the hospital. "Dedicated emergency department" is newly defined in the regulations at 42 CFR §489.24(b), as published in the September 9, 2003, *Federal Register* (68 *Federal Register* 53263).

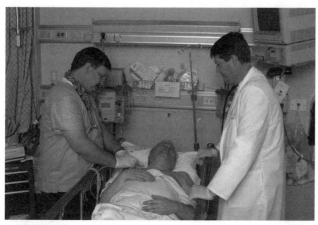

[T]he hospital must provide for an appropriate medical screening examination within the capability of the hospital's emergency department, including ancillary services routinely available to the emergency department, to determine whether or not an emergency medical condition . . . exists.[2]

The purpose, therefore, of the medical screening examination is to determine whether an individual has an emergency medical condition. All Medicare-participating hospitals are obligated to offer a medical screening examination to any individual who presents to the hospital's dedicated emergency department for evaluation and treatment of a medical condition, regardless of that person's insurance status or ability to pay for services rendered (**Figure 27-1**). If an individual is incompetent or incapacitated by illness or injury, the request may be made by anyone——a family member, neighbor, babysitter, police officer, hospital staff, or even EMS personnel. The revised regulations that took effect in November 2003 include **prudent layperson observer** language, which reinforces that anyone may make the request on an individual's behalf based on observations of the individual's behavior or appearance that would indicate the need to be screened and treated.[3]

If an emergency medical condition is discovered, the hospital is then obligated to provide stabilizing treatment within its capabilities, and if necessary transfer the patient to a higher-level facility that has the capability to treat the patient's emergency medical condition. Resolution of the emergency medical condition by the transferring hospital is not a prerequisite for transfer.

EMTALA is a federal statute, which means that it is applicable in all states and territories of the United States and supersedes any state or territorial law. The Centers for Medicare and Medicaid Services (CMS), a federal agency within the US Department of Health and Human Services, is responsible for drafting, disseminating, and enforcing EMTALA regulations. An EMTALA violation is a civil infraction punishable by monetary fines of up to $50,000 per violation, termination of the hospital's Medicare participation agreement, or both. Both physicians and hospitals can be — and have been — sanctioned for violating EMTALA.

Out-of-Hospital Transport

Hospital-Owned Ambulances

EMTALA stipulates that an individual has "come to the emergency department" when and where he or she enters a hospital-owned ambulance (or helicopter), even if the origin of the trip is many miles from the hospital.[4] Previously, the regulations required EMS to transport the individual to the hospital that owned the ambulance, even if it meant bypassing closer, more appropriate facilities. Under the revised regulations that went into effect November 10, 2003, however, a hospital-owned ambulance may now take the individual to another hospital, provided that this conforms to communitywide EMS protocols that require transport to the closest appropriate facility. This change in the regulations allows for more flexible and efficient use of resources to benefit communities.[5]

One important caveat: regardless of EMS protocols, an individual is deemed to have come to the emergency department of any hospital when the ambulance reaches that hospital's property, regardless of who owns the ambulance. However, for EMTALA to apply, *there must also be a concomitant request* for that individual to receive evaluation or treatment at that hospital. In practice, this means that an individual could be transported by ambulance to a small hospital that has a helipad, in anticipation of further transport by helicopter to a tertiary care facility (eg, a trauma center), without triggering an EMTALA obligation by the small hospital because there was no actual request for services at the small hospital.

EMS Communications

Has an individual who is being transported by a non–hospital-owned ambulance "come to the emergency department" of the hospital that provides medical direction to EMS personnel through its telemetry base station? This question has been answered differently by CMS and the courts. In two legal cases, the courts have held divergent interpretations of the EMTALA phrase "comes to the emergency department."

The US Court of Appeals, Seventh Circuit, ruled that it applies only to individuals who physically enter the hospital's emergency department. The Ninth Circuit, however, adopted the dictionary definition of "comes to" to conclude that the transport of individuals en route to an emergency department that is not on diversion satisfies the requirement of coming to the emergency department.[6,7] In both cases, the individuals were in respiratory distress, transported by non–hospital-owned ambulances, and diverted from going to the intended destination hospital. However, in the first case, the base station hospital was on formal diversion; in the second case, it was not. Therefore, a prudent policy would be for EMS personnel to transport individuals to the nearest appropriate hospital, regardless of whether it has the base station, unless that hospital is on diversion. In addition, the revised regulations permit a hospital-owned ambulance to transport an individual to a facility other than its own in accordance with communitywide EMS protocols, and when telemetry direction is provided by a physician who is not employed by or affiliated with the hospital that owns the ambulance.[8]

Ambulance Diversion

EMS providers are understandably concerned about their EMTALA obligations when overcrowded emergency departments divert ambulances to less-crowded facilities. A hospital that is on diversion due to a transient shortage of staff or beds or an overwhelming number of patients in its emergency department may legally request that a non–hospital-owned ambulance transport an individual elsewhere without risking an EMTALA violation.[9] However, if the ambulance crew ignores such a request and transports the individual to the emergency department anyway, the hospital is obligated to provide the EMTALA-mandated services.[10] The practice of having nurses meet ambulances at the emergency department door and direct them elsewhere is a flagrant EMTALA violation and should not be tolerated by any EMS provider. Once an ambulance is on hospital property and the request is made for examination or treatment, the hospital is obligated to medically screen the individual for an emergency medical condition and, if one is discovered, to treat and stabilize the condition within its capability and if necessary arrange for an appropriate transfer to another facility.

Multiple-Patient Transports

Under certain circumstances, an ambulance crew will pick up two individuals from the scene of an accident who request transport to different hospitals. It is permissible for an ambulance to take one individual to the first hospital and then continue on to the second hospital; EMTALA applies only when the individual comes to the emergency department *and* a request is made for examination or treatment of a medical condition at that emergency department.[11] Because the second individual requests treatment at a second hospital, the first facility is not obligated to treat him or her under EMTALA.

Interfacility Transfers

The term transfer is defined under EMTALA as "the movement (including the discharge) of an individual outside a hospital's facilities at the direction of any person employed by (or affiliated or associated, directly or indirectly, with) the hospital . . ."[12] Clearly, the transport of patients from one hospital to another meets the legal definition of transfer.

Requirements for Interfacility Transfers of Unstable Patients

There are only two conditions under which an unstable patient can be transferred under EMTALA: the existence of a valid *medical reason,* such as the lack of resources for treating the patient at the original facility, or the patient's *personal request.*[13] There are no other legally permissible transfers of unstable patients. If, for example, a patient wants to be transferred to a facility that is covered by his or her health insurance plan, it must be clearly documented in the medical record that the transfer is being effected at the *patient's* request. A nurse or physician should never document that the patient was transferred for "insurance reasons." In the case of a minor or an incompetent or incapacitated adult, the patient's legal guardian can request a transfer on the patient's behalf.

For a **medically indicated transfer** from the emergency department, the hospital (ie, the treating physician, as an agent of the hospital) is obligated to:

- Obtain the patient's written informed consent for transfer
- Certify that the medical benefits of receiving care at the other hospital outweigh the risks associated with the transfer
- Arrange an "appropriate" transfer, as defined by law[14]

In some situations, a patient's personal physician or managed care organization will request that the patient be transferred to another facility. Neither has the authority, alone, to force such a transfer. A **patient-requested transfer** must be just that: requested by the patient, or by the patient's guardian or power of attorney. The patient must *choose* to be transferred, knowing that the necessary medical services are available at the transferring hospital. The legal requirements necessary to effect a patient-requested transfer of an unstable patient are distinctly different from those of a medically indicated transfer. In this situation, the hospital is obligated to:

- Inform the patient of the hospital's obligations under EMTALA
- Inform the patient of the specific risks of transfer in an unstable condition, including the risks of ambulance transportation delays due to weather conditions or mechanical problems, and of the benefits of staying there to receive treatment
- Ascertain that the patient is competent to request transfer
- Obtain the patient's written informed consent for transfer to another facility, with an indication (by signature) that the patient or the patient's surrogate understands the hospital's obligations under EMTALA and the risks associated with the transfer
- Create a written document setting forth the patient's request for transfer and the reason for the transfer
- Arrange an "appropriate" transfer, as defined by law[14]

Figure 27-2 is a sample of a standardized transfer form that can be used to document all of the required elements of an interfacility patient transfer.

For an informed consent to be valid, the physician must explain in writing the hospital's obligation to a patient with an emergency medical condition, including the obligation to a woman in labor, and the risks and benefits to the patient based on clinical information available at the time of transfer, including the nonmedical risks (ie, those associated with ambulance or helicopter transport, such as mechanical breakdowns or crashes). For a medically indicated transfer, the physician also must certify that the benefits of the transfer outweigh any reasonably foreseeable risks. But for a patient-requested transfer of an unstable patient, such certification is not required — and not logical: by requesting transfer to another facility, the unstable patient is refusing treatment and essentially leaving against medical advice, and no physician could "certify" that as being in the patient's best interest.[15]

The transfer of an unstable patient to a facility with equal or lesser capabilities for treating the patient's emergency medical condition (unless it is patient requested) is a likely EMTALA violation.[16]

The EMTALA "reverse dumping" clause states that

a hospital that has specialized capabilities or facilities . . . shall not refuse to accept an appropriate transfer of an individual who requires such specialized capabilities or facilities if the hospital has the capacity to treat the individual.[17]

In this context, there are no geographic restrictions under EMTALA. Theoretically, under appropriate circumstances, a hospital in New York could be forced to accept a patient in transfer from a hospital in California. The one exception is that hospitals may refuse transfer requests from facilities outside the United States or its territories.

Definition of an Appropriate Transfer

There are five requirements for an appropriate transfer that must be met for all medically indicated transfers,[14] summarized as follows:

- The transferring hospital must do everything within its capabilities to stabilize the patient while waiting for the transfer to occur, in such a way as to reduce the risks to the individual's health and, in the case of a woman in labor, the health of the unborn child.
- The transferring hospital must arrange for another hospital to accept the patient in transfer. The receiving hospital must agree to accept the transfer if it has the capacity and capability to treat the patient's condition. The transfer must be accepted by a person who has the authority to do so on behalf of the receiving hospital.
- The transferring hospital must send copies of all medical records, diagnostic studies (eg, laboratory tests, radiology studies, ECGs), informed consent documents, and physician transfer certifications related to the emergency condition for which the patient is being treated.
- The transfer must be effected through the use of qualified personnel, equipment, and transport methods appropriate to the patient's clinical condition and sufficient to manage any foreseeable complications that could arise en route (**Figure 27-3**).
- The transfer must meet any other requirements that might be mandated by the Secretary of Health and Human Services in the interest of protecting the health and safety of transferred patients.

PHYSICIAN

Emergency Medical Condition (EMC) Identified: *(Mark appropriate box(es), then go to Section II)*

I. MEDICAL CONDITION: Diagnosis _____

☐ **No Emergency Medical Condition Identified:** This patient has been examined and an EMC has not been identified.

☐ **Patient Stable** - The patient has been examined and any medical condition stabilized such that, within reasonable clinical confidence, no material deterioration of this patient's condition is likely to result from or occur during transfer.

☐ **Patient Unstable** - The patient has been examined, an EMC has been identified and patient is not stable, but the transfer is medically indicated and in the best interest of the patient.
I have examined this patient and based upon the reasonable risks and benefits described below and upon the information available to me, I certify that the medical benefits reasonably expected from the provision of appropriate medical treatment at another facility outweigh the increased risk to this patient's medical condition that may result from effecting this transfer.

II. REASON FOR TRANSFER: ☐ Medically Indicated   ☐ Patient Requested _____
  ☐ On-call physician refused or failed to respond within a reasonable period of time.
      Physician Name _____ Address _____

III. RISK AND BENEFIT FOR TRANSFER:

Medical Benefits:	**Medical Risks:**
☐ Obtain level of care / service NA at this facility. ☐ Service _____ ☐ Benefits outweigh risks of transfer	☐ Deterioration of condition en route _____ ☐ Worsening of condition or death if you stay here. There is always risk of traffic delay/accident resulting in condition deterioration.

IV. Mode/Support/Treatment During Transfer as Determined by Physician – (Complete Applicable Items):

  Mode of transportation for transfer: ☐ BLS   ☐ ALS   ☐ Helicopter   ☐ Neonatal Unit   ☐ Private Car   ☐ Other _____
  Agency _____ Name/Title accompany hospital employee _____
  Support/Treatment during transfer: ☐ Cardiac Monitor   ☐ Oxygen – (Liters) _____   ☐ Pulse Oximeter   ☐ IV Pump
  ☐ IV Fluid _____ Rate _____   ☐ Restraints – Type _____   ☐ Other _____   ☐ None
  Radio on-line medical oversight *(If necessary):* ☐ Transfer Hospital   ☐ Destination Hospital   ☐ Other

V. Receiving Facility and Individual: The receiving facility has the capability for the treatment of this patient (including adequate equipment and medical personnel) and has agreed to accept the transfer and provide appropriate medical treatment.
Receiving Facility / Person accepting transfer _____ Time _____
Receiving MD _____
Transferring Physician Signature _____ Date/Time _____
Per Dr. _____ by _____ RN/ Qualified Medical Personnel Date/Time _____

NURSING

VI. ACCOMPANYING DOCUMENTATION – sent via: ☐ Patient/Responsible Party   ☐ Fax   ☐ Transporter
  ☐ Copy of Pertinent Medical Record   ☐ Lab/ EKG/ X-Ray   ☐ Copy of Transfer Form   ☐ Court Order
  ☐ Advance Directive   ☐ Other _____
  Report given (Person / title) _____
  Time of Transfer _____ Date _____ Nurse Signature _____ Unit _____
  Vital Signs Just Prior to Transfer T _____ Pulse _____ R _____ BP _____ Time _____

PATIENT

VII. PATIENT CONSENT TO "MEDICALLY INDICATED" OR "PATIENT REQUESTED" TRANSFER:

  ☐ I hereby **CONSENT TO TRANSFER** to another facility. I understand that it is the opinion of the physician responsible for my care that the benefits of transfer outweigh the risks of transfer. I have been informed of the risks and benefits upon which this transfer is being made.
  ☐ I hereby **REQUEST TRANSFER** to _____. I understand and have considered the hospital's responsibilities, the risks and benefits of transfer, and the physician's recommendation. I make this request upon my own suggestion and not that of the hospital, physician, or anyone associated with the hospital.

  The reason I request transfer is _____

Signature of ☐ Patient ☐ Responsible Person _____ Relationship _____

      Witness _____   Witness _____

TRANSFER FORM

White: Receiving Facility; **Yellow:** Medical Record; **Pink:** QA

Patient Name:

Date of Birth:

Medical Record Number:

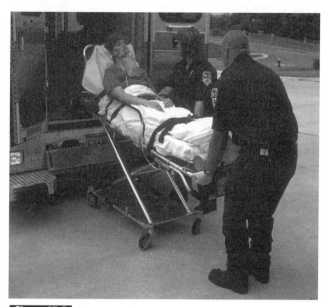

Figure 27-3 Only qualified personnel may transfer a patient.

Other Aspects of Interfacility Transfers

A patient transfer that is clearly not in the patient's best medical interests is an inappropriate transfer, and the proposed receiving facility is not obligated to accept such a patient in transfer. For example, if the requested receiving hospital is aware that the transferring hospital has the staff and resources available to stabilize an unstable patient, the requested hospital may refuse the transfer.[18] However, a hospital that refuses such a transfer, according to Bitterman, "had better be right." The receiving hospital might be better served by accepting the transfer and then telling the transferring hospital how to manage the patient's condition before transfer.[19]

If a hospital receives an inappropriately transferred patient, the hospital is obligated to report the transferring facility to CMS or the state survey agency.[20] Reporting is mandatory, and hospitals have been cited for failure to report inappropriate transfers.[21] The duty is imposed on the receiving hospital, but CMS expects hospitals to have policies requiring employees and staff physicians to report inappropriate transfers.[22] Therefore, EMS personnel who are involved in transfers they believe are inappropriate should report their concerns to the emergency department attending physician or charge nurse at the receiving hospital.

EMS system managers and medical directors must ensure that their transport policies are nondiscriminatory. For example, transporting an unstable HMO patient to the patient's HMO-participating hospital, bypassing a closer appropriate but nonparticipating facility, could be an EMTALA violation depending on the

patient's condition and other circumstances. In general, compliance with local or state-approved EMS transport policies is usually viewed as being compliant with EMTALA regulations. However, CMS reserves the right to review (retrospectively) hospital transport policies to determine whether they are discriminatory.[23]

Another aspect of conducting patient transfers that warrants mention is the interfacility transfer of stable patients. Recall the three basic elements of the EMTALA statute: the *screening* requirements apply to all individuals who "come to the emergency department" of Medicare-participating hospitals. The *stabilization* requirements apply to those in whom an emergency medical condition is discovered as a result of the screening exam. And the *transfer* requirements apply to those whose emergency medical conditions, for reasons dictated by law and regulations, will be treated at another hospital. Thus, the EMTALA transfer requirements are designed to protect unstable patients, not stable patients. Simply put by Bitterman, stable patients "can be transferred at any time, to any hospital, for any reason, including economic reasons, and EMTALA does not apply."[24] For example, transfer of a stable patient from a hospital that does not participate in the patient's managed care plan but is otherwise qualified to treat the patient is not prohibited under EMTALA, even if the transfer is solely for economic reasons. The patient's condition, however, must be stable; transfers of unstable patients for economic reasons are not permitted under EMTALA under any circumstances.

The transferring hospital must send copies of the patient's medical records and other documents related to the emergency medical condition along with the patient being transferred (ie, those documents that are available at the time of the transfer).[25]

Finally, even though EMTALA transfer requirements do not apply to the interfacility transport of stable patients, hospitals would be best served by having one transfer policy, procedure, and set of forms that it uses for *all* transfers. This approach ensures uniformity, reduces error, and protects the hospital — and its transferred patients.[26] Several types of documentation and forms and transfer orders might be used, but the transfer form in **Figure 27-2** is one that can be used for the transfer of any patient.

Summary

EMTALA provides a uniform guarantee of access to hospital-based emergency medical care for all individuals in the United States. The federally mandated requirements for a medical screening examination and, if necessary, stabilization and transfer must be applied in a nondiscriminatory manner to all persons seeking care in an emergency department. The EMS community has an essential role in fulfilling a hospital's EMTALA obligations through out-of-hospital transport and appropriate interfacility transfers. Through awareness of the EMTALA statute, EMS personnel can contribute to improved patient care while protecting hospitals from federal sanctions.

Author's Note: *Providing Emergency Care Under Federal Law: EMTALA,* by Robert A. Bitterman, MD, JD, FACEP, is a comprehensive resource on EMTALA and how it affects emergency medical care. It is available from the ACEP Bookstore (http://www.acep.org/bookstore). A supplement was published in April 2004 to explain the final rules and regulations that went into effect November 10, 2003. It is available as a download from the ACEP Web site.

References

1. Bitterman RA. *Providing Emergency Care Under Federal Law: EMTALA.* Dallas, Tex: American College of Emergency Physicians; 2000:15.
2. Section 1867 of the Social Security Act, Examination and treatment for emergency medical conditions and women in labor, 42 USC §1395dd(a).
3. Bitterman RA. *Supplement to Providing Emergency Care Under Federal Law: EMTALA.* Dallas, Tex: American College of Emergency Physicians; 2004:S12.
4. *Hernandez v Starr County Hospital District,* 30 F Supp 2d 970 (SD Tex 1999).
5. Bitterman RA. *Supplement to Providing Emergency Care Under Federal Law: EMTALA.* Dallas, Tex: American College of Emergency Physicians; 2004:S13–S14.
6. *Johnson v University of Chicago Hospitals,* 982 F2d 230 (7th Cir 1992).
7. *Arrington v Wong,* No. 98-17135 DC No. CV-98-00357-DAE.
8. 68 *Federal Register* 53263 (2003).
9. 42 CFR §489.24(b).
10. Bitterman RA. *Providing Emergency Care Under Federal Law: EMTALA.* Dallas, Tex: American College of Emergency Physicians; 2000:34.
11. Bitterman RA. *Providing Emergency Care Under Federal Law: EMTALA.* Dallas, Tex: American College of Emergency Physicians; 2000:38
12. 42 USC §1395dd(e)(4).
13. Bitterman RA. *Providing Emergency Care Under Federal Law: EMTALA.* Dallas, Tex: American College of Emergency Physicians; 2000:104–105.
14. 42 USC §1395dd(c)(2).
15. Bitterman RA. *Providing Emergency Care Under Federal Law: EMTALA.* Dallas, Tex: American College of Emergency Physicians; 2000:117.
16. HCFA interpretive guidelines, V-34; 1998. As cited in Bitterman RA. *Providing Emergency Care Under Federal Law: EMTALA.* Dallas, Tex: American College of Emergency Physicians; 2000:236.
17. 42 USC §1395dd(g).
18. 59 *Federal Register* 32105 (1994).
19. Bitterman RA. *Providing Emergency Care Under Federal Law: EMTALA.* Dallas, Tex: American College of Emergency Physicians; 2000:114.
20. 42 CFR §489.20(m).
21. 42 CFR §489.24(f); 42 CFR §489.53(a)(10) and (b)(1)(ii).
22. 59 *Federal Register* 32106 (1994). As cited in Bitterman RA. *Providing Emergency Care Under Federal Law: EMTALA.* Dallas, Tex: American College of Emergency Physicians; 2000:115.
23. HCFA interpretive guidelines, V-24; 1998. As cited in Bitterman RA. *Providing Emergency Care Under Federal Law: EMTALA.* Dallas, Tex: American College of Emergency Physicians; 2000:226.
24. Bitterman RA. *Providing Emergency Care Under Federal Law: EMTALA.* Dallas, Tex: American College of Emergency Physicians; 2000:117, citing *Green v Touro Infirmary,* 992 F2d 537 (5th Cir 1993); *Delaney v Cade,* 756 F Supp 1476 (D Kan 1991); *Cherukuri v Shalala,* 1999 FED App 0160P (6th Cir).
25. 42 USC §1395dd(c)(2)(C).
26. Bitterman RA. *Providing Emergency Care Under Federal Law: EMTALA.* Dallas, Tex: American College of Emergency Physicians; 2000:119.

Index

Photo Credits

Chapter 1

Chapter Opener: Campbell Fire Department Paramedics, 1970s. From left to right (standing) Gary Salmon, Al Lowder, Fred Van Hook, Fred Bailey, (kneeling) Mike Johnson, Rick Kinkaid, George Renshaw, and Ray Ravero. In 1974, the Campbell Fire Department gained statewide attention when it started the first paramedic program in Northern California. After a year of training at their own expense, eight men became certified paramedics. With a 1974 Chevrolet truck outfitted with compartments for a portable EKG, suction, a hospital radio, expanded medical kits, and the Hurst rescue tool, the paramedic Rescue Squad 25 was officially in service. Image 1974.01.0777, courtesy of The Campbell Historical Museums; 1-4 © Jeff Havlik/911 Pictures

Chapter 2

2-1 © Todd Hollis/AP Photo

Chapter 4

Opener Courtesy of the American Academy of Orthopaedic Surgeons; 4-1 Courtesy of California Highway Patrol. All rights reserved

Chapter 5

Opener © Keith Brofsky/Photodisc/Getty Images

Chapter 8

8-1 © Peter Fisher/911 Pictures

Chapter 9

9-1 Courtesy of Kevin Walsh, Forgotten NY Street Scenes (www.forgotten-ny.com); 9-2 Courtesy of George Roarty/Virginia Department of Emergency Management; 9-3 Courtesy of Comarco Wireless Technologies, Irvine, California

Chapter 10

10-1, 10-2, 10-4 Reprinted with permission of Medical Priority Consultants, Inc.; 10-5 The National Academies of Emergency Dispatch

Chapter 12

12-4 Task force of the American Heart Association, the European Resuscitation Council, the Heart and Stroke Foundation of Canada, and the Australian Resuscitation Council. *Ann Emerg Med.* 1991; 20(8): 862. Reprinted with permission from ACEP

Chapter 13

Opener Courtesy of Duke Life Flight; 13-1 Courtesy of Duke Life Flight

Chapter 14

Opener © Peter Fisher/911 Pictures; 14-1 Courtesy of Duke Life Flight

Chapter 15

15-3 Reprinted with permission from Singer JS, Ludwig S, eds. *Emergency Medical Services for Children: The Role of the Primary Care Provider.* Elk Grove Village, Ill: American Academy of Pediatrics; 1992

Chapter 16

Opener Courtesy of the American Academy of Orthopaedic Surgeons

Chapter 17

Opener Courtesy of Dave Saville/FEMA; 17-2 Mountain-Valley Emergency Medical Services Agency; 17-10 © Lou Romig, MD, 2002

Chapter 18

Opener Courtesy of Journalist 1st Class Monica Darby/US Navy; 18-1 © Linda Gheen; 18-8 Courtesy of Journalist 1st Class Monica Darby/US Navy

Chapter 19

Opener Courtesy of Journalist 1st Class Mark D. Faram/US Navy; 19-1 © Chikumo Chiaki/AP Photo; 19-2 Courtesy of Peter I. Dworsky, MPH, EMT-P

Chapter 20

Opener, 20-1, 20-2, 20-3, 20-4, 20-5, 20-6 Courtesy of Mary S. Bogucki, MD, PhD, FACEP

Chapter 22

Opener Courtesy of James Gathany/CDC

Chapter 23

Opener Courtesy of Rhonda Beck; 23-2 Courtesy of the American Academy of Orthopaedic Surgeons

Chapter 24

Opener Courtesy of the American Academy of Orthopaedic Surgeons; 24-3 Courtesy of Peter I. Dworsky, MPH, EMT-P

Chapter 25

25-1 Courtesy of Dr. Edwin P. Ewing, Jr./ CDC

Chapter 26

Opener © 2000 Craig Jackson/In the Dark Photography; 26-1 © Ken Hammond/USDA; 26-2 © 2000 Craig Jackson/In the Dark Photography

Chapter 27

27-3 Courtesy of the American Academy of Orthopaedic Surgeons

Unless otherwise indicated, photographs have been supplied by the Maryland Institute of Emergency Medical Services Systems. Photographs have also been supplied by the American College of Emergency Physicians and Jones and Bartlett Publishers.